Molecular Defects in Cardiovascular Disease

Naranjan S. Dhalla • Makoto Nagano
Bohuslav Ostadal

Editors

Molecular Defects in Cardiovascular Disease

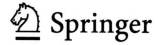 Springer

Editors
Naranjan S. Dhalla, PhD, MD (Hon)
Institute of Cardiovascular Sciences
St. Boniface General Hospital
Research Centre
Winnipeg, Canada
and
Department of Physiology
Faculty of Medicine
University of Manitoba
Winnipeg, Canada
nsdhalla@sbrc.ca

Makoto Nagano, MD, PhD
Jikei University School of Medicine
Tokyo, Japan
naganopr@st.catv.ne.jp

Bohuslav Ostadal, MD, DSc
Centre for Cardiovascular Research
Academy of Sciences
of the Czech Republic
Prague, Czech Republic
and
Institute of Physiology
Academy of Sciences
of the Czech Republic
Prague, Czech Republic
ostadal@biomed.cas.cz

ISBN 978-1-4419-7129-6   e-ISBN 978-1-4419-7130-2
DOI 10.1007/978-1-4419-7130-2
Springer New York Dordrecht Heidelberg London

Library of Congress Control Number: 2011933568

Printed on acid-free paper

Springer is part of Springer Science+Business Media (www.springer.com)

This book is dedicated in the memory of Kalwant (Ken) S. Dhalla for his untiring efforts to serve the cardiovascular community throughout the world during 1977–2010. This tribute to Ken Dhalla is accorded for his special talents in promoting collaborations and friendships within members of the International Society for Heart Research and the International Academy of Cardiovascular Sciences. Ken was a scholar, philosopher, and a great human being. His positive approach to see goodness in everybody and every event are truly being missed.

Preface

Cardiovascular disease is a major challenge for the health care system as it encompasses high levels of mortality and morbidity. Various cardiovascular complications, such as atherosclerosis, hypertension, and diabetes, are known to predispose the heart to become more susceptible to myocardial infarction and/or other pathological stimuli leading to the development of congestive heart failure. Not only is the cardiac muscle adversely affected, but also different risk factors are known to directly result in severe vascular abnormalities. It is generally considered that there occurs hormonal imbalance at initial stages of heart disease, and this results in the occurrence of some adaptive changes, including cardiac hypertrophy, for maintaining the normal status of the cardiovascular system. However, prolonged exposure of the body to diverse pathological stimuli ends up in the malfunction of cardiac and vascular myocytes. Despite a great deal of efforts, which have been made over the past 60 years, no satisfactory cure is available for the treatment of cardiovascular dysfunction associated with different types of heart disease. This state of affairs is primarily due to the lack of our knowledge concerning the mechanisms leading to cardiovascular dysfunction as well as the identification of specific targets for drug development and therapy. This problem is further complicated by the fact that cardiovascular defects are now being recognized as dependent upon the type as well as stage of the disease.

Recently, numerous studies are being directed for understanding the process of remodeling of cardiomyocytes and vascular myocytes to uncover the molecular mechanisms of cardiovascular dysfunction. In particular, various signal transduction systems, which affect the genetic machinery of the cell, are being explored in both cardiovascular health and disease. It is becoming clear that the occurrence of oxidative stress and the development of intracellular Ca^{2+}-overload, as well as metabolic derangements, play an important role in the activation of different proteases and phospholipases for the inhibition of subcellular organelle function. Furthermore, these mechanisms have also been discovered to alter the gene expression in both cardiomyocytes and vascular myocytes, and thus affect subcellular remodeling and activities of subcellular organelles. In particular, the functional groups of proteins in subcellular organelles become inactivated and/or protein content of different subcellular organelles, including sarcolemma, sarcoplasmic reticulum, mitochondria, myofibrils, and nucleus, as well as extracellular matrix become altered. These changes are then considered to result in abnormalities of cardiovascular function. The present book was, therefore, assembled to emphasize the significance of various molecular mechanisms which become defective and are thus associated with the genesis of cardiovascular dysfunction in different types of heart disease.

This book on "Molecular Defects in Cardiovascular Disease" is based on 27 invited articles from well-known investigators with distinct expertise in their fields of cardiovascular sciences. These articles have been arranged in three sections, namely: (a) Molecular Mechanisms in Heart Disease, (b) Cardiac Hypertrophy and Heart Failure, and (c) Hypertension and Diabetes. The first section is focused on general discussion for the role of intracellular Ca^{2+}-overload, oxidative stress, metalloproteases, regulation of intracellular electrolytes, hypoxic injury, and cell therapy for cardioprotection to emphasize the role of changes in molecular mechanisms for the development of cardiovascular dysfunction. The second section deals with metabolic derangements, Ca^{2+}-handling, and subcellular remodeling during the development of cardiac hypertrophy and heart failure with or without drug treatments. This section illustrates the role of a wide variety of molecular defects which may serve as targets associated with the transition of cardiac hypertrophy to heart failure. The third section in this book is mainly concerned with vascular defects which are associated with hypertension and diabetes. In addition, the importance of different hormones in the pathogenesis of hypertension and diabetic cardiomyopathy has been highlighted. Thus, the information outlined in this book can be seen to provide a multifaceted approach to find solutions of problems associated with cardiovascular dysfunction.

We are indeed grateful to Mrs. Eva Little and Dr. Vijayan Elimban for their help in the preparation of manuscripts for editing purposes. Our thanks are also due to Ms. Frances Louie and Mr. Ian Hayes, Springer New York, for their advice during the editorial process. It is hoped that this book containing state of the art articles will be valuable to students, fellows, scientists, clinicians, and surgeons for gaining insight into the molecular mechanisms of cardiovascular disease.

Winnipeg, Canada   Naranjan S. Dhalla
Tokyo, Japan   Makoto Nagano
Prague, Czech Republic   Bohuslav Ostadal

Contents

Contributors

Robert A. Ahokas Department of Obstetrics & Gynecology, University of Tennessee Health Science Center, Memphis, TN, USA

Gauri Akolkar Department of Biology, McMaster University, Hamilton, ON, Canada

Michael F. Allard Department of Pathology and Laboratory Medicine/James Hogg Research Centre, University of British Columbia, Vancouver, British Columbia, Canada

Madhu B. Anand-Srivastava Department of Physiology, Faculty of Medicine, University of Montreal, Montreal, Quebec, Canada

Andrea P. Babick Institute of Cardiovascular Sciences, St. Boniface General Hospital Research Centre, University of Manitoba, Winnipeg, Canada
Department of Physiology, Faculty of Medicine, University of Manitoba, Winnipeg, Canada

Luna Bhatta Department of Internal Medicine, SUNY Upstate Medical University, Syracuse, NY, USA
Veterans Affairs Medical Center, Syracuse, NY, USA

Syamal K. Bhattacharya Division of Cardiovascular Diseases, Department of Medicine, University of Tennessee Health Science Center, Memphis, TN, USA

Robert Carhart Department of Internal Medicine, SUNY Upstate Medical University, Syracuse, NY, USA

Subrata Chakrabarti Department of Pathology, University of Western Ontario, London, Ontario, Canada

Yaser Cheema Division of Cardiovascular Diseases, Department of Medicine, University of Tennessee Health Science Center, Memphis, TN, USA

Ryan H. Cunnington Department of Physiology, University of Manitoba and the Institute of Cardiovascular Sciences, St. Boniface General Hospital Research Centre, Winnipeg, MB, Canada

Jiazhen M. Dai Department of Pathology and Laboratory Medicine/Heart and Lung Institute, University of British Columbia, Vancouver, BC, Canada

Dipak K. Das Cardiovascular Research Center, University of Connecticut School of Medicine, Farmington, CT, USA

Naranjan S. Dhalla Institute of Cardiovascular Sciences, St. Boniface General Hospital Research Centre, Winnipeg, Canada

Department of Physiology, Faculty of Medicine, University of Manitoba, Winnipeg, Canada

Ian M.C. Dixon Department of Physiology, University of Manitoba and the Institute of Cardiovascular Sciences, St. Boniface General Hospital Research Centre, Winnipeg, MB, Canada

Josette M. Douville Department of Biochemistry and Medical Genetics, University of Manitoba and the Institute of Cardiovascular Sciences, St. Boniface General Hospital Research Centre, Winnipeg, MB, Canada

Vijayan Elimban Institute of Cardiovascular Sciences, St. Boniface General Hospital Research Centre, University of Manitoba, Winnipeg, Canada

Department of Physiology, Faculty of Medicine, University of Manitoba, Winnipeg, Canada

Larry Fliegel Department of Biochemistry, Faculty of Medicine, University of Alberta, Edmonton, Alberta, Canada

Timothy Ford Department of Internal Medicine, SUNY Upstate Medical University, Syracuse, NY, USA

Veterans Affairs Medical Center, Syracuse, NY, USA

Darren H. Freed Department of Surgery, Section of Cardiac Surgery, University of Manitoba, Winnipeg, MB, Canada

Department of Physiology, University of Manitoba, Winnipeg, MB, Canada

The Institute of Cardiovascular Sciences, St. Boniface General Hospital Research Centre, Winnipeg, MB, Canada

Ivan C. Gerling Division of Endocrinology, Department of Medicine, University of Tennessee Health Science Center, Memphis, TN, USA

Ashok K. Grover Department of Medicine, McMaster University, Hamilton, Ontario, Canada

Department of Biology, McMaster University, Hamilton, Ontario, Canada

Shivika Gupta Department of Physiology, University of Manitoba, Winnipeg, MB, Canada

The Institute of Cardiovascular Sciences, St. Boniface General Hospital Research Centre, Winnipeg, MB, Canada

Narasimman Gurusamy Cardiovascular Research Center, University of Connecticut School of Medicine, Farmington, CT, USA

Andrew J. Halayko Departments of Internal Medicine and Physiology, University of Manitoba, Winnipeg, MB, Canada

The Biology of Breathing Group, Manitoba Institute of Child Health, Winnipeg, MB, Canada

Grant M. Hatch Department of Pharmacology and Therapeutics, Biochemistry and Medical Genetics, Internal Medicine, Faculty of Medicine, Center for Research and Treatment of Atherosclerosis, Manitoba Institute of Child Health, University of Manitoba, Winnipeg, Canada

Stefan Hein Department of Cardiac Surgery, Kerckhoff Clinic, Bad Nauheim, Germany

Jagdip S. Jaswal Departments of Pediatrics and Pharmacology, Mazankowski Alberta Heart Institute, University of Alberta, Edmonton, AB, Canada

Bodh I. Jugdutt Division of Cardiology, Department of Medicine, University of Alberta and Hospitals, Edmonton, Alberta, Canada

P.J. Kadowitz Department of Pharmacology, Tulane University School of Medicine, New Orleans, LA, USA

Morris Karmazyn Department of Physiology and Pharmacology, The University of Western Ontario, London, Ontario, Canada

Chandrasekharan Cheranellore Kartha Division of Cardiovascular Disease Biology, Rajiv Gandhi Centre for Biotechnology, Trivandrum, India

Wendy Keung Departments of Pediatrics and Pharmacology, Mazankowski Alberta Heart Institute, University of Alberta, Edmonton, AB, Canada

Henk E.D.J. ter Keurs Department of Physiology and Biophysics, University of Calgary, Calgary, Alberta, Canada

Saisudha Koka Division of Cardiology, Department of Internal Medicine, Pauley Heart Center, Virginia Commonwealth University Medical Center, Richmond, VA, USA

F. Kolar Centre for Cardiovascular Research, Academy of Sciences of the Czech Republic, Prague, Czech Republic

Institute of Physiology, Academy of Sciences of the Czech Republic, Prague, Czech Republic

Sawa Kostin Max-Planck-Institute for Heart and Lung Research,
Bad Nauheim, Germany

Hani Kozman Department of Internal Medicine, SUNY Upstate
Medical University, Syracuse, NY, USA

Veterans Affairs Medical Center, Syracuse, NY, USA

Shilpa Kshatriya Department of Internal Medicine, SUNY Upstate
Medical University, Syracuse, NY, USA

Rakesh C. Kukreja Division of Cardiology, Department of Internal
Medicine, Pauley Heart Center, Virginia Commonwealth University
Medical Center, Richmond, VA, USA

Kan Liu Department of Internal Medicine, SUNY Upstate Medical
University, Syracuse, NY, USA

Veterans Affairs Medical Center, Syracuse, NY, USA

Gary D. Lopaschuk Departments of Pediatrics and Pharmacology,
University of Alberta, Mazankowski Alberta Heart Institute,
Edmonton, Alberta, Canada

Ashwani Malhotra Division of Nephrology, Department of Medicine,
Long Island Jewish Medical Center, New Hyde Park, NY, USA

D.B. McNamara Department of Pharmacology, Tulane University
School of Medicine, New Orleans, LA, USA

John H. McNeill Division of Pharmacology and Toxicology,
Faculty of Pharmaceutical Sciences, The University of British Columbia,
Vancouver, Canada

Leonard G. Meggs Department of Nephrology, Ochsner Clinic
Foundation, New Orleans, LA, USA

Robert Michiel Department of Internal Medicine, SUNY Upstate
Medical University, Syracuse, NY, USA

Veterans Affairs Medical Center, Syracuse, NY, USA

Partha Mukhopadhyay Laboratory of Physiologic Studies, NIAAA,
National Institute of Health, Bethesda, MD, USA

S.N. Murthy Department of Pharmacology, Tulane University
School of Medicine, New Orleans, LA, USA

I. Netuka Centre for Cardiovascular Research, Prague, Czech Republic

Institute for Clinical and Experimental Medicine, Prague, Czech Republic

Sarah O'Connor Department of Physiology, University of Manitoba
and the Institute of Cardiovascular Sciences, St. Boniface General
Hospital Research Centre, Winnipeg, MB, Canada

Bohuslav Ostadal Centre for Cardiovascular Research,
Prague, Czech Republic

Institute of Physiology, Academy of Sciences of the Czech Republic,
Prague, Czech Republic

I. Ostadalova Centre for Cardiovascular Research, Academy of Sciences of the Czech Republic, Prague, Czech Republic

Institute of Physiology, Academy of Sciences of the Czech Republic, Prague, Czech Republic

Raissa Perrault Department of Physiology, University of Manitoba and Canadian Centre for Agrifood Research in Health and Medicine, St. Boniface Hospital Research Centre, Winnipeg, Manitoba, Canada

Harikrishnan Sivadasanpillai Department of Cardiology, Sree Chitra Tirunal Institute for Medical Science and Technology, Trivandrum, India

Binil Raj Division of Cardiovascular Disease Biology, Rajiv Gandhi Center for Biotechnology, Trivandrum, India

Sunil G. Rattan Department of Physiology, University of Manitoba, Winnipeg, MB, Canada

The Institute of Cardiovascular Sciences, St. Boniface General Hospital Research Centre, Winnipeg, MB, Canada

Ali Salah Department of Internal Medicine, SUNY Upstate Medical University, Syracuse, NY, USA

Veterans Affairs Medical Center, Syracuse, NY, USA

Dedmer Schaafsma Departments of Internal Medicine and Physiology, University of Manitoba, Winnipeg, MB, Canada

The Biology of Breathing Group, Manitoba Institute of Child Health, Winnipeg, MB, Canada

Jutta Schaper Max-Planck-Institute for Heart and Lung Research, Bad Nauheim, Germany

Richard Schulz Departments of Pediatrics and Pharmacology, Cardiovascular Research Centre, Mazankowski Alberta Heart Institute, University of Alberta, Edmonton, AB, Canada

Atta U. Shahbaz Division of Cardiovascular Diseases, Department of Medicine, University of Tennessee Health Science Center, Memphis, TN, USA

Vijay Sharma Division of Pharmacology and Toxicology, Faculty of Pharmaceutical Sciences, The University of British Columbia, Vancouver, BC, Canada

Danish Siddiqui Department of Internal Medicine, SUNY Upstate Medical University, Syracuse, NY, USA

Veterans Affairs Medical Center, Syracuse, NY, USA

Dinender K. Singla Biomolecular Science Center, University of Central Florida, Orlando, FL, USA

Ashok K. Srivastava Laboratory of Cellular Signaling,
Montreal Diabetes Research Center, Research Center – Centre Hospitalier
de l'Université de Montréal (CRCHUM), Montréal, Québec, Canada
Department of Medicine, Université de Montréal, Montreal, Québec, Canada

Yao Sun Division of Cardiovascular Diseases, Department of Medicine,
University of Tennessee Health Science Center, Memphis, TN, USA

O. Szarszoi Centre for Cardiovascular Research, Institute for Clinical
and Experimental Medicine, Prague, Czech Republic

Paramjit S. Tappia Asper Clinical Research Institute, St. Boniface
Hospital Research and Department of Human Nutritional Sciences,
University of Manitoba, Winnipeg, Canada

John R. Ussher Departments of Pediatrics and Pharmacology,
Mazankowski Alberta Heart Institute, University of Alberta,
Edmonton, AB, Canada

George Vardatsikos Laboratory of Cellular Signaling, Montreal Diabetes
Research Center, Research Center – Centre Hospitalier de l'Université de
Montréal (CRCHUM), Montreal, Québec, Canada
Department of Medicine, Université de Montréal, Montreal, Québec, Canada

Himanshu Vashistha Department of Nephrology, Ochsner Clinic
Foundation, New Orleans, LA, USA

Daniel Villarreal Department of Internal Medicine, SUNY Upstate
Medical University, Syracuse, NY, USA
Veterans Affairs Medical Center, Syracuse, NY, USA

Wei Wang Departments of Pediatrics and Pharmacology,
Mazankowski Alberta Heart Institute, University of Alberta,
Edmonton, AB, Canada

Karl T. Weber Division of Cardiovascular Diseases, Department
of Medicine, University of Tennessee Health Science Center,
Memphis, TN, USA

Jeffrey T. Wigle Department of Biochemistry and Medical Genetics,
University of Manitoba and the Institute of Cardiovascular Sciences,
St. Boniface General Hospital Research Centre, Winnipeg, MB, Canada

Nermeen Youssef Departments of Pediatrics and Pharmacology,
Cardiovascular Research Centre, Mazankowski Alberta Heart Institute,
University of Alberta, Edmonton, AB, Canada

Peter Zahradka Department of Physiology, University of Manitoba and
Canadian Centre for Agrifood Research in Health and Medicine,
St. Boniface Hospital Research Centre, Winnipeg, Manitoba, Canada

Part I
Molecular Mechanisms in Heart Disease

Calcium Overloading-Induced Oxidative Stress-Mediated Cellular and Subcellular Remodeling

Yaser Cheema, Atta U. Shahbaz,
Syamal K. Bhattacharya, Robert A. Ahokas,
Yao Sun, Ivan C. Gerling, and Karl T. Weber

Abstract

A progressive loss of cardiomyocytes contributes to the heart's failure as a muscular pump. This includes the necrotic death of these cells, which are replaced by fibrous tissue (vis-à-vis apoptotic cell death). In the explanted failing heart, scattered foci of fibrosis are found throughout both ventricles, representing the major component of pathologic remodeling. Further evidence on the importance of cardiomyocyte necrosis relates to elevations in serum troponins, biomarkers of cellular disintegration that appear in patients having congestive heart failure (CHF) in the absence of ischemia–infarction or renal failure. The CHF syndrome has its origins rooted in neurohormonal activation, including the adrenergic nervous and renin–angiotensin–aldosterone systems, and secondary hyperparathyroidism. Effector hormones, including parathyroid hormone, contribute to cardiomyocyte necrosis based on a mitochondriocentric *signal-transducer–effector pathway* whose major components include the intracellular Ca^{2+} overloading-induced, oxidative stress-mediated opening of the mitochondria inner membrane permeability transition pore. An ensuing loss of ATP and organellar degeneration account for necrotic cell death. Herein, we focus on this pathway, as it relates to various acute and chronic stressor states: isoproterenol treatment, aldosterone–salt treatment, and the cardiomyopathy of the Syrian Hamster. Cumulative insights gathered from these models lead to the inevitable recognition as to the central role of mitochondria in cellular–subcellular remodeling. Toward this end, the efficacy and safety of mitochondria-targeted pharmaceuticals and/or nutriceuticals needs to be determined.

Keywords

Mitochondria • Cardiomyocytes • Calcium overloading • Oxidative stress • Neurohormones • Parathyroid hormone

K.T. Weber (✉)
Division of Cardiovascular Diseases,
Department of Medicine, University of Tennessee
Health Science Center, Memphis, TN, USA
e-mail: KTWeber@uthsc.edu

N.S. Dhalla, M. Nagano, B. Ostadal (eds.), *Molecular Defects in Cardiovascular Disease*,
DOI 10.1007/978-1-4419-7130-2_1, © Springer Science+Business Media, LLC 2011

Introduction

A progressive loss of cardiomyocytes, due to both necrotic and apoptotic cell death, contributes to the heart's failure as a muscular pump. Necrosis is considered a "dirty" form of cell death in which dying cells release their contents, including troponins, which stimulate the immune system [1–3]. An ensuing wound healing response is, therefore, invoked whereby inflammatory and fibroblast-like cell responses contribute to the appearance of fibrous tissue presenting morphologically as microscopic scars. Apoptosis, on the contrary, is a "sterile" form of cell death, where dying cells are rapidly scavenged by macrophages before they disintegrate, never losing their contents. Moreover, inflammatory cell and fibroblast responses are not invoked. Hence, there is no subsequent morphologic footprint of apoptosis.

In the explanted failing human heart, scattered foci of fibrous tissue are found throughout the ventricles, in which they represent the major component to the pathologic structural remodeling of myocardium [4]. This would suggest cardiomyocyte necrosis is likely to be an ongoing process which contributes to the progressive nature of heart failure. Further evidence in support of this putative pathophysiologic scenario is the appearance of elevated serum troponins that appear in patients hospitalized because of their congestive heart failure (CHF) [5–14]. Albeit modest in amount compared to the more marked elevations in serum troponins that accompany segmental myocardial infarction due to marked reductions in coronary blood flow, other factors account for cardiomyocyte necrosis in the setting of CHF. The identification and recognition of these factors are, therefore, critically important to designing optimal management strategies. Toward this end, understanding the pathophysiologic origins of CHF yielded significant insights.

CHF has its origins rooted in neurohormonal activation – a homeostatic response that has been inappropriately invoked and, when persistent, begets dyshomeostasis. Included in this hormonal onslaught of the heart and systemic tissues are effector hormones of the hypothalamic–pituitary–adrenal axis and the adrenergic nervous and renin–angiotensin–aldosteronism systems. In the case of the myocardium, this eventuates in cardiomyocyte necrosis whose pathogenesis is based on intracellular Ca^{2+} overloading-induced, oxidative stress-mediated opening of the mitochondria inner membrane permeability transition pore (mPTP) with ensuing organellar degeneration and consequent cell death. This mitochondriocentric *signal-transducer–effector pathway* has come to be recognized as the pathophysiologic substrate to cardiomyocyte necrosis in a diverse array of acute stressor states, including ischemia–reperfusion [15] and hypoxia–reoxygenation-related myocardial injury [16] and a hyperadrenergic state [17], that occurs in response to bodily injury, including head trauma, severe burns, myocardial infarction, and major cardiac surgery. Furthermore, this scenario applies to chronic stressor states, such as adriamycin treatment, diabetes, and the secondary aldosteronism of CHF [18–22].

Herein, we focus on excessive intracellular Ca^{2+} accumulation (EICA), as it relates to three different stressor states invoked in experimental animals: (a) isoproterenol treatment (Isop), which simulates an acute hyperadrenergic stressor state, (b) aldosterone–salt treatment (ALDOST), a chronic stressor state, such as CHF, in which EICA is primarily the result of secondary hyperparathyroidism with elevated circulating levels of a calcitropic hormone, parathyroid hormone (PTH), and (c) the cardiomyopathy of the Syrian hamster, where marked elevations in EICA occur due to hereditary δ-sarcoglycanopathy. A comparison of cardiac Ca^{2+} overloading in all the three experimental models described in this article is shown in Table 1.

The Signal-Transducer–Effector Pathway: A Historical Perspective

The Signal

Hans Selye [23] reported that normally adaptive neurohormonal responses, when activated inappropriately and persistently by a stressor

Table 1 A comparison of cardiac Ca^{2+} overloading between models

	Tissue total Ca^{2+} (nEq/mg FFDT)	Cytosolic free $[Ca^{2+}]_i$ (nM)	Mitochondrial free $[Ca^{2+}]_m$ (nM)	Mitochondrial total $[Ca^{2+}]_m$ (ng/mg mito. protein)
Control rats	3.78 ± 0.16	29 ± 4	80 ± 10	47.9 ± 4.9
Isop rats				
8 h	9.61 ± 0.52	–	183 ± 4	–
ALDOST rats				
Week 1	–	70 ± 5	–	89.5 ± 5.7
Week 4	5.42 ± 0.31	80 ± 5	140 ± 10	103.4 ± 10.4
Normal hamster				
7 Months	16.6 ± 1.0	–	–	118 ± 21
Dystrophic hamster				
7 Months	427.2 ± 75.9	–	–	564 ± 35

(e.g., extremes of temperature or treatment with a mineralocorticoid hormone, deoxycorticosterone), would lead to an adverse structural remodeling of systemic organs and the heart which he referred to as *diseases of adaptation*. Pathologic lesions that appeared included microscopic scarring indicative of parenchymal cell necrosis. Some years later, Albrecht Fleckenstein and coworkers [24, 25] hypothesized the hyperadrenergic state that accompanied an acute stressor state would lead to catecholamine-mediated EICA, particularly involving cardiac mitochondria and when coupled with the loss of high energy phosphate synthesis, led to the degeneration of these organelles followed by cardiomyocyte necrosis. Calcitropic hormones, such as PTH and vitamin D, were likewise incriminated in their conceptual framework of EICA-based cardiotoxicity. Toward this end, rodents were treated with Isop, either alone or in combination with verapamil, a calcium channel blocker, which prevented the documented intracellular Ca^{2+} overloading that accompanied Isop and as a result proved to be cardioprotective [24, 25].

Seminal studies, not only confirmatory to the Fleckenstein hypothesis but also provided additional insights, have emanated from different laboratories [26–29]. Isop or an oxidative product of epinephrine, namely, adrenochrome, is administered to intact animals or infused into isolated hearts. These findings identified the fundamental prerequisite of intracellular Ca^{2+} overloading, together with mitochondrial dysfunction and degeneration, as causative of cardiomyocyte necrosis and which could be prevented by cotreatment with either calcium channel blocker or a β-adrenergic receptor antagonist. Contemporaneous to these observations were a series of studies reported by Bhattacharya and coworkers who expanded on the EICA concept, including mitochondrial Ca^{2+} overloading, as contributing to the chronic stressor state found in the cardiomyopathic heart, as well as skeletal muscle and diaphragm, of Syrian hamsters [30–32].

Figure 1 depicts differences which exist between Ca^{2+} concentrations for the extra- and intracellular compartments of cardiomyocytes: (a) a 10,000-fold gradient between the extracellular compartment and cytosolic free Ca^{2+}, (b) a 10-fold gradient between cytosolic free Ca^{2+} and that present in the sarcoplasmic reticulum, and (c) a 1,000-fold gradient between cytosolic free and intramitochondrial Ca^{2+}. Mitochondria sequester Ca^{2+} to preserve this critical intracellular homeostasis within narrow physiologic thresholds during transient fluctuations in cytosolic Ca^{2+}. Persistent elevations in $[Ca^{2+}]_m$ eventually lead to the induction of oxidative stress.

The Transducer

The importance of oxidative stress with reactive oxygen (ROS) and nitrogen species, which overwhelm endogenous antioxidant defenses, would subsequently be identified as the *transducer* in

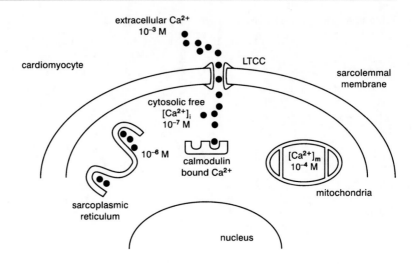

Fig. 1 A schematic representation of calcium found in the extracellular compartment and within the intracellular space of cardiomyocytes including cytosolic free, sarcoplasmic reticulum, and mitochondrial concentrations. See text for further discussion

the mitochondriocentric signal-transducer–effector pathway leading to cardiomyocyte necrosis. Mitochondrial Ca^{2+} overloading and the contribution of these organelles to the generation of oxidative stress represent a major source of ROS; cell membrane-bound NADPH oxidase is another. Furthermore, counterbalancing these oxidative damage mechanisms are endogenous antioxidant defenses, including Zn^{2+}, which are operative within the cytosol, mitochondria, and cell membrane. This capacity to detoxify reactive oxygen metabolites will prove cardioprotective provided these defenses are present in sufficient quantities [33].

The Effector

The *effector* component of this pathway has recently been localized to the mitochondrial inner membrane and recognized as its permeability transition pore (mPTP). Increased permeabilization, promoted by intracellular Ca^{2+} overloading and oxidative stress, leads to entry of low-molecular-weight solutes with ensuing osmotic swelling and degeneration [34, 35]. The important role of cyclophilin D, an isomerase of the mitochondrial matrix, to mPTP opening in the necrotic (vis-à-vis apoptotic) cell death pathway has been demonstrated in mice lacking this protein and through its pharmacologic inhibition by cyclosporine A [36, 37].

Isoproterenol and a Hyperadrenergic State

The Model

The acute stressor state induced by a single subcutaneous dose of Isop is accompanied by a dyshomeostasis of extra- and intracellular Ca^{2+} and Zn^{2+} involving diverse tissues [38]. In plasma, the appearance of ionized hypocalcemia and hypozincemia is concordant and appears within several hours and remain depressed before returning to control levels at 24 h. The genesis of ionized hypocalcemia provokes the parathyroid glands to secrete excessive amounts of parathyroid hormone, which in turn further promotes intracellular Ca^{2+} overloading (see Fig. 2) [20, 21, 39].

Shortly after Isop treatment, Rona et al. [40] found the sarcolemmal membrane of cardiomyocytes had become hyperpermeable, a feature that heralded impending cardiomyocyte death. The disrupted membrane facilitated entry of a monoclonal antibody directed at cardiac myosin. This allowed Benjamin et al. [41] and Tan and coworkers [42–44] to identify cardiomyocyte injury that occurred within hours of Isop treatment and where ensuing tissue repair accounted for the appearance of myocardial scarring days later, preferentially involving the subendocardium of the left ventricular (LV) apex and right ventricle (RV).

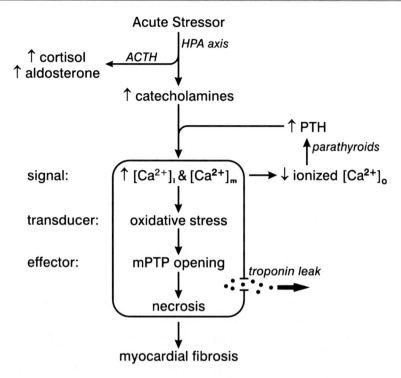

Fig. 2 An acute stressor state, such as bodily injury, is accompanied by an activation of the hypothalamic–pituitary–adrenal (HPA) axis with elevated circulating catecholamines and adrenocorticotropin (ACTH), which stimulates the release of cortisol and aldosterone from the adrenal glands. Catecholamines are responsible for intracellular Ca^{2+} overloading including cytosolic free $[Ca^{2+}]_i$ and mitochondrial $[Ca^{2+}]_m$ with a subsequent fall in plasma ionized $[Ca^{2+}]_o$. Hypocalcemia, in turn, provokes the parathyroid glands to release parathyroid hormone (PTH). It too contributes to intracellular Ca^{2+} overloading. In cardiomyocytes mitochondrial Ca^{2+} over- loading is accompanied by the induction of oxidative stress, which leads to the opening of the mitochondrial permeability transition pore (mPTP) and osmotic injury of these organelles. The necrosis of cardiomyocytes follows accompanied by the leak of troponins into the interstitial space and ultimate rise in plasma troponins, albeit a lesser rise than seen with an acute myocardial infarction due to a critical reduction in coronary blood flow. Cardiomyocytes lost to necrosis are replaced by fibrous tissue, or scarring, which preserves the structural integrity of myocardium. Adapted from Whitted AD, et al. Am J Med Sci. 2010;340:48–53

Intracellular Ca^{2+} Overloading

Following Isop, there is a preferential accumulation of Ca^{2+} within the LV apex (vis-à-vis the LV equator and base) and RV, whereas the tissue Zn^{2+} content declines and remains subnormal for 24 h [38]. This regional heterogeneity to intracellular Ca^{2+} accumulation that favors apical LV tissue is likely related to the high abundance of β_1-adrenergic receptors present at this site [45–47]. An alternate explanation would suggest that the binding affinity of β_1 receptors is greater at the LV apex [48]. In either scenario, this difference in β_1 receptor density or affinity innately relates to the apical to basal sequence of depolarization that occurs within the LV, allowing for a peristaltic-like pattern of contraction by the myocardium along the vertical axis contributing to the efficient propulsion of blood from its chamber into the aorta [49–51].

The EICA at the LV apex associated with Isop-induced injury is accompanied by an early induction of oxidative stress with a rise in 8-isoprostane at this site. Also contributory to the appearance of oxidative stress, when the rate of reactive oxygen and nitrogen species overwhelm their rate of elimination by endogenous antioxidant defenses, is the decline in tissue Zn^{2+} [52, 53]. Intracellular Zn^{2+}, acting as an antioxidant, is essential to the activity of Cu/Zn-superoxide dismutase, a metalloenzyme integral to these defenses and degradation of cytotoxic oxygen-rich intermediaries that appear in these tissues in response to intracellular Ca^{2+} overloading. The fall in cardiac tissue Zn^{2+} following Isop treatment contrasted to its rise in Zn^{2+} in cardiomyocytes that occurs in response to ischemia–reperfusion and the appearance of chronic stressor state associated with aldosterone–salt treatment [54–58]. A $ZnSO_4$ supplement given as pretreatment prior to Isop has been reported to be cardioprotective [59–61].

The predilection for cardiac injury and myocardial scarring following Isop that involves the LV apex [41, 62] is related to a preferential Ca^{2+} overloading at this site [38]. This importantly includes increased mitochondrial free $[Ca^{2+}]_m$ and the associated induction of oxidative stress by these organelles demonstrated by their increased H_2O_2 generation and 8-isoprostane concentration leading to consequent mPTP opening and ensuing cardiomyocyte necrosis [38]. In attenuating mitochondrial Ca^{2+} accumulation with mitochondria-targeted interventions, such as carvedilol, a β_1 receptor antagonist, or quercetin, a flavonoid with mitochondrial antioxidant properties, the greater propensity for mPTP opening in response to Isop was largely attenuated [38]. We would suggest these responses represent crucial mechanistic insights confirming that the proposed mitochondriocentric signal-transducer–effector pathway (see Fig. 2) begets cytotoxicity at the LV apex in response to a hyperadrenergic stressor state. Whether these findings are relevant to the predilection for hypokinesia of the apical segment of LV myocardium, termed apical ballooning or takotsubo cardiomyopathy that accompanies hyperadrenergic states remains uncertain [63–65]. However, carvedilol has proven effective in treating this particular form of cardiomyopathy [66].

In summary, the mitochondriocentric signal-transducer–effector pathway leading to LV apical injury and scarring of the endocardium in response to a single dose of Isop involves Ca^{2+} overloading of cardiac mitochondria, induction of oxidative stress, and increased opening potential of their inner membrane mPTP with discrete foci of necrosis and scarring. Persistent catecholamine excess with repeated dosing of Isop over days is accompanied by ongoing necrosis and fibrosis of the entire LV endocardium [41].

Aldosterone–Salt Treatment: A Chronic Stressor State

The Model

An osmotic minipump filled with aldosterone (ALDO) is implanted subcutaneously in uninephrectomized rats; it releases ALDO (0.75 µg/h) to raise plasma ALDO concentrations to levels found in patients with CHF [67]. Drinking water is fortified with 1% NaCl (ALDOST) to create inappropriate aldosteronism and 0.4% KCl to prevent ALDO-induced hypokalemia and cardiac pathology associated with K^+ dyshomeostasis alone [68]. Plasma renin activity and circulating AngII levels are each suppressed during ALDOST. The increment in Na^+ excretion that accompanies ALDOST is coupled with a marked augmentation in urinary and fecal excretion of Ca^{2+} and Mg^{2+}. Chronic inappropriate ALDOST is also accompanied by increased urinary and fecal excretory Zn^{2+} losses, hypozincemia, and a fall in plasma Cu/Zn-SOD activity [69]. Cotreatment with spironolactone, an ALDO receptor antagonist, attenuates the excretion of Ca^{2+}, Mg^{2+}, and Zn^{2+} at these sites [20, 69]. At week 4, ALDOST lesions appear for the first time in the heretofore normal heart as well as the systemic vasculature that includes the kidneys and mesentery [70]. Cardiac pathology in rats receiving ALDOST includes multiple foci of microscopic scarring, which is scattered throughout the right and left heart [70, 71].

Intracellular Ca^{2+} Overloading and SHPT

Our hypothesis for the induction of oxidative stress during ALDOST draws upon Fleckenstein's original concept that intracellular Ca^{2+} overloading of the heart is an integral and adverse pathophysiologic feature leading to myocardial necrosis [72]. In rats receiving chronic ALDOST, increased Ca^{2+} levels are found in the myocardium during weeks 1–4 accompanied by evidence of oxidative stress that includes increased levels of malondialdehyde and 8-isoprostane [20, 57, 73, 74].

The marked increase in urinary and fecal excretion of Ca^{2+} and Mg^{2+} during ALDOST leads to plasma ionized hypocalcemia and hypomagnesemia. The calcium-sensing receptor of the parathyroid glands responds with increased secretion of PTH with elevated plasma PTH levels at weeks 1–4 ALDOST [20] accompanied by bone resorption [75]. We, therefore, hypothesized the intracellular Ca^{2+} overloading and induction of oxidative stress that accompanies ALDOST leading to cardiomyocyte necrosis and fibrosis is inevitably mediated by the calcitropic hormone, PTH, and not aldosterone per se. PTH is known to regulate cardiomyocyte Ca^{2+} [39, 76, 77]. EICA in cardiomyocytes and consequent generation of reactive oxygen species (ROS) alters intracellular signaling events, including their perpetuation of intracellular Ca^{2+} overloading via L-type Ca^{2+} channel entry and inhibition of Ca^{2+} efflux by Ca^{2+}-ATPase [78, 79]. A Na^+/Ca^{2+} exchanger involved in regulating Na^+-dependent Ca^{2+} efflux from mitochondria may also be contributory [80, 81].

PTH-mediated early and persistent intracellular Ca^{2+} overloading is coupled to an induction of oxidative stress in diverse tissues, including cardiomyocytes and their mitochondria. Endogenous antioxidant defenses initially (week 1) neutralize oxygen metabolites, but ultimately (week 4) are overwhelmed by the persistent intracellular Ca^{2+} overloading [82]. In mitochondria, persistent Ca^{2+} overloading and oxidative stress lead to a nonphysiologic opening of the mPTP, with the ensuing osmotic-based structural and functional degeneration of these organelles that triggers the final common cell death pathway leading to cardiomyocyte necrosis [82].

A series of site-directed, sequential pharmacologic interventions targeted along the cellular–subcellular cascades to block downstream events leading to cardiomyocyte necrosis and myocardial scarring, including parathyroidectomy, were conducted and have been reviewed elsewhere [83]. These observations collectively validated our hypothesis regarding the pathologic sequelae of events leading to this structural remodeling of

myocardium in rats with chronic aldosteronism. We have not discounted a potential role for excess catecholamines that may accompany ALDOST.

Cytosolic free $[Zn^{2+}]_i$ in cardiac myocytes and total $[Zn^{2+}]_m$ concentration in mitochondria are concordantly increased with Ca^{2+} dyshomeostasis [57]. The rise in cardiomyocyte $[Zn^{2+}]_i$ is facilitated by the increased expression of membranous Zn^{2+} transporters. Increased $[Zn^{2+}]_i$ serves to augment the antioxidant defenses of cardiomyocytes, including their upregulation of MT-1 and activation of metal-responsive transcription factor (MTF)-1, which encodes genes related to various antioxidant defenses, such as Cu/Zn-SOD, MT-1, and glutathione synthase (see Fig. 3). Thus, intracellular Zn^{2+} loading in chronic aldosteronism is contemporaneous with intracellular Ca^{2+} overloading and relevant biomarkers of oxidative stress [58].

Pathophysiologically and in terms of innate redox states, Zn^{2+} appears to serve as antioxidant and Ca^{2+} as prooxidant. This concept propels the prospect of exploiting Zn^{2+} supplementation as a novel therapeutic strategy to uncouple the intrinsically coupled Ca^{2+} and Zn^{2+} dyshomeostasis in favor of increasing $[Zn^{2+}]_i$, thus enhancing the overall endogenous antioxidant defense capacity that simultaneously attenuate adverse myocardial remodeling. The efficacy of a Zn^{2+} supplement in augmenting intracellular $[Zn^{2+}]_i$, and thereby antioxidant defenses, in rats receiving ALDOST was explored using $ZnSO_4$ [57]. Cotreatment of ALDOST rats with $ZnSO_4$ prevented hypozincemia and a fall in plasma Cu/Zn-SOD activity, while significantly increasing cardiomyocyte cytosolic $[Zn^{2+}]_i$. It also attenuated the increase in biomarkers of oxidative stress, such as cardiac 8-isoprostane, and microscopic scarring.

In summary, these findings during ALDOST revalidate our view of the cellular–subcellular pathway leading to cardiomyocyte necrosis and the concept that increased tissue Zn^{2+} in the heart serves as an antioxidant, and intracellular Ca^{2+} overloading as prooxidant, in the genesis of cardiomyocyte necrosis. They further highlight the intrinsic codependency of these two biologically essential and dynamic divalent cations. An intrinsic coupling between intracellular Ca^{2+} and Zn^{2+} regulates the redox state of cardiac myocytes and mitochondria [58]. These cumulative salutary

Fig. 3 Our current understanding of the intrinsically coupled dyshomeostasis of Ca²⁺ and Zn²⁺ found in ALDOST. See text for details. Adapted from Kamalov G, et al. J Cardiovasc Pharmacol. 2009;53:414–23

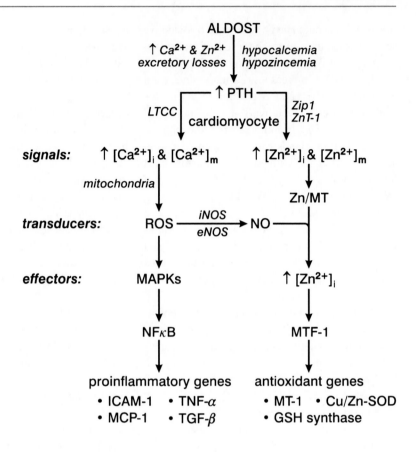

observations raise the therapeutic prospect that nutriceuticals capable of favorably influencing extra- and intracellular Ca²⁺ and Zn²⁺ balance, which is pivotal to combating oxidative injury, could prevent cardiac myocyte necrosis and myocardial scarring.

Cardiomyopathy of the Syrian Hamster

The Model

Membrane-mediated EICA and diminished cellular energetics with a progressive decline in contractility during 1–6 months of age with increasing mitochondrial Ca²⁺-overloading present in the myocardium, as well as diaphragm and skeletal muscle of the BIO-14.6 (analogous to CHF-146) strain dystrophic hamster (DH) are genetically predisposed to hereditary muscular dystrophy (HMD) and hypertrophic cardiomyopathy.

Intracellular Ca²⁺ Overloading

The BIO-14.6 strain of DH has been studied to elucidate the degree of EICA, other biochemical abnormalities, cardiac malfunction, and histological aberrations associated with the dystrophic pathophysiology in degenerating heart and muscles. DH demonstrated significant EICA: 21-fold in the myocardium, 3-fold in skeletal muscle, and 7-fold in the diaphragm. Histologically, Ca²⁺ deposition is evidenced by Ca²⁺-specific staining [30]. These profound EICA in dystrophic muscle from DH remains the highest reported in any living myofibers, and appears to be progressive in nature advancing with age and severity of the disease [31, 32].

Catecholamine and PTH-induced Ca overloading occurs in acute and chronic stressor states, such as in Isop-induced myocardial injury and ALDOST. Before the advent of Ca^{2+} channel blockers, it was thought that PTH may systemically act as an endogenous Ca^{2+} agonist, thus facilitating Ca^{2+} overloading in dystrophic tissues, albeit at PTH levels that are inappropriate even at normal to borderline elevated levels. Accordingly, young adult male DH with profound EICA was thyroparathyroidectomized and placed on daily subcutaneous L-thyroxine (TPTX) replacement. Following 55 days of TPTX, EICA in the heart, diaphragm, and rectus femoris was significantly reduced by 52, 25, and 43%, respectively, and necrosis and fibrosis attenuated without altering their Mg^{2+} content or plasma concentrations of Ca^{2+} or Mg^{2+}. Furthermore, none of these parameters were appreciably changed by TPTX in the age- and gender-matched controls [30].

Since Zn^{2+} is essential to antioxidant defenses and tissue repair, total Zn^{2+} concentrations were monitored in the cardiac and skeletal muscles in DH with advanced cardiomyopathy. Compared to controls and concomitant to EICA, total Zn^{2+} concentration was significantly increased in myocardium (30%), diaphragm (22%), and rectus femoris (82%) [84]. We hypothesized that Zn^{2+} may be cotransported with Ca^{2+} across the cellular membrane or substituted for Ca^{2+} in certain pathways. These observations suggest a possible reparative involvement of Zn^{2+} as an antioxidant in DH, as described in our models of ALDOST and Isop treatment.

Oral diltiazem, a Ca^{2+} channel blocker, was given to young adult male DH for 55 days to study its regulatory effect in modulating EICA in the dystrophic muscles, compared to those observed from the TPTX study. A marked reduction in EICA was noted in the diltiazem-treated group: 73% in the heart, 61% in diaphragm, and 48% in rectus femoris. Plasma creatine phosphokinase was also reduced significantly by 37%, together with a significant reduction in necrosis and Ca^{2+} deposition in the heart [85, 86]. Diltiazem also halted the high mortality and morbidity in DH. These findings implicate diltiazem to have potential therapeutic value in HMD.

Membrane-mediated EICA and diminished cellular energetics with low ATP content and cellular energy charge are invariably present in the dystrophic myocardium of DH [87] suggesting inherent mitochondrial functional deficits with Ca^{2+} overloading. Respiratory dysfunction and Ca^{2+} overloading of mitochondria harvested from the heart of young and old male DH were compared to those obtained from the age- and gender-matched normal hamsters. Mitochondria isolated in the absence of EDTA incorporated in the isolating medium (B_0 medium) revealed significantly poor coupling of oxidative phosphorylation, diminished stimulated oxygen consumption, and lower respiratory control ratios and ADP/O_2 ratios than those seen in controls. Incorporation of EDTA, a Ca^{2+} chelator (B_+ medium), reversed the mitochondrial malfunctions and simultaneously reduced the Ca^{2+} overloading in these dystrophic organelles [32]. Total Ca^{2+} concentration in the in vitro cardiac mitochondria from young and old dystrophic hamsters were significantly higher than their normal littermates, irrespective of the composition of the isolation medium and the age of the hamsters. Moreover, the dystrophic mitochondria isolated in B_+ medium had significantly lower Ca^{2+} concentration, and markedly improved oxidative phosphorylation, similar to those seen in cardiac mitochondria from controls. Furthermore, the total Ca^{2+} concentration of ventricular myocardium of both young and old DH, measured by atomic absorption spectroscopy, were significantly higher compared to controls, bearing a positive correlation with the Ca^{2+} overloading found in cardiac mitochondria of DH [32]. These findings suggest that mitochondrial dysfunction and Ca^{2+} overloading in DH may be reversible if membrane-mediated EICA is pharmacologically mitigated by diltiazem.

In summary, these cascading sequelae of intricate intracellular events in dystrophic myocardium directly influence the structural and functional integrity of cardiac mitochondria and appear to orchestrate the crucial pathogenic cellular–subcellular mechanism in the genesis of membrane-mediated EICA and oxidative stress-induced cardiomyocyte cell death. Cardiac EICA and the consequent mitochondrial Ca^{2+}

overloading predisposes to significant, but reversible, impairments in their oxidative phosphorylation and uncoupling that severely compromise ATP generation and adenine nucleotide translocase activity across the mitochondrial membrane. EICA and these inherent mitochondrial functional deficiencies can be effectively reversed by diltiazem [32, 88]. The potential efficacy of a Zn^{2+} supplement remains to be explored. Treatment with a cyclophilin inhibitor or deletion of the gene encoding it in rodents has rendered mitochondria insensitive to Ca^{2+} overloading-induced osmotic swelling to reduce attendant cardiomyocyte necrosis [89].

Conclusions

An ongoing loss of cardiomyocytes contributes to the progressive nature of the heart's failure as a muscular pump. Acute and chronic stressor states are associated with the loss of these cells. Herein, we reviewed the pathophysiologic basis to cardiomyocyte necrosis found in three different animal models: the acute stressor state that accompanies a single dose of Isop, the chronic stressor state found with 4 weeks of ALDOST, and the cardiomyopathy inherited by the Syrian hamsters. The mitochondriocentric signal-transducer–effector pathway leading to cardiomyocyte necrosis consists of calcitropic hormone-invoked, intracellular Ca^{2+} overloading-induced oxidative stress-mediated opening of the mPTP. This cellular–subcellular cascade eventuates in the dysfunction and structural degeneration of mitochondria and the ensuing necrotic death of cardiomyocytes. A natural wound healing response follows with a consequent replacement fibrosis, which is recognized as a major determinant to the adverse structural remodeling of the failing myocardium. Such microscopic scarring, while preserving the structural integrity of the myocardium, is not without adverse dysfunction of its mechanical and electrical behavior.

Cumulative insights gathered from these models, together with the mechanistic relevance of this pathophysiologic pathway in ischemia–reperfusion and hypoxia–reoxygenation forms of injury, as well as the cardiomyopathies that accompany diabetes and adriamycin treatment, lead to the inevitable recognition as to the central role of mitochondria as the determinant to the fate of cardiomyocytes. The potential of developing cardioprotective strategies that will salvage myocardium during stressor states and target mitochondria needs to be explored. Such interventions might encompass one or more diverse approaches: inhibiting their uptake of Ca^{2+}, modulating the equilibrium that exists between prooxidants generated and their detoxification by endogenous antioxidant defenses, and/or enhancing their resistance to mPTP opening. Toward this end, the efficacy and safety of mitochondria-targeted pharmaceuticals and/or nutriceuticals needs to be determined.

Acknowledgments This work was supported, in part, by NIH grants R01-HL73043 and R01-HL90867 (K.T.W.). Its contents are solely the responsibility of the authors and do not necessarily represent the official views of the NIH. The authors have no conflicts of interest to disclose.

References

1. Matzinger P. The danger model: a renewed sense of self. Science. 2002;296:301–5.
2. Gallucci S, Matzinger P. Danger signals: SOS to the immune system. Curr Opin Immunol. 2001;13:114–9.
3. Todryk SM, Melcher AA, Dalgleish AG, Vile RG. Heat shock proteins refine the danger theory. Immunology. 2000;99:334–7.
4. Beltrami CA, Finato N, Rocco M, et al. Structural basis of end-stage failure in ischemic cardiomyopathy in humans. Circulation. 1994;89:151–63.
5. Ishii J, Nomura M, Nakamura Y, et al. Risk stratification using a combination of cardiac troponin T and brain natriuretic peptide in patients hospitalized for worsening chronic heart failure. Am J Cardiol. 2002;89:691–5.
6. Kuwabara Y, Sato Y, Miyamoto T, et al. Persistently increased serum concentrations of cardiac troponin in patients with acutely decompensated heart failure are predictive of adverse outcomes. Circ J. 2007;71:1047–51.
7. Peacock 4th WF, De Marco T, Fonarow GC, et al. Cardiac troponin and outcome in acute heart failure. N Engl J Med. 2008;358:2117–26.
8. Zairis MN, Tsiaousis GZ, Georgilas AT, et al. Multimarker strategy for the prediction of 31 days cardiac death in patients with acutely decompensated chronic heart failure. Int J Cardiol. 2009;141:284–90.
9. Löwbeer C, Gustafsson SA, Seeberger A, Bouvier F, Hulting J. Serum cardiac troponin T in patients

hospitalized with heart failure is associated with left ventricular hypertrophy and systolic dysfunction. Scand J Clin Lab Invest. 2004;64:667–76.

10. Horwich TB, Patel J, MacLellan WR, et al. Cardiac troponin I is associated with impaired hemodynamics, progressive left ventricular dysfunction, and increased mortality rates in advanced heart failure. Circulation. 2003;108:833–8.

11. Sukova J, Ostadal P, Widimsky P. Profile of patients with acute heart failure and elevated troponin I levels. Exp Clin Cardiol. 2007;12:153–6.

12. Ilva T, Lassus J, Siirilä-Waris K, et al. Clinical significance of cardiac troponins I and T in acute heart failure. Eur J Heart Fail. 2008;10:772–9.

13. Sato Y, Nishi K, Taniguchi R, et al. In patients with heart failure and non-ischemic heart disease, cardiac troponin T is a reliable predictor of long-term echocardiographic changes and adverse cardiac events. J Cardiol. 2009;54:221–30.

14. Miller WL, Hartman KA, Burritt MF, et al. Profiles of serial changes in cardiac troponin T concentrations and outcome in ambulatory patients with chronic heart failure. J Am Coll Cardiol. 2009;54:1715–21.

15. Allard MF, Flint JD, English JC, et al. Calcium overload during reperfusion is accelerated in isolated hypertrophied rat hearts. J Mol Cell Cardiol. 1994;26:1551–63.

16. Kirshenbaum LA, Hill M, Singal PK. Endogenous antioxidants in isolated hypertrophied cardiac myocytes and hypoxia-reoxygenation injury. J Mol Cell Cardiol. 1995;27:263–72.

17. Nakayama H, Chen X, Baines CP, et al. Ca²⁺- and mitochondrial-dependent cardiomyocyte necrosis as a primary mediator of heart failure. J Clin Invest. 2007;117:2431–44.

18. Khullar M, Al-Shudiefat AA, Ludke A, et al. Oxidative stress: a key contributor to diabetic cardiomyopathy. Can J Physiol Pharmacol. 2010;88:233–40.

19. Cai L. Diabetic cardiomyopathy and its prevention by metallothionein: experimental evidence, possible mechanisms and clinical implications. Curr Med Chem. 2007;14:2193–203.

20. Chhokar VS, Sun Y, Bhattacharya SK, et al. Hyperparathyroidism and the calcium paradox of aldosteronism. Circulation. 2005;111:871–8.

21. Vidal A, Sun Y, Bhattacharya SK, et al. Calcium paradox of aldosteronism and the role of the parathyroid glands. Am J Physiol Heart Circ Physiol. 2006;290:H286–94.

22. Afzal N, Ganguly PK, Dhalla KS, et al. Beneficial effects of verapamil in diabetic cardiomyopathy. Diabetes. 1988;37:936–42.

23. Selye H. The general adaptation syndrome and the diseases of adaptation. J Clin Endocrinol. 1946;6:117–230.

24. Fleckenstein A, Kanke J, Döring HJ, et al. Key role of Ca in the production of noncoronarogenic myocardial necroses. Recent Adv Stud Cardiac Struct Metab. 1975;6:21–32.

25. Lossnitzer K, Janke J, Hein B, et al. Disturbed myocardial calcium metabolism: a possible pathogenetic factor in the hereditary cardiomyopathy of the Syrian hamster. Recent Adv Stud Cardiac Struct Metab. 1975;6:207–17.

26. Bier CB, Rona G. Mineralocorticoid potentiation of isoproterenol-induced myocardial injury: ultrastructural equivalent. J Mol Cell Cardiol. 1979;11:961–6.

27. Rona G, Boutet M, Huttner I. Reperfusion injury. A possible link between catecholamine-induced and ischemic myocardial alterations. Adv Myocardiol. 1983;4:427–39.

28. Yates JC, Taam GM, Singal PK, et al. Modification of adrenochrome-induced cardiac contractile failure and cell damage by changes in cation concentrations. Lab Invest. 1980;43:316–26.

29. Singal PK, Forbes MS, Sperelakis N. Occurrence of intramitochondrial Ca²⁺ granules in a hypertrophied heart exposed to adriamycin. Can J Physiol Pharmacol. 1984;62:1239–44.

30. Palmieri GM, Nutting DF, Bhattacharya SK, et al. Parathyroid ablation in dystrophic hamsters. Effects on Ca content and histology of heart, diaphragm, and rectus femoris. J Clin Invest. 1981;68:646–54.

31. Bhattacharya SK, Crawford AJ, Pate JW. Electrocardiographic, biochemical, and morphologic abnormalities in dystrophic hamsters with cardiomyopathy. Muscle Nerve. 1987;10:168–76.

32. Bhattacharya SK, Johnson PL, Thakar JH. Reversal of impaired oxidative phosphorylation and calcium overloading in the in vitro cardiac mitochondria of CHF-146 dystrophic hamsters with hereditary muscular dystrophy. J Neurol Sci. 1993;120:180–6.

33. Singal PK, Kirshenbaum LA. A relative deficit in antioxidant reserve may contribute in cardiac failure. Can J Cardiol. 1990;6:47–9.

34. Li Y, Johnson N, Capano M, et al. Cyclophilin-D promotes the mitochondrial permeability transition but has opposite effects on apoptosis and necrosis. Biochem J. 2004;383:101–9.

35. Basso E, Fante L, Fowlkes J, et al. Properties of the permeability transition pore in mitochondria devoid of Cyclophilin D. J Biol Chem. 2005;280:18558–61.

36. Baines CP, Kaiser RA, Purcell NH, et al. Loss of cyclophilin D reveals a critical role for mitochondrial permeability transition in cell death. Nature. 2005;434:658–62.

37. Nakagawa T, Shimizu S, Watanabe T, et al. Cyclophilin D-dependent mitochondrial permeability transition regulates some necrotic but not apoptotic cell death. Nature. 2005;434:652–8.

38. Shahbaz AU, Zhao T, Zhao W, et al. Calcium and zinc dyshomeostasis during isoproterenol-induced acute stressor state. Am J Physiol Heart Circ Physiol. 2011;300(2):H636–44.

39. Smogorzewski M, Zayed M, Zhang YB, et al. Parathyroid hormone increases cytosolic calcium concentration in adult rat cardiac myocytes. Am J Physiol. 1993;264:H1998–2006.

40. Boutet M, Hüttner I, Rona G. Permeability alteration of sarcolemmal membrane in catecholamine-induced cardiac muscle cell injury. In vivo studies with fine

structural diffusion tracer horse radish peroxidase. Lab Invest. 1976;34:482–8.

41. Benjamin IJ, Jalil JE, Tan LB, et al. Isoproterenol-induced myocardial fibrosis in relation to myocyte necrosis. Circ Res. 1989;65:657–70.

42. Tan LB, Burniston JG, Clark WA, et al. Characterization of adrenoceptor involvement in skeletal and cardiac myotoxicity induced by sympathomimetic agents: toward a new bioassay for beta-blockers. J Cardiovasc Pharmacol. 2003;41:518–25.

43. Goldspink DF, Burniston JG, Ellison GM, et al. Catecholamine-induced apoptosis and necrosis in cardiac and skeletal myocytes of the rat in vivo: the same or separate death pathways? Exp Physiol. 2004;89: 407–16.

44. Burniston JG, Ellison GM, Clark WA, et al. Relative toxicity of cardiotonic agents: some induce more cardiac and skeletal myocyte apoptosis and necrosis in vivo than others. Cardiovasc Toxicol. 2005;5: 355–64.

45. Lathers CM, Levin RM, Spivey WH. Regional distribution of myocardial β-adrenoceptors in the cat. Eur J Pharmacol. 1986;130:111–7.

46. Myslivecek J, Nováková M, Palkovits M, et al. Distribution of mRNA and binding sites of adrenoceptors and muscarinic receptors in the rat heart. Life Sci. 2006;79:112–20.

47. Gengo PJ, Sabbah HN, Steffen RP, et al. Myocardial beta adrenoceptor and voltage sensitive calcium channel changes in a canine model of chronic heart failure. J Mol Cell Cardiol. 1992;24:1361–9.

48. Upsher ME, Weiss HR. Heterogeneous distribution of beta adrenoceptors in the dog left ventricle. J Mol Cell Cardiol. 1986;18:657–60.

49. Rushmer RF, Thal N. The mechanics of ventricular contraction; a cinefluorographic study. Circulation. 1951;4(2):219–28.

50. Sedmera D, Reckova M, Bigelow MR, et al. Developmental transitions in electrical activation patterns in chick embryonic heart. Anat Rec A Discov Mol Cell Evol Biol. 2004;280:1001–9.

51. Buchalter MB, Rademakers FE, Weiss JL, et al. Rotational deformation of the canine left ventricle measured by magnetic resonance tagging: effects of catecholamines, ischaemia, and pacing. Cardiovasc Res. 1994;28:629–35.

52. Mathew BM, Kumar S, Ahmad MS, et al. A temporal profile of myocardial zinc changes after isoproterenol induced cardiac necrosis. Jpn Circ J. 1978;42:353–7.

53. Ahmad M, Salahuddin, Mathew BM, et al. Effect of extent of myocardial damage on the behavior of myocardial zinc in albino rats. Adv Myocardiol. 1980;2: 171–6.

54. McIntosh R, Lee S, Ghio AJ, et al. The critical role of intracellular zinc in adenosine A_2 receptor activation induced cardioprotection against reperfusion injury. J Mol Cell Cardiol. 2010;49:41–7.

55. Chanoit G, Lee S, Xi J, et al. Exogenous zinc protects cardiac cells from reperfusion injury by targeting mitochondrial permeability transition pore through

56. Lee S, Chanoit G, McIntosh R, et al. Molecular mechanism underlying Akt activation in zinc-induced cardioprotection. Am J Physiol Heart Circ Physiol. 2009;297:H569–75.

57. Gandhi MS, Deshmukh PA, Kamalov G, et al. Causes and consequences of zinc dyshomeostasis in rats with chronic aldosteronism. J Cardiovasc Pharmacol. 2008;52:245–52.

58. Kamalov G, Deshmukh PA, Baburyan NY, et al. Coupled calcium and zinc dyshomeostasis and oxidative stress in cardiac myocytes and mitochondria of rats with chronic aldosteronism. J Cardiovasc Pharmacol. 2009;53:414–23.

59. Chvapil M, Owen JA. Effect of zinc on acute and chronic isoproterenol induced heart injury. J Mol Cell Cardiol. 1977;9:151–9.

60. Singal PK, Kapur N, Dhillon KS, et al. Role of free radicals in catecholamine-induced cardiomyopathy. Can J Physiol Pharmacol. 1982;60:1390–7.

61. Singal PK, Dhillon KS, Beamish RE, et al. Protective effect of zinc against catecholamine-induced myocardial changes electrocardiographic and ultrastructural studies. Lab Invest. 1981;44:426–33.

62. Rona G. Catecholamine cardiotoxicity. J Mol Cell Cardiol. 1985;17:291–306.

63. Zielen P, Klisiewicz A, Januszewicz A, et al. Pheochromocytoma-related 'classic' takotsubo cardiomyopathy. J Hum Hypertens. 2010;24:363–6.

64. Gastwirth VG, Yang HS, Steidley DE, et al. Dobutamine stress-induced cardiomyopathy in an orthotopic heart transplant patient. J Heart Lung Transplant. 2009;28:968–70.

65. Margey R, Diamond P, McCann H, et al. Dobutamine stress echo-induced apical ballooning (Takotsubo) syndrome. Eur J Echocardiogr. 2009;10:395–9.

66. Nykamp D, Titak JA. Takotsubo cardiomyopathy, or broken-heart syndrome. Ann Pharmacother. 2010; 44:590–3.

67. Brilla CG, Janicki JS, Weber KT. Impaired diastolic function and coronary reserve in genetic hypertension: role of interstitial fibrosis and medial thickening of intramyocardial coronary arteries. Circ Res. 1991;69:107–15.

68. Darrow DC, Miller HC. The production of cardiac lesions by repeated injections of desoxycorticosterone acetate. J Clin Invest. 1942;21:601–11.

69. Thomas M, Vidal A, Bhattacharya SK, et al. Zinc dyshomeostasis in rats with aldosteronism. Response to spironolactone. Am J Physiol Heart Circ Physiol. 2007;293:H2361–6.

70. Sun Y, Zhang J, Lu L, et al. Aldosterone-induced inflammation in the rat heart. Role of oxidative stress. Am J Pathol. 2002;161:1773–81.

71. Brilla CG, Pick R, Tan LB, et al. Remodeling of the rat right and left ventricle in experimental hypertension. Circ Res. 1990;67:1355–64.

72. Fleckenstein A, Frey M, Fleckenstein-Grun G. Consequences of uncontrolled calcium entry and its

inactivation of glycogen synthase kinase-3β. Am J Physiol Heart Circ Physiol. 2008;295:H1227–33.

prevention with calcium antagonists. Eur Heart J. 1983;4(Suppl H):43–50.

73. Ahokas RA, Sun Y, Bhattacharya SK, et al. Aldosteronism and a proinflammatory vascular phenotype. Role of Mg^{2+}, Ca^{2+} and H_2O_2 in peripheral blood mononuclear cells. Circulation. 2005;111:51–7.

74. Ahokas RA, Warrington KJ, Gerling IC, et al. Aldosteronism and peripheral blood mononuclear cell activation. A neuroendocrine-immune interface. Circ Res. 2003;93:e124–35.

75. Chhokar VS, Sun Y, Bhattacharya SK, et al. Loss of bone minerals and strength in rats with aldosteronism. Am J Physiol Heart Circ Physiol. 2004;287:H2023–6.

76. Rampe D, Lacerda AE, Dage RC, et al. Parathyroid hormone: an endogenous modulator of cardiac calcium channels. Am J Physiol. 1991;261(6 Pt 2):H1945–50.

77. Perna AF, Smogorzewski M, Massry SG. Effects of verapamil on the abnormalities in fatty acid oxidation of myocardium. Kidney Int. 1989;36:453–7.

78. Massry SG, Smogorzewski M. Mechanisms through which parathyroid hormone mediates its deleterious effects on organ function in uremia. Semin Nephrol. 1994;14:219–31.

79. Touyz RM. Reactive oxygen species as mediators of calcium signaling by angiotensin II: implications in vascular physiology and pathophysiology. Antioxid Redox Signal. 2005;7:1302–14.

80. Palty R, Silverman WF, Hershfinkel M, et al. NCLX is an essential component of mitochondrial Na^+/Ca^{2+} exchange. Proc Natl Acad Sci USA. 2010;107:436–41.

81. Kuo TH, Zhu L, Golden K, et al. Altered Ca^{2+} homeostasis and impaired mitochondrial function in cardiomyopathy. Mol Cell Biochem. 2002;238:119–27.

82. Kamalov G, Ahokas RA, Zhao W, et al. Temporal responses to intrinsically coupled calcium and zinc dyshomeostasis in cardiac myocytes and mitochondria during aldosteronism. Am J Physiol Heart Circ Physiol. 2010;298:H385–94.

83. Zia AA, Kamalov G, Newman KP, et al. From aldosteronism to oxidative stress: the role of excessive intracellular calcium accumulation. Hypertens Res. 2010;33(11):1091–101.

84. Crawford AJ, Bhattacharya SK. Excessive intracellular zinc accumulation in cardiac and skeletal muscles of dystrophic hamsters. Exp Neurol. 1987;95:265–76.

85. Bhattacharya SK, Palmieri GM, Bertorini TE, et al. The effects of diltiazem in dystrophic hamsters. Muscle Nerve. 1982;5:73–8.

86. Johnson PL, Bhattacharya SK. Regulation of membrane-mediated chronic muscle degeneration in dystrophic hamsters by calcium-channel blockers: diltiazem, nifedipine and verapamil. J Neurol Sci. 1993;115:76–90.

87. Fedelesova M, Dhalla NS. High energy phosphate stores in the hearts of genetically dystrophic hamsters. J Mol Cell Cardiol. 1971;3:93–102.

88. Bhattacharya SK, Johnson PL, Thakar JH. Reversal of impaired oxidative phosphorylation and calcium overloading in the skeletal muscle mitochondria of CHF-146 dystrophic hamsters. Mol Chem Neuropathol. 1998;34:53–77.

89. Millay DP, Sargent MA, Osinska H, et al. Genetic and pharmacologic inhibition of mitochondrial-dependent necrosis attenuates muscular dystrophy. Nat Med. 2008;14:442–7.

Intracellular MMP-2: Role in Normal and Diseased Hearts

Nermeen Youssef and Richard Schulz

Abstract

Matrix metalloproteinase (MMP)-2 is an abundant protease found in all cells of the heart and is well known for its role in extracellular matrix remodeling. Its biological actions in physiological processes such as angiogenesis and heart development, as well as in cardiac pathologies such as ischemia–reperfusion injury and heart failure, have been significantly expanded, as it is now understood to have specific targets and actions inside the cardiac myocyte. MMP-2 localizes to the nucleus, mitochondria, caveolae, and especially the sarcomere of cardiac myocytes. 72-kDa MMP-2 is directly activated by oxidative stress, especially by peroxynitrite, in a mechanism not requiring proteolytic removal of its propeptide. Studies from our laboratory have identified novel intracellular substrates for it including troponin I, titin, myosin light chain-1, α-actinin, glycogen synthase kinase-3β, and poly (ADP-ribose) polymerase. The proteolysis of the sarcomeric proteins by MMP-2 rapidly follows reperfusion of ischemic heart muscle and contributes to myocardial stunning injury, which can be ameliorated by MMP inhibitors. Other intracellular targets are yet to be discovered, and each provides new mechanisms by which MMP-2 can affect cardiac contractile function. MMP inhibitors may become therapeutic drugs for the treatment of heart diseases associated with enhanced oxidative stress.

Keywords

Matrix metalloproteinase-2 • Extracellular matrix • Gelatinase • Oxidative stress • Phosphorylation • TIMP • MMP inhibitors • Caveolin-1 • Doxycycline • Peroxynitrite • Troponin I • Titin • Myosin light chain-1 • Cytoskeleton • α-Actinin • Glycogen synthase kinase-3β • Sarcomere • Ischemia–reperfusion • Glutathiolation • Stunning

R. Schulz (✉)
Departments of Pediatrics and Pharmacology,
Cardiovascular Research Centre, Mazankowski Alberta
Heart Institute, University of Alberta,
Edmonton, AB, Canada
e-mail: richard.schulz@ualberta.ca

N.S. Dhalla, M. Nagano, B. Ostadal (eds.), *Molecular Defects in Cardiovascular Disease*,
DOI 10.1007/978-1-4419-7130-2_2, © Springer Science+Business Media, LLC 2011

Introduction

Proteases are known to be pivotal regulators of many vital physiological and pathological processes. Their activation or deactivation is a key step in preventing or effecting disease. They play key roles in cardiovascular diseases, from caspases in cardiac cell death, to renin and angiotensin-converting enzyme in hypertension, and to matrix metalloproteinases (MMPs) in ischemic and inflammatory heart disease. Known primarily for their ability to proteolyze extracellular matrix proteins, MMPs have been extensively studied in the past 50 years following their discovery. Their proteolytic activity was later found to be central in several physiological as well as pathological processes in the human body. MMP-2 is found in almost all cells and is particularly known to be involved in cardiovascular pathologies related to enhanced oxidative stress such as ischemia–reperfusion (IR) injury. Contrary to the common idea that MMP-2 is only an extracellular protease, compelling evidence shows that there are new biological roles for it inside the cell. Acute changes in myocardial contractile function are caused by MMP-2's intracellular localization and ability to cleave specific proteins important in regulating the contractile function of the heart. In this chapter, we discuss some of the novel intracellular roles of MMP-2 that are thus far known in normal and diseased hearts.

MMPs

MMPs are a family of structurally related zinc-dependent endopeptidases. MMP activity was first discovered in 1962 by Gross and Lapiere as a collagen-digesting enzyme involved in tail resorption during the morphogenesis of tadpoles into frogs [1]. This discovery opened the doors to a new field of research focusing mainly on the biological actions of these proteases to proteolytically remodel the extracellular matrix. Such research explained how several physiological remodeling processes such as angiogenesis, embryogenesis [2], uterine involution [3], bone and connective tissue turnover, to name a few, require the extracellular matrix degrading properties of MMPs. In addition to that, MMPs have been shown to play a part in several pathologies including aortic aneurysms [4], cancer [5], and several inflammatory diseases including periodontitis [6] and arthritis [7].

MMPs are referred to numerically from MMP-1 to MMP-28. In the past, they were conventionally grouped according to their substrates, primary structure, or subcellular localizations into the following: gelatinases (MMP-2 and-9), collagenases (MMP-1, -8 and -13), stromelysins (MMP-7 and -26), matrilysins (MMP-3, -10 and -11), metalloelastases (MMP-12), and membrane-type MMPs (MMP-14-16 and MMP-23-25). MMP-4, -5, and -6 are not unique MMPs, since they turned out to be either MMP-2 or MMP-3. The mammalian homologue of MMP-18 has not been found yet [8]. In cardiovascular disease, MMP-2 appears to be of greater significance compared to other MMPs, based on its elevated activity in hypertension, heart failure, and ischemic and inflammatory heart diseases. We refer here to useful and extensive reviews on the intracellular [9] and extracellular [10] actions of MMPs in the heart. This chapter, however, focuses solely on the more recently discovered intracellular roles of MMP-2 in the heart.

MMP-2

MMP-2, previously known as gelatinase A or type IV collagenase, is expressed in almost all cell types. It proteolyzes denatured collagen (gelatin) and intact collagen type IV, both of which are core components of the basement membrane. MMP-2 is abundantly expressed in the heart tissue, particularly in the vasculature, cardiomyocytes, and fibroblasts [11–14].

Structure

MMP-2 as with other MMPs is synthesized as a 72-kDa inactive zymogen or "pro-MMP" (see Fig. 1). At its N terminus, it contains an

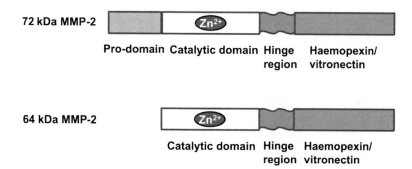

Fig. 1 Schematic structure of 72 and 64 kDa MMP-2. The figure shows the 72 kDa form of MMP-2 containing the prodomain, the catalytic domain, the hinge region and the hemopexin/vitronectin domain. The catalytic domain contains a zinc ion that is essential for MMP-2's activity. The figure also shows the 64 kDa form of MMP-2 where the prodomain has been removed by the action of other proteases

autoinhibitory, hydrophobic propeptide domain that shields the catalytic site of the enzyme. The catalytic site contains a zinc ion that is essential for its activity. The presence of a second structural zinc ion in addition to two or three calcium ions has been suggested [15].

Regulation of MMP-2

A well-studied component of the activation of pro-MMPs is the necessity to disrupt the coordination bond between the cysteine sulfhydryl of the propeptide domain and the zinc ion in the catalytic domain, creating a "cysteine switch" [16]. In the case of MMP-2, this can take place through proteolytic cleavage and removal of the propeptide domain of the full-length 72-kDa enzyme by action of membrane-type-1 MMP (MMP-14), in conjunction with tissue inhibitor of metalloproteinase-2 (TIMP-2), to yield an enzymatically active 64-kDa enzyme [17] (see Fig. 1). However, far less attention has been given to what is likely a very important alternative mechanism of MMP-2 activation, independent of the proteolytic removal of the propeptide domain, by specific disruption of the cysteine–zinc bond by reactive oxygen/nitrogen species (vide infra).

The activity of MMP-2 is regulated at several different levels depending on the type of stimulus. It can be regulated through: (1) changes in gene transcription and translation, (2) posttranslational modifications such as glutathiolation and phosphorylation, (3) interaction with endogenous inhibitors known as the tissue inhibitors of metalloproteinases (TIMPs), and (4) interaction with caveolin-1 in cell membrane caveolae.

Transcription and Translational Changes

It was believed that MMP-2 is a constitutive enzyme; however, it is now known that its expression can be induced. The promoter region of the MMP-2 gene does not contain a TATA box, contrary to that of MMP-9, and allows for multiple transcription sites. MMP-2 transcription occurs by binding of transcription factors to a downstream GC box. The MMP-2 promoter does not contain a proximal AP-1-binding site; however, studies investigating regulation of its transcription revealed a functional AP-1 consensus binding sequence [18]. At the mRNA level, MMP-2 expression in cardiac and vascular smooth muscle cells is upregulated in response to hypoxic conditions, angiotensin II, endothelin-1, interleukin-1β, or high glucose [18–21]. MMP-2 expression in human macrovascular endothelial cells was found to be notably increased upon reoxygenation following hypoxia [22], in hearts after IR injury [23] and in congestive heart failure [24]. In addition to that, protein and mRNA levels of MMP-2 are significantly increased upon signaling by proinflammatory cytokines [25].

Oxidative Stress

Studies from our lab and others have shown that it is not necessary for the full-length 72-kDa MMP-2 to lose its propeptide domain to become an active protease. Activation can also take place upon exposure to reactive oxygen/nitrogen species such as peroxynitrite ($ONOO^-$), an important mediator of oxidative stress injury [26]. In a reaction requiring $ONOO^-$ and glutathione, the cysteine–zinc bond in the cysteine switch is disrupted without cleavage of the propeptide domain [27–29]. Okamoto et al. [27] demonstrated that low concentrations of $ONOO^-$ caused S-glutathiolation of the cysteine residue in the PRCGVPD sequence in the MMP-1, -8 and -9 propeptide domain (highly conserved among MMPs) and enhanced their enzymatic activity. Our lab found that 0.3–10 µM $ONOO^-$ activated 72-kDa MMP-2, whereas >100 µM inhibited activity [29]. Fliss and Ménard showed that H_2O_2 modulated a 3 inc metalloprotein, metallothionein, activity in a similar manner, whereby 4 µM activated MMP-2 and 10–50 µM inhibited enzyme activity [30]. Both the responses of MMP-2 to $ONOO^-$ and H_2O_2 suggest a biphasic response to oxidative stress through different posttranslational modifications of the protein and subsequent configurational changes controlling access to the catalytic zinc ion [29].

Phosphorylation

Phosphorylation of serine, threonine, and/or tyrosine residues is an important means to regulate the activity of some proteins. We investigated whether MMP-2 is a phosphorylated protein and if its phosphorylation status affects its enzymatic activity. Recombinant human MMP-2 and native MMP-2 secreted from HT1080 human fibrosarcoma cells were found to be phosphorylated [31]. The activity of MMP-2 after its dephosphorylation with alkaline phosphatase was enhanced, whereas phosphorylation with protein kinase C in vitro reduced its activity. We identified five phosphorylation sites on residues with side chains accessible on the surface of MMP-2 (S32, S160, T250, S365, and Y271); however, the exact phosphorylation sites in vivo are yet unknown. In the setting of IR injury, isolated rat hearts perfused with okadaic acid, an inhibitor

of protein phosphatase 2A, showed improved recovery following reperfusion and reduced loss of troponin I (TnI), an MMP-2 substrate (vide infra), which is an important regulator of actin–myosin interaction. This observation may be attributed to the effect of inhibiting the action of protein phosphatase 2A on MMP-2 to keep MMP-2 in a more phosphorylated and hence, less active state [32]. The protein kinases and phosphatases controlling MMP-2 phosphorylation status in vivo are yet unknown. A study by Nyalendo et al. [33] showed that MMP-14 is phosphorylated and inhibition of its phosphorylation reduced tumor cell proliferation in mice. However, the effect of MMP-14 phosphorylation on its activity is unknown. Figure 2 is a diagram that shows activation pathways of MMP-2 and how this may be further modified by MMP-2 phosphorylation.

TIMPs

Tissue inhibitors of metalloproteinases (TIMPs) are endogenous inhibitors of MMP activity. The TIMP family consists of four known members, TIMP-1 through TIMP-4 [34]. They bind to MMPs in a 1:1 stoichiometric ratio, thereby inhibiting their activity. TIMPs do not show particular specificity toward various MMPs, nonetheless TIMP-2 shows some preferential inhibition of MMP-2 and TIMP-1 with MMP-9 [35]. All TIMPs are constitutively expressed in the heart and vasculature [14]. TIMP-4 protein is abundant in the heart and is localized to the sarcomere within cardiac myocytes in the same subcellular compartment as MMP-2, a fact that implies TIMP-4's likely protective activity against the detrimental actions of MMP-2 in oxidative stress [36, 37]. TIMP-3, on the contrary, is tightly bound to the extracellular matrix where it is exclusively localized [38]. Its level is lowered in the hearts of in mice with heart failure [39] and in aortas of patients with thoracic aortic aneurysms [40].

Caveolin-1

A recently discovered additional means to regulate MMP-2 activity is through its interaction with caveolin-1. A portion of cellular MMP-2 was found to be localized within caveolae of

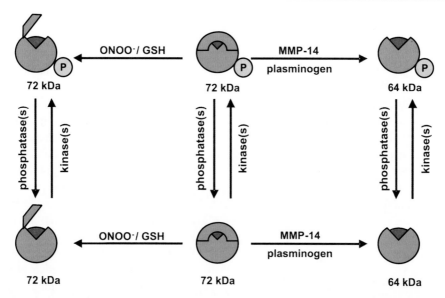

Fig. 2 Different modes of regulation and activation of MMP-2. The 72 kDa form of MMP-2 can be activated by MMP-14 or plasminogen via cleavage of its prodomain to yield the 64 kDa form. 72 kDa MMP-2 can also be activated by exposure to ONOO⁻ in the presence of cellular glutathione without losing the pro-domain. MMP-2 is also a phosphoprotein with several identified phosphorylation sites and whose activity is further modulated by its phosphorylation status [31]. However, the kinases and phosphatases involved in its in vivo regulation are unknown

cardiomyocytes [13, 41] and endothelial cells [42]. Caveolae are invaginations of the cell membrane that regulate cytoplasmic signaling proteins and transport of macromolecules in and out of the cell [43]. We showed that MMP-2 colocalizes with caveolin-1 in cardiac myocytes, an integral membrane protein found within lipid rafts on the inner leaflet of the cell membrane. Hearts from caveolin-1 knockout mice show elevated myocardial MMP-2 activity compared to wild-type control hearts. A peptide containing the caveolin scaffolding domain from caveolin-1 or caveolin-3 inhibited MMP-2 activity in vitro [41]. Despite these findings, we did not find impaired cardiac contractile function in isolated working hearts from young (6–8 week old) mice, either in response to physiological (preload) or pharmacological (isoproterenol) challenges [44]. We speculate that the caveolin-1–MMP-2 interaction may be a means to control the activity of the portion of MMP-2 that is plasma-membrane-bound [41]; however, more work in this area needs to be done.

Pharmacological MMP Inhibitors

Most pharmacological inhibitors of MMP-2 act by chelating the zinc ion in the enzyme's catalytic site [45]. Such MMP inhibitors include batimastat, marimastat, GM-6001 (ilomastat/gelardin), *o*-phenanthroline, PD-166793 [46], and ONO-4817 [47]. Although these compounds selectively inhibit MMP activity in comparison to their lack of action on other protease classes, they do not preferentially inhibit a single MMP. In addition, the tetracycline antibiotics, dependent upon their ability to chelate divalent cations, have proved to be effective inhibitors of MMPs. In investigating their structure–activity relationship, Golub and coworkers synthesized chemically modified tetracyclines which maintained their ability to inhibit MMPs but were devoid of antimicrobial activity [48]. Of the tetracyclines, the most potent MMP inhibitor belonging to this family is doxycyline [49] followed by minocycline. The latter is a more lipophilic molecule and thus exploited for its ability to cross the blood–brain barrier for treatment of neurodegenerative diseases. Studies have demonstrated that doxycycline preferentially inhibits MMP-2, -9, and MMP-8 in comparison to MMP-1 and it has no effect on either MMP-3 or -7 [50]. In vivo doxycycline was found to inhibit MMP activity at a plasma concentration lower than that required for its antibacterial effect [51]. This led to the development of an FDA and Health Canada approved, subantimicrobial dose formulation of doxycycline (doxycycline hyclate, 20 mg b.i.d) approved for the treatment of periodontitis (Periostat®).

Physiological Roles of MMP-2 in the Heart

Before discussing the role of MMP-2 in heart disease, we would first like to shed light on some of its few known physiological roles in the heart. MMP-2 appears to have a crucial role in embryonic heart development [2] including angiogenesis [52], valve development, and heart tube formation [53]. To exemplify the importance of MMP-2 in heart development, Linask et al. used an MMP-2 neutralizing antibody or the MMP inhibitor ilomastat to inhibit MMP-2 in developing chick embryos. This caused severe heart tube defects, cardia bifida, and a disruption in the looping direction, which suggested a key role of MMP-2 in cell migration and remodeling required for normal heart development [53]. MMP-2 knockout mice survive at birth and are viable as adults; however, they display significantly retarded growth in comparison to the wild-type controls [54]. These studies, however, have only focussed on the extracellular matrix degrading actions of MMP-2.

Intracellular MMP-2

In studying IR injury in perfused rat hearts, Cheung et al. found a significantly enhanced release of 72-kDa MMP-2 which peaked in the first 2–5 min of reperfusion [55]. This release of

MMP-2 activity during reperfusion was enhanced with increasing duration of ischemia and showed a negative correlation with the recovery of contractile function during reperfusion. Addition of semi-purified MMP-2 to the perfusion buffer diminished contractile recovery of the heart following IR injury, whereas a neutralizing MMP-2 antibody or the MMP inhibitors o-phenanthroline or doxycycline improved the recovery of contractile function in reperfusion. Looking at these findings one finds compelling evidence for a role of MMP-2 in IR injury. We suggested that the release of MMP-2 from heart tissue reflects its preceding activation for example by ONOO⁻, the biosynthesis of which peaks in the first minute of reperfusion as shown in the same isolated rat heart model [56]. Thus MMP-2 resident within cardiomyocytes is rapidly activated by ONOO⁻ stress and its proteolytic activity may have cleaved intracellular targets prior to its release from cells, the latter a means to reduce overall intracellular proteolytic stress. These findings [55] suggested that MMP-2 may be acting in a different way other than on extracellular matrix proteins to reduce the recovery of cardiac mechanical function as changes in the extracellular matrix were absent in a similar model of acute myocardial stunning injury [57]. A paper by Spinale's group studying the activation of MMPs in failing hearts showed the localization of MMP-2 to the sarcomere in isolated left ventricular myocytes [24]. Although the authors did not discuss this finding it was one of the clues that led us to consider a possible and novel intracellular role of MMP-2 in cardiac myocytes independent of its actions on the extracellular matrix. In the next section we describe the discovery of intracellular biological MMP-2 actions in the heart by its proteolysis of novel intracellular targets and discuss how this is relevant to heart pathology.

Troponin I

Although TnI, an important regulatory protein in the contractile machinery of the heart, is known to be rapidly proteolyzed during acute IR injury, the exact protease(s) involved in this, despite some evidence for calpain, was unclear [58]. Using immunogold electron microscopy we showed that MMP-2 was localized to the sarcomere in cardiac myocytes. TnI was highly susceptible to the proteolytic action of MMP-2 in vitro, and subjecting isolated rat hearts to acute IR injury diminished myocardial TnI content, an effect that was blocked by MMP inhibitors. We provided evidence that myocardial stunning injury is caused in part by MMP-2 mediated TnI proteolysis. This study was the first to recognize an intracellular biological role of any MMP as well as identify the first intracellular target of MMP-2 in cardiomyocytes as TnI. In hearts overexpressing a constitutively active MMP-2 in myocardial specific fashion there were marked derangements in the sarcomere, including TnI degradation and reduced contractile function [59, 60].

Other Sarcomeric Targets of MMP-2 Beyond TnI

Myosin Light Chain-1

Following the same line of thought, since MMP-2 could be localized on the sarcomere, then the possibility of it targeting other sarcomeric proteins was not unlikely. Myosin light chain-1 (MLC-1) is a sarcomeric protein and a blood serum marker of the severity of myocardial infarction [61]. MLC-1 was found to be proteolytically degraded in a canine model of myocardial infarction [62], and this was confirmed in isolated rat hearts subjected to global IR injury [63]; however, the enzyme responsible for its cleavage was unknown. We subjected isolated rat hearts to IR injury to test if MLC-1 degradation was due to its cleavage by MMP-2. We took a pharmacoproteomic approach to find myocardial proteins that may be cleaved by MMP activity. The hearts were treated with or without MMP inhibitors (o-phenanthroline or doxycycline) and 2D gel electrophoresis was performed on myocardial extracts to look at changes in protein spot density. We only considered those changes in spot density to be worthy of further analysis if they changed as a result of IR injury and were then normalized in extracts from

hearts treated with the MMP inhibitors. We identified spots meeting these criteria using mass spectroscopy as MLC-1 degradation products. Moreover, colocalization of MLC-1 and MMP-2 on the thick myofilaments of the sarcomere was demonstrated by immunogold electron microscopy, immunoprecipitation experiments and isolation of purified thick myofilament fractions [64]. The loss in contractile function and MLC-1 content after IR injury was reduced in hearts treated with the MMP inhibitors. MLC-1 is thus another contractile protein element that could be protected by inhibiting MMP activity in oxidative stress injury to the heart.

Titin

Titin is the largest known mammalian protein (3,000–4,000 kDa) and is found in striated muscles, both cardiac and skeletal. It spans nearly half the length of the sarcomere, from the Z-disk to the M-line region. It consists of elastic segments in the I band region, which allows it to act as a molecular spring that helps maintain the structural and functional stability of the myocyte [65]. Titin is also the molecular superstructure on which sarcomeric proteins are assembled during sarcomerogenesis in embryonic myocytes. In cardiac muscle titin is of vast importance since it is a determinant of both diastolic and systolic function and the Frank–Starling mechanism of the heart [66]. We showed in rat and human myocardium that MMP-2 colocalizes with titin mainly near the Z-disk region of the cardiac sarcomere. Cleavage of titin in perfused rat hearts subjected to IR injury or in skinned cardiomyocytes incubated with MMP-2 was prevented with MMP inhibitors o-phenanthroline or ONO-4817 [67]. Titin degradation in hearts was abolished in MMP-2 knockout mice subjected to IR in vivo. Thus MMP-2 plays an important role in titin homeostasis, which directly affects the contractile function of the heart at the sarcomeric level.

Cytoskeletal Targets

α-Actinin is a cytoskeletal protein found at the Z line of the sarcomere. It connects actin filaments in adjacent sarcomeres and thus serves as a pivotal protein in transmitting the force generated by the actin–myosin complex. α-Actinin was shown to activate myosin-ATPase in vitro; therefore, any disturbance in its homeostasis would directly alter the activity of the ATPase and as a result lead to contractile dysfunction [68]. Some clues lead us to test the possibility that MMP-2 might target α-actinin in IR: (a) myocardial levels of some cytoskeletal proteins including α-actinin were reduced after IR injury [63, 64], and (b) immunohistochemistry and confocal microscopy for MMP-2 and α-actinin in cardiac muscle suggested a close subcellular localization [12].

Perfused rat hearts subjected to 15 min ONOO⁻ infusion showed a significant decline in contractile function and α-actinin content, an effect blocked by MMP inhibitors [69]. No significant changes in the protein levels of other cytoskeletal proteins (desmin and αII-spectrin) were observed. In vitro, α-actinin was most susceptible to MMP-2 degradation followed by desmin, whereas αII-spectrin was resistant [70]. A limitation of the study was the use of 64-kDa MMP-2 in the in vitro degradation experiments, and not 72-kDa MMP-2 activated by ONOO⁻ and glutathione. Therefore, the in vitro results and their interpretation may not truly reflect the exact susceptibility of cytoskeletal proteins to degradation by MMP-2 in vivo.

Nuclear Targets

While investigating the subcellular localization of MMP-2 in cardiac myocytes with immunogold electron microscopy we came across additional, unexpected findings. MMP-2 staining was not only exclusive to the sarcomere, as there was evidence of staining in mitochondria and nuclei of cardiac myocytes as well [11]. Interestingly, the nuclear matrix has similarities to that of the extracellular matrix, and important cellular processes such as apoptosis [71] and cell cycle regulation [72] all involve proteolysis of nuclear matrix proteins. Si-Tayeb and colleagues have also shown that the truncated form of MMP-3 is localized in the nucleus, whereas the full-length enzyme is cytosolic [73].

Kwan et al. showed that nuclear extracts purified from either human hearts or rat livers exhibited both MMP-2 as well as MMP-9 activity. We found that both MMP-2 and MMP-9 have a nuclear localization sequence at the C-terminal of MMP-2. Both TIMP-2 and doxycycline reduced the gelatinolytic activities seen in these nuclear extracts [74]. The study also showed that poly (ADP-ribose) polymerase, an enzyme that repairs DNA strand breaks and is present in the nuclear matrix, is susceptible to MMP-2 proteolysis in vitro. Interestingly, DNA strand breaks are caused by ONOO⁻ [75], which can also activate 72-kDa MMP-2 [29]. When DNA damage occurs, PARP uses NAD⁺ and ATP to repair this. However, under severe ONOO⁻ stress, excessive activation of PARP may cause it to deplete metabolites essential for cell survival. We speculated that MMP-2 may play dual roles in the nucleus under oxidative stress, one may be protective by reducing PARP levels to preserve cell energy requirements, and the other is detrimental whereby MMP-2 removal of PARP prevents it from repairing damaged DNA strands [74]. Much further investigation is still needed to identify the role of MMP-2 in the nucleus in both normal and stress conditions.

Other Targets

Glycogen synthase kinase (GSK)-3 is a serine/threonine kinase abundantly expressed in eukaryotes and is important in regulating glycogen metabolism. One of its isoforms, GSK-3β, is pivotal in regulating processes such as cell cycle, apoptosis and cell polarity [76]. GSK-3β is susceptible to proteolysis during oxidative stress and is, therefore, dysregulated. Work by Kandasamy et al. showed that incubation of MMP-2 with GSK-3β resulted in the time and concentration dependent cleavage of GSK-3β. The cleavage product was shown to be lacking the N-terminal of the enzyme as shown by mass spectroscopy. The activity of GSK-3β was significantly enhanced upon incubation with MMP-2 and this was prevented by the MMP inhibitors GM-6001 or ONO-4817. This study showed that GSK-3β may be a target of MMP-2 and that MMP-2 mediates its activity through cleaving the N-terminal of GSK-3β

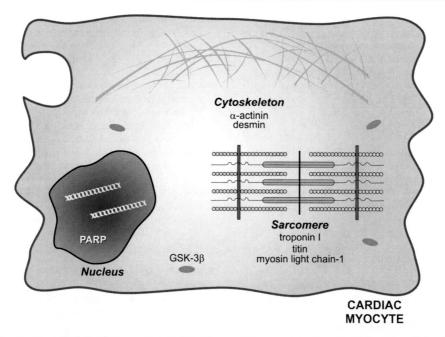

Fig. 3 Thus far identified intracellular targets of MMP-2 in cardiac myocytes. Shown are the: (1) sarcomeric targets of MMP-2: troponin I, titin and myosin light chain-1; (2) cytoskeletal targets: α-actinin and desmin; (3) possible nuclear target poly (ADP-ribose) polymerase (PARP), and (4) the cytosolic target glycogen synthase kinase (GSK)-3β

which contains the autoinhibitory phosphoserine 9 residue. H_2O_2 stimulated GSK-3β activity in cardiomyoblasts and this was prevented with MMP inhibitors [77]. This may suggest that MMP-2 mediated cleavage and activation of GSK-3β may be an additional means whereby MMP-2 contributes to oxidative stress-induced cardiac dysfunction.

Conclusions

MMP-2 is abundant in the normal heart. In cardiomyocytes it is localized to discrete subcellular compartments including the sarcomere, nuclei, mitochondria, and caveolae. It is activated within the cell as a rapid (seconds to minutes time scale) response to enhanced oxidative stress. It is in close proximity to specific proteins within the cell which it selectively proteolyzes as a result of oxidative stress. Figure 3 gives a summary of the thus far known intracellular targets of MMP-2 in cardiomyocytes. The extensive yet incomplete body of knowledge on its activation, regulation and inhibition in both normal physiology and in disease states has added MMP-2 to the list of proteases critical in heart disease both for in its intracellular and extracellular actions. Why MMP-2 is localized to the sarcomere at the core of the contractile apparatus is a puzzle that needs solving. The discovery of intracellular targets of MMP-2 encourages us to further identify new biological roles of MMP-2 inside the cell as the cardiac myocyte is not the only cell where intracellular MMP-2 is found. This knowledge will help in the design of tailored pharmacological inhibitors of MMP-2 that may provide safe and effective drugs to treat cardiac diseases.

Acknowledgments We thank Dawne Colwell for graphics. Studies from the Schulz lab have been generously supported by the Canadian Institutes for Health Research, the Heart and Stroke Foundation of Alberta, NWT and Nunavut, and the Alberta Heritage Foundation for Medical Research.

References

1. Gross J, Lapiere CM. Collagenolytic activity in amphibian tissues: a tissue culture assay. Proc Natl Acad Sci USA. 1962;48:1014–22.
2. Vu TH, Werb Z. Matrix metalloproteinases: effectors of development and normal physiology. Genes Dev. 2000;14:2123–33.
3. Sellers A, Woessner Jr JF. The extraction of a neutral metalloproteinase from the involuting rat uterus, and its action on cartilage proteoglycan. Biochem J. 1980;189:521–31.
4. Thompson M, Cockerill G. Matrix metalloproteinase-2: the forgotten enzyme in aneurysm pathogenesis. Ann NY Acad Sci. 2006;1085:170–4.
5. Deryugina EI, Quigley JP. Matrix metalloproteinases and tumor metastasis. Cancer Metastasis Rev. 2006; 25:9–34.
6. Beutner EH, Triftshauser C, Hazen SP. Collagenase activity of gingival tissue from patients with periodontal disease. Proc Soc Exp Biol Med. 1966;121:1082–5.
7. Mohammed FF, Smookler DS, Khokha R. Metalloproteinases, inflammation, and rheumatoid arthritis. Ann Rheum Dis. 2003;62:ii43–7.
8. Ra HJ, Parks WC. Control of matrix metalloproteinase catalytic activity. Matrix Biol. 2007;26:587–96.
9. Schulz R. Intracellular targets of matrix metalloproteinase-2 in cardiac disease: rationale and therapeutic approaches. Annu Rev Pharmacol Toxicol. 2007;47: 211–42.
10. Spinale FG. Myocardial matrix remodeling and the matrix metalloproteinases: influence on cardiac form and function. Physiol Rev. 2007;87:1285–342.
11. Wang W, Schulze CJ, Suarez-Pinzon WL, et al. Intracellular action of matrix metalloproteinase-2 accounts for acute myocardial ischemia and reperfusion injury. Circulation. 2002;106:1543–9.
12. Coker ML, Doscher MA, Thomas CV, et al. Matrix metalloproteinase synthesis and expression in isolated LV myocyte preparations. Am J Physiol. 1999;277: H777–87.
13. Cho WJ, Chow AK, Schulz R, et al. Matrix metalloproteinase-2, caveolins, focal adhesion kinase and c-kit in cells of the mouse myocardium. J Cell Mol Med. 2007;11:1069–86.
14. Nuttall RK, Sampieri CL, Pennington CJ, et al. Expression analysis of the entire MMP and TIMP gene families during mouse tissue development. FEBS Lett. 2004;563:129–34.
15. Whittaker M, Floyd CD, Brown P, et al. Design and therapeutic application of matrix metalloproteinase inhibitors. Chem Rev. 1999;99:2735–76.
16. Van Wart HE, Birkedal-Hansen H. The cysteine switch: a principle of regulation of metalloproteinase activity with potential applicability to the entire matrix metalloproteinase gene family. Proc Natl Acad Sci USA. 1990;87:5578–82.
17. Cao J, Sato H, Takino T, et al. The C-terminal region of membrane type matrix metalloproteinase is a functional transmembrane domain required for pro-gelatinase A activation. J Biol Chem. 1995;270:801–5.
18. Bergman MR, Cheng S, Honbo N, et al. A functional activating protein 1 (AP-1) site regulates matrix metalloproteinase 2 (MMP-2) transcription by cardiac cells through interactions with JunB-Fra1 and JunB-FosB heterodimers. Biochem J. 2003;369:485–96.
19. Galis ZS, Muszynski M, Sukhova GK, et al. Enhanced expression of vascular matrix metalloproteinases induced in vitro by cytokines and in regions of human atherosclerotic lesions. Ann NY Acad Sci. 1995;748: 501–7.
20. Siwik DA, Chang DL, Colucci WS. Interleukin-1beta and tumor necrosis factor-alpha decrease collagen synthesis and increase matrix metalloproteinase activity in cardiac fibroblasts in vitro. Circ Res. 2000;86: 1259–65.
21. Uzui H, Harpf A, Liu M, et al. Increased expression of membrane type 3-matrix metalloproteinase in human atherosclerotic plaque: role of activated macrophages and inflammatory cytokines. Circulation. 2002;106: 3024–30.
22. Ben-Yosef Y, Lahat N, Shapiro S, et al. Regulation of endothelial matrix metalloproteinase-2 by hypoxia/ reoxygenation. Circ Res. 2002;90:784–91.
23. Alfonso-Jaume MA, Bergman MR, Mahimkar R, et al. Cardiac ischemia-reperfusion injury induces matrix metalloproteinase-2 expression through the AP-1 components FosB and JunB. Am J Physiol Heart Circ Physiol. 2006;291:H1838–46.
24. Spinale FG, Coker ML, Heung LJ, et al. A matrix metalloproteinase induction/activation system exists in the human left ventricular myocardium and is upregulated in heart failure. Circulation. 2000;102:1944–9.
25. Mountain DJ, Singh M, Menon B, et al. Interleukin-1beta increases expression and activity of matrix metalloproteinase-2 in cardiac microvascular endothelial cells: role of PKCalpha/beta1 and MAPKs. Am J Physiol Cell Physiol. 2007;292:C867–75.
26. Pacher P, Beckman JS, Liaudet L. Nitric oxide and peroxynitrite in health and disease. Physiol Rev. 2007;87:315–424.
27. Okamoto T, Akaike T, Sawa T, et al. Activation of matrix metalloproteinases by peroxynitrite-induced protein S-glutathiolation via disulfide S-oxide formation. J Biol Chem. 2001;276:29596–602.
28. Okamoto T, Akaike T, Nagano T, et al. Activation of human neutrophil procollagenase by nitrogen dioxide and peroxynitrite: a novel mechanism for procollagenase activation involving nitric oxide. Arch Biochem Biophys. 1997;342:261–74.
29. Viappiani S, Nicolescu AC, Holt A, et al. Activation and modulation of 72kDa matrix metalloproteinase-2

by peroxynitrite and glutathione. Biochem Pharmacol. 2009;77:826–34.

30. Fliss H, Menard M. Oxidant-induced mobilization of zinc from metallothionein. Arch Biochem Biophys. 1992;293:195–9.

31. Sariahmetoglu M, Crawford BD, Leon H, et al. Regulation of matrix metalloproteinase-2 (MMP-2) activity by phosphorylation. FASEB J. 2007;21:2486–95.

32. Sariahmetoglu M, Skrzypiec M, Leon H, et al. Phosphorylation status of matrix metalloproteinase-2 and potentialrole in myocardial ischemia-reperfusion injury. Circlation, 2004; 110: III-267 (abstract).

33. Nyalendo C, Sartelet H, Gingras D, et al. Inhibition of membrane-type 1 matrix metalloproteinase tyrosine phosphorylation blocks tumor progression in mice. Anticancer Res. 2010;30:1887–95.

34. Baker AH, Edwards DR, Murphy G. Metalloproteinase inhibitors: biological actions and therapeutic opportunities. J Cell Sci. 2002;115:3719–27.

35. Goldberg GI, Strongin A, Collier IE, et al. Interaction of 92-kDa type IV collagenase with the tissue inhibitor of metalloproteinases prevents dimerization, complex formation with interstitial collagenase, and activation of the proenzyme with stromelysin. J Biol Chem. 1992;267:4583–91.

36. Schulze CJ, Wang W, Suarez-Pinzon WL, et al. Imbalance between tissue inhibitor of metalloproteinase-4 and matrix metalloproteinases during acute myocardial ischemia-reperfusion injury. Circulation. 2003;107:2487–92.

37. Cox MJ, Hawkins UA, Hoit BD, et al. Attenuation of oxidative stress and remodeling by cardiac inhibitor of metalloproteinase protein transfer. Circulation. 2004;109:2123–8.

38. Pavloff N, Staskus PW, Kishnani NS, et al. A new inhibitor of metalloproteinases from chicken: ChIMP-3. A third member of the TIMP family. J Biol Chem. 1992;267:17321–6.

39. Fedak PW, Smookler DS, Kassiri Z, et al. TIMP-3 deficiency leads to dilated cardiomyopathy. Circulation. 2004;110:2401–9.

40. Ikonomidis JS, Jones JA, Barbour JR, et al. Expression of matrix metalloproteinases and endogenous inhibitors within ascending aortic aneurysms of patients with Marfan syndrome. Circulation. 2006;114:I365–70.

41. Chow AK, Cena J, El-Yazbi AF, et al. Caveolin-1 inhibits matrix metalloproteinase-2 activity in the heart. J Mol Cell Cardiol. 2007;42:896–901.

42. Puyraimond A, Fridman R, Lemesle M, et al. MMP-2 colocalizes with caveolae on the surface of endothelial cells. Exp Cell Res. 2001;262:28–36.

43. Gratton JP, Bernatchez P, Sessa WC. Caveolae and caveolins in the cardiovascular system. Circ Res. 2004;94:1408–17.

44. Chow AK, Daniel EE, Schulz R. Cardiac function is not significantly diminished in hearts isolated from young caveolin-1 knockout mice. Am J Physiol Heart Circ Physiol. 2010;299:H1183–9.

45. Birkedal-Hansen H, Moore WG, Bodden MK, et al. Matrix metalloproteinases: a review. Crit Rev Oral Biol Med. 1993;4:197–250.

46. Peterson JT. Matrix metalloproteinase inhibitor development and the remodeling of drug discovery. Heart Fail Rev. 2004;9:63–79.

47. Yamada A, Uegaki A, Nakamura T, et al. ONO-4817, an orally active matrix metalloproteinase inhibitor, prevents lipopolysaccharide-induced proteoglycan release from the joint cartilage in guinea pigs. Inflamm Res. 2000;49:144–6.

48. Golub LM, McNamara TF, D'Angelo G, et al. A non-antibacterial chemically-modified tetracycline inhibits mammalian collagenase activity. J Dent Res. 1987;66:1310–4.

49. Lee HM, Ciancio SG, Tuter G, et al. Subantimicrobial dose doxycycline efficacy as a matrix metalloproteinase inhibitor in chronic periodontitis patients is enhanced when combined with a non-steroidal anti-inflammatory drug. J Periodontol. 2004;75:453–63.

50. Smith Jr GN, Mickler EA, Hasty KA, et al. Specificity of inhibition of matrix metalloproteinase activity by doxycycline: relationship to structure of the enzyme. Arthritis Rheum. 1999;42:1140–6.

51. Golub LM, Lee HM, Ryan ME, et al. Tetracyclines inhibit connective tissue breakdown by multiple non-antimicrobial mechanisms. Adv Dent Res. 1998;12:12–26.

52. Roy R, Zhang B, Moses MA. Making the cut: protease-mediated regulation of angiogenesis. Exp Cell Res. 2006;312:608–22.

53. Linask KK, Manisastry S, Han M. Cross talk between cell-cell and cell-matrix adhesion signaling pathways during heart organogenesis: implications for cardiac birth defects. Microsc Microanal. 2005;11:200–8.

54. Itoh T, Ikeda T, Gomi H, et al. Unaltered secretion of beta-amyloid precursor protein in gelatinase A (matrix metalloproteinase 2)-deficient mice. J Biol Chem. 1997;272:22389–92.

55. Cheung PY, Sawicki G, Wozniak M, et al. Matrix metalloproteinase-2 contributes to ischemia-reperfusion injury in the heart. Circulation. 2000;101:1833–9.

56. Yasmin W, Strynadka KD, Schulz R. Generation of peroxynitrite contributes to ischemia-reperfusion injury in isolated rat hearts. Cardiovasc Res. 1997;33:422–32.

57. Lonn E, Factor SM, Van Hoeven KH, et al. Effects of oxygen free radicals and scavengers on the cardiac extracellular collagen matrix during ischemia-reperfusion. Can J Cardiol. 1994;10:203–13.

58. Bolli R, Marban E. Molecular and cellular mechanisms of myocardial stunning. Physiol Rev. 1999;79:609–34.

59. Bergman MR, Teerlink JR, Mahimkar R, et al. Cardiac matrix metalloproteinase-2 expression independently induces marked ventricular remodeling and systolic dysfunction. Am J Physiol Heart Circ Physiol. 2007;292:H1847–60.

60. Wang GY, Bergman MR, Nguyen AP, et al. Cardiac transgenic matrix metalloproteinase-2 expression

directly induces impaired contractility. Cardiovasc Res. 2006;69:688–96.

61. Yamada T, Matsumori A, Tamaki S, et al. Myosin light chain I grade: a simple marker for the severity and prognosis of patients with acute myocardial infarction. Am Heart J. 1998;135:329–34.

62. Tsuchida K, Kaneko K, Yamazaki R, et al. Degradation of cardiac structural proteins induced by reperfusion in the infarcted myocardium. Res Commun Chem Pathol Pharmacol. 1986;53:195–202.

63. Van Eyk JE, Powers F, Law W, et al. Breakdown and release of myofilament proteins during ischemia and ischemia/reperfusion in rat hearts: identification of degradation products and effects on the pCa-force relation. Circ Res. 1998;82:261–71.

64. Sawicki G, Leon H, Sawicka J, et al. Degradation of myosin light chain in isolated rat hearts subjected to ischemia-reperfusion injury: a new intracellular target for matrix metalloproteinase-2. Circulation. 2005;112: 544–52.

65. Granzier HL, Labeit S. The giant protein titin: a major player in myocardial mechanics, signaling, and disease. Circ Res. 2004;94:284–95.

66. Fukuda N, Granzier HL, Ishiwata S, et al. Physiological functions of the giant elastic protein titin in mammalian striated muscle. J Physiol Sci. 2008;58:151–9.

67. Ali M, Cho W, Hudson B, Kassiri Z, et al. Titin is a target of MMP-2: implications in myocardial ischemia/reperfusion injury. Circulation. 2010;122:2039–47.

68. Malhotra A, Margossian SS, Slayter HS. Physicochemical properties of rat and dog cardiac alpha-actinin. Biochim Biophys Acta. 1986;874:347–54.

69. Wang W, Sawicki G, Schulz R. Peroxynitrite-induced myocardial injury is mediated through matrix metalloproteinase-2. Cardiovasc Res. 2002; 53:165–74.

70. Sung MM, Schulz CG, Wang W, et al. Matrix metalloproteinase-2 degrades the cytoskeletal protein alpha-actinin in peroxynitrite mediated myocardial injury. J Mol Cell Cardiol. 2007;43:429–36.

71. Martelli AM, Bareggi R, Bortul R, et al. The nuclear matrix and apoptosis. Histochem Cell Biol. 1997; 108:1–10.

72. Georgi AB, Stukenberg PT, Kirschner MW. Timing of events in mitosis. Curr Biol. 2002;12:105–14.

73. Si-Tayeb K, Monvoisin A, Mazzocco C, et al. Matrix metalloproteinase 3 is present in the cell nucleus and is involved in apoptosis. Am J Pathol. 2006;169: 1390–401.

74. Kwan JA, Schulze CJ, Wang W, et al. Matrix metalloproteinase-2 (MMP-2) is present in the nucleus of cardiac myocytes and is capable of cleaving poly (ADP-ribose) polymerase (PARP) in vitro. FASEB J. 2004;18:690–2.

75. Pacher P, Schulz R, Liaudet L, et al. Nitrosative stress and pharmacological modulation of heart failure. Trends Pharmacol Sci. 2005;26:302–10.

76. Grimes CA, Jope RS. The multifaceted roles of glycogen synthase kinase 3beta in cellular signaling. Prog Neurobiol. 2001;65:391–426.

77. Kandasamy AD, Chow AK, Ali MA, et al. Matrix metalloproteinase-2 and myocardial oxidative stress injury: beyond the matrix. Cardiovasc Res. 2009;83: 698–706.

Control of the Mesenchymal-Derived Cell Phenotype by Ski and Meox2: A Putative Mechanism for Postdevelopmental Phenoconversion

Ryan H. Cunnington, Josette M. Douville, Jeffrey T. Wigle, Darren H. Freed, Dedmer Schaafsma, Sarah O'Connor, Shivika Gupta, Sunil G. Rattan, Andrew J. Halayko, and Ian M.C. Dixon

Abstract

The developing mesenchyme gives rise to a diverse host of important cell types, including fibroblasts, endothelial and smooth muscle cells. In postnatal tissues, stromal cells continue to differentiate into subtypes with specific functions, e.g., fibroblasts to myofibroblasts, but the molecular signals that govern their phenoconversion are incompletely understood. Herein, we provide a review of the function of c-Ski (Ski) and Meox2 transcription factors and provide a rationale to support our suggestion that these factors trigger the phenoconversion of "undifferentiated" parenchymal and stromal cells to variants with novel function. As phenoconversion events underlie both normal organ function and the pathogenesis of disease including cardiac fibrosis, we have developed a novel hypothesis to facilitate a clearer understanding of their underlying mechanisms.

Keywords

Ski • Meox2 • Myofibroblast • Cell phenotype • Airway smooth muscle • Endothelium • EMT

Introduction

In normal development, the mesenchyme gives rise to a diverse host of important cell types, including fibroblasts, endothelial and smooth muscle cells. The range of cell phenotypes within these broadly defined groups is large. For example, the current definition of a fibroblast *per se* is more or less limited to their mesenchymal derivation and residence in the extracellular matrix (matrix) of organs, but does not distinguish between fibroblasts from different organs. Nonetheless, the discovery of topographic and organ-specific fibroblastic phenotypes highlights their broad diversity among organ types and even to the topography within a given organ [1, 2]. While postdevelopment differentiation of these mesenchymal cells

I.M.C. Dixon (✉)
Department of Physiology, University of Manitoba and the Institute of Cardiovascular Sciences, St. Boniface General Hospital Research Centre, Winnipeg, MB, Canada
e-mail: idixon@sbrc.ca

N.S. Dhalla, M. Nagano, B. Ostadal (eds.), *Molecular Defects in Cardiovascular Disease*,
DOI 10.1007/978-1-4419-7130-2_3, © Springer Science+Business Media, LLC 2011

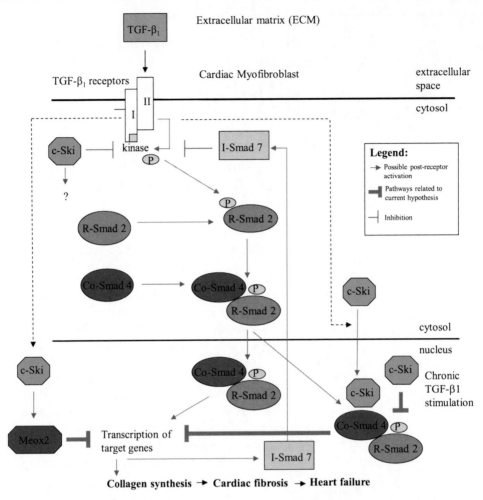

Fig. 1 Canonical R-Smad signaling and the putative role of Ski in cardiac myofibroblasts. Schematic representation of integrated Smad signaling in cardiac myofibroblasts in response to TGF-β_1 stimulation. Receptor-activated Smad2 (R-Smad2) is phosphorylated by TβRI which potentiates enhanced synthesis of fibrillar collagens. Inhibition of R-Smad function occurs in the presence of nuclear localized and cytosolic Ski, likely by interference with the CoSmad4-Smad2 dimer function in the myofibroblast nucleus (disrupting bridge model of inhibition) and by inhibition of TβRI, respectively. Ski induces expression of the Meox2 homeobox transcription factor, which we propose inhibits TGF-β_1 induced phenoconversion of fibroblasts to myofibroblasts

to derivatives and specific subphenotypes is a generally accepted phenomenon, the molecular signals that govern their phenoconversion are incompletely understood. Recent work has led to an improved understanding of the importance of (1) transcription factors and (2) homeobox regulator genes in the control of mesenchymal phenotype, including c-Ski (Ski – a phosphorylated protooncogene transcription factor known to inhibit canonical TGF-β_1 signaling) and Meox2, respectively. Herein, we provide a rationale to

support a putative phenotype switching function for a novel Ski-Meox2 pathway in mesenchyme-derived cells in health and disease.

The c-Ski protooncoprotein is a known inhibitor of TGF-β_1 signaling (Fig. 1) and has recently been shown to function as a potent regulator of cardiac myofibroblast function [3]. Cardiac fibroblasts are relatively quiescent cells that do not contribute to rapid matrix remodeling and also highly express markers such as the Meox1 and Meox2 homeobox transcription factors (Fig. 2). Conversely,

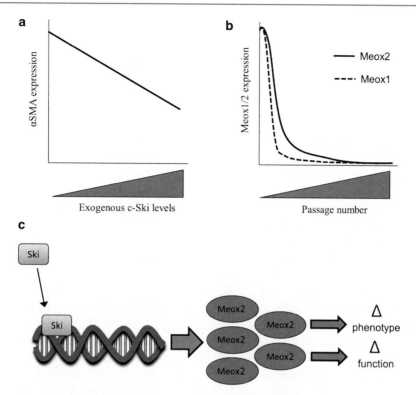

Fig. 2 (**a**) Ski overexpression diminishes myofibroblast phenotype observed through reduced expression of α-smooth muscle actin (αSMA), and (**b**) Meox1 and Meox2 mRNA expression is decreased with increasing passage number of cells. (**c**) Proposed mechanism for (1) Ski-mediated alteration of myofibroblast phenotype and function changes with fibroblast to myofibroblast transition, and (2) Ski exerts a marked effect on Meox2 mRNA expression and myofibroblast phenotype

cardiac myofibroblasts are phenoconverted fibroblasts that exhibit marked expression of α-smooth muscle actin (αSMA) among other markers [3, 4]. Cardiac myofibroblasts are able to (1) contract like smooth muscle cells and (2) secrete matrix and focal adhesion proteins [4, 5]. They migrate to the infarct zone, restoring cellularity to the region of heart that has undergone massive dropout of parenchymal muscle cells [6]. Their contraction allows for direct matrix remodeling by physical reorientation of matrix proteins, e.g., collagen fibrils, scar contraction, and activation of latent TGF-β_1 [7–11].

While fibrosis contributes to the development of heart failure, and R-Smads may regulate collagen secretion and myofibroblast contractility, the mechanisms for Ski-mediated inhibition of R-Smad signaling are not well understood. Our recent work indicates the following: (1) a causal

link exists between increased Ski expression and decreased collagen secretion and contractility in myofibroblasts [3]; (2) conversion of fibroblasts to myofibroblasts is associated with reduced Meox2 expression; and (3) increased Ski expression reduces αSMA while increasing Meox2 expression (Fig. 2) [3]. Rapid collagen deposition and net turnover by myofibroblasts is a hallmark of early infarct scar formation and in chronic remodeling of the matrix, which are pivotal to the pathogenesis of post myocardial infarction (post-MI) heart failure [12–14]. Our past and current research is based on our hypothesis that an imbalance between R-Smads and Ski may trigger fibrosis and contribute to ongoing remodeling in post-MI congestive heart failure (Fig. 1). A corollary of this hypothesis is that Ski may function, in part, by regulating Meox2 gene expression, itself a modulator of phenotype. Thus, in the current paper, we present the evidence to support a link between Ski, Meox2 and myofibroblast phenotype and function. A review of TGF-β_1/Smad signaling as well as the known and putative roles for Ski and Meox2 in mesenchymal-derived cells is offered.

Canonical TGF-β_1 Signaling

TGF-β_1 signaling from cell-surface receptors to nucleus is transduced by Smads and their DNA-binding partners [15–27]. TGF-β_1 receptor type I and II (TβRI and TβRII respectively) are Ser/Thr kinase class proteins and signal through receptor-regulated Smads (R-Smad2 or –3) by recognition/phosphorylation steps [28, 29]. Canonical TGF-β_1 signaling in fibroblasts of healthy hearts is the sum of different stimulatory (R-Smads) and inhibitory proteins such as Ski and I-Smad7 [3, 13, 25, 26, 30–32]. R-Smads are key receptor-regulated proteins that bind several known DNA-binding coactivators [25–27, 33] as well as the Ski corepressor [3], and this binding is stabilized by Co-Smad4 [34]. Smad7 binds to and facilitates the degradation of the TβRI receptor, thereby turning off the receptor kinase and inhibiting R-Smad function [35, 36]. Rapid phosphorylation of R-Smad2 occurs within 5 min of exposure to low-dose TGF-β_1 *in vitro,* and its chronic phosphorylation *in vivo* is associated with post-MI heart failure [12, 31]. Myofibroblasts populate the infarct scar and the interstitial space of noninfarcted heart and express high levels of matrix and focal adhesion proteins [4, 37]. In the failing heart, we observe diminished I-Smad7 expression and speculate that R-Smads in cardiac myofibroblasts may override Ski function and that this imbalance contributes to increased matrix production. Smad proteins control multiple systems in mammalian cells [25, 26] and regulate collagen metabolism in cardiac myofibroblasts [12–14, 31].

Ski is highly expressed in myofibroblasts populating the healed infarct scar vs. noninfarcted control tissue, and in the fibroblasts that are phenoconverted to myofibroblasts in culture [3]. In our *in vitro* experiments, Ski localizes to and is retained in the nuclei of myofibroblasts following TGF-β_1 stimulation where it inhibits Smad function. In myofibroblasts of the post-MI heart, Ski is predominant in the cytoplasm. The mechanisms responsible for this subcellular redistribution are yet to be determined. Our most recent results provide us with a causal relationship between acutely increased Ski (95 kDa form) expression leading to modulation of myofibroblast phenotype, and function [3]. This includes demonstrating a direct effect of increased Ski on maintaining Meox2 homeobox expression.

The Biology of Smads and Ski

As mentioned above, phosphorylated R-Smads complex with common Smad4 (Co-Smad4) and translocate to the nucleus [29, 38–40] (Fig. 1). A Smad complex bound to nuclear DNA is able to recruit either coactivators (e.g., p300) or corepressors (e.g., Ski), respectively [15, 18, 20, 25, 41–50]. R-Smad function depends upon localization of R-Smad to the nucleus. This activation is extensively regulated [25], and R-Smad activation has been linked to activation of collagen genes [51, 52]. Genes that are transcriptionally responsive to Smads contain Smad-binding elements (SBE) in their promoter regions [53, 54]. Endogenous inhibitors of R-Smads include I-Smad7 and nuclear Smad corepressors (e.g., Ski and SnoN), and they either competitively inhibit TβRI-mediated phosphorylation of R-Smads or stabilize inactive Smad complexes on DNA, respectively [35, 42, 46, 55–58].

Using cardiac myofibroblasts, we have observed that Ski acts as a negative regulator of R-Smads [3]. Ski, a phosphoprotein and cellular homologue of v-Ski [59], is widely expressed among tissues and highly conserved among human, *Xenopus*, and mouse [60–62]. It is important in morphological transformation and growth of chicken embryo fibroblasts, as well as for cellular differentiation [59, 63]. Ski induces myogenic differentiation in avian fibroblasts [59, 64], and muscle terminal differentiation in mouse myoblasts by transcriptional activation of myogenin [65]. Ski "knockout" mice exhibit defects in CNS and skeletal muscle development [66]. Ski may bind DNA directly but also binds a number of transcription factors and may function as either a coactivator or a corepressor depending on its binding partner [59, 64, 67, 68].

Ski incorporates into DNA-binding complexes of Smad proteins and may negatively regulate TGF-β_1 responsive transcriptional activation through recruitment of HDAC complexes [69]. Ski-mediated "trapping" of inactive Smad2–Smad4 complexes to DNA is a means by which it inhibits TGF-β_1 signaling, and this depends upon Smad4 binding [46]. R-Smad2 and -3 also interact with Ski in a ligand-dependent manner [15, 47, 70]. Similar to Smad7, c-Ski has been recently shown to directly bind and block the function of TβRI [71]. This binding by Ski blocks the nuclear translocation of the activated SMAD complexes to the nucleus, thereby inhibiting SMAD signaling.

The function of Ski appears to depend on the cell type assayed. Classically defined as a nuclear factor, Ski binds specific DNA motifs for transcriptional repression [69, 72–74]. Ski may also function as a coactivator in cells expressing NF1 [75]. Although the control of Ski expression/localization is unclear, its pluripotency implicates its participation in both physiologic and pathophysiologic processes.

Despite new advances in the biology of Ski, its effects on cardiac myofibroblast phenotype, migration, and proliferation are still unclear. Fibroblasts from various organs display wide diversity, topographic differentiation, and positional "memory" [1]. In post-MI hearts, Ski induction may depend upon the type and stage of failure, as we have observed with other regulatory proteins [76].

Smad Signaling and Extracellular Matrix (Matrix) Remodeling

The myocardial matrix, which is comprised of fibrillar collagens, proteoglycans, fibronectins, laminin, and others, is an organized network that is intimately associated with cardiac function. The matrix is tethered to myocytes and nonmyocytes alike (via focal adhesion complexes and integrins) and serves to direct, transmit, and distribute myocyte-generated contractile force [77, 78]. Other functions include regulation of cell death, gene expression, and parenchymal cell differentiation

[79, 80]. Nonetheless, elevated fibrillar collagen expression in heart disease may be responsible for changing heart function based on its adverse influence on myocardial stiffness [81–83]. Pathological cardiac hypertrophy is associated with interstitial and perivascular fibrosis in the remnant heart or as replacement fibrosis for necrosed muscle [84–86]. Ongoing collagen remodeling may contribute to decompensated cardiac function in the stage of severe heart failure [76, 87].

TGF-β_1 modulates expression of fibrillar collagens [88–91] and is associated with matrix remodeling in heart [12, 13, 92]. Thus, a pathogenic role for elevated levels of TGF-β_1 in common cardiac diseases (e.g., post-MI cardiac hypertrophy and failure) that are marked by matrix remodeling and eventual global cardiac fibrosis has been established [5, 12, 13, 31, 93], and abnormal expression of R-Smads is observed in the remnant myocardium and infarct scar of experimental hearts [12, 76, 85, 94]. By activating postreceptor R-Smads, TGF-β_1 stimulates matrix deposition and influences matrix remodeling by stimulating myofibroblast contraction. Myofibroblast contraction also imparts mechanical strain or tension into existing extracellular matrix, which is known to decrease susceptibility of pre–existing collagen matrices to degradation by collagenases or MMP-1 action [95–97]. To complement earlier data that highlights Ski's role in muscle differentiation [65], we have shown that in cardiac myofibroblasts Ski functions as a R-Smad repressor in primary cardiac cells [3]. The pattern of R-Smads, I-Smad7, and Ski expression in progressive post-MI heart failure is unique, as the pathogenesis of different types of heart failure are themselves unique [13, 98, 99].

Effects of TGF-β_1 on Cardiac Myofibroblasts

In mammalian tissues, fibroblasts exhibit marked organ-specific phenotypic diversity [1]. Fibroblasts are abundant in the heart [86], while wound healing/interstitial cardiac fibrosis is mediated by phenotypic derivative myofibroblasts [37, 100–102]. When not affected by senescence

[103], cardiac myofibroblasts are highly synthetic [104], expressing α-smooth muscle actin (αSMA), vimentin, TGF-β receptors, fibrillar collagens [12–14, 31, 92, 100, 105–108], DDR2, fibronectin ED-A, myocardin, and focal adhesion components including vinculin, paxillin, and tensin [3]. The myofibroblast phenotype is induced by TGF-β_1 and in vitro culture seeding at low density [3, 4, 109–111]. We have demonstrated the predominance of myofibroblasts in the infarct scar in post-MI rats and in cultured adult cells [4, 37]; adult myofibroblasts are phenotypically stable [110]. Increasing evidence suggests that circulating progenitor cells of bone marrow origin contribute to the cardiac myofibroblast pool, in particular post-MI and in experimental myocarditis. We have observed the myofibroblast phenotype in bone marrow stromal cells derived from humans and rats in vitro. These cells are responsive to TGF-β in similar manner to cardiac myofibroblasts and express Ski (unpublished observations). Further work is required to determine the role of Ski in this mesenchymal cell type.

TGF-β_1 mediates cell growth and differentiation, tissue wound repair, and extracellular matrix production [112–114], including regulation of fibrillar collagens [89–91, 101, 115]. TGF-β_1 signaling is active in the normal and hypertrophied myocardium [12, 85, 94, 113, 116, 117]. We have shown that acute TGF-β_1 treatment stimulates myofibroblast contraction and inhibits low-serum mediated proliferation of these cells [5, 31]. Abnormal TGF-β_1 ligand expression is linked to cardiac fibrosis [118]. TGF-β_1 signaling is mediated by Smads [17–25, 33]. We suggest that in post-MI heart, myofibroblasts are chronically exposed to abnormally high TGF-β_1 levels and that this exposure may be linked to loss of normal Ski localization as well as Ski regulation of myofibroblast function by an unidentified mechanism [3, 13, 31].

Mesenchyme Homeobox 2 Regulation of Cell Cycle

Meox2 is expressed in embryonic and adult vascular smooth muscle, cardiac muscle, and endothelial cells [119, 120]. Meox1 and Meox2

are 95% identical at the amino acid level within the homeodomain, but there is little sequence conservation outside of this region. Meox2 regulates the growth of VSMCs and cardiomyocytes in vitro and in vivo [121, 122]. This hypothesis was supported by studies of Meox2 in cultured VSMCs and fibroblasts that demonstrated that ectopic Meox2 arrested cells in the G_1 phase of the cell cycle and blocked their migration [121, 123]. Meox2 blocks proliferation via induction of the p21 cyclin dependent kinase (CDK) inhibitor [121]. Meox2 has been shown to directly regulate p21 transcription by binding to regulatory sites in the p21 promoter [124, 125].

Meox2 is quickly downregulated in response to mitogen stimulation in vitro [126] and in vivo vessel injury [127]. This reduction in Meox2 expression in VSMCs allows for cell cycle progression and is associated with the phenotypic switch of VSMCs from the differentiated contractile phenotype to the less differentiated synthetic phenotype that occurs during atherogenesis and restenosis [128]. Ectopic expression of Meox2 is able to prevent this phenotypic switch, thereby preventing vessel occlusion [129, 130].

In addition to its effect on the cell cycle, Meox2 overexpression has also been shown to be pro-apoptotic in vitro and in vivo under conditions of mitogen stimulation. Ectopic Meox2 expression in either proliferating VSMCs or MEFs stimulated with growth factors induces apoptosis within 48 h [131].

Meox2 and TGF-β_1 Signaling

Recent results have linked Meox2 and TGF-β_1 signaling. In adventitial fibroblasts, Meox2 blocked the pro-proliferative and proinflammatory actions of TGF-β_1 signaling [132] Meox2 was shown to enhance TGF-β_1 induced reduction in epithelial cell proliferation [124]. This study also demonstrates that Meox2 binds to Smad2, -3, and -4. In contrast to its enhancement of the antiproliferative effects of TGF-β_1, Meox2 blocked TGF-β_1 induced epithelial to mesenchymal transition (EMT) [124]. EMT has been well described in embryonic development and cancer where it has been associated with increased tumor motility and metastasis [133]. Both EMT and endothelial to mesenchymal transition (EndMT) can give rise to myofibroblasts [134, 135]. In a recent study, Meox2 has been shown to be a target of the miR221/ZEB2 pathway [136]. ZEB2, also known as Smad interacting protein (SIP1), is a two-handed zinc finger transcription factor that functions as a transcriptional repressor to potentiate EMT by decreasing expression of cell adhesion proteins [137, 138]. In addition, ZEB2 binds to regulatory regions of Meox2 to decrease its expression [136]. The miR200 family targets ZEB2 and its family member ZEB1 and thereby blocks EMT. miR221 was shown to increase Meox2 expression via its downregulation of ZEB2 [136]. In summary, Meox2 functions to block the action of TGF-β_1 in different cell types; however, whether it serves this role in cardiac myofibroblasts is unknown.

Why Is the Regulation of Fibroblast to Myofibroblast Transition Important?

The majority of proliferating cells in the surviving myocardium and infarct scar are fibroblasts and myofibroblasts [4, 139–141]. While fibroblasts maintain minimal matrix turnover in normal myocardium, damaged myocardium is characterized by the presence of myofibroblasts in the infarct and eventually in the adjacent borderzone muscle. The latter cells generate matrix that is useful for strengthening the infarcted heart, but eventually contributes to net accumulation of excessive collagen, e.g., fibrosis. Normally, the cardiac matrix participates in active restoration of sarcomeric length, via release of stored potential energy in matrix proteins [142, 143]. Overt fibrosis contributes to abnormal cardiac function by increasing myocardial stiffness [144]. Collagen types I and III (fibrillar collagens) are the most abundant proteins in the matrix [142, 143, 145, 146]. We have shown that altered matrix synthesis and deposition participates in the development of heart failure [76, 85, 94, 147–149]. Clinical or

experimental results from this lab [4, 12, 76, 147, 150–152] and others [86, 92, 153] provide evidence of fibrosis in the left ventricle remote to the infarct site with increased myocardial stiffness and increased cross-linking of collagen fibrils [81–83, 150, 154]. The regulation of collagen expression by Smads and Ski is established [3, 4, 13, 31, 85].

Although scar formation is completed at 3 weeks post-MI [155], myofibroblasts, the dominant cell type in the infarct scar [100, 139, 156], remain active even 8 weeks post-MI [76, 87, 139], and collagen content may continually increase over months [155, 157]. These cells may persist in the infarct scar in post-MI patients for many years, even decades, after the initial insult [87, 140, 158]. Limited fibrosis in the healing infarct scar [103] may help to preserve ventricular function, as the new scar tissue selectively resists circumferential deformation [139, 140, 158, 159], and myofibroblasts are the major source of R-Smad expression [85] leading to this fibrosis. Myofibroblasts produce isometric tension within granulation tissue *in vivo* and in culture [160, 161]. Tension is exerted at the level of focal adhesions (FAs), which connect cells to matrix [109]. Myofibroblast contraction confers matrix distortion in wound healing [161] as the tensile force opposes retractile forces and promotes scar contraction in the post-MI heart [7, 8].

Whether Ski functions via induction of Meox2 to regulate myofibroblast phenotype e.g., back to the fibroblast phenotype, and myofibroblast function either *in vitro* or in post-MI hearts is essentially an untested question. However, our preliminary data suggest that Ski is a regulator of various aspects of myofibroblast function in vitro and that Meox2 expression is induced by Ski (Fig. 2). Thus, a putative link between the function of Ski and the expression of Meox2 exists and may serve to control myofibroblast function *in vitro* and *in vivo* in post-MI heart failure. Based on our recently published data and other preliminary results from our lab (Fig. 2), we suggest that c-Ski (Ski) regulates the myofibroblast phenotype both *in vitro* (two-dimensional cultured cells plated on stiff or incompressible matrix) and *in vivo* in the post-MI heart. Further work is needed to provide a definitive answer to this intriguing possibility.

TGF-β and Smooth Muscle Phenotype: Transcription and Protein Translation

Phenotypic plasticity occurs in differentiated smooth muscle cells and is defined as the reversible modulation and maturation of individual myocytes both *in vitro* and *in vivo* [162–164]. Phenotype switching requires changes in the expression of phenotype-specific genes and the subsequent accumulation of the proteins that they encode. A number of recognized molecular markers are abundant in contractile phenotype smooth muscle cells; in particular intracellular contractile apparatus- and cytoskeleton-associated proteins, including smooth muscle myosin heavy chain (smMHC), SM22, calponin, and αSMA [162, 165]. Conversely, the content of nonmuscle MHC, L-caldesmon, vimentin, alpha/beta-protein kinase C (PKC), and CD44 homing cellular adhesion molecule is augmented in proliferative smooth muscle cells [165]. Studying expression of these proteins provides a useful tool for the investigation of smooth muscle function in tissue biopsies taken from the vasculature or other hollow organs, including the airways.

TGF-β is a potent inducer of a hypertrophic and hypercontractile phenotype in mesenchymal cells, that can promote Serum Response Factor (SRF)-dependent gene transcription through activation of Smad signaling [50, 166, 167]. TGF-β, via TβRI and TβRII induces phosphorylation and nuclear translocation of "regulatory" Smad-2, -3, and -4. Regulatory Smads can bind with nuclear SRF to promote smooth-muscle-specific gene transcription, whereas Smad-7 counteracts this effect [167]. Of note, caveolin-1 appears to suppress TGF-β induced regulatory-Smad activation, suggesting a regulatory role for caveolae in TGF-β-induced myocyte phenotype expression.

Recent studies revealed potential roles of microRNAs (miRs) in the regulation of smooth muscle phenotype. Thus, in vascular smooth muscle it was shown that miR-26a counteracts

TGF-β induced differentiation, which was associated with reduced Smad-1 and -4 gene expression [168]. In separate studies, it was demonstrated that Platelet Derived Growth Factor (PDGF)-BB induces microRNA24 (miR24), which in turn leads to a downregulation of Tribbles-like protein-3 (Trb3). Trb3 promotes degradation of Smad ubiquitin-regulatory factor-1 (Smurf1), and as such facilitates TGF-β signaling. PDGF-induced repression of Trb3 coincided with a reduced expression of Smad proteins and decreased TGF-β signaling, promoting a synthetic smooth muscle phenotype. Conversely, inhibition of miR24 diminished downregulation of Trb3 as well as the prosynthetic activity of the PDGF-signaling pathway [169]. Altogether, an important role for miRs in regulating Smad-associated signaling in smooth muscle seems evident.

PI3K-Akt1 signaling may control SRF-mediated transcription of smooth-muscle-specific genes as well through the phosphorylation of Foxo4 forkhead transcription factor [170]. In its unphosphorylated state Foxo4 binds to nuclear myocardin and inhibits its interaction with SRF, thereby dampening transcription of smooth-muscle-specific genes. Phosphorylation of Foxo4 by Akt1 releases a suppressive mechanism by allowing myocardin–SRF binding, which activates transcription of smooth-muscle-specific genes.

The transcripts from smooth-muscle-specific genes need to be translated into proteins to impact on myocyte phenotype and function. Protein translation is under control of several pathways that converge at the level of the ribosome, and a number of these are required for smooth muscle maturation. Mature smooth muscle cells express elevated levels of active, phosphorylated kinases with known effects on protein translation, including PI3K, Akt1, mTOR (mammalian target of rapamycin), and p70 ribosomal S6 kinase [171]. Pharmacological inhibition of PI3K and mTOR is sufficient to prevent p70 ribosomal S6 kinase activation and accumulation of smooth-muscle-specific proteins [171]. Furthermore, active mTOR can phosphorylate and activate 4E-BP1, a protein that binds to and activates the eukaryotic initiation factor, eIF4, which initiates protein translation and contractile protein accumulation [172]. Activation of these PI3K dependent signaling pathways is required for TGF-β and insulin-induced smooth muscle maturation [166, 173], indicating that in addition to SRF dependent gene transcription, the translation of smooth-muscle-specific proteins is tightly regulated by specific intracellular signaling pathways.

Conclusions

The canonical TGF-β/Smad signal is an important mediator of phenotype modulation in mesenchymal cells; however, the precise molecular mechanisms that underlie mesenchymal phenoconversion remain poorly understood. These events are critical in the pathology of various disease etiologies. For example, phenoconversion to the myofibroblastic cell marks a significant event in cardiac wound healing ultimately resulting in heart failure. To date, there has been no specific evidence to test for the existence of the hypothetical link between Ski and Meox2 proteins in modulating mesenchymal cell phenoconversion. Ski and Meox2 are remarkably similar with respect to some aspects of function, and as they both associate with Smads, it is logical to expect that they serve in parallel or even common signaling pathways. Our recent work points to the Ski–Meox2 pathway as a novel negative regulator of the myofibroblastic phenotype. This new insight into phenoconversion raises the possibility of a mode of precise control of this complex process and also opens an avenue for the therapeutic treatment in myofibroblast-related pathologies including cardiac fibrosis of various types.

Acknowledgments This work was supported by a Heart and Stroke Foundation of Manitoba Grant-in-Aid (I.M.C.D.), the Canadian Institutes of Health Research (I.M.C.D. and J.T.W.), and the St. Boniface Hospital Research Foundation (I.M.C.D. and D.H.F.). A.J.H. holds a Canada Research Chair in Airway Cell and Molecular Biology. D.S. is supported by a CIHR fellowship and a CIHR/HSFC IMPACT strategic training program grant in pulmonary and cardiovascular research. R.H.C. is supported by a CIHR-RPP graduate scholarship. S.O. and J.M.D. are supported by an ICS studentship.

References

1. Chang HY, Chi JT, Dudoit S, et al. Diversity, topographic differentiation, and positional memory in human fibroblasts. Proc Natl Acad Sci USA. 2002;99:12877–82.
2. Kalluri R, Zeisberg E. Controlling angiogenesis in heart valves. Nat Med. 2006;12:1118–9.
3. Cunnington RH, Wang B, Bathe KL, et al. Antifibrotic properties of c-Ski and its regulation of cardiac myofibroblast contractililty and phenotype. Am J Physiol. 2011;200:C176–86.
4. Santiago JJ, Dangerfield AL, Rattan SG, et al. Cardiac fibroblast to myofibroblast differentiation in vivo and in vitro: expression of focal adhesion components in neonatal and adult rat ventricular myofibroblasts. Dev Dyn. 2010;239:1573–84.
5. Drobic V, Cunnington RH, Bedosky KM, et al. Differential and combined effects of cardiotrophin-1 and TGF-beta on cardiac myofibroblast proliferation and contraction. Am J Physiol Heart Circ Physiol. 2007;293:H1053–64.
6. Norman D. An exploration of two opposing theories of wound contraction. J Wound Care. 2004;13: 138–40.
7. Lijnen P, Petrov V, Fagard R. Transforming growth factor-beta 1-mediated collagen gel contraction by cardiac fibroblasts. J Renin Angiotensin Aldosterone Syst. 2003;4:113–8.
8. Grinnell F. Fibroblasts, myofibroblasts, and wound contraction. J Cell Biol. 1994;4:401–4.
9. Arany PR, Flanders KC, Kobayashi T, et al. Smad3 deficiency alters key structural elements of the extracellular matrix and mechanotransduction of wound closure. Proc Natl Acad Sci USA. 2006;103: 9250–5.
10. Wipff PJ, Rifkin DB, Meister JJ, et al. Myofibroblast contraction activates latent TGF-beta1 from the extracellular matrix. J Cell Biol. 2007;179: 1311–23.
11. Wang J, Chen H, Seth A, et al. Mechanical force regulation of myofibroblast differentiation in cardiac fibroblasts. Am J Physiol Heart Circ Physiol. 2003;285:H1871–81.
12. Hao J, Wang B, Jones SC, et al. Interaction between angiotensin II and Smad proteins in fibroblasts in failing heart and in vitro. Am J Physiol Heart Circ Physiol. 2000;279:H3020–30.
13. Wang B, Hao J, Jones SC, et al. Decreased Smad 7 expression contributes to cardiac fibrosis in the infarcted rat heart. Am J Physiol Heart Circ Physiol. 2002;282:H1685–96.
14. Freed DH, Cunnington RH, Dangerfield AL, et al. Emerging evidence for the role of cardiotrophin-1 in cardiac repair in the infarcted heart. Cardiovasc Res. 2005;65:782–92.
15. Xu W, Angelis K, Danielpour D, et al. Ski acts as a co-repressor with Smad2 and Smad3 to regulate the

response to type beta transforming growth factor. Proc Natl Acad Sci USA. 2000;97:5924–9.

16. Kokura K, Kim H, Shinagawa T, et al. The Ski-binding protein C184M negatively regulates tumor growth factor-beta signaling by sequestering the Smad proteins in the cytoplasm. J Biol Chem. 2003;278:20133–9.

17. Massague J, Hata A, Liu F. Tgf-beta signalling through the Smad pathway. Trends Cell Biol. 1997;7:187–92.

18. Wrana J, Pawson T. Signal transduction. Mad about SMADs. Nature. 1997;388:28–9.

19. Nakao A, Roijer E, Imamura T, et al. Identification of Smad2, a human Mad-related protein in the transforming growth factor beta signaling pathway. J Biol Chem. 1997;272:2896–900.

20. Chen X, Rubock MJ, Whitman M. A transcriptional partner for MAD proteins in TGF-beta signalling. Nature. 1996;383:691–6.

21. Zhou S, Zawel L, Lengauer C, et al. Characterization of human FAST-1, a TGF beta and activin signal transducer. Mol Cell. 1998;2:121–7.

22. Chen YG, Hata A, Lo RS, et al. Determinants of specificity in TGF-beta signal transduction. Genes Dev. 1998;12:2144–52.

23. Derynck R, Zhang Y, Feng XH. Smads: transcriptional activators of TGF-beta responses. Cell. 1998;95:737–40.

24. Massague J. TGF-beta signal transduction. Annu Rev Biochem. 1998;67:753–91.

25. Wrana JL. Regulation of Smad activity. Cell. 2000;100:189–92.

26. Park SH. Fine tuning and cross-talking of TGF-beta signal by inhibitory Smads. J Biochem Mol Biol. 2005;38:9–16.

27. Brown KA, Pietenpol JA, Moses HL. A tale of two proteins: differential roles and regulation of Smad2 and Smad3 in TGF-beta signaling. J Cell Biochem. 2007;101:9–33.

28. Zhang Y, Feng X, We R, et al. Receptor-associated Mad homologues synergize as effectors of the TGF-beta response. Nature. 1996;383:168–72.

29. Macias-Silva M, Abdollah S, Hoodless PA, et al. MADR2 is a substrate of the TGFbeta receptor and its phosphorylation is required for nuclear accumulation and signaling. Cell. 1996;87:1215–24.

30. Dixon IMC, Wang B, Bedosky K, et al. Regulatory role of TGF-b in cardiac myofibroblast function and post-MI cardiac fibrosis: key role of Smad7 and c-Ski. In: Srivastava AKA-S, Madhu B, editors. Advances in biochemistry in health and disease (ABHD) – focus on signal transduction in cardiovascular system in health and disease, vol. 3. New York: Springer; 2008.

31. Wang B, Omar A, Angelovska T, et al. Regulation of collagen synthesis by inhibitory Smad7 in cardiac myofibroblasts. Am J Physiol Heart Circ Physiol. 2007;293:H1282–90.

32. Cunnington RH, Nazari M, Dixon IMC. c-Ski, Smurf2 and Arkadia as regulators of TGF-b

signaling: new targets for managing myofibroblast function and cardiac fibrosis. Can J Physiol Pharmacol. 2009;87:764–72.

33. Li P, Wang D, Lucas J, et al. Atrial natriuretic peptide inhibits transforming growth factor beta-induced Smad signaling and myofibroblast transformation in mouse cardiac fibroblasts. Circ Res. 2008;102:185–92.

34. Chen X, Weisberg E, Fridmacher V, et al. Smad4 and FAST-1 in the assembly of activin-responsive factor. Nature. 1997;389:85–9.

35. Christian JL, Nakayama T. Can't get no SMADisfaction: Smad proteins as positive and negative regulators of TGF-beta family signals. Bioessays. 1999;21:382–90.

36. Chong PA, Lin H, Wrana JL, et al. An expanded WW domain recognition motif revealed by the interaction between Smad7 and the E3 ubiquitin ligase Smurf2. J Biol Chem. 2006;281:17069–75.

37. Peterson DJ, Ju H, Hao J, et al. Expression of Gi-2 alpha and Gs alpha in myofibroblasts localized to the infarct scar in heart failure due to myocardial infarction. Cardiovasc Res. 1999;41:575–85.

38. Lagna G, Hata A, Hemmati-Brivanlou A, et al. Partnership between DPC4 and SMAD proteins in TGF-beta signalling pathways. Nature. 1996; 383:832–6.

39. Wrana JL. The secret life of Smad4. Cell. 2009;136:13–4.

40. Dupont S, Mamidi A, Cordenonsi M, et al. FAM/USP9x, a deubiquitinating enzyme essential for TGFbeta signaling, controls Smad4 monoubiquitination. Cell. 2009;136:123–35.

41. Heldin CH, Miyazono K, ten Dijke P. TGF-beta signalling from cell membrane to nucleus through SMAD proteins. Nature. 1997;390:465–71.

42. Massague J, Wotton D. Transcriptional control by the TGF-beta/Smad signaling system. EMBO J. 2000;19:1745–54.

43. Ueki N, Hayman MJ. Direct interaction of Ski with either Smad3 or Smad4 is necessary and sufficient for Ski-mediated repression of transforming growth factor-beta signaling. J Biol Chem. 2003; 278:32489–92.

44. Luo K, Stroschein SL, Wang W, et al. The Ski oncoprotein interacts with the Smad proteins to repress TGFbeta signaling. Genes Dev. 1999; 13:2196–206.

45. Luo K. Ski and SnoN: negative regulators of TGF-beta signaling. Curr Opin Genet Dev. 2004; 14:65–70.

46. Suzuki H, Yagi K, Kondo M, et al. c-Ski inhibits the TGF-beta signaling pathway through stabilization of inactive Smad complexes on Smad-binding elements. Oncogene. 2004;23:5068–76.

47. Akiyoshi S, Inoue H, Hanai J, et al. c-Ski acts as a transcriptional co-repressor in transforming growth factor-beta signaling through interaction with smads. J Biol Chem. 1999;274:35269–77.

48. Prunier C, Pessah M, Ferrand N, et al. The oncoprotein Ski acts as an antagonist of transforming

growth factor-beta signaling by suppressing Smad2 phosphorylation. J Biol Chem. 2003;278: 26249–57.

49. Qiu P, Ritchie RP, Fu Z, et al. Myocardin enhances Smad3-mediated transforming growth factor-beta1 signaling in a CArG box-independent manner: Smad-binding element is an important cis element for SM22alpha transcription in vivo. Circ Res. 2005;97:983–91.

50. Qiu P, Feng XH, Li L. Interaction of Smad3 and SRF-associated complex mediates TGF-beta1 signals to regulate SM22 transcription during myofibroblast differentiation. J Mol Cell Cardiol. 2003;35: 1407–20.

51. Vindevoghel L, Kon A, Lechleider RJ, et al. Smad-dependent transcriptional activation of human type VII collagen gene (COL7A1) promoter by transforming growth factor-beta. J Biol Chem. 1998;273:13053–7.

52. Vindevoghel L, Lechleider RJ, Kon A, et al. SMAD3/4-dependent transcriptional activation of the human type VII collagen gene (COL7A1) promoter by transforming growth factor beta. Proc Natl Acad Sci USA. 1998;95:14769–74.

53. Zawel L, Dai JL, Buckhaults P, et al. Human Smad3 and Smad4 are sequence-specific transcription activators. Mol Cell. 1998;1:611–7.

54. Chen S, Kulik M, Lechleider RJ. Smad proteins regulate transcriptional induction of the SM22alpha gene by TGF-beta. Nucleic Acids Res. 2003; 31:1302–10.

55. Hayashi H, Abdollah S, Qiu Y, et al. The MAD-related protein Smad7 associates with the TGFbeta receptor and functions as an antagonist of TGFbeta signaling. Cell. 1997;89:1165–73.

56. Imamura T, Takase M, Nishihara A, et al. Smad6 inhibits signalling by the TGF-beta superfamily. Nature. 1997;389(6651):622–6.

57. Nakao A, Afrakhte M, Moren A, et al. Identification of Smad7, a TGFbeta-inducible antagonist of TGF-beta signalling. Nature. 1997;389:631–5.

58. Whitman M. Signal transduction. Feedback from inhibitory SMADs. Nature. 1997;389:549–51.

59. Li Y, Turck CM, Teumer JK, et al. Unique sequence, ski, in Sloan-Kettering avian retroviruses with properties of a new cell-derived oncogene. J Virol. 1986;57:1065–72.

60. Ludolph DC, Neff AW, Parker MA, et al. Cloning and expression of the axolotl proto-oncogene ski. Biochim Biophys Acta. 1995;1260:102–4.

61. Nomura N, Sasamoto S, Ishii S, et al. Isolation of human cDNA clones of ski and the ski-related gene, sno. Nucleic Acids Res. 1989;17:5489–500.

62. Sleeman JP, Laskey RA. Xenopus c-ski contains a novel coiled-coil protein domain, and is maternally expressed during development. Oncogene. 1993;8:67–77.

63. Reed JA, Bales E, Xu W, et al. Cytoplasmic localization of the oncogenic protein Ski in human cutaneous melanomas in vivo: functional implications for

transforming growth factor beta signaling. Cancer Res. 2001;61:8074–8.

64. Stavnezer E, Barkas AE, Brennan LA, et al. Transforming Sloan-Kettering viruses generated from the cloned v-ski oncogene by in vitro and in vivo recombinations. J Virol. 1986;57:1073–83.

65. Zhang H, Stavnezer E. Ski regulates muscle terminal differentiation by transcriptional activation of Myog in a complex with Six1 and Eya3. J Biol Chem. 2009;284:2867–79.

66. Sutrave P, Kelly AM, Hughes SH. Ski can cause selective growth of skeletal muscle in transgenic mice. Genes Dev. 1990;4:1462–72.

67. Nicol R, Stavnezer E. Transcriptional repression by v-Ski and c-Ski mediated by a specific DNA binding site. J Biol Chem. 1998;273:3588–97.

68. Nagase T, Mizuguchi G, Nomura N, et al. Requirement of protein co-factor for the DNA-binding function of the human ski proto-oncogene product. Nucleic Acids Res. 1990;18:337–43.

69. Nomura T, Khan MM, Kaul SC, et al. Ski is a component of the histone deacetylase complex required for transcriptional repression by Mad and thyroid hormone receptor. Genes Dev. 1999;13: 412–23.

70. Sun Y, Liu X, Eaton EN, Lane WS, et al. Interaction of the Ski oncoprotein with Smad3 regulates TGF-beta signaling. Mol Cell. 1999;4:499–509.

71. Ferrand N, Atfi A, Prunier C. The oncoprotein c-ski functions as a direct antagonist of the transforming growth factor-{beta} type I receptor. Cancer Res. 2010;70:8457–66.

72. Dahl R, Kieslinger M, Beug H, et al. Transformation of hematopoietic cells by the Ski oncoprotein involves repression of retinoic acid receptor signaling. Proc Natl Acad Sci USA. 1998;95:11187–92.

73. Kokura K, Kaul SC, Wadhwa R, et al. The Ski protein family is required for MeCP2-mediated transcriptional repression. J Biol Chem. 2001;276:34115–21.

74. Tokitou F, Nomura T, Khan MM, et al. Viral ski inhibits retinoblastoma protein (Rb)-mediated transcriptional repression in a dominant negative fashion. J Biol Chem. 1999;274:4485–8.

75. Tarapore P, Richmond C, Zheng G, et al. DNA binding and transcriptional activation by the Ski oncoprotein mediated by interaction with NFI. Nucleic Acids Res. 1997;25:3895–903.

76. Ju H, Zhao S, Tappia PS, Panagia V, et al. Expression of Gqalpha and PLC-beta in scar and border tissue in heart failure due to myocardial infarction. Circulation. 1998;97:892–9.

77. Caulfield JB, Borg TK. The collagen network of the heart. Lab Invest. 1979;40:364–72.

78. Ott HC, Matthiesen TS, Goh SK, et al. Perfusion-decellularized matrix: using nature's platform to engineer a bioartificial heart. Nat Med. 2008; 14:213–21.

79. Birchmeier C, Birchmeier W. Molecular aspects of mesenchymal-epithelial interactions. Annu Rev Cell Biol. 1993;9:511–40.

80. Simon-Assmann P, Kedinger M, De Arcangelis A, et al. Extracellular matrix components in intestinal development. Experientia. 1995;51:883–900.

81. Makino N, Hata T, Sugano M, et al. Regression of hypertrophy after myocardial infarction is produced by the chronic blockade of angiotensin type 1 receptor in rats. J Mol Cell Cardiol. 1996;28:507–17.

82. Jalil JE, Doering CW, Janicki JS, et al. Fibrillar collagen and myocardial stiffness in the intact hypertrophied rat left ventricle. Circ Res. 1989;64:1041–50.

83. Thiedemann KU, Holubarsch C, Medugorac I, Jacob R. Connective tissue content and myocardial stiffness in pressure overload hypertrophy. A combined study of morphologic, morphometric, biochemical, and mechanical parameters. Basic Res Cardiol. 1983;78:140–55.

84. Bartosova D, Chvapil M, Korecky B, et al. The growth of the muscular and collagenous parts of the rat heart in various forms of cardiomegaly. J Physiol (Lond). 1969;200:285–95.

85. Hao J, Ju H, Zhao S, Junaid A, et al. Elevation of expression of Smads 2, 3, and 4, decorin and TGF-beta in the chronic phase of myocardial infarct scar healing. J Mol Cell Cardiol. 1999;31:667–78.

86. Weber KT, Brilla CG. Pathological hypertrophy and cardiac interstitium. Fibrosis and renin-angiotensin-aldosterone system. Circulation. 1991;83:1849–65.

87. Cleutjens JP, Blankesteijn WM, Daemen MJ, et al. The infarcted myocardium: simply dead tissue, or a lively target for therapeutic interventions. Cardiovasc Res. 1999;44:232–41.

88. Roberts AB, McCune BK, Sporn MB. TGF-beta: regulation of extracellular matrix. Kidney Int. 1992;41:557–9.

89. Ignotz RA, Massague J. Transforming growth factor-beta stimulates the expression of fibronectin and collagen and their incorporation into the extracellular matrix. J Biol Chem. 1986;261:4337–45.

90. Butt RP, Bishop JE. Mechanical load enhances the stimulatory effect of serum growth factors on cardiac fibroblast procollagen synthesis. J Mol Cell Cardiol. 1997;29:1141–51.

91. Roberts AB, Heine UI, Flanders KC, et al. Transforming growth factor-beta. Major role in regulation of extracellular matrix. Ann NY Acad Sci. 1990;580:225–32.

92. Weber KT. Fibrosis, a common pathway to organ failure: angiotensin II and tissue repair. Semin Nephrol. 1997;17:467–91.

93. Thompson NL, Bazoberry F, Speir EH, et al. Transforming growth factor beta-1 in acute myocardial infarction in rats. Growth Factors. 1988;1:91–9.

94. Dixon IMC, Hao J, Reid NL, et al. Effect of chronic AT1 receptor blockade on cardiac smad overexpression in hereditary cardiomyopathic hamsters. Cardiovasc Res. 2000;46:286–97.

95. Follonier Castella L, Gabbiani G, et al. Regulation of myofibroblast activities: calcium pulls some strings behind the scene. Exp Cell Res. 2010; 316:2390–401.

96. Bhole AP, Flynn BP, Liles M, et al. Mechanical strain enhances survivability of collagen micronetworks in the presence of collagenase: implications for load-bearing matrix growth and stability. Philos Transact A Math Phys Eng Sci. 2009;367:3339–62.

97. Flynn BP, Bhole AP, Saeidi N, et al. Mechanical strain stabilizes reconstituted collagen fibrils against enzymatic degradation by mammalian collagenase matrix metalloproteinase 8 (MMP-8). PLoS One. 2010;5:e12337.

98. Hunter JJ, Chien KR. Signaling pathways for cardiac hypertrophy and failure. N Engl J Med. 1999;341:1276–83.

99. Stiles GL. Multifunctional G proteins. Searching for functions in the heart [editorial; comment]. Circulation. 1996;94:602–3.

100. Sun Y. Local angiotensin II and myocardial fibrosis. In: Zanchetti A et al., editors. Hypertension and the heart. New York: Plenum; 1997. p. 55–61.

101. Powell DW, Mifflin RC, Valentich JD, et al. Myofibroblasts. I. Paracrine cells important in health and disease. Am J Physiol Cell Physiol. 1999;277:C1–9.

102. Eghbali M, Czaja MJ, Zeydel M, et al. Collagen chain mRNAs in isolated heart cells from young and adult rats. J Mol Cell Cardiol. 1988;20:267–76.

103. Jun JI, Lau LF. The matricellular protein CCN1 induces fibroblast senescence and restricts fibrosis in cutaneous wound healing. Nat Cell Biol. 2010;12:676–85.

104. Frangogiannis NG, Smith CW, Entman ML. The inflammatory response in myocardial infarction. Cardiovasc Res. 2002;53:31–47.

105. Sun Y, Cleutjens JP, Diaz-Arias AA, et al. Cardiac angiotensin converting enzyme and myocardial fibrosis in the heart. Cardiovasc Res. 1994;28:1423–32.

106. Sun Y, Weber KT. Angiotensin II receptor binding following myocardial infarction in the rat. Cardiovasc Res. 1994;28:1623–8.

107. Hildebrand A, Romaris M, Rasmussen LM, et al. Interaction of the small interstitial proteoglycans biglycan, decorin and fibromodulin with transforming growth factor beta. Biochem J. 1994;302:527–34.

108. Raizman JE, Komljenovic J, Chang R, et al. The participation of the Na^+-Ca^{2+} exchanger in primary cardiac myofibroblast migration, contraction, and proliferation. J Cell Physiol. 2007;213:540–51.

109. Dugina V, Fontao L, Chaponnier C, et al. Focal adhesion features during myofibroblastic differentiation are controlled by intracellular and extracellular factors. J Cell Sci. 2001;114:3285–96.

110. Masur SK, Dewal HS, Dinh TT, et al. Myofibroblasts differentiate from fibroblasts when plated at low density. Proc Natl Acad Sci USA. 1996;93: 4219–23.

111. Evans RA, Tian YC, Steadman R, et al. TGF-beta1-mediated fibroblast-myofibroblast terminal differentiation-the role of smad proteins. Exp Cell Res. 2003;282:90–100.

112. Brand T, Schneider MD. Transforming growth factor-beta signal transduction. Circ Res. 1996;78:173–9.

113. Brand T, Schneider MD. The TGF beta superfamily in myocardium: ligands, receptors, transduction, and function. J Mol Cell Cardiol. 1995;27:5–18.

114. Kingsley DM. The TGF-beta superfamily: new members, new receptors, and new genetic tests of function in different organisms. Genes Dev. 1994;8:133–46.

115. Inagaki Y, Truter S, Ramirez F. Transforming growth factor-beta stimulates alpha 2(I) collagen gene expression through a cis-acting element that contains an Sp1-binding site. J Biol Chem. 1994;269: 14828–34.

116. Sadoshima J, Izumo S. Molecular characterization of angiotensin II–induced hypertrophy of cardiac myocytes and hyperplasia of cardiac fibroblasts. Critical role of the AT1 receptor subtype. Circ Res. 1993;73:413–23.

117. Ohta K, Kim S, Hamaguchi A, et al. Role of angiotensin II in extracellular matrix and transforming growth factor-beta 1 expression in hypertensive rats. Eur J Pharmacol. 1994;269:115–9.

118. Brooks WW, Conrad CH. Myocardial fibrosis in transforming growth factor beta(1)heterozygous mice. J Mol Cell Cardiol. 2000;32:187–95.

119. Skopicki HA, Lyons GE, Schatteman G, et al. Embryonic expression of the Gax homeodomain protein in cardiac, smooth, and skeletal muscle. Circ Res. 1997;80:452–62.

120. Wu Z, Guo H, Chow N, et al. Role of the MEOX2 homeobox gene in neurovascular dysfunction in Alzheimer disease. Nat Med. 2005;11:959–65.

121. Smith RC, Branellec D, Gorski DH, et al. p21CIP1-mediated inhibition of cell proliferation by overexpression of the gax homeodomain gene. Genes Dev. 1997;11:1674–89.

122. Fisher SA, Siwik E, Branellec D, et al. Forced expression of the homeodomain protein Gax inhibits cardiomyocyte proliferation and perturbs heart morphogenesis. Development. 1997;124:4405–13.

123. Witzenbichler B, Kureishi Y, Luo Z, et al. Regulation of smooth muscle cell migration and integrin expression by the Gax transcription factor. J Clin Invest. 1999;104:1469–80.

124. Valcourt U, Thuault S, Pardali K, et al. Functional role of Meox2 during the epithelial cytostatic response to TGF-beta. Mol Oncol. 2007;1:55–71.

125. Chen Y, Leal AD, Patel S, et al. The homeobox gene GAX activates p21WAF1/CIP1 expression in vascular endothelial cells through direct interaction with upstream AT-rich sequences. J Biol Chem. 2007;282:507–17.

126. Gorski DH, LePage DF, Patel CV, et al. Molecular cloning of a diverged homeobox gene that is rapidly down-regulated during the G0/G1 transition in vascular smooth muscle cells. Mol Cell Biol. 1993;13:3722–33.

127. Weir L, Chen D, Pastore C, et al. Expression of gax, a growth arrest homeobox gene, is rapidly down-regulated in the rat carotid artery during the proliferative response to balloon injury. J Biol Chem. 1995;270:5457–61.

128. Markmann A, Rauterberg J, Vischer P, et al. Expression of transcription factors and matrix genes in response to serum stimulus in vascular smooth muscle cells. Eur J Cell Biol. 2003;82:119–29.

129. Maillard L, Van Belle E, Smith RC, et al. Percutaneous delivery of the gax gene inhibits vessel stenosis in a rabbit model of balloon angioplasty. Cardiovasc Res. 1997;35:536–46.

130. Maillard L, Van Belle E, Tio FO, et al. Effect of percutaneous adenovirus-mediated Gax gene delivery to the arterial wall in double-injured atheromatous stented rabbit iliac arteries. Gene Ther. 2000;7:1353–61.

131. Perlman H, Luo Z, Krasinski K, et al. Adenovirus-mediated delivery of the Gax transcription factor to rat carotid arteries inhibits smooth muscle proliferation and induces apoptosis. Gene Ther. 1999;6:758–63.

132. Liu P, Zhang C, Feng JB, et al. Cross talk among Smad, MAPK, and integrin signaling pathways enhances adventitial fibroblast functions activated by transforming growth factor-beta1 and inhibited by Gax. Arterioscler Thromb Vasc Biol. 2008;28:725–31.

133. Ansieau S, Morel AP, Hinkal G, et al. Twisting an embryonic transcription factor into an oncoprotein. Oncogene. 2010;29:3173–84.

134. Zeisberg EM, Tarnavski O, Zeisberg M, et al. Endothelial-to-mesenchymal transition contributes to cardiac fibrosis. Nat Med. 2007;13:952–61.

135. Larsson O, Diebold D, Fan D, et al. Fibrotic myofibroblasts manifest genome-wide derangements of translational control. PLoS One. 2008;3:e3220.

136. Chen Y, Banda M, Speyer CL, et al. Regulation of the expression and activity of the antiangiogenic homeobox gene GAX/MEOX2 by ZEB2 and microRNA-221. Mol Cell Biol. 2010;30:3902–13.

137. Comijn J, Berx G, Vermassen P, et al. The two-handed E box binding zinc finger protein SIP1 downregulates E-cadherin and induces invasion. Mol Cell. 2001;7:1267–78.

138. Vandewalle C, Comijn J, De Craene B, et al. SIP1/ZEB2 induces EMT by repressing genes of different epithelial cell-cell junctions. Nucleic Acids Res. 2005;33:6566–78.

139. Peterson DJ, Ju H, Jianming Hao PM, Chapman D, Dixon IMC. Expression of Gia2 and Gsa in myofibroblasts localized to the infarct scar in heart failure due to myocardial infarction. Cardiovasc Res. 1998;41:575–85.

140. Cleutjens JP, Verluyten MJ, Smits JF, et al. Collagen remodeling after myocardial infarction in the rat heart. Am J Pathol. 1995;147:325–38.

141. van Krimpen C, Schoemaker RG, Cleutjens JP, et al. Angiotensin I converting enzyme inhibitors and cardiac remodeling. Basic Res Cardiol. 1991;86 Suppl 1:149–55.

142. Robinson TF, Factor SM, Sonnenblick EH. The heart as a suction pump. Sci Am. 1986;254:84–91.

143. Robinson TF, Cohen-Gould L, Factor SM. Skeletal framework of mammalian heart muscle. Arrangement of inter- and pericellular connective tissue structures. Lab Invest. 1983;49:482–98.

144. Brown L. Cardiac extracellular matrix: a dynamic entity. Am J Physiol Heart Circ Physiol. 2005;289:H973–4.

145. Bashey RI, Martinez Hernandez A, Jimenez SA. Isolation, characterization, and localization of cardiac collagen type VI. Associations with other extracellular matrix components. Circ Res. 1992; 70:1006–17.

146. Weber KT, Jalil JE, Janicki JS. Myocardial collagen remodeling in pressure overload hypertrophy. A case for interstitial heart disease. Am J Hypertens. 1989;2:931–40.

147. Ju H, Zhao S, Davinder SJ, et al. Effect of AT1 receptor blockade on cardiac collagen remodeling after myocardial infarction. Cardiovasc Res. 1997; 35:223–32.

148. Pelouch V, Dixon IM, Golfman L, et al. Role of extracellular matrix proteins in heart function. Mol Cell Biochem. 1993;129:101–20.

149. Dixon IMC, Reid NL, Ju H. Angiotensin II and TGF-b in the development of cardiac fibrosis, myocyte hypertrophy, and heart failure. Heart Fail Rev. 1997;2:107–16.

150. Pelouch V, Dixon IM, Sethi R, et al. Alteration of collagenous protein profile in congestive heart failure secondary to myocardial infarction. Mol Cell Biochem. 1993;129:121–31.

151. Liu KZ, Jackson M, Sowa MG, et al. Modification of the extracellular matrix following myocardial infarction monitored by FTIR spectroscopy. Biochim Biophys Acta. 1996;1315:73–7.

152. Dixon IMC, Ju H, Jassal DS, et al. Effect of ramipril and losartan on collagen expression in right and left heart after myocardial infarction. Mol Cell Biochem. 1996;165:31–45.

153. Weber KT. Extracellular matrix remodeling in heart failure: a role for de novo angiotensin II generation. Circulation. 1997;96:4065–82.

154. Dixon IMC, Ju H, Reid NL. The role of angiotensin II in post-translational regulation of fibrillar collagens in fibrosed and failing rat heart. In: Dhalla NS, Zahradka P, Dixon IMC, Beamish RE, editors. Angiotensin II receptor blockade: physiological and clinical implications. Boston: Kluwer Academic; 1998. p. 471–98.

155. Fishbein MC, Maclean D, Maroko PR. Experimental myocardial infarction in the rat: qualitative and quantitative changes during pathologic evolution. Am J Pathol. 1978;90:57–70.

156. Sun Y, Weber KT. Angiotensin converting enzyme and myofibroblasts during tissue repair in the rat heart. J Mol Cell Cardiol. 1996;28:851–8.

157. Jugdutt BI, Amy RW. Healing after myocardial infarction in the dog: changes in infarct hydroxyproline and topography. J Am Coll Cardiol. 1986;7: 91–102.

158. Willems IE, Havenith MG, De Mey JG, et al. The alpha-smooth muscle actin-positive cells in healing human myocardial scars. Am J Pathol. 1994;145:868–75.

159. Holmes JW, Nunez JA, Covell JW. Functional implications of myocardial scar structure. Am J Physiol. 1997;272:H2123–30.

160. Serini G, Gabbiani G. Mechanisms of myofibroblast activity and phenotypic modulation. Exp Cell Res. 1999;250:273–83.

161. Tomasek JJ, Gabbiani G, Hinz B, et al. Myofibroblasts and mechano-regulation of connective tissue remodelling. Nat Rev Mol Cell Biol. 2002;3:349–63.

162. Owens GK. Regulation of differentiation of vascular smooth muscle cells. Physiol Rev. 1995;75:487–517.

163. Halayko AJ, Solway J. Molecular mechanisms of phenotypic plasticity in smooth muscle cells. J Appl Physiol. 2001;90:358–68.

164. Hirota JA, Nguyen TT, Schaafsma D, et al. Airway smooth muscle in asthma: phenotype plasticity and function. Pulm Pharmacol Ther. 2009;22:370–8.

165. Halayko AJ, Salari H, Ma X, et al. Markers of airway smooth muscle cell phenotype. Am J Physiol Lung Cell Mol Physiol. 1996;270:L1040–51.

166. Goldsmith AM, Bentley JK, Zhou L, et al. Transforming growth factor-beta induces airway smooth muscle hypertrophy. Am J Respir Cell Mol Biol. 2006;34:247–54.

167. Camoretti-Mercado B, Fernandes DJ, Dewundara S, et al. Inhibition of transforming growth factor beta-enhanced serum response factor-dependent transcription by SMAD7. J Biol Chem. 2006; 281:20383–92.

168. Leeper NJ, Raiesdana A, Kojima Y, et al. MicroRNA-26a is a novel regulator of vascular smooth muscle cell function. J Cell Physiol. 2011;226:1035–43.

169. Chan MC, Hilyard AC, Wu C, et al. Molecular basis for antagonism between PDGF and the TGFbeta family of signalling pathways by control of miR-24 expression. EMBO J. 2010;29:559–73.

170. Liu ZP, Wang Z, Yanagisawa H, et al. Phenotypic modulation of smooth muscle cells through interaction of Foxo4 and myocardin. Developmental Cell. 2005;9:261–70.

171. Halayko AJ, Kartha S, Stelmack GL, et al. Phophatidylinositol-3 kinase/mammalian target of rapamycin/p70S6K regulates contractile protein accumulation in airway myocyte differentiation. Am J Respir Cell Mol Biol. 2004;31:266–75.

172. Zhou L, Goldsmith AM, Bentley JK, et al. 4E-binding protein phosphorylation and eukaryotic initiation factor-4E release are required for airway smooth muscle hypertrophy. Am J Respir Cell Mol Biol. 2005;33:195–202.

173. Schaafsma D, McNeill KD, Stelmack GL, et al. Insulin increases the expression of contractile phenotypic markers in airway smooth muscle. Am J Physiol Cell Physiol. 2007;293:C429–39.

Elevated Na+–H+ Exchanger Expression and Its Role in Myocardial Disease

Larry Fliegel

Abstract

The mammalian Na+–H+ exchanger isoform 1 (NHE1) is a plasma membrane protein that regulates intracellular pH in the myocardium by removing one intracellular hydrogen ion in exchange for one extracellular sodium ion. While NHE1 regulates intracellular pH, it is also involved in the damage that occurs to the myocardium with ischemia and reperfusion. Additionally, NHE1 levels are elevated in cardiac diseases such as hypertrophy, and NHE1 inhibition can reduce ischemia–reperfusion damage and prevent heart hypertrophy in animal models. Recently, it has been demonstrated that elevation of NHE1 levels occurs in several kinds of hearts disease. Surprisingly, the effect of elevation of these levels is varied, sometimes having beneficial and sometimes detrimental effects.

Keywords

Acidosis • Apoptosis • Hypertrophy • Ischemia • MAP kinase • Membrane • NHE1 • Na+–H+ exchanger • pH regulation

Introduction

The mammalian Na+–H+ exchanger (NHE) is a membrane protein that removes one intracellular hydrogen ion in exchange for one extracellular sodium ion. It is ubiquitously expressed in mammalian cells and is widespread throughout the animal kingdom. NHE plays a critical role in intracellular pH (pHi) regulation protecting cells from acidification as well as regulating cell volume and sodium fluxes (reviewed in [1]). One family of ten isoforms of NHE exist; however, the NHE isoform 1 (NHE1) is the only plasma membrane isoform expressed in the myocardium [2–7]. NHE1 is of special importance in the myocardium as it is implicated in both myocardial damage from ischemia–reperfusion injury, and heart hypertrophy (see below and reviewed in [8]). NHE1 consists of a membrane domain that transports ions and a cytosolic domain that modulates activity of the

L. Fliegel (✉)
Department of Biochemistry, Faculty of Medicine, University of Alberta, Edmonton, Alberta, Canada
e-mail: lfliegel@ualberta.ca

N.S. Dhalla, M. Nagano, B. Ostadal (eds.), *Molecular Defects in Cardiovascular Disease*, DOI 10.1007/978-1-4419-7130-2_4, © Springer Science+Business Media, LLC 2011

membrane domain and is a target of various forms of regulation (reviewed in [9]).

NHE Structure and Subtypes

Human NHE1 is an 815 amino acid protein. The first 500 residues are predicted to be 12 transmembrane spanning segments, and the remaining residues constitute a cytosolic intracellular regulatory domain [10–12] (Fig. 1). It should be noted, however, that there is recently some doubt about the transmembrane organization [13]. NHE1 forms homodimers in vivo, although the individual protein subunits can function independently of each other [14, 15]. The structure of a bacterial sodium hydrogen antiporter has been determined [16], but it is not very homologous with NHE1 and is part of a different NHE family with different characteristics including electrogenic transport [17]. The family of mammalian NHE-like proteins includes ten commonly known isoforms (NHE1-10) each the product of a different gene and with different tissue distributions and physiological roles (reviewed in [9, 18]). The first type cloned was named NHE1 [19], and it is ubiquitously expressed in mammalian cells. NHE1 was also identified by our laboratory as the predominant plasma membrane isoform in the myocardium

[3]. It has been shown to be concentrated along intercalated disks and transverse tubule system of heart cells [20]. Heart cells lack the plasma membrane isoforms NHE2–5. NHE2–4 are expressed mainly in the kidney and gastrointestinal tract [21–23]. NHE5 is found in the brain [24], while NHE6–9 are localized to intracellular organelle membranes, such as endosomes, mitochondria, and the Golgi apparatus [25, 26], NHE10 is expressed in osteoclasts [27]. The protein identity of the various isoforms varies from 25 to 70%; however, all share a common predicted secondary structure [7]. A more distant family of two mammalian cation proton antiporters is made of NHA1 and NHA2, and these proteins may be involved in mediating hypertension [28, 29]. Similarly, a splice variant of NHE1 has also been suggested to be important in hypertension [30].

Importance of NHE and pH Regulation in the Myocardium

NHE is important in pHi regulation in the myocardium. Myocardial energy production generates protons and the negative membrane potential of the plasma membrane tends to accumulate protons within the cytosol (Fig. 2). Decreased pHi inhibits contractility. NHE1 removes these

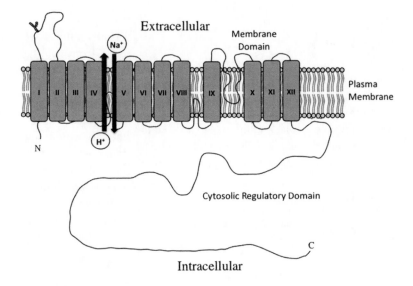

Fig. 1 Simplified schematic diagram of the Na$^+$–H$^+$ exchanger. The membrane domain of approximately 500 amino acids catalyzes the exchange of one intracellular H$^+$ in exchange for one extracellular Na$^+$. The intracellular cytosolic domain of approximately 315 amino acids regulates the membrane domain

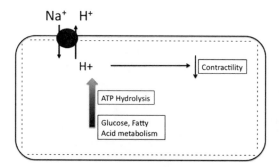

Fig. 2 Illustration of the role of the Na⁺–H⁺ exchanger in myocardial metabolism. The Na⁺–H⁺ exchanger removes protons generated as a result of metabolism or ATP hydrolysis. Excess protons are inhibitory to cardiac contractility. The negative membrane potential tends to retain intracellular protons

protons. At low pHi (pH ≤ 6.5), the exchanger is maximally active and at higher pH's activity is reduced or negligible. However, the pH dependence can be shifted toward the more alkaline range by α1-adrenergic stimulation and by hormones such as endothelin [31, 32]. Our laboratory has shown that MAP kinase-dependent pathways are important in this response [33, 34]. NHE1 is normally the key mechanism of proton removal with HCO$_3$-based transporters contributing to a lesser degree from recovery from intracellular acidosis [35–41].

NHE1 Physiological and Pathological Roles (in Other Tissues)

NHE1 has several roles in many cell types (see [7, 9, 17, 42] for reviews). Knockout of NHE1 from cells shows that NHE1 plays a role in growth, especially in the presence of more acidic media [43]. Similarly, NHE1-deficient mice demonstrated decreased postnatal growth and ataxia and epileptic-like seizures [44, 45]. NHE1 is also important in cell cycle progression [46, 47], while NHE1 is additionally permissive in cell differentiation which we [48] and others [49] demonstrated. The involvement of NHE1 in cell growth and differentiation suggests that the protein is important in normal developmental processes. NHE1 also modifies apoptosis. In mouse β-cells,

trophic factor withdrawal triggers pHi dysregulation and apoptosis. NHE1 is activated leading to cellular alkalinization and progression of apoptosis [50]. We showed that this activation is through p38-dependent phosphorylation of the NHE1 tail [50]. NHE1-dependent alkalinization plays a pivotal role in the development of a transformed phenotype of malignant cells, and inhibition of NHE1 prevents or reduces such development [51–53]. Additionally, in breast cancer cells NHE1 activation is key in their cell invasion activity [54–56].

Pathological Roles of NHE1 in the Myocardium

NHE1 contributes to several types of myocardial disease. The best known is the role of NHE1 in ischemia–reperfusion damage in the myocardium [57–60]. During ischemia, anaerobic glycolysis occurs, resulting in the increased production of protons. These serve to activate NHE1. The activated NHE1 exchanges the more H⁺i for extracellular Na⁺. This leads to a rapid accumulation of sodium in the cell [57–60]. The high sodium concentration drives an increase in Ca^{2+} via reversal of the activity of the Na⁺–Ca^{2+} exchanger. This results in an increased level of intracellular Ca^{2+}, which triggers various pathways leading to cell death (Fig. 3). Hundreds of preclinical studies have shown that inhibition of NHE1 during ischemia and reperfusion protects the myocardium from calcium overload (see [60, 61] for reviews). In various animal models, NHE1 inhibitors such as cariporide, amiloride, and EMD 85131 have proven to be cardioprotective [62–64]. Activation of NHE1 regulatory pathways is also important in NHE1-mediated damage to the myocardium, and this results in further detrimental activity of the NHE1 protein [65].

NHE1 Is Important in Cardiac Hypertrophy

Preclinical studies have shown directly that NHE1 inhibition prevents cardiac hypertrophy including in vivo in rats subjected to myocardial

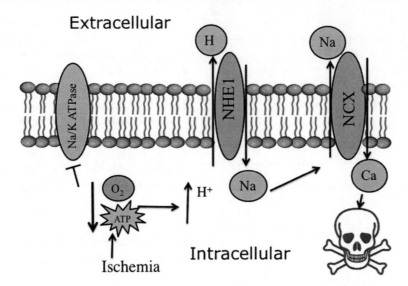

Fig. 3 Series of events leading to myocardial injury through the Na⁺–H⁺ exchanger. Ischemia leads to an increase in intracellular protons and decrease in ATP levels. This causes an increase in intracellular protons and the decrease in cellular ATP levels is inhibitory to the Na⁺–K⁺ ATPase. Excess intracellular protons are removed by the Na⁺–H⁺ exchanger, which results in an increase in intracellular sodium. This is removed by the reverse mode of the Na⁺–Ca²⁺ exchanger, resulting in an increase in intracellular calcium. This leads to cell damage including necrosis and apoptosis

infarction [66, 67], in mice with guanylyl cyclase-A receptor knockout [68] and in vitro in isolated cardiomyocytes [69]. NHE1 is activated by MAP kinases and protein kinase C-dependent pathways, which are important in hypertrophic and remodeling processes [34, 70]. We demonstrated that the effect of the hypertrophic agonist aldosterone can be blocked by NHE1 inhibition [69] as can stretch-induced hypertrophy [71]. Prevention of increases in intracellular Na⁺ is a possible mechanism by which NHE1 inhibition prevents hypertrophy [72, 73].

NHE1 Is Important in Apoptosis in the Myocardium

Studies in animals and humans have shown that in addition to necrosis, apoptosis significantly contributes to myocyte loss following myocardial infarction [74–77] including results suggesting that apoptosis is a critical form of cell death in infarcted human myocardium [78]. Much of the detrimental effects of NHE1 in hypoxia-reoxygenation are mediated through apoptosis. Inhibition of NHE1 activity via the specific inhibitor cariporide results in decreased apoptosis in isolated cardiomyocytes [79] and in fibroblasts [80]. In addition, inhibition of NHE1 activity before ischemia has been shown to reduce myocardial apoptosis in isolated rat hearts [81, 82], in mouse hearts [83] and in pacing-induced heart failure in rabbits [84]. Humphreys et al. [85] also reported that in an ischemic rat model, the NHE1 inhibitor cariporide reduced apoptosis and this was associated with a significantly higher ratio of (antiapoptotic) Bcl-2 to (pro-apoptotic) Bax [83, 85]. Regulation of NHE1 has been implicated in NHE1 induced apoptosis in the myocardium [86, 87]. Recently, we have shown that amino acids Ser⁷²⁶ and Ser⁷²⁹ are involved in critical regulation of NHE1 causing apoptosis [88]; however, in cardiac myocytes we showed that amino acids Ser⁷⁷⁰ and Ser⁷⁷¹ are more important in regulation of NHE1 [65].

NHE1 Inhibition for Treatment of Other Cardiovascular Conditions

Aside from the general conditions of hypertrophy and ischemia–reperfusion damage, a number of specific cardiovascular conditions have been examined and are briefly summarized. NHE1 inhibitors have for example, been useful in inhibiting diabetic vascular hypertrophy [89, 90] and prevent alterations in coronary endothelial function in streptozotocin-induced diabetes [91]. NHE1 is also known to play an important role in ischemia–reperfusion injury in the central nervous system where NHE1 inhibition is beneficial [92]. Studies have shown the NHE1 inhibition has potent antifibrillatory and antiarrhythmic effects in dogs and rats [93, 94]. These effects extend to other species where NHE1 inhibition has been shown to an effective intervention for resuscitation from ventricular fibrillation [95]. In addition, NHE1 inhibition has been shown to be a better protective agent than ischemic preconditioning in some trials [96, 97]. It has been suggested that NHE1 inhibitors may be of use during cardiac surgery, including being of use in hearts subjected to prolonged hypothermic storage [98]. Kim et al. [99, 100] also showed that NHE1 inhibition was beneficial in improving the outcome in a canine transplantation model. Inhibition of NHE1 has also been shown to be protective in models of cardiac resuscitation [101]. NHE1 inhibition may additionally be useful in treatment of circulatory shock as NHE-1 inhibition attenuated ischemic myocardial hypercontracture and cardiovascular decompensation, and delayed the onset of hypovolemic circulatory shock in a porcine model of circulatory shock [102]. Overall, it can be said that inhibition of NHE1 activity has many and varied beneficial cardiovascular effects in a large number of models.

Clinical Trials

Despite all the success with inhibition of NHE1 in preclinical experiments, trials with NHE1 inhibitors have not been very successful. Large-scale studies with several inhibitors in various types of myocardial infarctions and treatments have given mostly disappointing results (see [87] for review). Rupprecht et al. [103] tested effects of cariporide in a small trial of patients with myocardial infarction who received coronary angioplasty. They found some beneficial effects on ejection fraction, wall-motion abnormalities and enzyme release. A larger scale two-stage trial [104] with eniporide treatment of myocardial infarction showed a dose-dependent effect to reduce enzyme release, indicating reduced infarction. However, in a second later stage of the trial there was no beneficial effect and an overall negative effect. The reason for the discrepancy between the beneficial effects in pre-clinical trials and the negative effects in clinical trials may be because NHE inhibition is required early in ischemia, rather than in reperfusion as was the case in the clinical trials [87]. The GUARDIAN trial [105], had some more positive results. In patients undergoing coronary artery bypass graft surgery analysis of subgroups showed that cariporide was beneficial. Treatment with the inhibitor in this trial was early, which may account for its beneficial effect in this study [87]. The EXPEDITION trial tested if pre-ischemic inhibition of NHE1 by cariporide reduces myocardial injury in patients with coronary artery bypass graft surgery. Cariporide reduced myocardial infarction but it also had adverse side effects and increasing cerebrovascular events significantly. This resulted in the study being terminated early [87, 105]. Another study [106] tested the efficacy of the NHE inhibitor zoniporide on reducing cardiovascular events in patients undergoing non-cardiac vascular surgery. There was no beneficial effect and this has been attributed to a lack of myocardial reperfusion, which is required for beneficial NHE inhibitors to access the myocardium [87, 106].

NHE1 Is Elevated in Myocardial Disease

A variety of studies have shown that NHE1 protein expression and activity increases in the myocardium in response to stimuli that occur in the disease

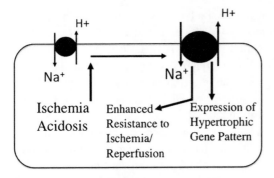

Fig. 4 Chronic stimuli increase Na⁺–H⁺ exchanger activity. Chronic stimulation by ischemia, acidosis, or other factors can cause an elevation in Na⁺–H⁺ exchanger messenger RNA levels, activity, and protein levels. This can lead to expression of a hypertrophic gene pattern but can also lead to enhanced resistance to ischemia–reperfusion damage

state. Early experiments showed that NHE1 message levels are elevated in hearts subjected to ischemia followed by reperfusion. In addition, treatment of primary cultures of neonatal rat myocytes with low external pH increased NHE1 activity [107]. Further studies showed that ischemia with or without reperfusion increase NHE1 levels in the disease state [108]. Interestingly, human sarcolemmal NHE1 activity was elevated in recipient hearts with chronic end stage heart failure, even though protein abundance was not increased [109] suggesting that the protein is activated (Fig. 4).

Aside from ischemia–reperfusion, the expression level and activity of NHE1 are elevated in a variety of cardiovascular diseases, including in hypertensive, hypertrophied, or diabetic myocardium [69, 110–112]. Both NHE1 message levels and protein levels have been shown to be elevated in these models. In aldosterone-induced hypertrophy, inhibition of NHE1 activity prevented the effect of aldosterone on inducing cardiac hypertrophy [69].

Transgenic Models of Elevated NHE1 Show Hypertrophy, but Surprisingly, Resistance to Ischemia Reperfusion

Because of the known elevation in the levels of NHE1 that occur in myocardial disease, a number of studies have examined transgenic mice with

elevation of the levels of the NHE1 protein. We first examined the effect of NHE1 overexpression in mice hearts subjected to subjected to 20 min of ischemia followed by 40 min of reperfusion. Surprisingly, contractility after ischemia reperfusion, improved in NHE1-overexpressing hearts (Fig. 4). In addition, NMR spectroscopy revealed that NHE1 overexpressor hearts contained higher ATP levels during early reperfusion and there was no difference in Na⁺ accumulation during between transgenic and WT hearts. Cariporide, the NHE1 inhibitor, equivalently protected both WT and NHE1-overexpressing hearts. Similar results were later shown by Cook et al. [113] who also showed that NHE1 overexpression induced an ER stress response in mouse myocardium, which might afford protection against ischemia–reperfusion-induced injury. We also suggested that a possible explanation for the beneficial effects is that basal activity of NHE1 is not rate-limiting in causing damage during ischemia–reperfusion, therefore increasing the level of NHE1 does not enhance injury and can have some small protective effects [114].

While overexpression of NHE1 may have some beneficial effects with ischemia and reperfusion, it has other detrimental effects. In a different transgenic model, Nakamura et al. [115] demonstrated that overexpression of an activated NHE1 led to cardiac hypertrophy and eventually to heart failure. Intracellular Na⁺ levels were elevated, as were both diastolic and systolic calcium levels. This study found that the Ca²⁺-dependent prohypertrophic molecules calcineurin and CaMKII were highly activated in these transgenic hearts. More recently we examined transgenic mice that had an elevation of either wild-type NHE1 protein or had an elevation of hyperactive NHE1 protein [116]. We found that mice with hyperactive NHE1 developed hypertrophy, including elevated heart weight-to-body weight ratio and increased cross-sectional area of the cardiomyocytes, interstitial fibrosis, as well as depressed cardiac function. Mice which expressed only wild-type NHE1 had modest changes in gene expression whereas mice expressing hyperactive NHE1 had a very strong transcriptional response. The most significant changes in gene expression were elevations in message levels of genes involved in cardiac hypertrophy, cardiac necrosis/cell death, and cardiac infarction. Secreted phosphoprotein 1 and its signaling pathways were notably upregulated in mice with hyperactive NHE1. This study demonstrated that expression of activated NHE1 elicits specific pathways of gene activation in the myocardium that lead to cardiac hypertrophy, cell death, and infarction (Fig. 4).

Conclusions

It is clear that NHE1 has a number of detrimental effects on the myocardium and is involved in the cardiac pathologies of ischemia–reperfusion damage and cardiac hypertrophy. NHE1 inhibition has not yet proven to be a useful clinical tool. Whether more specific NHE1 inhibitors can be developed, which could be useful clinically for treatment of ischemic heart disease, has still to be determined. It is of interest that elevation of NHE1 levels has some cardioprotective effects. Whether this is due to elevation of ER stress proteins or through other cardioprotective mechanisms should be investigated. Animal models have been able to achieve almost total inhibition of NHE1 protein activity, while this may be difficult to obtain in humans with treatment with inhibitors. Is it possible that clinical studies have achieved only partial inhibition of the Na⁺–H⁺ exchanger in humans and that the inhibition is both not effective enough to prevent calcium overload and also abrogates some other beneficial activities of the protein? Further studies are required to answer this question. The detrimental effects of elevation of NHE1 levels, in causing cardiac hypertrophy, are of significant interest. Since NHE1 inhibitors prevent myocardial hypertrophy in preclinical studies, NHE1 inhibition for treatment of myocardial hypertrophy remains a potential clinical target.

References

1. Fliegel L. The Na⁺/H⁺ exchanger isoform 1. Int J Biochem Cell Biol. 2005;37:33–7.
2. Fliegel L, Dyck JRB, Wang H, et al. Cloning and analysis of the human myocardial Na⁺/H⁺ exchanger. Mol Cell Biochem. 1993;125:137–43.
3. Fliegel L, Sardet C, Pouysségur J, et al. Identification of the protein and cDNA of the cardiac Na⁺/H⁺ exchanger. FEBS Lett. 1991;279:25–9.
4. Fliegel L. Functional and cellular regulation of the myocardial Na⁺/H⁺ exchanger. J Thromb Thrombolysis. 1999;8:9–14.
5. Orlowski J, Kandasamy RA, Shull GE. Molecular cloning of putative members of the Na⁺/H⁺ exchanger gene family. J Biol Chem. 1992;267:9331–9.
6. Takaichi K, Wang D, Balkovetz DF, et al. Cloning, sequencing, and expression of Na⁺/H⁺ antiporter cDNAs from human tissues. Am J Physiol Cell Physiol. 1992;262:C1069–76.
7. Orlowski J, Grinstein S. Diversity of the mammalian sodium/proton exchanger SLC9 gene family. Pflugers Arch. 2004;447:549–65.
8. Karmazyn M, Gan T, Humphreys RA, et al. The myocardial Na⁺–H⁺ exchange. Structure, regulation, and its role in heart disease. Circ Res. 1999;85:777–86.
9. Malo ME, Fliegel L. Physiological role and regulation of the Na⁺/H⁺ exchanger. Can J Physiol Pharmacol. 2006;84:1081–95.
10. Sardet C, Franchi A, Pouysségur J. Molecular cloning, primary structure, and expression of the human growth factor-activatable Na⁺/H⁺ antiporter. Cell. 1989;56:271–80.
11. Wakabayashi S, Pang T, Su X, et al. A novel topology model of the human Na⁺/H⁺ exchanger isoform 1. J Biol Chem. 2000;275:7942–9.
12. Kyte J, Doolittle RF. A simple method for displaying the hydropathic character of a protein. J Mol Biol. 1982;157:105–32.
13. Landau M, Herz K, Padan E, et al. Model structure of the Na⁺/H⁺ exchanger 1 (NHE1): functional and clinical implications. J Biol Chem. 2007;282: 37854–63.
14. Fliegel L, Haworth RS, Dyck JRB. Characterization of the placental brush border membrane Na⁺/H⁺ exchanger: Identification of thiol-dependent transitions in apparent molecular size. Biochem J. 1993;289: 101–7.
15. Fafournoux P, Noel J, Pouysségur J. Evidence that Na⁺/H⁺ exchanger isoforms NHE1 and NHE3 exist as stable dimers in membranes with a high degree of specificity for homodimers. J Biol Chem. 1994;269: 2589–96.
16. Hunte C, Screpanti E, Venturi M, et al. Structure of a Na⁺/H⁺ antiporter and insights into mechanism of action and regulation by pH. Nature. 2005; 435:1197–202.
17. Brett CL, Donowitz M, Rao R. Evolutionary origins of eukaryotic sodium/proton exchangers. Am J Physiol Cell Physiol. 2005;288:C223–39.
18. Putney LK, Denker SP, Barber DL. The changing face of the Na⁺/H⁺ exchanger, NHE1: structure, regulation, and cellular actions. Annu Rev Pharmacol Toxicol. 2002;42:527–52.
19. Sardet C, Franchi A, Pouysségur J. Molecular cloning of the growth-factor-activatable human Na⁺/H⁺ antiporter. Cold Spring Harb Symp Quant Biol. 1988;LIII: 1011–8.

20. Petrecca K, Atanasiu R, Grinstein S, et al. Subcellular localization of the Na$^+$/H$^+$ exchanger NHE1 in rat myocardium. Am J Physiol Heart Circ Physiol. 1999;276:H709–17.

21. Malakooti J, Dahdal RY, Schmidt L, et al. Molecular cloning, tissue distribution, and functional expression of the human Na$^+$/H$^+$ exchanger NHE2. Am J Physiol Gen Physiol. 1999;277:G383–90.

22. Amemiya M, Loffing J, Lotscher M, et al. Expression of NHE-3 in the apical membrane of rat renal proximal tubule and thick ascending limb. Kidney Int. 1995;48:1206–15.

23. Biemesderfer D, Pizzonia J, Abu-Alfa A, et al. NHE3: a exchanger isoform of renal brush border. Am J Physiol Ren Physiol. 1993;265:F736–42.

24. Baird NR, Orlowski J, Szabo EZ, et al. Molecular cloning, genomic organization, and functional expression of Na$^+$/H$^+$ exchanger isoform 5 (NHE5) from human brain. J Biol Chem. 1999;274:4377–82.

25. Nakamura N, Tanaka S, Teko Y, et al. Four Na$^+$/H$^+$ exchanger isoforms are distributed to Golgi and post-Golgi compartments and are involved in organelle pH regulation. J Biol Chem. 2005;280:1561–72.

26. Numata M, Petrecca K, Lake N, et al. Identification of a mitochondrial Na$^+$/H$^+$ exchanger. J Biol Chem. 1998;273:6951–9.

27. Lee SH, Kim T, Park ES, et al. NHE10, an osteoclast-specific member of the Na$^+$/H$^+$ exchanger family, regulates osteoclast differentiation and survival [corrected]. Biochem Biophys Res Commun. 2008; 369:320–6.

28. Xiang M, Feng M, Muend S, et al. A human Na$^+$/H$^+$ antiporter sharing evolutionary origins with bacterial NhaA may be a candidate gene for essential hypertension. Proc Natl Acad Sci USA. 2007;104:18677–81.

29. Schushan M, Xiang M, Bogomiakov P, et al. Model-guided mutagenesis drives functional studies of human NHA2, implicated in hypertension. J Mol Biol. 2010;396:1181–96.

30. Zerbini G, Maestroni A, Breviario D, et al. Alternative splicing of NHE-1 mediates Na–Li countertransport and associates with activity rate. Diabetes. 2003;52: 1511–8.

31. Karmazyn M, Moffat MP. Role of Na/H exchange in cardiac physiology and pathophysiology: mediation of myocardial reperfusion injury by the pH paradox. Cardiovasc Res. 1993;27:915–24.

32. Haworth RS, Avkiran M. Receptor-mediated regulation of the cardiac sarcolemmal Na$^+$/H$^+$ exchanger. Mechanisms and (patho)physiological significance. In: Karmazyn M, Avkiran M, Fliegel L, editors. The Na$^+$/H$^+$ exchanger, from molecular to its role in disease. Boston: Kluwer; 2003. p. 191–209.

33. Moor AN, Fliegel L. Protein kinase mediated regulation of the Na$^+$/H$^+$ exchanger in the rat myocardium by MAP-kinase-dependent pathways. J Biol Chem. 1999;274:22985–92.

34. Moor AN, Gan XT, Karmazyn M, et al. Activation of Na$^+$/H$^+$ exchanger-directed protein kinases in the ischemic and ischemic-reperfused rat myocardium. J Biol Chem. 2001;27:16113–22.

35. Liu S, Piwnica-Worms D, Lieberman M. Intracellular pH regulation in cultured embryonic chick heart cells. Na$^+$-dependent Cl$^-$/HCO$_3$$^-$ exchange. J Gen Physiol. 1990;96:1247–69.

36. Lagadic-Gossmann D, Buckler KJ, Vaughan-Jones RD. Role of bicarbonate in pH recovery from intracellular acidosis in the guinea-pig ventricular myocyte. J Physiol. 1992;458:361–84.

37. Lagadic-Gossmann D, Vaughan-Jones RD, Buckler KJ. Adrenaline and extracellular ATP switch between two modes of acid extrusion in the guinea-pig ventricular myocyte. J Physiol. 1992;458:385–407.

38. Dart C, Vaughan-Jones RD. Na$^+$–HCO$_3$$^-$ symport in the sheep cardiac purkinje fibre. J Physiol. 1992;451:365–85.

39. Grace AA, Kirschenlohr HL, Metcalfe JC, et al. Regulation of intracellular pH in the perfused heart by external HCO$_3$$^-$ and Na$^+$–H$^+$ exchange. Am J Physiol Heart Circ Physiol. 1993;265:H289–98.

40. Vandenberg JI, Metcalfe JC, Grace AA. Mechanisms of pHi recovery after global ischemia in the perfused heart. Circ Res. 1993;72:993–1003.

41. Vandenberg JI, Metcalfe JC, Grace AA. Intracellular pH recovery during respiratory acidosis in perfused hearts. Am J Physiol. 1994;266:C489–97.

42. Meima ME, Mackley JR, Barber DL. Beyond ion translocation: structural functions of the sodium–hydrogen exchanger isoform-1. Curr Opin Nephrol Hypertens. 2007;16:365–72.

43. Pouyssegur J, Sardet C, Franchi A, et al. A specific mutation abolishing Na$^+$/H$^+$ antiport activity in hamster fibroblasts precludes growth at neutral and acidic pH. Proc Natl Acad Sci USA. 1984;81:4833–7.

44. Bell SM, Schreiner CM, Schultheis PJ, et al. Targeted disruption of the murine Nhe1 locus induces ataxia, growth retardation, and seizures. Am J Physiol Cell Physiol. 1999;276:C788–95.

45. Cox GA, Lutz CM, Yang C-L, et al. Sodium/hydrogen exchanger gene defect in slow-wave epilepsy mice. Cell. 1997;91:139–48.

46. Putney LK, Barber DL. Na–H exchange-dependent increase in intracellular pH times G2/M entry and transition. J Biol Chem. 2003;278:44645–9.

47. Putney LK, Barber DL. Expression profile of genes regulated by activity of the Na–H exchanger NHE1. BMC Genomics. 2004;5:46–59.

48. Wang H, Singh D, Fliegel L. The Na$^+$/H$^+$ antiporter potentiates growth and retinoic- acid induced differentiation of P19 embryonal carcinoma cells. J Biol Chem. 1997;272:26545–9.

49. Rao GN, Sardet C, Pouyssegur J, et al. Na$^+$/H$^+$ antiporter gene expression increases during retinoic acid-induced granulocytic differentiation of HL60 cells. J Cell Physiol. 1992;151:361–6.

50. Khaled AR, Moor AN, Li A, et al. Trophic factor withdrawal: p38 mitogen-activated protein kinase activates NHE1, which induces intracellular alkalinization. Mol Cell Biol. 2001;21:7545–57.

51. Reshkin SJ, Bellizzi A, Caldeira S, et al. Na$^+$/H$^+$ exchanger-dependent intracellular alkalinization is an early event in malignant transformation and plays an

essential role in the development of subsequent transformation-associated phenotypes. FASEB J. 2000;14:2185–97.

52. McLean LA, Roscoe J, Jorgensen NK, et al. Malignant gliomas display altered pH regulation by NHE1 compared with nontransformed astrocytes. Am J Physiol Cell Physiol. 2000;278:C676–88.

53. Rich IN, Worthington-White D, Garden OA, et al. Apoptosis of leukemic cells accompanies reduction in intracellular pH after targeted inhibition of the Na⁺/H⁺ exchanger. Blood. 2000;95:1427–34.

54. Reshkin SJ, Bellizzi A, Albarani V, et al. Phosphoinositide 3-kinase is involved in the tumor-specific activation of human breast cancer cell Na⁺/H⁺ exchange, motility, and invasion induced by serum deprivation. J Biol Chem. 2000;275:5361–9.

55. Cardone RA, Bagorda A, Bellizzi A, et al. Protein kinase A gating of a pseudopodial-located RhoA/ROCK/p38/NHE1 signal module regulates invasion in breast cancer cell lines. Mol Biol Cell. 2005; 16:3117–27.

56. Paradiso A, Cardone RA, Bellizzi A, et al. The Na⁺–H⁺ exchanger-1 induces cytoskeletal changes involving reciprocal RhoA and Rac1 signaling, resulting in motility and invasion in MDA-MB-435 cells. Breast Cancer Res. 2004;6:R616–28.

57. Allen DG, Xiao XH. Role of the cardiac Na⁺/H⁺ exchanger during ischemia and reperfusion. Cardiovasc Res. 2003;57:934–41.

58. Lazdunski M, Frelin C, Vigne P. The sodium/hydrogen exchange system in cardiac cells. Its biochemical and pharmacological properties and its role in regulating internal concentrations of sodium and internal pH. J Mol Cell Cardiol. 1985;17:1029–42.

59. Avkiran M. Protection of the ischaemic myocardium by Na⁺/H⁺ exchange inhibitors: potential mechanisms of action. Basic Res Cardiol. 2001;96:306–11.

60. Karmazyn M, Sawyer M, Fliegel L. The Na⁺/H⁺ exchanger: a target for cardiac therapeutic intervention. Curr Drug Targets Cardiovasc Haematol Disord. 2005;5:323–35.

61. Avkiran M, Marber MS. Na⁺/H⁺ exchange inhibitors for cardioprotective therapy: progress, problems and prospects. J Am Coll Cardiol. 2002;39:747–53.

62. Karmazyn M. Amiloride enhances post ischemic recovery: possible role of Na⁺/H⁺ exchange. Am J Physiol Heart Circ Physiol. 1988;255:H608–15.

63. Scholz W, Albus U, Counillon L, et al. Protective effects of HOE642, a selective sodium–hydrogen exchange subtype 1 inhibitor, on cardiac ischaemia and reperfusion. Cardiovasc Res. 1995;29:260–8.

64. Gumina RJ, Mizumura T, Beier N, et al. A new sodium/hydrogen exchange inhibitor, EMD 85131, limits infarct size in dogs when administered before or after coronary artery occlusion. J Pharmacol Exp Ther. 1998;286:175–83.

65. Coccaro E, Karki P, Cojocaru C, et al. Phenylephrine and sustained acidosis activate the neonatal rat cardiomyocyte Na⁺/H⁺ exchanger through phosphorylation of amino acids Ser770 and Ser771. Am J Physiol Heart Circ Physiol. 2009;297:H846–58.

66. Kusumoto K, Haist JV, Karmazyn M. Na⁺/H⁺ exchange inhibition reduces hypertrophy and heart failure after myocardial infarction in rats. Am J Physiol Heart Circ Physiol. 2001;280:H738–45.

67. Yoshida H, Karmazyn M. Na⁺/H⁺ exchange inhibition attenuates hypertrophy and heart failure in 1-wk postinfarction rat myocardium. Am J Physiol Heart Circ Physiol. 2000;278:H300–4.

68. Kilic A, Velic A, De Windt LJ, et al. Enhanced activity of the myocardial Na⁺/H⁺ exchanger NHE-1 contributes to cardiac remodeling in atrial natriuretic peptide receptor-deficient mice. Circulation. 2005;112: 2307–17.

69. Karmazyn M, Liu Q, Gan XT, et al. Aldosterone increases NHE-1 expression and induces NHE-1-dependent hypertrophy in neonatal rat ventricular myocytes. Hypertension. 2003;42:1171–6.

70. Karmazyn M. Role of NHE-1 in cardiac hypertrophy and heart failure. In: Karmazyn M, Avkiran M, Fliegel L, editors. The Na⁺/H⁺ exchanger, from molecular to its role in disease. Boston: Kluwer; 2003. p. 211–9.

71. Cingolani HE, Alvarez BV, Ennis IL, et al. Stretch-induced alkalinization of feline papillary muscle: an autocrine-paracrine system. Circ Res. 1998;83: 775–80.

72. Cingolani HE, Ennis IL. Sodium–hydrogen exchanger, cardiac overload, and myocardial hypertrophy. Circulation. 2007;115:1090–100.

73. Dulce RA, Hurtado C, Ennis IL, et al. Endothelin-1 induced hypertrophic effect in neonatal rat cardiomyocytes: involvement of Na⁺/H⁺ and Na⁺/Ca²⁺ exchangers. J Mol Cell Cardiol. 2006;41:807–15.

74. Dumont EA, Reutelingsperger CP, Smits JF, et al. Real-time imaging of apoptotic cell-membrane changes at the single-cell level in the beating murine heart. Nat Med. 2001;7:1352–5.

75. Kajstura J, Cheng W, Reiss K, et al. Apoptotic and necrotic myocyte cell deaths are independent contributing variables of infarct size in rats. Lab Invest. 1996;74:86–107.

76. Dumont EA, Hofstra L, van Heerde WL, et al. Cardiomyocyte death induced by myocardial ischemia and reperfusion: measurement with recombinant human annexin-V in a mouse model. Circulation. 2000;102:1564–8.

77. Saraste A, Pulkki K, Kallajoki M, et al. Apoptosis in human acute myocardial infarction. Circulation. 1997;95:320–3.

78. Veinot JP, Gattinger DA, Fliss H. Early apoptosis in human myocardial infarcts. Hum Pathol. 1997;28: 485–92.

79. Sun HY, Wang NP, Halkos ME, et al. Involvement of Na⁺/H⁺ exchanger in hypoxia/re-oxygenation-induced neonatal rat cardiomyocyte apoptosis. Eur J Pharmacol. 2004;486:121–31.

80. Jung YS, Kim MY, Kim MJ, et al. Pharmacological profile of KR-33028, a highly selective inhibitor of Na⁺/H⁺ exchanger. Eur J Pharmacol. 2006;535: 220–7.

81. Chakrabarti S, Hoque AN, Karmazyn M. A rapid ischemia-induced apoptosis in isolated rat hearts and

its attenuation by the sodium–hydrogen exchange inhibitor HOE 642 (cariporide). J Mol Cell Cardiol. 1997;29:3169–74.

82. Javadov S, Choi A, Rajapurohitam V, et al. NHE-1 inhibition-induced cardioprotection against ischaemia/reperfusion is associated with attenuation of the mitochondrial permeability transition. Cardiovasc Res. 2008;77:416–24.

83. Garg S, Hofstra L, Reutelingsperger C, et al. Apoptosis as a therapeutic target in acutely ischemic myocardium. Curr Opin Cardiol. 2003;18:372–7.

84. Aker S, Snabaitis AK, Konietzka I, et al. Inhibition of the Na$^+$/H$^+$exchanger attenuates the deterioration of ventricular function during pacing-induced heart failure in rabbits. Cardiovasc Res. 2004;63:273–82.

85. Humphreys RA, Haist JV, Chakrabarti S, et al. Orally administered NHE1 inhibitor cariporide reduces acute responses to coronary occlusion and reperfusion. Am J Physiol Heart Circ Physiol. 1999;276:H749–57.

86. Maekawa N, Abe J, Shishido T, et al. Inhibiting p90 ribosomal S6 kinase prevents Na$^+$–H$^+$ exchanger-mediated cardiac ischemia-reperfusion injury. Circulation. 2006;113:2516–23.

87. Avkiran M, Cook AR, Cuello F. Targeting Na$^+$/H$^+$ exchanger regulation for cardiac protection: a RSKy approach? Curr Opin Pharmacol. 2008;8(2):133–40.

88. Grenier AL, Abu-ihweij K, Zhang G, et al. Apoptosis-induced alkalinization by the Na$^+$/H$^+$ exchanger isoform 1 is mediated through phosphorylation of amino acids Ser726 and Ser729. Am J Physiol Cell Physiol. 2008;295:C883–96.

89. Dilley RJ, Farrelly CA, Allen TJ, et al. Diabetes induces Na/H exchange activity and hypertrophy of rat mesenteric but not basilar arteries. Diab Res Clin Pract. 2005;70:201–8.

90. Little PJ, Dilley RJ. Role of Na–H exchanger in vascular remodelling in diabetes. In: Karmazyn M, Avkiran M, Fliegel L, editors. The Na$^+$/H$^+$ exchanger, from molecular to its role in disease. Boston: Kluwer; 2003. p. 159–75.

91. Vial G, Dubouchaud H, Couturier K, et al. Na$^+$/H$^+$ exchange inhibition with cariporide prevents alterations of coronary endothelial function in streptozotocin-induced diabetes. Mol Cell Biochem. 2008; 310:93–102.

92. Phillis JW, Pilitsis JG, O'Regan MH. The potential role of the Na$^+$/H$^+$ exchanger in ischemia/reperfusion injury of the central nervous system. In: Karmazyn M, Avkiran M, Fliegel L, editors. The Na$^+$/H$^+$ exchanger, from molecular to its role in disease. Boston: Kluwer; 2003. p. 177–89.

93. Gumina RJ, Daemmgen J, Gross GJ. Inhibition of the Na$^+$/H$^+$ exchanger attenuates phase 1b ischemic arrhythmias and reperfusion-induced ventricular fibrillation. Eur J Pharmacol. 2000;396:119–24.

94. Aye NN, Komori S, Hashimoto K. Effects and interaction, of cariporide and preconditioning on cardiac arrhythmias and infarction in rat in vivo. Br J Pharmacol. 1999;127:1048–55.

95. Gazmuri RJ, Ayoub IM, Hoffner E, et al. Successful ventricular defibrillation by the selective sodium–hydrogen exchanger isoform-1 inhibitor cariporide. Circulation. 2001;104:234–9.

96. Gumina RJ, Gross GJ. If ischemic preconditioning is the gold standard, has a platinum standard of cardioprotection arrived? Comparison with NHE inhibition. J Thromb Thrombolysis. 1999;8: 39–44.

97. Gumina RJ, Buerger E, Eickmeier C, et al. Inhibition of the Na$^+$/H$^+$ exchanger confers greater cardioprotection against 90 minutes of myocardial ischemia than ischemic preconditioning in dogs. Circulation. 1999;100:2519–26, discussion 469–472.

98. Myers ML, Karmazyn M. Improved cardiac function after prolonged hypothermic ischemia with the exchange Na$^+$/H$^+$ inhibitor HOE 694. Ann Thorac Surg. 1996;61:1400–6.

99. Kim YI, Herijgers P, Laycock SK, et al. Na$^+$/H$^+$ exchange inhibition improves long-term myocardial preservation. Ann Thorac Surg. 1998;66:436–42.

100. Kim YI, Herijgers P, Van Lommel A, et al. Na$^+$/H$^+$ exchange inhibition improves post-transplant myocardial compliance in 4-hour stored donor hearts. Cardiovasc Surg. 1998;6:67–75.

101. Gazmuri RJ, Ayoub IM. NHE-1 inhibition: a potential new treatment for resuscitation from cardiac arrest. In: Karmazyn M, Avkiran M, Fliegel L, editors. The Na$^+$/H$^+$ exchanger, from molecular to its role in disease. Boston: Kluwer; 2003. p. 291–308.

102. Wu D, Arias J, Bassuk J, et al. Na$^+$/H$^+$ exchange inhibition delays the onset of hypovolemic circulatory shock in pigs. Shock. 2008;29:519–25.

103. Rupprecht HJ, vom Dahl J, Terres W, et al. Cardioprotective effects of the Na$^+$/H$^+$ exchange inhibitor cariporide in patients with acute anterior myocardial infarction undergoing direct PTCA. Circulation. 2000;101:2902–8.

104. Zeymer U, Suryapranata H, Monassier JP, et al. The Na$^+$/H$^+$ exchange inhibitor eniporide as an adjunct to early reperfusion therapy for acute myocardial infarction. Results of the evaluation of the safety and cardioprotective effects of eniporide in acute myocardial infarction (ESCAMI) trial. J Am Coll Cardiol. 2001;38:1644–50.

105. Boyce SW, Bartels C, Bolli R, et al. Impact of sodium–hydrogen exchange inhibition by cariporide on death or myocardial infarction in high-risk CABG surgery patients: results of the CABG surgery cohort of the GUARDIAN study. J Thorac Cardiovasc Surg. 2003;126:420–7.

106. Fleisher LA, Newman MF, St. Aubin LB, et al. Efficacy of zoniporide, an Na/H exchange ion inhibitor, for reducing perioperative cardiovascular events in vascular surgery patients. J Cardiothorac Vasc Anesth. 2005;19:570–6.

107. Dyck JRB, Maddaford T, Pierce GN, et al. Induction of expression of the sodium–hydrogen exchanger in rat myocardium. Cardiovasc Res. 1995;29:203–8.

108. Gan XT, Chakrabarti S, Karmazyn M. Modulation of Na$^+$/H$^+$ exchange isoform 1 mRNA expression in isolated rat hearts. Am J Physiol Heart Circ Physiol. 1999;277:H993–8.

109. Yokoyama H, Gunasegaram S, Harding S, Avkiran M. Sarcolemmal Na$^+$/H$^+$ exchanger activity and expression in human ventricular myocardium. J Am Coll Cardiol. 2000;36:534–40.

110. Chen L, Gan XT, Haist JV, et al. Attenuation of compensatory right ventricular hypertrophy and heart failure following monocrotaline-induced pulmonary vascular injury by the Na$^+$–H$^+$ exchange inhibitor cariporide. J Pharmacol Exp Ther. 2001;298:469–76.

111. Engelhardt S, Hein L, Keller U, et al. Inhibition of Na$^+$–H$^+$ exchange prevents hypertrophy, fibrosis, and heart failure in beta(1)-adrenergic receptor transgenic mice. Circ Res. 2002;90:814–9.

112. Jandeleit-Dahm K, Hannan KM, Farrelly CA, et al. Diabetes-induced vascular hypertrophy is accompanied by activation of Na$^+$–H$^+$ exchange and prevented by Na$^+$–H$^+$ exchange inhibition. Circ Res. 2000;87:1133–40.

113. Cook AR, Bardswell SC, Pretheshan S, et al. Paradoxical resistance to myocardial ischemia and age-related cardiomyopathy in NHE1 transgenic mice: a role for ER stress? J Mol Cell Cardiol. 2009;46:225–33.

114. Imahashi K, Mraiche F, Steenbergen C, et al. Overexpression of the Na$^+$/H$^+$ exchanger and ischemia-reperfusion injury in the myocardium. Am J Physiol Heart Circ Physiol. 2007;292:H2237–47.

115. Nakamura TY, Iwata Y, Arai Y, et al. Activation of Na$^+$/H$^+$ exchanger 1 is sufficient to generate Ca^{2+} signals that induce cardiac hypertrophy and heart failure. Circ Res. 2008;103:891–9.

116. Xue J, Mraiche F, Zhou D, et al. Elevated myocardial Na$^+$/H$^+$ exchanger isoform 1 activity elicits gene expression that leads to cardiac hypertrophy. Physiol Genomics. 2010;42:374–83.

Impact of Perinatal Chronic Hypoxia on Cardiac Tolerance to Acute Ischemia

Bohuslav Ostadal, I. Ostadalova, F. Kolar, I. Netuka, and O. Szarszoi

Abstract

Perinatal period is critical for the normal cardiac development, and different interventions imposed on the heart may significantly influence myocardial structure and function. Perinatal hypoxemia, although transient, may thus have serious early and late consequences on the cardiovascular system. Epidemiological and experimental studies have repeatedly suggested a possible link between perinatal hypoxia and increased sensitivity to ischemia/reperfusion (I/R) injury in adults. The mechanisms of this increased susceptibility are not known at present. It has been found that prenatal chronic hypoxia sensitizes the apoptosis pathway in the adult male heart in response to I/R stimulation. In addition, cardiac heat shock proteins (Hsp) 70 expression was significantly lower in prenatal hypoxic hearts than in controls; this fact may play a role in the increased susceptibility of the adult heart to I/R injury. The decreased eNOS levels in adult prenatal hypoxic hearts may also contribute to their increased sensitivity. These studies suggest that chronic hypoxic exposure during early development may cause in utero or neonatal programming of several genes which can play an important role in the increased susceptibility of the adult male heart to I/R injury. Furthermore, it has been observed in the rat model that late myocardial effects of chronic hypoxia, experienced in early life, may be sex-dependent. Unlike in males, perinatal exposure to chronic hypoxia significantly increased cardiac tolerance to acute I/R injury in adult females, expressed as the lower incidence of ischemic arrhythmias, decreased infarct size, decreased cardiac enzyme release, and increased postischemic recovery of left ventricular function. It was suggested that these sex-dependent changes may be due to differences in fetal programming

B. Ostadal (✉)
Centre for Cardiovascular Research,
Prague, Czech Republic

Institute of Physiology, Academy of Sciences
of the Czech Republic, Prague, Czech Republic
e-mail: ostadal@biomed.cas.cz

N.S. Dhalla, M. Nagano, B. Ostadal (eds.), *Molecular Defects in Cardiovascular Disease*,
DOI 10.1007/978-1-4419-7130-2_5, © Springer Science+Business Media, LLC 2011

of PKCε gene expression, which play a pivotal role in cardioprotection; down-regulation of PKCε function was observed in the hearts of adult male offspring only. These results would have important clinical implications, since cardiac sensitivity to oxygen deprivation in adult patients may be significantly influenced by perinatal hypoxia in a sex-dependent manner.

Keywords

Perinatal period • Fetal heart • Neonatal heart • Cardiac development • Mitochondrial development • Chronic hypoxia • Cardiac tolerance to ischemia • Infarct size • Arrhythmias • Barker's concept • Ischemia/reperfusion injury • Prenatal hypoxia • Early postnatal hypoxia • Late effects of perinatal hypoxia • Sex-dependent changes

Introduction

Human epidemiological studies have shown a clear association of adverse intrauterine environment and an increased risk of ischemic heart disease in later adult life [1]. Of all these stresses to which the fetus is subjected, perhaps the most important and clinically relevant is that of hypoxia [2]. The fetus may experience prolonged hypoxic stress under many different conditions, including pregnancy at high altitude, pregnancy with anemia, placental insufficiency, cord compression, and heart, lung, and kidney disease. There is clear evidence of a link between hypoxia and fetal intrauterine growth restriction: human studies at high altitude suggest that hypoxia per se, independent of maternal nutrition, causes fetal growth restriction, resulting in low birth weight and altered body shape at birth [3].

One of the most common insults during early stages of postnatal ontogenetic development is hypoxemia due to congenital cyanotic heart defects or pulmonary disease secondary to prematurity. Such hypoxemia may persist for several weeks or months until surgical repair of the structural defects or improvement in pulmonary function makes the individual normoxemic [4]. Epidemiological studies clearly show that the number of adult patients undergoing surgery for congenital cyanotic defects has increased significantly [5]. Moreover, this group of patients is growing older and is approaching the age characterized by significantly increased risk of serious cardiovascular diseases, such as hypertension and ischemic heart disease. Therefore, it can be expected that more such patients will require diagnostic or therapeutic catheterization or cardiac surgery.

Under these conditions, the question of the presumed cardiovascular impact of perinatal hypoxia will be of considerable importance [6]. The aim of the present survey was, therefore, to summarize the data available on the impact of perinatal chronic hypoxia on cardiac tolerance to acute oxygen deprivation in adults. Because clinical and experimental studies suggest that there may be a sex difference in the cardiac tolerance to ischemia, particular attention was paid to the comparison of effects of perinatal hypoxia on adult male and female hearts.

Perinatal Critical Developmental Period

To study the late effects of early disturbances, the theory of critical developmental periods, introduced already in 1921 by Stockard [7], should be revived. According to this idea the tissues are most sensitive to injury during the period of intense growth. The intervention during this critical period can modify the structure and function of this particular tissue or organ. The consequences of an intervention during the critical developmental period can appear after a period of latency, either spontaneously or induced by some other insults.

Perinatal period represents a typical example of such developmentally decisive critical period. The fetus makes numerous adaptations to ensure normal development in spite of its low arterial PO_2, which corresponds to an altitude of 8,000 m ("Mt. Everest in utero") [8]. Among these adaptations are polycythemia, leftward shift of the dissociation curve, fetal hemoglobin, a high cardiac output, and low arterial blood pressure, which help provide adequate oxygen and nutrient delivery to the developing tissues. Fetal heart operates at near maximum levels and is very sensitive to increases in afterload.

The major changes in oxygen saturation can be observed during delivery. Within the short period of time mammalian fetus (and its heart) comes from the hypoxic environment with low PO_2 and low oxygen saturation into the normal atmosphere, arterial saturation increases more than three times. As a consequence of these dramatic changes at birth, mammalian hearts meet suddenly with an extremely high reactive oxygen species (ROS) concentration. The delivery is, furthermore, accompanied by the transition from the amniotic fluid to the air, by the marked decrease of the ambient temperature, and by the termination of placental nutrition. This transition requires appropriate physiological adaptations: onset of pulmonary respiration, transition from fetal to neonatal circulation, switching-on of thermoregulation, and increase of basal metabolic rate. Very important is the change of nutrition: trans-placental supply is interrupted and mother's milk nutrition is not yet fully developed [9]. The neonatal heart can probably use ROS for the increase of protein degradation which permits utilization of amino acids, necessary for the maintenance of energy homeostasis during neonatal starvation [9–11].

The early postnatal period is characterized by further adaptation to postnatal living conditions: relative heart weight significantly increases [12, 13], proliferation of myocytes (hyperplasia) is replaced by hypertrophic growth [14], rapid rate of coronary capillary formation occurs [15], cardiac mitochondrial function and calcium handling change substantially [16, 17], and contractility increases; cardiac sensitivity to the increasing concentration of calcium is the highest [13] (for review, see ref. [18]). Hemodynamic parameters are stepwise approaching the adult values (blood pressure and heart rate). The changes are very fast: e.g., the contractile response to low extracellular sodium differs in rats even day-by-day during the first week of life [19]. The whole period is characterized by intensive body growth [20]. In conclusion, it is obvious that the perinatal period is critical for normal cardiac development, and different interventions imposed on the heart may significantly influence myocardial structure and function.

Effect of Prenatal Chronic Hypoxia on Cardiac Development

As mentioned above, chronic hypoxia during the course of pregnancy is one of the common insults to fetal development and is thought to be associated with fetal intrauterine growth retardation. Experimental studies have demonstrated that reduced fetal oxygen or nutrient supply influence heart development. In fetal sheep, long-term hypoxemia (natural altitude 3,820 m, 110 days) reduced cardiac output and contractility [21], increased lactate dehydrogenase and citrate synthase [22] and resulted in cardiac hypertrophy [23, 24]. In this connection it may be of interest to mention that undernutrition increased cardiac expression of several genes that regulate hypertrophy and remodeling by midgestation [25]. Bae et al. [26] have observed that maternal chronic hypoxia (10.5% oxygen, 7 days) increased the hypoxia-inducible factor (HIF) 1α and increased apoptotic cell death in fetal rat hearts. The increased cell death may lead to asymmetric cardiac enlargement. Although the mechanisms underlying hypoxia-induced apoptosis are not clear and are likely to be multiplex, the above study demonstrated that apoptosis was associated with an increase in Fas receptors and decrease in Bcl-2 proteins. In addition, chronic hypoxia significantly suppressed expression of heat shock protein (Hsp) 70 and differentially regulated β-adrenoreceptor (AR) subtypes in the fetal heart. There was no difference in β_2-AR protein levels between the control and hypoxic heart but β_1-AR protein levels were significantly increased in the hypoxic group. Recently, Patterson et al. [27] observed that hypoxic treatment of pregnant rats from days 15 to 21 of gestation resulted in significant decrease in protein kinase (PKC) ϵ protein and mRNA in fetal hearts. These findings demonstrate a direct effect of hypoxia on cardiac gene expression, linking fetal hypoxia to possible pathophysiological consequences in the heart of adult offspring.

The population-based prospective cohort study has studied fetal hemodynamic adaptive changes related to intrauterine growth retardation [28]. Fetal growth characteristics and fetal circulation variables were assessed with ultrasound and Doppler examinations in 1,215 healthy women. It has been observed that decreased fetal growth is associated with cardiac remodeling and changes of cardiac output, consistent with gradual increase in afterload and compromised arterial compliance. These changes have already begun to occur before the stage of clinically apparent fetal growth restriction. These data imply that limitation of either oxygen or nutrient supply to the fetus produces functional and structural changes in the neonatal heart. However, less is known regarding the persistence and long-term consequences of these changes and their possible contribution to the increased risk of cardiovascular disease in later life.

Effect of Early Postnatal Chronic Hypoxia on Cardiac Development

In the chronically hypoxic newborn mammals, body growth is blunted [29]. Neonatal growth retardation during moderate (15% O_2) or severe (10% O_2) hypoxic exposure can be almost entirely attributed to the effects of hypoxia on the newborn, and is not mediated by the maternal response [30]. The faulty maternal lactation and limited food availability to the suckling are not the primary mechanisms of the neonatal growth retardation in chronic hypoxia, as was suggested by the observations that the cellular responses to hypoxia differ from those of experimental starvation [31].

In this connection it is necessary to mention that nutritional status markedly influences cardiac development. Slow-growing pups confer smaller cardiomyocyte length and volume [32], accompanied by qualitative changes of the subcellular structures. The development of α_1- and β-AR is retarded, and the resulting receptor deficit probably contributes to reduced responsiveness to adrenergic stimulation [33, 34]. These changes are connected with alterations of cardiac ornithine decarboxylase activity [35]. Moreover, we have observed [36] that the number of cardiomyocytes in both the right and left ventricular myocardium was significantly lower in slow-growing weanling rats. Early postnatal nutritional modification also altered protein remodeling in the immature myocardium: concentration of collagenous proteins in slow-growing rats significantly decreased [37]. Furthermore, undernutrition markedly decreased the basal values of left ventricular pressure and contractility in 3-week-old rats [38]; data on younger animals are, unfortunately, lacking.

Mild (19% O_2) or moderate levels of 1-week hypoxic exposure significantly increased cardiac weight and DNA synthesis in neonatal rats [30]. This suggests that hypoxia can truly stimulate cardiac muscle cell multiplication as has been demonstrated in neonatal rats exposed to sideropenic anemia [39, 40] or to low oxygen atmosphere [41, 42]. In neonatal animals exposed to high altitude the cardiac enlargement and activation of DNA synthesis was significantly more expressed in the right ventricular myocardium. The mechanisms behind the hypoxia-induced cardiac hyperplasia are unclear but it is possible that they relate to the greater cardiac work caused by the higher cardiac output, blood viscosity, and pulmonary vascular resistance.

As has been mentioned in the Introduction, chronic hypoxia is the main pathophysiological feature of hypoxemic congenital heart disease. Timing of corrective surgery is critically important, with early surgery desirable to promote more normal development. Many children undergoing cardiac surgery in the first year of life exhibit varying degrees of cyanotic heart disease where the myocardium is chronically perfused with hypoxic blood. We have observed [43] metabolic

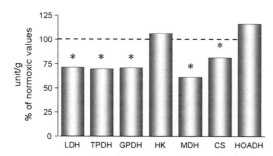

Fig. 1 Energy-supplying enzymes in the right atrium of children with tetralogy of Fallot and with normoxemic heart diseases (expressed as % of normoxemic values). *LDH* lactate dehydrogenase, *TPDH* triosephosphate dehydrogenase, *GPDH* glycerol-3-phosphate dehydrogenase, *HK* hexokinase, *MDH* malate dehydrogenase, *CS* citrate synthase, *HOADH* 3-hydroxyacyl-CoA dehydrogenase. *Statistically significant difference ($p < 0.01$) from normoxemic values. Data from ref. [43], reprinted with permission from ref. [69]

adaptation to chronic hypoxia in the myocardium of children with cyanotic congenital cardiac malformations (see Fig. 1). The capacity of the aerobic energy metabolism was significantly reduced in hypoxic hearts as compared with normoxic patients. Understanding the mechanisms by which cyanotic congenital heart disease modifies the myocardium and how the modifications impact on the cardiac tolerance to ischemia may provide insight into the treatments for limiting myocardial damage during cardiac surgery [44]. Unfortunately, so far the clinical data are missing. Moreover, to date no experimental model is available that adequately mimics chronic perfusion of immature hearts with hypoxic blood, caused by congenital cyanotic defects. Therefore, similar models as in adults, i.e., chronic hypoxia simulated in the normobaric or hypobaric chamber, are being used in experimental studies performed during early stages of ontogenetic development [45, 46].

Perinatal Chronic Hypoxia and Cardiac Tolerance to Ischemia

Cardiac tolerance of the immature heart to oxygen deficiency is significantly higher as compared with the adult myocardium; myocardial infarction is extremely rare during early ontogenetic development. Riva and Hearse [47] observed that age-dependent changes in resistance to global ischemia in the isolated rat heart showed a biphasic pattern with increasing tolerance from 5 to 23 days of age, followed by a decline to adulthood. Detailed analysis of the tolerance of the isolated rat heart to global ischemia during the first week of life has revealed a significant decrease from day 1 to 7 [48], suggesting a possible triphasic pattern of the ontogenetic development of cardiac sensitivity to ischemia. The sensitivity of neonatal myocardium may be species-dependent; Baker et al. [49] have shown that the neonatal pig heart is more susceptible to ischemia than the neonatal rabbit heart.

The mechanisms of the higher resistance of the immature heart to oxygen deprivation have not yet been satisfactorily clarified. For the explanation of this fact, the above-mentioned physiological changes during perinatal period should be taken into consideration, particularly the transition from the "Mt. Everest" to the sea level. The reason of the higher tolerance during further development can be still only hypothetical. It may be speculated that an explanation of the phenomenon lies in the greater anaerobic glycolytic capacity, higher glycogen reserves of the immature heart [50] or amino acid utilization by transamination [51]. Moreover, the ATP metabolic pathways change during development [52]; the immature heart is better equipped to ATP synthesis than to its breakdown, the situation that might be advantageous in conditions of low substrate availability. The immature heart thus suffers less ischemic injury after the same ischemic insult. Another factor that may contribute to the increased tolerance of the immature heart is the age-related change in calcium handling [17]: the relative contribution of transsarcolemmal calcium influx and calcium release from the sarcoplasmic reticulum varies significantly during development. The contraction of the immature myocardium, where the sarcoplasmic reticulum is not fully developed, depends to a large extent on the fluxes of calcium across sarcolemma [53]. Calcium overload, common in the adult myocardium, was not described in the immature heart.

Still unclear is the role of mitochondria in the developmental changes of cardiac tolerance to oxygen deprivation, in spite of the fact that mitochondria are responsible for cellular oxygen handling. Mitochondrial oxidative phosphorylation is not completely developed in the rat heart at birth; cardiac maturation during the first postnatal week is characterized by increasing content and specific activity of cytochrome c oxidase and enhanced flux of adenine nucleotides across the inner mitochondrial membrane [54, 55]. We have shown previously [16] that the content of cytochromes in cardiac mitochondria increased two-fold between birth and day 30, similarly as the expression of adenine nucleotide translocase 1. Moreover, in newborn animals, a single population of mitochondria with relatively high mitochondrial membrane potential (MMP) was observed. Starting with the weaning period, a second population of mitochondria with significantly lower MMP occurs. The collapse of MMP due to the opening of a high-conductance mitochondrial permeability transition pore (MPTP) has been implicated in the molecular mechanisms associated with ischemia/reperfusion (I/R) injury of the adult heart [56, 57]. We have observed, however, significant ontogenetic differences in the role of MPTP in the I/R injury. Whereas the blockade of MPTP by sanglifehrin in perfused rat heart had a protective effect on I/R-induced damage in the adult myocardium as already demonstrated [58], it had no effect in the neonatal heart [59]. For the explanation of this difference, a modified amount of cyclophilin receptors or lower sensitivity of MPTP in the neonatal heart to pore opening factors has to be taken into consideration. Furthermore, we found [59] that in cardiac mitochondria isolated from neonatal rats Ca^{2+}-dependent and cyclosporine-sensitive MPTP is less sensitive to Ca^{2+} ions as compared with adults. We can only speculate that its lower sensitivity to the calcium-induced swelling may be related to the higher ischemic tolerance of the neonatal heart. All these results support the view that cardiac mitochondria are deeply involved in the regulation of cardiac tolerance to oxygen deprivation during ontogenetic development.

Adaptation of the adult hearts to chronic hypoxia confers long-lasting cardiac protection against I/R injury. This phenomenon has been demonstrated both in human populations living at high altitude (for review, see ref. [60]) and in many animal studies (for review, see ref. [61]). Hearts adapted to chronic hypoxia exhibit decreased infarct size [62], increased postischemic recovery of contractile function [63], and decreased incidence and severity of ischemic and reperfusion arrhythmias [64, 65]. Protective mechanisms include K_{ATP}, oxygen free radicals, NO, different protein kinases, opioids, and erythropoietin; however, other factors cannot be excluded [66].

In this connection the question arises whether adaptation to chronic hypoxia can further increase the already high ischemic tolerance of the immature heart. However, only a few authors have compared tolerance to oxygen deprivation in chronically hypoxic versus normoxic immature myocardium. We have observed [67] that chronic hypoxia, simulated in the barochamber, results in similarly enhanced cardiac resistance in rats exposed to chronic hypoxia either from the fourth day of postnatal life or in adulthood. Similarly, Baker et al. [49] demonstrated that adaptation to chronic hypoxia increased the tolerance of the developing rabbit heart. However, it follows from our results [68] (see Fig. 2) that the protective effect of chronic hypoxia is absent in newborn rats; exposure of pregnant rats to simulated intermittent hypobaric hypoxia failed to improve cardiac ischemic tolerance in newborns. Early postnatal exposure to chronic hypoxia increased cardiac tolerance to acute ischemia already by the end of the first postnatal week [68]. Decreasing tolerance to ischemic insult during early postnatal life is thus counteracted by the development of endogenous protection. These results suggest that we might be dealing with the more general biological phenomenon: the already high resistance of the cardiac muscle cannot be further increased by different protective mechanisms. A similar situation as in the immature mammalian heart can be observed also in highly tolerant hearts of pokilotherms or in the myocardium of young females [69].

Overwhelming majority of studies, analyzing the possible mechanisms of cardiac adaptation to chronic hypoxia, deals, unfortunately, exclusively with the adult myocardium (for review, see ref. [66]).

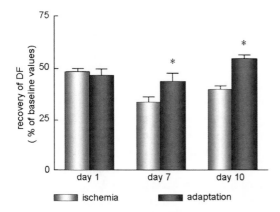

Fig. 2 Tolerance of the isolated perfused neonatal rat heart to acute ischemia (expressed as the recovery of the developed force – DF) in controls and in animals adapted to chronic hypoxia. *Statistically significant difference ($p < 0.01$) between both groups. Data from ref. [68], reprinted with permission from ref. [69]

We have shown previously [68] that blockade of mitochondrial K_{ATP} channels with 5-hydroxyde-canoate completely abolished the cardioprotective effect of adaptation to chronic hypoxia also in neonatal rats; a similar effect was observed after the blockade of NO by L-NAME. It seems, therefore, that both mitochondrial K_{ATP} channels and NO may play an important role in the mechanisms of adaptation of the immature heart to chronic hypoxia. Furthermore, it has been shown that also angiotensin II is involved in the mechanisms of adaptation of the immature heart to chronic hypoxia. The chronic blockade of angiotensin II type 1 receptors (AT_1) by irbesartan completely abolished the cardioprotective effect of chronic hypoxia [70]. The involvement of AT_1 receptor pathway in the adaptive responses of the immature hearts to chronic hypoxia should be taken into consideration in the treatment of children suffering from cyanotic congenital heart disease.

Effect of Perinatal Chronic Hypoxia on Cardiac Tolerance to Ischemia/ Reperfusion Injury in Adult Males

Perinatal hypoxemia, although transient, may have serious late consequences on the adult cardiovascular system. This fact is in accordance with Barker's concept [71] of fetal and neonatal programming, which is based on epidemiological studies showing that perinatal pathogenetic factors may be linked with the development of adult cardiovascular diseases. In the recent years, the development of Barker's hypothesis opened the field for extensive research into the fetal origin of adult diseases. The association between low birth weight, which reflects intrauterine nutritional status and the development of adult diseases, has been confirmed in many studies for coronary heart disease [72]. One of the first was the Hertfordshire cohort study (15,756 men and women [73]), demonstrating that the death from coronary heart disease decreased twofold with higher birth weights. A longitudinal cohort study of 70,297 nurses in United States has provided strong evidence of association between low birth weight and increased risk of nonfatal cardiovascular disease [74]. Furthermore, Swedish study [75] performed on 14,611 babies delivered at the Uppsala Academic Hospital during 1915–1929 was followed up to the end of 1995. This study provides by far the most convincing evidence of a real association between body size at birth and mortality from ischemic heart disease in men, which cannot be methodological artifact or socio-economic confounding. Size at birth and birth weight are, however, not the only cardiovascular risk factors: catch-up growth during infancy and childhood has been associated also with increased risk of adult coronary heart disease [76].

Recent study by Crispi et al. [77] provides direct clinical evidence that children (age 5 years) with fetal growth restriction show changes in cardiac morphology, subclinical cardiac longitudinal dysfunction, and arterial remodeling, all of which increase linearly with the severity of growth restriction and are independent of gestational age at the delivery, lipid profile, or body mass index. These findings support the existence of direct cardiac programming in fetal growth restriction and suggest a new mechanistic pathway for the association between fetal growth and cardiovascular disease. Fetal growth restriction affects 5–10% of all newborns, and therefore the finding of the above study concerns thousands of children each year. The importance of early identification and intervention in pediatric risk factors for cardiovascular diseases is now well established [28].

Experimental studies on the late effects of chronic hypoxia on cardiac tolerance to hypoxia and ischemia are unfortunately not concise; moreover most of them have used exclusively males. Furthermore, they differ in the critical ontogenetic period studied (prenatal, perinatal, and early postnatal), intensity, and duration of hypoxia. Nevertheless, animal studies have repeatedly suggested a possible link between early hypoxia and increased risk of cardiovascular disease in offspring. Li et al. [78] have found that prenatal chronic hypoxia (10% O_2, from day 15 to 21 of gestation) significantly increases the sensitivity of the adult 6-month-old rat heart to ischemia/reperfusion injury, as indicated by increased myocardial infarct size and decreased postischemic recovery of left ventricular function. However, in their later study on 2-month-old animals [79], ischemia/reperfusion caused a comparable degree of infarction in prenatal hypoxic and control rats. These contradictory results suggest possible age-dependent changes in cardiac tolerance to oxygen deprivation induced by early exposure to chronic hypoxia. Another explanation may be the different duration of ischemia; prolongation may mask the potential differences in ischemic injury. We have observed that alternative end point – ischemic arrhythmias and LDH release – were able to differentiate the degree of ischemic insult already in 3-month-old rats [6]. Xu et al. [80] have demonstrated that prenatal hypoxia induced in 4-month-old rats left and right ventricular enlargement, increased the expression of collagen I and III, increased the ratio of beta and alpha myosin heavy chain protein, and decreased the matrix metalloproteinase activity. Cardiac remodeling was consistent with the diastolic dysfunction and increased sensitivity to I/R injury. According to Peyronnet et al. [81], perinatal exposure of rats to hypoxia exerts adverse effects on the development of the autonomic nervous system related to cardiovascular events and increased hemodynamic response under stress conditions in adults. Furthermore, Rohlicek et al. [4] observed that adult rats made hypoxemic neonatally showed a markedly greater cardiac output response to acute hypoxia than controls. This may be due to altered myocardial function and/or changes in the autonomic nervous system response to acute hypoxemia. Similarly, Hampl and Herget [82] and Hampl et al. [83] have shown that perinatal hypoxia increases the susceptibility to hypoxic pulmonary hypertension later in life.

The developmental mechanisms of the increased susceptibility of the adult hearts to I/R injury are not known at present. Li et al. [78] have observed that I/R-induced apoptosis was 44% higher in the hearts of rats that had experienced prenatal chronic hypoxia compared with control animals. This finding was in agreement with the results of myocardial infarction, which showed a 56% increase in prenatal hypoxic hearts. Consistent with the increased apoptosis, the ratio of cleaved form to pro-form of caspase-3 was significantly higher in hypoxic hearts after I/R, indicating increased caspase-3 activity. Taken together, these results suggest that prenatal chronic hypoxia sensitizes the apoptosis pathway in the adult heart in response to I/R stimulation. In addition, they have found [79] that cardiac Hsp70 expression was significantly lower in hypoxic hearts than in the controls. It has been well documented that Hsp70 plays an important role in protection against I/R injury and that the degree of postischemic functional recovery correlates with the absolute Hsp70 tissue contents [84]. It can be, therefore, assumed that decreased Hsp70 levels play a key role in the increased susceptibility of the adult heart to I/R injury in prenatal hypoxic animals. These results suggest that down-regulation of the Hsp70 gene in the fetal heart by chronic hypoxia (see above) has lasting and life-long importance. The finding of decreased eNOS levels in adult prenatal hypoxic hearts suggests their contribution to the increased susceptibility to I/R injury. One of the potential mechanisms for NO's cardioprotective effect is likely to be its beneficial effect on postischemic coronary flow. Moreover, they have found that prenatal hypoxia did not change β_1-AR levels but significantly increased β_2-AR in the adult left ventricle. In addition, it increased $G_s\alpha$ but decreased $G_i\alpha$ protein. These studies suggest that chronic hypoxic exposure during early development may cause in utero or neonatal programming of several genes which may play important roles in the increased susceptibility of the adult male heart to I/R injury.

Perinatal Hypoxia-Induced Sex-Dependent Changes in Heart Susceptibility to Ischemia/ Reperfusion Injury in Adults

Clinical and experimental studies suggest that there may be sex differences in the cardiac tolerance to ischemia. Hearts of adult males usually have a higher susceptibility to myocardial injury than hearts of females (for review, see ref. [69]). In this connection the question arises whether the effects of perinatal hypoxia on cardiac tolerance to ischemia differ in adult males and females. We have observed in the rat model that late myocardial effects of hypoxemia, experienced in early life, may be sex-dependent (see Fig. 3). Perinatal exposure to chronic hypoxia significantly increased cardiac tolerance to acute I/R injury in adult female rats, expressed as the lower incidence of ischemic arrhythmias; the effect on arrhythmias in males was the opposite [6]. Similar sex-dependent effect of early hypoxia was later confirmed by Xue and Zhang [2]. They have observed that prenatal hypoxia significantly decreased postischemic recovery of left ventricular function, increased cardiac enzyme release, and infarct size in adult male but not in female rats.

Gender differences in the long-term effects of perinatal hypoxia on the response of the pulmonary circulation were studied by Hampl and Herget [82] and Hampl et al. [83]. They found that perinatal hypoxia had a permanent consequence of elevated right to left ventricular weight ratio in females only; this result is consistent with our finding of a persistent right ventricular hypertrophy in females exposed to chronic hypoxia. Moreover, ovariectomy at a very young age greatly augmented the effects of perinatal hypoxia in females, so that pulmonary arterial pressure in adulthood was significantly increased. They have concluded that, during maturation, ovaries exert a

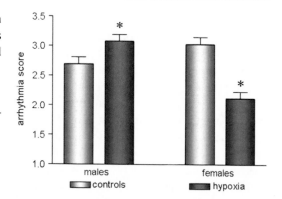

Fig. 3 Arrhythmia score over 30-min coronary artery occlusion in control and perinatal hypoxic group. *Statistically significant difference ($p < 0.01$) between control and perinatal hypoxic group. Data from ref. [6], reprinted with permission from ref. [69]

protective influence against permanent consequences of perinatal hypoxia in lung vessels.

The question remains of the cause of the sex difference in cardiac sensitivity to ischemia (for review, see ref. [69]). A large body of evidence indicates that estrogen is involved in sex-related mechanisms of cardiac tolerance to ischemia. Along with their well-known "genomic" effects, additional processes termed "nongenomic" occur rapidly and independently of protein synthesis [85]. Among the many pathways that can modify the sex-dependent susceptibility to ischemic injury is NO [86], sarcolemmal [87], and mitochondrial K_{ATP} channels [88], protein kinase B (Akt) and protein kinase Cε levels [89], tumor necrosis factor α [80], Ca^{2+} loading [90], or mitochondrial production of H_2O_2 [91]. Nevertheless, the cardiovascular system is influenced not only by estrogens, but at least by one additional player – androgens. Similarly to estrogens, androgens are present in both sexes, albeit at different concentrations and ratios. However, the influence of testosterone on cardiovascular system is still controversial; experimental studies have shown its positive as well as negative effect on cardiac sensitivity to oxygen deprivation.

Recently, two studies have analyzed the possible mechanisms involved in prenatal hypoxia-induced sex-dependent changes in cardiac tolerance to ischemia in adults. According to Xue and Zhang [2], these changes are due to differences in fetal programming of PKCε gene expression which plays a pivotal role in cardioprotection against I/R injury [92, 93]; down-regulation of PKCε function was observed in the hearts of adult male offspring only. Patterson et al. [27] have found that chronic hypoxia during gestation downregulated PKCε expression in the developing heart through an epigenetic modification. They found sex differences in methylation of specificity protein (SP) 1 binding sites and PKCε transcription. Hypoxia-induced methylation was significantly greater in the heart of male fetuses. This sex difference may be according to Patterson et al. [27] caused in part by the greater expression of estrogen receptors α and β in the heart of female fetuses. The finding that both estrogen receptors α and β interacted with the SP1 binding sites at the PKCε promoter in the fetal heart suggests a possible mechanism for the increased protection of SP1 binding sites and PKCε transcription in the female hearts in response to hypoxic stress. Although it may be difficult to translate the present findings directly into the humans, the possibility that fetal hypoxia may result in sex-dependent programming of specific genes in the offspring with the consequence of increased cardiac susceptibility to I/R provides an experimental finding worthy of investigation in human.

Conclusions

Our present focus on the immature heart is driven by clinical urgency: ischemic heart disease is no more the disease of the fifth and older decades but its origin as well as risk factors is present already during early phases of ontogenetic development. Among them perinatal hypoxemia, although transient, may have serious late consequences on the adult cardiovascular system. Experimental and clinical studies have shown an association between perinatal hypoxia and increased risk of ischemic disease in later adult life; moreover, this late effect of perinatal hypoxia may be sex-dependent. The results support the hypothesis that perinatal hypoxia is a primary programming stimulus in the heart, leading to changes in cardiac tolerance to acute oxygen deprivation in later adult life. This fact would have important clinical implications: (1) cardiac sensitivity to oxygen deprivation in adult patients may be significantly influenced by perinatal hypoxia and (2) the observed sex differences suggest that the management of the diseased human male and female heart should be different.

Acknowledgments This study was supported by grants MSMT 1 M0510 and AVOZ 50110509.

References

1. Barker DJ, Osmond C, Golding J, et al. Growth in utero, blood pressure in childhood and adult life, and mortality from cardiovascular disease. BMJ. 1989; 298:564–7.
2. Xue Q, Zhang L. Prenatal hypoxia causes a sex-dependent increase in heart susceptibility to ischaemia and reperfusion injury in adult male offspring: role of protein kinase Cε. J Pharmacol Exp Therap. 2009;330:624–32.
3. Giussani DA, Phillips PS, Anstee S, et al. Effects of altitude versus economic status on birth weight and body shape at birth. Pediatr Res. 2001;49:490–4.
4. Rohlicek CV, Matsuoka T, Saiki C. Cardiovascular response to acute hypoxemia in adult rats hypoxemic neonatally. Cardiovasc Res. 2002;53:263–70.
5. Nollert G, Fischlein T, Bouterwek S, et al. Long-term survival in patients with repair of tetralogy of Fallot: 36-year follow-up of 490 survivors of the first year after surgical repair. J Am Coll Cardiol. 1997;30: 1374–83.
6. Netuka I, Szarszoi O, Maly J, et al. Effect of perinatal hypoxia on cardiac tolerance to acute ischaemia in adult male and female rats. Clin Exp Pharmacol Physiol. 2006;33:714–9.
7. Krecek J. The weanling period as a critical period of development. In: Krecek J, editor. The post-natal development of phenotype. Prague: Academia; 1970. p. 33–44.
8. Eastman NJ. Mount Everest in utero. President's address. Am J Obstet Gynecol. 1954;67:701–11.
9. Kuma A, Hatano M, Matsui M, et al. The role of autophagy during the early neonatal starvation period. Nature. 2004;432:1032–6.
10. Mühlfeld C, Singer D, Engelhardt N, et al. Electron microscopy and microcalorimetry of the postnatal rat heart (*Rattus norvegicus*). Comp Biochem Physiol A Mol Integr Physiol. 2005;141:310–8.
11. Ostadalova I, Charvatova Z, Wilhelm J. Lipofuscin-like pigments in the rat heart during early postnatal development: effect of selenium supplementation. Physiol Res. 2010;59:881–6.
12. Ostadal B, Wachtlova M, Bily J, et al. Weight of the heart in the rats before and after birth. Physiol bohemoslov. 1967;16:111–9.

13. Ostadalova I, Kolar F, Ostadal B, et al. Early postnatal development of contractile performance and responsiveness to Ca^{2+}, verapamil and ryanodine in the isolated rat heart. J Mol Cell Cardiol. 1993;25:733–40.

14. Li F, Wang X, Capasso JM, et al. Rapid transition of cardiac myocytes from hyperplasia to hypertrophy during postnatal development. J Mol Cell Cardiol. 1996;28:1737–46.

15. Rakusan K. Vascularization of the heart during normal and pathological growth. Adv Org Biol. 1999;7: 130–53.

16. Skarka L, Bardova K, Brauner P, et al. Expression of mitochondrial uncoupling protein 3 and adenine nucleotide translocase 1 genes in developing rat heart: putative involvement in control of mitochondrial membrane potential. J Mol Cell Cardiol. 2003;35:321–30.

17. Nijjar MS, Dhalla NS. Biochemical basis of calcium handling in developing myocardium. In: Ostadal B, Nagano M, Takeda N, Dhalla NS, editors. The developing heart. Philadelphia, P.A.: Lippincott; 1997. p. 189–217.

18. Ostadal B, Ostadalova I, Dhalla NS. Development of cardiac sensitivity to oxygen deficiency: comparative and ontogenetic aspects. Physiol Rev. 1999;79: 635–59.

19. Ostadalova I, Ostadal B, Kolar F. Effect of prenatal hypoxia on contractile performance and responsiveness to Ca^{2+} in the isolated perinatal rat heart. Physiol Res. 1995;44:135–7.

20. Babicky A, Ostadalova I, Parizek J, et al. Initial solid food intake and growth of young rats in nests of different sizes. Physiol Bohemoslov. 1973;22:557–66.

21. Gilbert RD. Fetal myocardial responses to long-term hypoxemia. Comp Biochem Physiol. 1998;3:669–74.

22. Ohtsuka T, Gilbert RD. Cardiac enzyme activities in fetal and adult pregnant and non pregnant sheep exposed to high altitude hypoxemia. J Appl Physiol. 1995;79:1286–9.

23. Murotsuki J, Challis JR, Han VK, et al. Chronic fetal placental embolization and hypoxaemia cause hypertension and myocardial hypertrophy in fetal sheep. Am J Physiol Regul Integr Comp Physiol. 1997;272: R201–7.

24. Martin C, Yu AY, Jiang BH, et al. Cardiac hypertrophy in chronically anemic fetal sheep: increased vascularization is associated with increased myocardial expression of vascular endothelial growth factor and hypoxia-inducible factor 1. Am J Obstet Gynecol. 1998;178:527–34.

25. Han HC, Austin KJ, Nathanielsz PVV, et al. Maternal nutrient restriction alters gene expression in the ovine fetal heart. J Physiol. 2004;555:111–21.

26. Bae S, Xiao Y, Li G, et al. Effect of maternal chronic hypoxic exposure during gestation on apoptosis in fetal rat heart. Am J Physiol Heart Circ Physiol. 2003; 285:H983–90.

27. Patterson AJ, Chen M, Xue Q, et al. Chronic prenatal hypoxia induces epigenetic programming of PKCε gene expression in rat hearts. Circulation Res. 2010; 107:365–73.

28. Verburg BO, Jaddoe VW, Wladimiroff JW, et al. Fetal hemodynamic adaptive changes related to intrauterine growth: the generation R study. Circulation. 2008;117: 649–59.

29. Chvojkova Z, Ostadalova I, Ostadal B. Low body weight and cardiac tolerance to ischemia in neonatal rats. Physiol Res. 2005;54:357–62.

30. Mortola JP, Xu L, Lauzon A-M. Body growth, lung and heart weight, and DNA content in newborn rats exposed to different levels of chronic hypoxia. Can J Physiol Pharmacol. 1990;68:1590–4.

31. Naye RL. Organ and cellular development in mice growing at simulated high altitude. Lab Invest. 1966;15:700–6.

32. Bai SL, Campbell SE, Moore JA, et al. Influence of age, growth, and sex on cardiac myocyte size and number in rats. Anat Rec. 1990;226:207–12.

33. Bell JM, Slotkin TA. Postnatal nutritional status influences development of cardiac adrenergic receptor binding sites. Brain Res Bull. 1988;21:893–6.

34. Ostadalova I, Ostadal B. Ontogenetic differences in isoproterenol induced [85] Sr uptake in the myocardium. In: Nagano M, Takeda N, Dhalla NS, editors. The cardiomyopathic heart. New York: Raven; 1994. p. 395–400.

35. Bell JM, Whitmore WL, Queen KL, et al. Biochemical determinants of growth sparing during neonatal deprivation or enhancement: ornithine decarboxylase, polyamines, and macromolecules in brain regions and heart. Pediatr Res. 1987;22:599–604.

36. Brodsky VY, Pelouch V, Arefyeva AM, et al. Lack of proportionality between gene dosage and total muscle protein content in the rat heart. Int J Dev Biol. 1992; 36:339–42.

37. Pelouch V, Kolar F, Milerova M, et al. Effect of preweaning nutritional state on the cardiac protein profile and functional performance of the rat heart. Mol Cell Biochem. 1997;177:221–8.

38. Dowell RT, Martin AF. Perinatal nutritional modification of weanling rat heart contractile protein. Am J Physiol Heart Circ Physiol. 1984;247:H967–72.

39. Rakusan K, Poupa O. Differences in capillary supply of hypertrophied and hyperplastic hearts. Cardiologia. 1966;49:293–8.

40. Neffgen F, Korecky B. Cellular hyperplasia and hypertrophy in cardiomegalies induced by anaemia in young and adult rats. Circulation Res. 1972;30: 104–13.

41. Hollenberg M, Honbo N, Samorodin AJ. Effects of hypoxia on cardiac growth in neonatal rats. Am J Physiol. 1976;231:1445–50.

42. Wachtlova M, Mares V, Ostadal B. DNA synthesis in the ventricular myocardium of young rats exposed to intermittent high altitude (IHA) hypoxia. Virchows Arch B Cell Path. 1977;24:335–42.

43. Samanek M, Bass A, Ostadal B, et al. Effect of hypoxaemia on enzymes supplying myocardial energy in children with congenital heart disease. Int J Cardiol. 1989;25:265–70.

44. Fitzpatrick CM, Shi Y, Hutchins WC, et al. Cardioprotection in chronically hypoxic rabbits on

exposure to normoxia: role of NOS and K_{ATP} channels. Am J Physiol Heart Circ Physiol. 2005;288:H62–8.

45. Ostadal B, Kolar F. Cardiac ischemia: from injury to protection. Boston: Kluwer Academic; 1999.

46. Ostadal B, Netuka I, Maly J, et al. Gender differences in cardiac ischemic injury and protection-experimental aspects. Exp Biol Med. 2009;234:1011–9.

47. Riva A, Hearse DJ. Age-dependent changes in myocardial succeptibility to ischemic injury. Cardioscience. 2009;4:85–92.

48. Ostadalova I, Ostadal B, Kolar F, et al. Tolerance to ischemia and ischaemic preconditioning in neonatal rat heart. J Mol Cell Cardiol. 1998;30:857–65.

49. Baker EJ, Boerboom LE, Olinger GN, et al. Tolerance of the developing heart to ischemia: impact of hypoxemia from birth. Am J Physiol. 1998;268:H1165–73.

50. Hoerter J. Changes in the sensitivity to hypoxia and glucose deprivation in the isolated perfused rabbit heart during perinatal development. Pflugers Arch. 1976;363:1–6.

51. Julia P, Young PP, Buckberg GD, et al. Studies of myocardial protection in the immature heart. II. Evidence for importance of amino acid metabolism in tolerance to ischemia. J Thorac Cardiovasc Res. 1990;100:888–95.

52. Hohl CM. Effect of respiratory inhibition and ischemia on nucleotide metabolism in newborn swine cardiac myocytes. In: Ostadal B, Nagano M, Takeda N, Dhalla NS, editors. The developing heart. Philadelphia, PA: Lippincott; 1997. p. 393–406.

53. Vetter R, Studer R, Reinecke H, et al. Reciprocal changes in the postnatal expression of the sarcolemmal Na^+-Ca^{2+}-exchanger and SERCA2 in rat heart. J Mol Cell Cardiol. 1995;27:1689–701.

54. Schagger H, Noack H, Halangk W, et al. Cytochrome c oxidase in developing rat heart. Enzymic properties and amino-terminal sequences suggest identity of the fetal heart and the adult liver isoform. Eur J Biochem. 1995;230:235–41.

55. Drahota Z, Milerova M, Stieglerova A, et al. Developmental changes of cytochrome c oxidase and citrate synthase in rat heart homogenate. Physiol Res. 2004;53:119–22.

56. Di Lisa F, Bernardi P. Mitochondrial function as a determinant of recovery or death in cell response to injury. Mol Cell Biochem. 1998;184:379–91.

57. Di Lisa F, Bernardi P. Mitochondrial function and myocardial aging. A critical analysis of the role of permeability transition. Cardiovasc Res. 2006;66: 222–32.

58. Di Lisa F, Menabo R, Canton M, et al. Opening of the mitochondrial permeability transition pore causes depletion of mitochondrial and cytosolic NAD^+ and is a causative event in the death of myocytes in postischemic reperfusion of the heart. J Biol Chem. 2001;276: 2571–5.

59. Milerova M, Charvatova Z, Skarka L, et al. Neonatal cardiac mitochondria and ischemia/reperfusion injury. Mol Cell Biochem. 2010;335:147–53.

60. Heath D, Williams DR. High altitude medicine and pathology. Oxford: Oxford University Press; 1995.

61. Ostadal B, Kolar F. Cardiac adaptation to chronic high altitude hypoxia. Respir Physiol Neurobiol. 2007; 158:224–36.

62. Neckar J, Papousek F, Novakova O, et al. Cardioprotective effects of chronic hypoxia and ischaemic preconditioning are not additive. Basic Res Cardiol. 2002;97:161–7.

63. Neckar J, Szarszoi O, Koten L, et al. Effects of mitochondrial K_{ATP} modulators on cardioprotection induced by chronic high altitude hypoxia in rats. Cardiovasc Res. 2002;55:567–75.

64. Asemu G, Papousek F, Ostadal B, et al. Adaptation to high altitude hypoxia protects the rat heart against ischemia-induced arrhythmias. Involvement of mitochondrial KATP channel. J Mol Cell Cardiol. 1999;31:821–31.

65. Szarszoi O, Asemu G, Ostadal B, et al. Effects of melatonin on ischemia and reperfusion injury of the rat heart. Cardiovasc Drugs Ther. 2001;15:251–7.

66. Kolar F, Ostadal B. Molecular mechanisms of cardiac protection by adaptation to chronic hypoxia. Physiol Res. 2004;53 Suppl 1:S3–13.

67. Ostadal B, Kolar F, Pelouch V, et al. Ontogenetic differences in cardiopulmonary adaptation to chronic hypoxia. Physiol Res. 1995;44:45–51.

68. Ostadalova I, Ostadal B, Jarkovska D, et al. Ischemic preconditioning in chronically hypoxic neonatal rat heart. Pediatr Res. 2002;52:561–7.

69. Ostadal B, Ostadalova I, Kolar F, et al. Ontogenetic development of cardiac tolerance to oxygen deprivation – possible mechanisms. Physiol Res. 2009;58 Suppl 2:S1–12.

70. Rakusan K, Chvojkova Z, Oliviero P, et al. ANG II type 1 receptor antagonist irbesartan inhibits coronary angiogenesis stimulated by chronic intermittent hypoxia in neonatal rats. Am J Physiol Heart Circ Physiol. 2007;292:H1–8.

71. Barker DJ. In utero programming of cardiovascular disease. Theriogenology. 2000;53:555–74.

72. Sallout B, Walker M. The fetal origin of adult disease. J Obstet Gynaecol. 2003;23:555–60.

73. Osmond C, Barker DJP, Winter PD, et al. Early growth and death from cardiovascular disease in women. BMJ. 1993;307:1519–24.

74. Rich-Edwards JW, Stampfer MJ, Manson JE, et al. Birth weight and risk of cardiovascular disease in a cohort of women followed up since 1976. BMJ. 1997;315:396–400.

75. Leon DA, Lithell HO, Vagero D, et al. Reduced fetal growth rate and increased risk of death from ischaemic heart disease: cohort study of 15 000 Swedish men and women born 1915–1929. BMJ. 1998;317: 241–5.

76. Eriksson JG, Forsen T, Toumilehto J, et al. Catch-up growth in childhood and death from coronary heart disease: longitudinal study. BMJ. 1999;318: 427–31.

77. Crispi F, Bijnens B, Figueras F, et al. Fetal growth restriction results in remodeled and less efficient hearts in children. Circulation. 2010;121:2427–36.

78. Li G, Xiao Y, Estrella JL, et al. Effect of fetal hypoxia on heart susceptibility to ischemia and reperfusion injury in the adult heart. J Soc Gynecol Investig. 2003;10:265–74.

79. Li G, Bae S, Zhang L. Effect of prenatal hypoxia on heat stress-mediated cardioprotection in adult rat heart. Am J Physiol Heart Circ Physiol. 2004;286:1712–9.

80. Xu Y, Williams SJ, O'Brien D, et al. Hypoxia or nutrient restriction during pregnancy in rats leads to progressive cardiac remodeling and impairs postischemic recovery in adult male offspring. FASEB J. 2006;20: 1251–3.

81. Peyronnet J, Dalmaz Y, Ehrstrom M. Long-lasting adverse effects of prenatal hypoxia on developing autonomic nervous system and cardiovascular parameters in rats. Pflugers Arch. 2002;443:858–65.

82. Hampl V, Herget J. Perinatal hypoxia increases hypoxic pulmonary vasoconstriction in adult rats recovering from chronic exposure to hypoxia. Am Rev Respir Dis. 1990;142:619–24.

83. Hampl V, Bibova J, Ostadalova I, et al. Gender differences in the long-term effects of perinatal hypoxia on pulmonary circulation in rats. Am J Physiol Lung Cell Mol Physiol. 2003;285:L386–92.

84. Snoeckx LH, Cornelussen RN, Van Nieuwenhoven FA, et al. Heat shock proteins and cardiovascular pathophysiology. Physiol Rev. 2001;81:1461–97.

85. Di Lisa F. A female way to protect the heart. Say NO to calcium. Circ Res. 2006;98:298–300.

86. Sun J, Picht E, Ginsburg KS, et al. Hypercontractile female hearts exhibit increased S-nitrosylation of the L-type Ca^{2+} channel alpha 1 subunit and reduced ischemia-reperfusion injury. Circ Res. 2006;98: 403–11.

87. Johnson MS, Moore RL, Brown DA. Sex differences in myocardial infarct size are abolished by sarcolemmal K_{ATP} channel blocade in rat. Am J Physiol Heart Circ Physiol. 2006;290:H2644–7.

88. Lee TM, Su SF, Tsai CC, et al. Cardioprotective effects of 17 beta-estradiol produced by activation of mitochondrial ATP-sensitive K^+ channels in canine hearts. J Mol Cell Cardiol. 2000;32:1147–58.

89. Bae S, Zhang L. Gender differences in cardioprotection against ischemia/reperfusion injury in adult rat hearts: focus on Akt and protein kinase C signaling. J Pharmacol Exp Therap. 2005;315:1125–35.

90. Cross HR, Murphy E, Steenbergen C. Ca^{2+} loading and adrenergic stimulation reveal male/female differences in susceptibility to ischemia-reperfusion injury. Am J Physiol Heart Circ Physiol. 2002;283: H481–9.

91. Lagranha CJ, Deschamps A, Aponte A, et al. Sex differences in the phosphorylation of mitochondrial proteins result in reduced production of reactive oxygen species and cardioprotection in females. Circ Res. 2010;106:1681–91.

92. Murriel CL, Mochly-Rosen D. Opposing roles of delta and epsilon PKC in cardiac ischemia and reperfusion: targeting the apoptotic machinery. Arch Biochem Biophys. 2003;420:246–54.

93. Kolar F, Novak F, Neckar J, et al. Role of protein kinases in chronic intermittent hypoxia-induced cardioprotection. In: Xi L, Serebrovskaya TV, editors. Intermittent hypoxia. New York: Nova Science; 2009. p. 213–30.

Stem Cell, MicroRNA and Redox Cycling

Partha Mukhopadhyay, Narasimman Gurusamy, and Dipak K. Das

Abstract

Mobilization and homing of the hematopoietic stem cells appear to be regulated by mechanism involving redox cycling. Stem cells are localized inside bone marrow in a strictly hypoxic environment and must move to the injury site that is subjected to oxidative environment. Cytokines and adhesion molecules control stem cell mobilization through a redox-regulated process. The major hitch in stem cell therapy includes the life of the stem cells after the stem cell therapy; most cells do not survive beyond 24–72 h. Sudden exposure of the stem cells from the hypoxic melieu into the oxidative environment likely causes severe injury to the cells. FoxO-SirT network appears to be intimately involved in redox-regulated stem cell homeostasis, while their differentiation process is regulated by redox factor protein-1, Ref-1. Lack of oxygen [hypoxia], specifically controlled hypoxia can stimulate the growth of the stem cells in their niche, and HIF-1α plays a significant role in their maintenance and homing mechanism. Recently, resveratrol, a polyphenolic phytoalexin, prolonged the survival of the stem cells as evidenced by active proliferation and differentiation of the cells even after 4 months of cell therapy. The enhancement of stem cell survival was shown to be due to the ability of resveratrol to maintain a reduced tissue environment by over-expressing Nrf2 and Ref-1 in rat heart up to 6 months resulting in an enhancement of the regeneration of the adult cardiac stem cells as evidenced by increased cell survival and differentiation leading to improved cardiac function. Expression of stromal cell-derived factor (SDF) and myosin conclusively demonstrated homing of stem cells in the infracted myocardium, its regeneration leading to improvement of cardiac function.

D.K. Das (✉)
Cardiovascular Research Center,
University of Connecticut School of Medicine,
Farmington, CT, USA
e-mail: ddas@neuron.uchc.edu

N.S. Dhalla, M. Nagano, B. Ostadal (eds.), *Molecular Defects in Cardiovascular Disease*,
DOI 10.1007/978-1-4419-7130-2_6, © Springer Science+Business Media, LLC 2011

Keywords

Cardiac stem cells • Resveratrol • Redox • Nrf2 • Ref-1 • NFkB • Heart • Ischemia

Introduction

The rapidly expanding fields of stem cell biology and its potential role in cardiac repair process have stimulated the investigators to explore the molecular mechanisms of stem cell mobilization and homing. Existing reports indicate cardiac chimerism resulting from the migration of primitive cells from the recipients to the grafted heart [1]. In this study, the authors showed that as compared with the ventricles of the control hearts, the ventricles of the transplanted hearts had higher number of cells, which were positive for C-kit and Sca-1. More recent studies suggest that cytokines and adhesion molecules might be involved in the stem cell homing process. The continuous presence of CD34+ cells in the peripheral blood during the steady-state hematopoiesis support the role of adhesion molecules in the homing process [2]. Most of the adhesion molecules are believed to be members of β_1 and β_2 integrin, selectin and super immunoglobulin [3, 4]. l-Selectin that is responsible for the contact of leukocytes with endothelium is highly expressed on CD34+ progenitor cells, suggesting its role for homing [5]. Very late antigen-4 (VLA-4) is expressed on circulating CD34+ cells residing in the bone marrow, suggesting a role of VLA-4 on the release and circulating the CD34+ cells [6, 7]. Leukocyte function-associated molecule-1 (LFA-1) and CD18/CD11a also play a role in the interaction between CD34+ hematopoietic progenitor cells and bone marrow cells [5].

Similar to the adhesive molecules many cytokines are likely to be involved in stem cell mobilization. For example, a number of cytokines including IL-3, IL-8, IL-11, Flt-3 and stem cell factor (SCF) have been implicated for the mobilization of CD34+ cells [8, 9]. However, G-CSF and GM-CSF are best known for the mobilization of peripheral blood stem cell [10, 11].

These factors are involved in the differentiation of progenitor cells into granulocytes and monocytes, respectively.

There is no doubt that the success of stem cell therapy depends largely on the efficiency of the hematopoietic stem cells to home to bone marrow. Despite the role of cytokines and adhesive molecules in stem cell mobilization, exact mechanisms remain unclear. Interestingly, signal transduction pathways leading to cytokine expression and inflammatory response are redox-regulated. For example, downregulation of intracellular glutathione level is associated with the enhancement of oxidative stress-mediated inflammation and is differentially involved in controlling redox-dependent cytokine regulation [12]. In another study, thioredoxin reduced cysteine residues of transcription factors in the nucleus to regulate their DNA binding and transactivation activities. Upon TNFα stimulation and subsequent generation of ROS, thioredoxin becomes oxidized and releases ASK-1 [13]. In another related study, an alteration of cytokine response was found to be related with activation of redox-dependent transcription factors [14].

From the above discussion, it should be clear that the principle factors of stem cell mobilization, cytokines and adhesion molecules are redox-regulated. Thus, it may be speculated that homing mechanisms of stem cell are also redox-regulated. In fact, a handful number of papers recently appeared that could substantiate this hypothesis. For example, a recent study showed impaired endothelial progenitor cell function in response to the oxidative stress [15]. Another study demonstrated a positive role of ROS in the regulation of normal and neoplastic hematopoiesis [16]. Another related study revealed that thioredoxin mediates redox regulation of the embryonic stem cell transcription factor Oct-4 [17]. More recently, it is found that the production of ROS is greatly stimulated by the inhibition of Ref-1, which ultimately results in induced differentiation of adult cardiac stem cells [18].

The purpose of this review is to discuss the potential redox regulation of stem cell biology and how the redox signaling can potentiate a homing mechanism leading to the repair of the injured cells.

Redox Regulation of Stem Cells in Regeneration of Infarcted Myocardium

ROS in Stem Cell Biology

A growing body of evidence supports the notion that stem cells possess the ability to cope with oxygen overload through an unique adaptive mechanism by which they can upregulate their own antioxidant defense system [19]. Hematopoietic stem cells are located in a hypoxic environment inside the bone marrow where they remain quiescent. Upon mobilization, they are exposed to oxygenic environment, which potentiates proliferation and differentiation [20, 21]. Most cells and tissues exhibit alterations in their antioxidant reserve and capacity to undergo redox cycling during different stages of differentiation. Antioxidant protection abilities of the progenitor cells are highly amplified under stress enhancing their ability to exert resistance against oxidative stress [22]. ROS has been utilized by the embryonic stem cells as transducers of mechanical strain-induced cardiovascular differentiation [23]. A recent study showed that shear stress increased lysine acetylation of histone H3 at position 14, serine phosphorylation at position 10 and lysine methylation at position 79 [24]. Shear stress-induced phosphorylation of Flk-1 is shown in Flk-positive embryonic stem cells in a recent study [25]. Interestingly enough, shear stress-mediated angiogenic response is redox-regulated. Indeed, a recent study demonstrated redox regulation of the members of MAP kinase pathway including ERK1,2, JNK and p38MAPK, which potentiate a signaling cascade for the initiation of cardiovascular differentiation of embryonic stem cells [23]. In another

study, ROS was found to exert deleterious effects of oxidative stress on hematopoietic stem cells self-renewal and identifies p38MAPK as a key mediator of ROS-induced stem cell lifespan shortening [26].

A continuous increase in ROS activity was demonstrated during the time course of differentiation of embryonic stem cells [27]. A NADPH oxidase like enzyme was identified as a source of ROS in embryonic stem cell-derived embryoid bodies, which appeared to interfere with diverse signaling cascades, thereby affecting stem cell differentiation. A subsequent study showed that upregulation of HIF-1α at the gene and protein levels led to an increase in VEGF activity, which is critical for vasculogenesis in embryonic stem cells [23, 28].

Manipulation of subcellular p53 localization in response to endogenous ROS is efficiently done by Sirt1 for the regulation of apoptosis and Nanog expression in mouse embryonic stem cells [29]. The authors showed that SirT1 blocks nuclear translocation of cytoplasmic p53 in response to endogenous ROS and triggers mitochondrial-dependent apoptosis in mouse embryonic stem cells. Nanog expression of SirT1$^{-/-}$ embryonic stem cells clearly revealed an accelerated sensitivity to ROS and a simultaneous p53-mediated repression of Nanog expression, suggesting that ROS is important for stem cell maintenance in culture. Interestingly, it is FoxO-deficient hematopoietic stem cells that have a significant increase in ROS, suggesting that there might be a link between ROS and cell cycle activities [30]. In this study, FoxO-deficient mice exhibited marked reduction in the lineage-negative Sca1$^+$ and c-Kit$^+$ compartment that contains hematopoietic stem cells. In concert, there was a significant increase in ROS in FoxO-deficient stem cells compared to wild-type cells correlating with changes in gene expression that regulate ROS. N-Acetyl cysteine, a cell-permeable antioxidant, reduced FoxO-deficient stem cell phenotype and corrected the deficiencies in cell cycle regulation.

Several recent studies have indicated that oxidative stress can regulate FoxOs through a Ral/Jnk-dependent mechanism [31]. Conditional deletion of some members of FoxO reduced hematopoietic stem cell lineages simultaneously reducing resistance to oxidative stress [30]. Another recent study showed that FoxO3 is specifically required for induction of proteins, which regulate redox signaling in murine erythrocytes [32]. Accordingly, the animals lacking FoxO3 in hematopoietic cells undergo sudden death when exposed to ROS, which also reduces the amount of ROS scavenging enzymes [32]. FoxO-deficient hematopoietic stem cells are subjected to increased amount of oxidative stress and undergo apoptosis. Several studies suggest crucial roles of FoxOs and ROS as signaling network partners in hematopoietic stem cell homoeostasis [33].

Redox Regulation of Stem Cell Proliferation and Differentiation

Stem cells are usually sheltered in a stable microenvironment called niches, which preserve the survival and replication potential of stem cells in an organ [34, 35]. ROS are known to play a major role in induction of the exit of hematopoietic stem cells from the niche in bone marrow. Redox effector protein-1 (Ref-1) plays an essential role in DNA repair and redox regulation of several transcription factors. In a recent study, we examined the role of Ref-1 in maintaining the redox status and survivability of adult cardiac stem cells challenged with subtoxic level of H_2O_2 under inhibition of Ref-1 by RNA interference. Treatment with low concentration of H_2O_2 in mouse embryonic stem cells is shown to induce the components of NADPH oxidase and vital cardiac transcriptional regulators such as Nkx2.5, MEF2C and GATA4 [18, 36]. When adult cardiac stem cells are treated with low concentration of H_2O_2 (10 µM) under the inhibition of Ref-1, the amount of ROS production was tremendously increased via activation of components of NAPDH oxidase such as p22 phox, p47 phox and Nox4, leading to the differentiation (increased expression of Nkx2.5, MEF2C, GATA4 and α-sarcomeric actinin) and cell death by apoptosis. In this study, the involvement of ROS in the induction of cardiac differentiation was confirmed

by pretreating cardiac stem cells with N-acetyl-l-cysteine, a scavenger of ROS, which abolished the Ref-1 inhibition-mediated induction of NADPH oxidase components, and cardiac differentiation transcription factors. Moreover, a role for phosphatidylinositol-3-kinase has been identified in ROS-mediated cardiac differentiation of embryonic stem cells [37]. These results indicate that Ref-1 plays an important role in maintaining the redox status of cardiac stem cells and protects from oxidative injury-mediated cell death and differentiation [18].

Simultaneous occurrence of apoptosis and differentiation has been observed during embryonic stem cell differentiation [38, 39]. Tumor suppressor protein p53 regulates cell cycle checkpoint, differentiation and induces cell apoptosis. p53 was shown to be involved in the simultaneous induction of apoptosis and differentiation [40, 41]. Induction of endogenous p53 is found to be associated with differentiation in mouse-cultured keratinocytes, mouse embryonic stem cells, hematopoietic and muscle cells [42]. High level of p53 was found in undifferentiated embryonic stem cells, and it was decreased as differentiation proceeds [43, 44]. The addition of retinoic acid, a physiological regulator of embryonic development, onto murine embryonic stem cells caused an increase in the level of p53 followed by accelerated neural differentiation and apoptosis [45]. Redox-dependent and redox-independent mechanisms have been shown to regulate p53 [46]. Ref-1 is a potent activator of p53 [47]. The activation of survival signaling kinase Akt inhibits p53, whereas pro-apoptotic stimuli-induced p53 inhibits Akt [48]. When the cardiac stem cells are treated with low concentration of H_2O_2, the level of p53 is decreased than normal cellular levels. H_2O_2 treatment under Ref-1 inhibition almost completely abolished the activation of survival signaling molecule Akt; at the same time the level of p53 was significantly higher than normal levels leading to an enhanced level of ROS production and ROS-mediated cell death and differentiation. The above findings thus indicate that p53 plays an important role in determining the fine balance between growth, differentiation and cell death (Fig. 1) [18].

Fig. 1 Ref-1-mediated redox signaling protects stem cells. (**a**) Addition of pro-oxidants like hydrogen peroxide at low concentration induces redox signaling mediated through Ref-1 and Akt leading to the survival of stem cells. (**b**) Treatment with low concentration of hydrogen peroxide under inhibition of Ref-1 induced the level of reactive oxygen species, and the level of NADPH leading to p53-mediated apoptosis and differentiation in adult cardiac stem cells

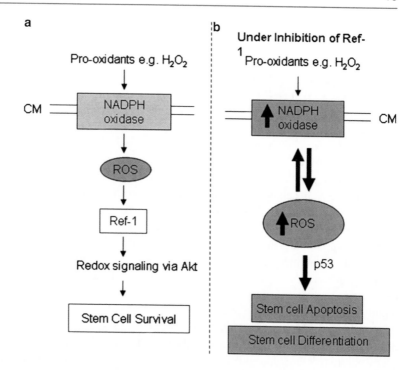

Hypoxic Regulation of Stem Cell Differentiation

Hypoxic preconditioning has been found to extrapolate the potency of mesenchymal stem cells to repair infarcted myocardium, which was attributed to reduced cell death and apoptosis of implanted cells and increased angiogenesis/revascularization [49]. In vivo and in vitro studies have showed an enhancement in the expression of pro-survival and pro-angiogenic factors including hypoxia-inducible factor 1, angiopoietin-1, vascular endothelial growth factor and its receptor, Flk-1, erythropoietin, Bcl-2 and Bcl-xL with a simultaneous decrement in caspase-3 activation in these cells in response to hypoxic preconditioning compared to their normoxic counterpart. Transplantation of normoxic versus hypoxic mesenchymal stem cells after myocardial infarction (MI) resulted in comparable increment in angiogenesis as well as enhanced morphologic and functional benefits of stem cell therapy in the latter group. Another study demonstrated that the quiescent stem cells survive in hypoxic niches of hematopoietic tissue with the corresponding

increase in the mitochondrial number [50, 51]. The authors were able to demonstrate that the activated stem cells move to less hypoxic areas close to the niches, and in better oxygenated areas, they would undergo proliferation and differentiation. In another related study, culture of mesenchymal stem cells in conditions of low oxygen increased expression of c-Met and migration rate in response to chemoattractant gradients [52]. To demonstrate in vivo efficacy the scientists administered control mesenchymal stem cells, and mesenchymal stem cells that have been preconditioned for 24 h by hypoxia to mice having undergone femoral artery ligation. The mesenchymal stem cells were administered intra-arterially. While both groups had positive response, increased vascularity and reduced limb loss were observed in the groups that received mesenchymal stem cells that were preconditioned with hypoxia.

Recently, specific signaling pathways such as Notch and the expression of transcription factors such as Oct4 that control stem cell self-renewal and multipotency are shown to be activated by HIFs [53]. In another recent study, exposing embryoid bodies derived from embryonic stem cells to ambient oxygen at or below 5% resulted in stabilization as well as an increased transcription of hypoxic responsive genes such as HIF-1α [54]. Interestingly enough, HIF-1α expression peaked to the highest level after 48 h of hypoxia and then declined to undetectable levels in spite of continued hypoxic exposure.

Consistent with this report, a study demonstrated that prolonged hypoxia in conjunction with serum deprivation caused massive human mesenchymal stem cell death [55]. Indeed, transplantation of mesenchymal stem cells into ischemic heart causes over 99% cell death within 96 h [55]. In contrast, neonatal cardiomyocytes grafted into a vascular bed survived better than cells transplanted into ischemic tissues [56]. To resolve this problem, a study was undertaken to modify mesenchymal stem cells with a hypoxia-regulated HO-1 plasmid to enhance the survival of stem cells in acute MI heart. In this study, mesenchymal stem cells collected from bone marrow were transfected with either HO-1 or LacZ plasmids. The MSCHO-1 group had higher expression of HO-1 and a twofold reduction in the number of terminal deoxynucleotidyl transferase-mediated deoxyuridine triphosphate in situ nick end labeling-positive cells compared to that of the MSCLacZ group, in the ischemic myocardium. Seven days after implantation, not only the survival in MSCHO-1 was fivefold greater than that of the MSCLacZ group but MSCHO-1 also attenuated postischemic left ventricular remodeling with an enhancement in the functional recovery of infarcted hearts 2 weeks after MI [57].

Redox Regulation of Stem Cell Mobilization

The importance of redox regulation of stem cells is increasingly realized as ROS have been implicated in pathological, biological and physiological control of stem cell maintenance and mobilization. ROS are of particular importance for maintaining a critical balance between preservation of the stem cells in an undifferentiated state and mobilization of the cells to the site [homing] where they can undergo differentiation process [58].

It is now believed that homeostatic regulation of hematopoietic stem cells is fine-tuned by redox signaling, which include their maintenance, proliferation, differentiation, mobilization and finally homing [59].

As mentioned earlier, stem cells can survive better under lower oxygen atmosphere. For example, the self-renewal potential of the hematopoietic stem cells is higher in the low-oxygenic osteoblastic niche [60]. The hematopietic stem cells present in the low-oxygenic niche express a higher level of Notch1, N-cadherin, calcium receptor, telomerase, Bcrp and p21, and express lower level of p38 MAPK, p53 and mTOR [60]. On the other hand, hematopoietic stem cells in the high ROS population express higher level of p38 MAPK and mTOR, where treatment with an antioxidant, a p38 MAPK inhibitor or rapamycin, an inhibitor of mTOR, restores the function of hematopietic stem cells in the high ROS population [60]. These results indicate that ROS-related signaling plays an important role in the preservation of stem cells, self-renewal potential, and relatively enhanced proliferation of the stem cells at lower oxygen may be due to their adaptation to hypoxic condition in original niche bone marrow, where oxygen concentration is relatively low [60]. Interestingly, antioxidants can enhance the self-renewal of hematopoietic stem cells through ataxia telangiectasia-mutated (ATM) gene, which maintains [delete] genomic stability by activating a key cell cycle checkpoint in response to DNA damage, telomeric instability or oxidative stress [61]. Ito et al. [61] have also shown that ATM-mediated inhibition of oxidative stress potentiates the self-renewal capacity of hematopoietic stem cells. Yalcin et al. [62] have shown that Forkhead transcription factor Foxo3 represses ROS via regulation of ATM, and thus maintains the stem cell pool.

Both mobilization and homing of the stem cells appear to be redox-regulated. The important growth factors VEGF and erythropoietin that can mobilize stem cells are certainly under the control of redox regulation [58, 63]. The homing of stem cells to bone marrow is mediated by the binding of chemokine stromal cell-derived factor-1 (SDF-1) to CXCR4 receptor present on the circulating cells [64]. Ceradini et al. [65] have shown that reduced oxygen tension-mediated expression of HIF-1 regulates and induces the expression of SDF-1 in the regenerating ischemic tissues. A recent study showed that uncoupling of endothelial nitric oxide synthase (eNOS) resulting in superoxide anion formation caused diabetic endothelial dysfunction, while eNOS regulated mobilization and vascular repair of endothelial progenitor cells [66]. Urao et al. [67] have shown that hindlimb ischemia increased the production of ROS and Nox2 in bone marrow mononuclear cells, where Nox-2-derived ROS play an important role in the mobilization, homing and angiogenic capacity of stem or progenitor cells, leading to the revascularization of ischemic tissue. Piccoli et al. [68] have shown that bone marrow-derived hematopoietic stem or progenitor cells express multiple isoforms of NADPH oxidase such as NOX1, NOX2 and NOX4 and its regulatory subunits such as p22, p40, p47, p67, rac1, rac2, NOXO1 and NOXA1. The activation of NOX isoforms facilitates the fine tuning of the ROS level, which balances the self-renewal and differentiation in stem cells [68].

MicroRNA as Regulator of Resveratrol-Mediated Cardioprotection

Emerging of MicroRNA

The rapid pace of outstanding findings in the RNA interference research followed by the completion of human genome project leads to the development of critical tools to understand the basic processes of life and disease. One of the key discoveries is microRNA (miRNA), which includes over thousands from many species and these were identified by bioinformatics, genetics and molecular biology approach. Genes for miRNAs are an essential component of the genetic program of all species, most of them also being evolutionarily conserved [69]. The first report of RNA silencing was found to be in plant system [70] but the fundamental study is carried out in

Caenorhabditis elegans where a gene loci lin-4 is found to be the regulator of developmental gene expression [71]. Molecules like resveratrol regulate the expression of mRNA genes in heart by direct or indirect mechanisms. miRNAs are the mature form of processed pre-miRNA. Pre-miRNAs are processed by Drosha from bigger polyadenylated transcripts, known as pri-miRNA, in the nucleus and export to cytoplasm by Exportin 5 [72]. Further maturation of pre-miRNA to miRNA occurs in both nucleus and cytoplasm through Dicer and other protein complexes (Fig. 2). miRNAs target their mRNA by base pairing complimentary sequence located mainly at 3′UTR (untranslated region). miRNAs also target 5′UTR or coding regions of mRNA [73, 74]. In addition to sequence-specific targeting of mRNA, miRNA function as a ribonucleoprotein complex (miRNPs), also known as miRISCs (miRNA-induced silencing complex). Key components of miRISCs include AGO (Argonaute) and GW182 (glycine-tryptophan repeat-containing protein family). Mature miRNAs are generally thought to be stable due its small size, however, they are prone to degradation by both 5′ to 3′ and 3′ to 5′ exoribonucleases present in cells [75, 76]. miRNA stability is also determined by its sequence complexity [77]. miRNAs are well known for its role as inhibitor of protein synthesis and thus interfering with target protein molecules. Recently miRNAs were also shown to activate protein synthesis [74, 78, 79].

MicroRNA in Cardiovascular Health

Cardiovascular diseases are complex process involving different cell types including cardiomyocytes, fibroblasts, endothelial cells, smooth muscle cells, neurons and various blood cells. The signatures of miRNA are different in those cell types and thus can be explained based on specific disease models. Cardiac fibroblasts take the lead role in the development of many diseases like cardiomyopathy, hypertension, MI, chronic cardiomyopathy and regulate the cardiac extracellular matrix components [80–82]. The dysfunction of miRNA metabolism leads to hypertrophy

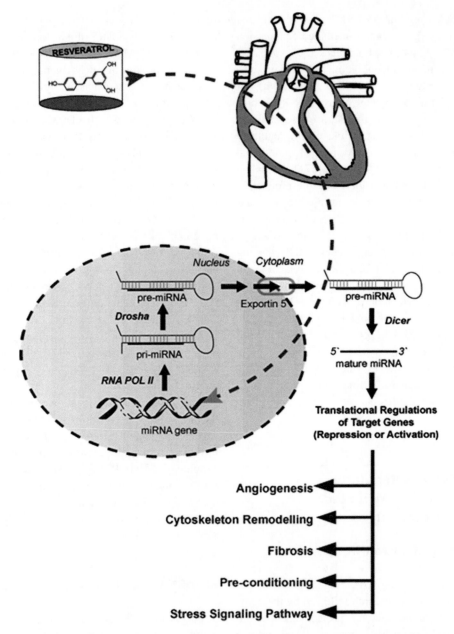

Fig. 2 Mechanism of MicroRNA-mediated cardioprotection by resveratrol. Resveratrol targets miRNA gene and after synthesis by RNA Polymerase II (RNA POL II), primary transcripts of miRNA (pri-miRNA) are recognized by Drosha and Pasha which excise the hairpin precursor generating precursor miRNA (pre-miRNA). These are transported to cytoplasm by Exportin 5 and further processed by Dicer to mature ~23 nt miRNAs. Mature miRNAs associated with Argonaute and other factors lead to the targeted translational regulation. Release from Argonaute or absence of protection machinery leaves miRNAs prone to degradation by exoribonuclease. miRNAs modulate translation either by repression or activation although the mechanism is different. The target genes of miRNAs include various cardiac molecular functions as described

and ventricular fibrosis [83]. Cardiac-specific overexpression of miR-208 resulted in cardiac hypertrophy, whereas genetic deletion of miR-208 blunted the hypertrophic response and decreased interstitial fibrosis following aortic banding [84, 85]. Dysregulation of miRNA (miR-29) family was observed in acute MI model, and knocking down of the miRNA resulted in reduced collagen expression in fibroblasts [86]. Increased expression of miR-21, miR-214 and miR-224, and reduced expression of miR-29b and miR-149 are also found in MI [86]. Similar studies with microarray and northern blot analyses lead to the discovery of miR-21 overexpression in failing heart and miR-21 observed to regulate ERK–MAP kinase pathways [87]. CTGF, a key player in fibrosis, is regulated at posttranslational level by miR-133 and miR-30 [88]. In Ischemic heart disease, miR-1 has been shown to be upregulated in human studies, and overexpression studies in rat correlate miR-1 expression with arrhythmogenesis, cardiac conduction disturbance and membrane potential abnormality [89]. Another miRNA (miR-133), encoded by the same loci of miR-1, induced myoblast proliferation in vitro and is shown to proliferate skeletal as well as cardiac muscle after overexpression in *Xenopus* embryos [90]. Hypoxia-inducible factor (HIF-1α) is the transcription factor involved in cardiac hypoxia and is beneficial to the treatment of ischemic injury [91]. Hypoxia-induced HIF-1α upregulation is partly regulated by a miRNA, miR-199 [92]. Bcl2, a key regulator of apoptosis by mitochondrial pathway, is regulated by miR-1 and miR-15 family [93]. miR-92a is present in endothelial cells and is upregulated upon induction of ischemia and knockdown of miR-92a resulted in improved recovery after MI due to accelerated vessel growth [94]. miR-320 regulates heat shock proteins (HSPs) and HSPs mediate cardioprotection against ischemic condition in heart [95]. Ischemic preconditioning of bone marrow-derived mesenchymal stem cells improved by their survival following engraftment in the infarcted heart and miR-210 has crucial role in the process [96].

Role of MicroRNA in Resveratrol-Mediated Cardioprotection

Recent real-time PCR-based array studies with resveratrol demonstrate unique expression pattern for resveratrol pretreated hearts. Differential expression of over 50 miRNAs is observed in ex vivo ischemia reperfused (IR) heart; some of

them are previously implicated [97]. Based on computational analyses, the target genes for the differentially expressed miRNAs include genes of various molecular functions such as metal ion binding, transcription factors and cytoskeleton remodeling which may play a key role in reducing IR injury. IR samples pretreated with resveratrol or its commercial formulation reverse the up- or downregulation in IR samples in the opposite direction in more than 50% of differentially expressed miRNAs, and either resveratrol or its commercial formulation, but not both, reverse the up- or downregulation compared to IR control in 20% of miRNAs. There is a significant upregulation of miR-21 expression with resveratrol. miR-21 is shown to regulate the ERK–MAP kinase signaling pathway in cardiac fibroblasts, which has impacts on global cardiac structure and function [87]. It has been shown earlier that resveratrol triggers MAPK signaling pathway as a preconditioning mechanism [98]. FOXO1 is regulated by miR-27a in cancer cells, whereas VEGF is modulated by miR-20b through HIF-1α [99, 100]. SIRT1 is observed to be regulated by miR-9 in stem cells and miR-199 in cardiomyocyte [92, 101]. Both miRNAs are modulated in resveratrol-treated rat heart. Complex statistical analyses such as principal component analyses reveal that the IR samples pretreated with resveratrol are remarkably similar to vehicle sample in terms of miRNA gene expression [97]. These results are indeed of utmost importance, as they document that resveratrol can protect the ischemic heart by restoring the IR-induced upregulation or downregulation of gene expression. Future studies will be based on the mechanistic action and stability of miRNAs. Further detailed in vivo and in vitro studies like targeting those miRNAs followed by loss/gain of function will able to explore the complex mechanism underlying the cardioprotection by resveratrol.

Conclusions

The process of stem cells maintenance and growth in their niche appears to be regulated by controlled hypoxia and HIF-1α, while the mobilization and homing is controlled by cytokines and/or adhesive molecules, which are driven by redox signaling that in turn appears to be regulated by redox-controlled FoxO-SirT network. miRNAs regulate target gene mostly by translational repression and sometimes through translational activation. Resveratrol regulates miRNA expression in healthy heart and ischemic-reperfused heart. Future detailed studies based on this approach and analyses will pave the way for the development of novel therapeutic intervention for cardioprotection in acute IR injury. As more studies of the importance of miRNA appear in publication database, a tremendous impulse is generated for the feasibility of its therapeutic potential. There are some limitations to this process. First of all, the mechanism of action for miRNA is still unfolding and more information is required such as how it is transported, metabolized and targets the specific as well as nonspecific genes. Other limitation is related to the stability of miRNAs and administration at high dose based on animal studies and related toxic effect (if any) in targeted or nontargeted tissue delivery. Currently several modified versions of antisense oligonucleotides, commonly known as antagomirs or anti-miRs, are available. These include 2′-O-methoxy ethyl/phosphorothioate, locked nucleic acid and hairpin inhibitors [102–104]. Another important aspect of miRNAs in cardiovascular research is its potential use as biomarker of cardiovascular disease [105–107]. More insights of miRNAs are required before it is actually implemented in clinical use.

Acknowledgements This study was supported in part by NIH HL 34360, HL 33889 and HL 22559.

References

1. Quaini F, Urbanek K, Beltrami AP, et al. Chimerism of the transplanted heart. N Engl J Med. 2002;346:5–15.
2. Kronenwett R, Martin S, Haas R. The role of cytokines and adhesion molecules for mobilization of peripheral blood stem cells. Stem Cells. 2000;18:320–30.
3. Kinashi T, Springer TA. Adhesion molecules in hematopoietic cells. Blood Cells. 1994;20(1):25–44.
4. Carlos TM, Harlan JM. Leukocyte-endothelial adhesion molecules. Blood. 1994;84:2068–101.

5. Mohle R, Murea S, Kirsch M, et al. Differential expression of L-selectin, VLA-4, and LFA-1 on CD34+ progenitor cells from bone marrow and peripheral blood during G-CSF-enhanced recovery. Exp Hematol. 1995;23:1535–42.
6. Lichterfeld M, Martin S, Burkly L, et al. Mobilization of CD34+ haematopoietic stem cells is associated with a functional inactivation of the integrin very late antigen 4. Br J Haematol. 2000;110:71–81.
7. Yamaguchi M, Ikebuchi K, Hirayama F, et al. Different adhesive characteristics and VLA-4 expression of CD34+ progenitors in G0/G1 versus S+G2/M phases of the cell cycle. Blood. 1998;92:842–8.
8. Laterveer L, Lindley IJ, Heemskerk DP, et al. Rapid mobilization of hematopoietic progenitor cells in rhesus monkeys by a single intravenous injection of interleukin-8. Blood. 1996;87:781–8.
9. Maurer AM, Liu Y, Caen JP, et al. Ex vivo expansion of megakaryocytic cells. Int J Hematol. 2000;71:203–10.
10. Duhrsen U, Villeval JL, Boyd J, et al. Effects of recombinant human granulocyte colony-stimulating factor on hematopoietic progenitor cells in cancer patients. Blood. 1988;72:2074–81.
11. Gazitt Y. Recent developments in the regulation of peripheral blood stem cell mobilization and engraftment by cytokines, chemokines, and adhesion molecules. J Hematother Stem Cell Res. 2001;10:229–36.
12. Haddad JJ. Redox regulation of pro-inflammatory cytokines and IkappaB-alpha/NF-kappaB nuclear translocation and activation. Biochem Biophys Res Commun. 2002;296:847–56.
13. Liu H, Nishitoh H, Ichijo H, et al. Activation of apoptosis signal-regulating kinase 1 (ASK1) by tumor necrosis factor receptor-associated factor 2 requires prior dissociation of the ASK1 inhibitor thioredoxin. Mol Cell Biol. 2000;20:2198–208.
14. Wilmanski J, Siddiqi M, Deitch EA, et al. Augmented IL-10 production and redox-dependent signaling pathways in glucose-6-phosphate dehydrogenase-deficient mouse peritoneal macrophages. J Leukoc Biol. 2005;78:85–94.
15. Case J, Ingram DA, Haneline LS. Oxidative stress impairs endothelial progenitor cell function. Antioxid Redox Signal. 2008;10:1895–907.
16. Ghaffari S. Oxidative stress in the regulation of normal and neoplastic hematopoiesis. Antioxid Redox Signal. 2008;10:1923–40.
17. Guo Y, Einhorn L, Kelley M, et al. Redox regulation of the embryonic stem cell transcription factor oct-4 by thioredoxin. Stem Cells. 2004;22:259–64.
18. Gurusamy N, Mukherjee S, Lekli I, et al. Inhibition of Ref-1 stimulates the production of reactive oxygen species and induces differentiation in adult cardiac stem cells. Antioxid Redox Signal. 2009;11:589–600.
19. Li Z, Li L. Understanding hematopoietic stem-cell microenvironments. Trends Biochem Sci. 2006;31:589–95.

20. Kopp HG, Avecilla ST, Hooper AT, et al. The bone marrow vascular niche: home of HSC differentiation and mobilization. Physiology (Bethesda). 2005;20: 349–56.

21. Haneline LS. Redox regulation of stem and progenitor cells. Antioxid Redox Signal. 2008;10:1849–52.

22. Dernbach E, Urbich C, Brandes RP, et al. Antioxidative stress-associated genes in circulating progenitor cells: evidence for enhanced resistance against oxidative stress. Blood. 2004;104:3591–7.

23. Schmelter M, Ateghang B, Helmig S, et al. Embryonic stem cells utilize reactive oxygen species as transducers of mechanical strain-induced cardiovascular differentiation. FASEB J. 2006;20:1182–4.

24. Illi B, Scopece A, Nanni S, et al. Epigenetic histone modification and cardiovascular lineage programming in mouse embryonic stem cells exposed to laminar shear stress. Circ Res. 2005;96:501–8.

25. Yamamoto K, Sokabe T, Watabe T, et al. Fluid shear stress induces differentiation of Flk-1-positive embryonic stem cells into vascular endothelial cells in vitro. Am J Physiol Heart Circ Physiol. 2005;288: H1915–24.

26. Ito K, Hirao A, Arai F, et al. Reactive oxygen species act through p38 MAPK to limit the lifespan of hematopoietic stem cells. Nat Med. 2006;12:446–51.

27. Sauer H, Rahimi G, Hescheler J, et al. Role of reactive oxygen species and phosphatidylinositol 3-kinase in cardiomyocyte differentiation of embryonic stem cells. FEBS Lett. 2000;476:218–23.

28. Wartenberg M, Donmez F, Ling FC, et al. Tumor-induced angiogenesis studied in confrontation cultures of multicellular tumor spheroids and embryoid bodies grown from pluripotent embryonic stem cells. FASEB J. 2001;15:995–1005.

29. Han MK, Song EK, Guo Y, et al. SIRT1 regulates apoptosis and Nanog expression in mouse embryonic stem cells by controlling p53 subcellular localization. Cell Stem Cell. 2008;2:241–51.

30. Tothova Z, Kollipara R, Huntly BJ, et al. FoxOs are critical mediators of hematopoietic stem cell resistance to physiologic oxidative stress. Cell. 2007;128: 325–39.

31. Essers MA, Weijzen S, de Vries-Smits AM, et al. FOXO transcription factor activation by oxidative stress mediated by the small GTPase Ral and JNK. EMBO J. 2004;23:4802–12.

32. Marinkovic D, Zhang X, Yalcin S, et al. Foxo3 is required for the regulation of oxidative stress in erythropoiesis. J Clin Investig. 2007;117:2133–44.

33. Tothova Z, Gilliland DG. FoxO transcription factors and stem cell homeostasis: insights from the hematopoietic system. Cell Stem Cell. 2007;1: 140–52.

34. Hosokawa K, Arai F, Yoshihara H, et al. Function of oxidative stress in the regulation of hematopoietic stem cell-niche interaction. Biochem Biophys Res Commun. 2007;363:578–83.

35. Spradling A, Drummond-Barbosa D, Kai T. Stem cells find their niche. Nature. 2001;414:98–104.

36. Angkeow P, Deshpande SS, Qi B, et al. Redox factor-1: an extra-nuclear role in the regulation of endothelial oxidative stress and apoptosis. Cell Death Differ. 2002;9:717–25.

37. Allen RG, Venkatraj VS. Oxidants and antioxidants in development and differentiation. J Nutr. 1992; 122(3 Suppl):631–5.

38. Beltrami AP, Barlucchi L, Torella D, et al. Adult cardiac stem cells are multipotent and support myocardial regeneration. Cell. 2003;114:763–76.

39. Beckman BS, Balin AK, Allen RG. Superoxide dismutase induces differentiation of Friend erythroleukemia cells. J Cell Physiol. 1989;139:370–6.

40. Almog N, Rotter V. Involvement of p53 in cell differentiation and development. Biochim Biophys Acta. 1997;1333:F1–27.

41. Bachelder RE, Ribick MJ, Marchetti A, et al. p53 inhibits alpha 6 beta 4 integrin survival signaling by promoting the caspase 3-dependent cleavage of AKT/PKB. J Cell Biol. 1999;147:1063–72.

42. Gottlieb TM, Leal JF, Seger R, et al. Cross-talk between Akt, p53 and Mdm2: possible implications for the regulation of apoptosis. Oncogene. 2002;21: 1299–303.

43. Keren-Tal I, Suh BS, Dantes A, et al. Involvement of p53 expression in cAMP-mediated apoptosis in immortalized granulosa cells. Exp Cell Res. 1995; 218:283–95.

44. Eizenberg O, Faber-Elman A, Gottlieb E, et al. p53 plays a regulatory role in differentiation and apoptosis of central nervous system-associated cells. Mol Cell Biol. 1996;16:5178–85.

45. Sabapathy K, Klemm M, Jaenisch R, et al. Regulation of ES cell differentiation by functional and conformational modulation of p53. EMBO J. 1997;16: 6217–29.

46. Ostrakhovitch EA, Cherian MG. Role of p53 and reactive oxygen species in apoptotic response to copper and zinc in epithelial breast cancer cells. Apoptosis. 2005;10:111–21.

47. Jayaraman L, Murthy KG, Zhu C, et al. Identification of redox/repair protein Ref-1 as a potent activator of p53. Genes Dev. 1997;11:558–70.

48. Liu B, Chen Y, St Clair DK. ROS and p53: a versatile partnership. Free Radic Biol Med. 2008;44: 1529–35.

49. Hu X, Yu SP, Fraser JL, et al. Transplantation of hypoxia-preconditioned mesenchymal stem cells improves infarcted heart function via enhanced survival of implanted cells and angiogenesis. J Thorac Cardiovasc Surg. 2008;135:799–808.

50. Cipolleschi MG, Dello Sbarba P, et al. The role of hypoxia in the maintenance of hematopoietic stem cells. Blood. 1993;82:2031–7.

51. Rajasekhar VK, Vemuri MC. Stem cells, hypoxia and hypoxia-inducible factors. In: Rajasekhar VK, Vemuri MC, editors. Regulatory networks in stem cells. New York: Humana; 2009. p. 211–31.

52. Rosova I, Dao M, Capoccia B, et al. Hypoxic preconditioning results in increased motility and improved

therapeutic potential of human mesenchymal stem cells. Stem Cells. 2008;26:2173–82.

53. Keith B, Simon MC. Hypoxia-inducible factors, stem cells, and cancer. Cell. 2007;129:465–72.

54. Cameron CM, Harding F, Hu WS, et al. Activation of hypoxic response in human embryonic stem cell-derived embryoid bodies. Exp Biol Med (Maywood). 2008;233:1044–57.

55. Potier E, Ferreira E, Meunier A, et al. Prolonged hypoxia concomitant with serum deprivation induces massive human mesenchymal stem cell death. Tissue Eng. 2007;13:1325–31.

56. Ivanovic Z, Dello Sbarba P, Trimoreau F, et al. Primitive human HPCs are better maintained and expanded in vitro at 1 percent oxygen than at 20 percent. Transfusion. 2000;40:1482–8.

57. Tang YL, Tang Y, Zhang YC, et al. Improved graft mesenchymal stem cell survival in ischemic heart with a hypoxia-regulated heme oxygenase-1 vector. J Am Coll Cardiol. 2005;46:1339–50.

58. Csete M. Oxygen in the cultivation of stem cells. Ann NY Acad Sci. 2005;1049:1–8.

59. Saretzki G, Armstrong L, Leake A, et al. Stress defense in murine embryonic stem cells is superior to that of various differentiated murine cells. Stem Cells. 2004;22:962–71.

60. Jang YY, Sharkis SJ. A low level of reactive oxygen species selects for primitive hematopoietic stem cells that may reside in the low-oxygenic niche. Blood. 2007;110:3056–63.

61. Ito K, Hirao A, Arai F, et al. Regulation of oxidative stress by ATM is required for self-renewal of haematopoietic stem cells. Nature. 2004;431:997–1002.

62. Yalcin S, Zhang X, Luciano JP, et al. Foxo3 is essential for the regulation of ataxia telangiectasia mutated and oxidative stress-mediated homeostasis of hematopoietic stem cells. J Biol Chem. 2008;283:25692–705.

63. Rabbany SY, Heissig B, Hattori K, et al. Molecular pathways regulating mobilization of marrow-derived stem cells for tissue revascularization. Trends Mol Med. 2003;9:109–17.

64. Peled A, Grabovsky V, Habler L, et al. The chemokine SDF-1 stimulates integrin-mediated arrest of CD34+ cells on vascular endothelium under shear flow. J Clin Investig. 1999;104:1199–211.

65. Ceradini DJ, Kulkarni AR, Callaghan MJ, et al. Progenitor cell trafficking is regulated by hypoxic gradients through HIF-1 induction of SDF-1. Nat Med. 2004;10:858–64.

66. Thum T, Fraccarollco D, Schultheiss M, et al. Endothelial nitric oxide synthase uncoupling impairs endothelial progenitor cell mobilization and function in diabetes. Diabetes. 2007;56:666–74.

67. Urao N, Inomata H, Razvi M, et al. Role of nox2-based NADPH oxidase in bone marrow and progenitor cell function involved in neovascularization induced by hindlimb ischemia. Circ Res. 2008;103:212–20.

68. Piccoli C, D'Aprile A, Ripoli M, et al. Bone-marrow derived hematopoietic stem/progenitor cells express multiple isoforms of NADPH oxidase and produce constitutively reactive oxygen species. Biochem Biophys Res Commun. 2007;353:965–72.

69. Ambros V. The functions of animal microRNAs. Nature. 2004;431:350–5.

70. Hamilton AJ, Baulcombe DC. A species of small antisense RNA in posttranscriptional gene silencing in plants. Science. 1999;286:950–2.

71. Olsen PH, Ambros V. The lin-4 regulatory RNA controls developmental timing in Caenorhabditis elegans by blocking LIN-14 protein synthesis after the initiation of translation. Dev Biol. 1999;216:671–80.

72. Hammond SM. Dicing and slicing: the core machinery of the RNA interference pathway. FEBS Lett. 2005;579:5822–9.

73. Rigoutsos I. New tricks for animal microRNAs: targeting of amino acid coding regions at conserved and nonconserved sites. Cancer Res. 2009;69:3245–8.

74. Orom UA, Nielsen FC, Lund AH. MicroRNA-10a binds the 5′UTR of ribosomal protein mRNAs and enhances their translation. Mol Cell. 2008;30:460–71.

75. Kai ZS, Pasquinelli AE. MicroRNA assassins: factors that regulate the disappearance of miRNAs. Nat Struct Mol Biol. 2010;17:5–10.

76. Krol J, Loedige I, Filipowicz W. The widespread regulation of microRNA biogenesis, function and decay. Nat Rev Genet. 2010;11:597–610.

77. Bail S, Swerdel M, Liu H, et al. Differential regulation of microRNA stability. RNA. 2010;16:1032–9.

78. Buchan JR, Parker R. Molecular biology. The two faces of miRNA. Science. 2007;318:1877–8.

79. Vasudevan S, Steitz JA. AU-rich-element-mediated upregulation of translation by FXR1 and Argonaute 2. Cell. 2007;128:1105–18.

80. Mukhopadhyay P, Rajesh M, Batkai S, et al. CB1 cannabinoid receptors promote oxidative stress and cell death in murine models of doxorubicin-induced cardiomyopathy and in human cardiomyocytes. Cardiovasc Res. 2010;85:773–84.

81. Raman SV. The hypertensive heart. An integrated understanding informed by imaging. J Am Coll Cardiol. 2010;55:91–6.

82. Jellis C, Martin J, Narula J, et al. Assessment of nonischemic myocardial fibrosis. J Am Coll Cardiol. 2010;56:89–97.

83. Da Costa Martins PA, Bourajjaj M, Gladka M, et al. Conditional dicer gene deletion in the postnatal myocardium provokes spontaneous cardiac remodeling. Circulation. 2008;118:1567–76.

84. van Rooij E, Sutherland LB, Qi X, et al. Control of stress-dependent cardiac growth and gene expression by a microRNA. Science. 2007;316:575–9.

85. Callis TE, Pandya K, Seok HY, et al. MicroRNA-208a is a regulator of cardiac hypertrophy and conduction in mice. J Clin Investig. 2009;119:2772–86.

86. van Rooij E, Sutherland LB, Thatcher JE, et al. Dysregulation of microRNAs after myocardial

infarction reveals a role of miR-29 in cardiac fibrosis. Proc Natl Acad Sci USA. 2008;105:13027–32.

87. Thum T, Gross C, Fiedler J, et al. MicroRNA-21 contributes to myocardial disease by stimulating MAP kinase signalling in fibroblasts. Nature. 2008;456: 980–4.

88. Duisters RF, Tijsen AJ, Schroen B, et al. miR-133 and miR-30 regulate connective tissue growth factor: implications for a role of microRNAs in myocardial matrix remodeling. Circ Res. 2009;104:170–8.

89. Yang B, Lin H, Xiao J, et al. The muscle-specific microRNA miR-1 regulates cardiac arrhythmogenic potential by targeting GJA1 and KCNJ2. Nat Med. 2007;13:486–91.

90. Chen JF, Mandel EM, Thomson JM, et al. The role of microRNA-1 and microRNA-133 in skeletal muscle proliferation and differentiation. Nat Genet. 2006;38:228–33.

91. Loor G, Schumacker PT. Role of hypoxia-inducible factor in cell survival during myocardial ischemia-reperfusion. Cell Death Differ. 2008;15:686–90.

92. Rane S, He M, Sayed D, et al. Downregulation of miR-199a derepresses hypoxia-inducible factor-1alpha and Sirtuin 1 and recapitulates hypoxia preconditioning in cardiac myocytes. Circ Res. 2009;104:879–86.

93. Tang Y, Zheng J, Sun Y, et al. MicroRNA-1 regulates cardiomyocyte apoptosis by targeting Bcl-2. Int Heart J. 2009;50:377–87.

94. Bonauer A, Dimmeler S. The microRNA-17-92 cluster: still a miRacle? Cell Cycle. 2009;8:3866–73.

95. Ren XP, Wu J, Wang X, et al. MicroRNA-320 is involved in the regulation of cardiac ischemia/reperfusion injury by targeting heat-shock protein 20. Circulation. 2009;119:2357–66.

96. Kim HW, Haider HK, Jiang S, et al. Ischemic preconditioning augments survival of stem cells via miR-210 expression by targeting caspase-8-associated protein 2. J Biol Chem. 2009;284:33161–8.

97. Mukhopadhyay P, Mukherjee S, Ahsan K, et al. Restoration of altered microRNA expression in the ischemic heart with resveratrol. PLoS One. 2010; 5(12):e15705.

98. Das S, Tosaki A, Bagchi D, et al. Potentiation of a survival signal in the ischemic heart by resveratrol through p38 mitogen-activated protein kinase/mitogen- and stress-activated protein kinase 1/cAMP response element-binding protein signaling. J Pharmacol Exp Ther. 2006;317:980–8.

99. Cascio S, D'Andrea A, Ferla R, et al. miR-20b modulates VEGF expression by targeting HIF-1 alpha and STAT3 in MCF-7 breast cancer cells. J Cell Physiol. 2010;224:242–9.

100. Guttilla IK, White BA. Coordinate regulation of FOXO1 by miR-27a, miR-96, and miR-182 in breast cancer cells. J Biol Chem. 2009;284:23204–16.

101. Saunders LR, Sharma AD, Tawney J, et al. miRNAs regulate SIRT1 expression during mouse embryonic stem cell differentiation and in adult mouse tissues. Aging (Albany NY). 2010;2:415–31.

102. Huynh C, Segura MF, Gaziel-Sovran A, et al. Efficient in vivo microRNA targeting of liver metastasis. Oncogene. 2010. doi:10.1038/onc.2010.523.

103. Elmen J, Lindow M, Schutz S, et al. LNA-mediated microRNA silencing in non-human primates. Nature. 2008;452:896–9.

104. Vermeulen A, Robertson B, Dalby AB, et al. Double-stranded regions are essential design components of potent inhibitors of RISC function. RNA. 2007;13: 723–30.

105. Fichtlscherer S, De Rosa S, Fox H, et al. Circulating microRNAs in patients with coronary artery disease. Circ Res. 2010;107:677–84.

106. Kumarswamy R, Anker SD, Thum T. MicroRNAs as circulating biomarkers for heart failure: questions about MiR-423-5p. Circ Res. 2010;106:e8. author reply e9.

107. Wang GK, Zhu JQ, Zhang JT, et al. Circulating microRNA: a novel potential biomarker for early diagnosis of acute myocardial infarction in humans. Eur Heart J. 2010;31:659–66.

Cardiac Cell Therapy: Present and Future

Dinender K. Singla

Abstract

End stage heart failure following myocardial infarction is a major health problem despite significant improvement in treatment intervention. Heart transplantation is the only option to treat end stage heart failure patients, however; the supply needed has severe shortage. Therefore, cell transplantation has gained significant interest as a future treatment of various heart diseases including myocardial infarction. Optimal cell type for complete cardiac regeneration is still needed as clinical trials using adult stem cell transplantation so far did not show long-term significant improvement in cardiac function. Moreover, there are concerns over the differentiation of adult stem cells into cardiac cell types. Embryonic stem cells can be used for cell transplantation but their potential in clinical trial has been hampered due to their characteristics of teratoma formation. Furthermore, beneficial effects observed in clinical and experimental studies that may be associated with released autocrine or paracrine factors following cell transplantation is another major area of current investigation discussed in this review.

Keywords

Myocardial infarction • Heart regeneration • Factors released from stem cells • Teratoma • Cell transplantation

Introduction

Cardiovascular diseases remain a major health problem [1] despite significant advances in diagnostics, treatment interventions and therapeutics. Blockage of coronary artery initiates myocardial infarction (MI), which leads to adverse ventricular remodeling. This process

D.K. Singla (✉)
Biomolecular Science Center, University of Central Florida, Orlando, FL, USA
e-mail: dsingla@mail.ucf.edu

N.S. Dhalla, M. Nagano, B. Ostadal (eds.), *Molecular Defects in Cardiovascular Disease*,
DOI 10.1007/978-1-4419-7130-2_7, © Springer Science+Business Media, LLC 2011

involves apoptotic and necrotic cell death of cardiac myocytes, endothelial and vascular smooth muscle cells. This gives rise to the formation of both interstitial and vascular fibrosis that ultimately deteriorates cardiac function [2, 3]. These changes result in rearrangement of myocardial tissue in response to altered working conditions [2, 3]. Importantly, adverse ventricular remodeling begins within hours of the MI which is generally initiated by a series of cytokines and inflammatory factors being released by inflammatory cells such as macrophages. The Most abundantly examined cytokine, TGFβ1, has been shown to stimulate cardiac fibroblast proliferation, convert interstitial fibroblasts into myofibroblasts and accelerate ventricular remodeling of the extracellular matrix (ECM) leading to a net accumulation of matrix metalloproteins [2–4]. Increased synthesis of collagen proteins in the infarcted heart is associated with post-MI fibrosis. Moreover, the complex process of the development of fibrosis is also associated with concurrent ECM degradation through activation of matrix metalloproteinases (MMPs) and urokinase plasminogen activator and its inhibitor, PAI-1 [2–4].

Various angiotensin-converting enzyme inhibitors and antioxidant drugs are currently used to treat MI patients. In the case of end stage heart failure patients, the last resort remains as heart transplantation [2–4]. However, heart transplantation supply is severely inadequate compared with the number of patients waiting in the hospitals. Therefore, recent progress in basic science research points to the potential of cell transplantation as a therapeutic option to treat injured myocardium [5, 6].

Recent experimental studies have documented the formation of cardiomyocytes and other heart cell types from transplanted bone marrow stem cells, cardiac stem cells (CSCs) and embryonic stem (ES) cells as well as the migration of primitive cells to the heart [5, 6]. Furthermore, several transplanted cell types, including ES cells, were shown to improve myocardial function [5, 6]. However, the most appropriate donor cell types for cell therapy remain uncertain.

Embryonic Stem Cells Differentiate into Cardiomyocytes in the Cell Culture

ES cells are derived from the inner cell mass (ICM) of the preimplantation blastocyst of various species including human and mouse [6, 7]. Isolated ES cells have shown to be pluripotent as they were able to propagate without differentiation in cell culture while preserving their potential to differentiate into all three embryonic germ layers such as ectoderm, endoderm and mesoderm [6, 7]. Moreover, these pluripotent cells have been differentiated into derivatives of representative of all three embryonic germ layers in the cell culture system [6, 7]. This is achieved by the generation of embryoid bodies (EBs) [6, 7], which are cell aggregates of ES cells. For example, EB cells generated from both human and mouse ES cells demonstrated their potential to differentiate into all three major heart cells [8, 9]. These interesting studies have shown the proof of principle to generate heart cells in the cell culture system, however the amount of newly differentiated cardiac cell types remains significantly low compared with cell number required for complete cardiac regeneration. A large amount of resources have been used to enhance derived cardiac myocyte differentiation from both human and mouse ES cells including use of various growth factors/cytokine treatment strategies [10]. In this regard, our published data show that treatment of mouse CGR8 ES cells to cytokine, required for embryonic cardiogenesis, TGF-β2 significantly increased spontaneous and rhythmically beating cardiomyocytes [8]. Similarly, bone morphogenic proteins (BMP2), fibroblast growth factor 2 (FGF2), vitamin A and C treatment to ES cells have also been shown to enhance the differentiation of beating cardiac myocytes [11].

Cell Therapy

Over the past 15 years, both embryonic and adult stem cell transplantation to treat heart disease have been studied in a variety of animal models

[6, 12–15]. Demonstration of successful engraftment in injured myocardium has made cell transplantation a means to replace dysfunctional myocardium and the treatment of heart failure a potential realistic possibility [6, 12–15]. One rationale underlying this approach is that regeneration of injured myocardium with new heart cell types will improve the mechanical properties of the infarcted region. Different cell types have been studied with varied potentials of regeneration including skeletal myoblasts, smooth muscle cells, fetal and embryonic cardiomyocytes, bone marrow stromal and hematopoietic stem cells, iPS cells and mouse ES cells [6, 12–15]. These cell transplantation studies have shown significant improvement in cardiac function despite often limited regeneration, i.e., regeneration that is insufficient to compensate for cell loss due to apoptosis and/or necrosis [6, 12–15]. The amount of regeneration has varied significantly depending in part on the number and type of cell transplantation [6, 12–15].

This animal studies data generated an interest in clinical testing of these autologous skeletal muscle cells or BMS cells for cell therapy in patients [6, 12–15]. Adult stem cells transplanted in patients have resulted in improvement in global cardiac function [15]. Noticeably, these clinical trials suggest that transplantation of autologous BMS cells into the myocardium of MI patients improves LV ejection fraction (EF) at 6 months; however, enthusiasm in these studies were significantly lowered when improved function was not statistically significant the 18-month follow-up [15]. Moreover, cell transplantation data in these patients have usually been performed in association with surgical or percutaneous revascularization, therefore, this remains completely unknown whether slightly improved cardiac functions in these patients are due to cell transplantation. In contrast, other studies showed no significant improvement in cardiac function following adult stem cell transplantation in patients [15]. Moreover, bone marrow stem cell applications remain controversial because optimization is needed in cell type transplantation, patient population selection criteria and their follow-up procedures.

Next, CSCs are another stem cell population residing in the heart which can be optimized for cardiac regeneration. These are undifferentiated, self-renewing, clonogenic and capable of differentiating into all three major heart cell types both in vitro and in vivo [16–18]. These cells have been identified and characterized as resident cells in the heart of mice [19], rat [16] and humans [20]. This would be most important and intriguing to develop strategies to promote translocation of resident CSCs from the storage site to the injury and their differentiation into heart cell types. We also demonstrate that there is significant increase in CSC activation and differentiation into cardiac myocytes positive with c-kit marker and cardiac α-actin following ES cell-conditioned medium transplantation post-MI (unpublished data, Singla Lab).

Moreover, transplantation of undifferentiated ES cells labeled with GFP/β-gal demonstrated engraftment and differentiation into all three major heart cells (cardiomyocytes, endothelial and vascular smooth muscle) at 2-week post-MI [9]. Similarly, transplanted ES cells in the infarcted hearts of mouse, rat and sheep exhibit differentiation into cardiomyocytes up to 12-weeks post-MI [21]. Interestingly, as expected transplanted ES cells in the infarcted hearts of mouse, rat and sheep have been shown to improve cardiac function [9, 13, 21–23]. However, the actual amount of engraftment and differentiation into cardiomyocytes varies in different animal models, noticeably, irrespective of variation in cardiac myocyte differentiation; the amount of newly differentiated cells is limited. Therefore, this is urgently needed to refine the cell transplantation strategies to improve engraftment and differentiation. However, among the various options to enhance cardiac regeneration, the most frequent attempt was to use appropriate growth factors to induce differentiation of ES cells in the cell culture system. These cell culture studies have yielded exciting improvement in cardiac myocyte differentiation. However, it remains to be clearly demonstrated whether growth factor-primed ES cells used for cell transplantation can enhance engraftment, cardiac myocyte differentiation and ultimately better regeneration in the infarcted heart.

Undifferentiated mouse ES cells primed with insulin growth factor-1 subsequently transplanted into infarcted mouse hearts enhanced cardiac myocyte differentiation along with associated improvement in cardiac function compared with unprimed ES cells [24]. Another set of growth factors, such as TGF-β and FGF, and primed ES cells were transplanted into infarcted mouse hearts. Data obtained from this study suggest that TGF-β growth factor demonstrated most effective increase in the donor cell engraftment, cardiac myocyte differentiation, increase in the expression of connexin-43 and improved cardiac function [25]. Moreover, recent cell transplant studies suggest that donor cell death following transplantation is a major limiting factor for cell survival, engraftment and differentiation. Apoptosis has been shown following transplantation of dopaminergic neurons for Parkinson's disease, islet cells for diabetes mellitus and skeletal myoblasts for muscular dystrophy [25–29]. Similarly, transplantation of neonatal or adult cardiomyocytes into injured myocardium is associated with significant apoptosis, necrosis or both [30, 31]. Correspondingly, transplantation of cardiomyocytes transfected with the antiapoptotic gene Akt decreases donor cell death following transplantation [31]. Thus, mesenchymal stem cells (MSCs) transfected with the Akt gene (Akt-MSCs) have better survival compared with wild-type MSC cells [32, 33].

Cardiac Remodeling and Fibrosis Following Stem Cell Transplantation

MI leads to cardiac remodeling, a complex, dynamic and time-dependent phenomenon characterized by (a) death of cardiac myocytes, endothelial and vascular smooth muscle cells, which is associated with interstitial and vascular fibrosis; (b) fibrosis, which is associated with increased collagen synthesis and caused by various cytokines, proteins and growth factors [2–4, 34–37]. These alterations in the depletion of cardiac myocyte cells and replacement with fibroblasts

result in the rearrangement of myocardial tissue in response to meet the demand of the working heart [2–4, 34–37]. Importantly, the development and progression of remodeling includes migration of macrophages, neutrophils and mast cells (inflammatory cells), which produce cytokines and growth factors that stimulate cardiac fibroblast proliferation and accelerate cardiac remodeling of the ECM which ultimately accumulates large amount of ECM [2–4, 34–37]. In the development of cardiac fibrosis, parallel ECM degradation occurs via activation of MMPs and urokinase plasminogen activator and its inhibitor PAI-1 [2–4, 34–41]. During endogenous fibrinolysis post-MI, tPA converts plasminogen into the active enzyme plasmin that plays a direct role in ECM degradation [38–41]. PAI-1 mRNA has been shown to be expressed in cardiomyocytes post-MI. PAI-1 is involved in remodeling and fibrosis by inhibiting the activation of MMPs as well as plasmin generation [38–41]. A recent study suggests that PAI-1 knockout mice develop less myocardial and perivascular fibrosis compared with wild-type mice post-MI, suggesting a direct role of PAI-1 in the development and progression of fibrosis [41]. Post-MI remodeling can be divided into early and late phases. Early remodeling (24–96 h) involves coagulation necrosis (myofibrillar hypereosinophilia and loss of nuclei), myocyte cell loss, enhanced ECM degradation, cytokine production, inflammation and infiltration of neutrophils [3, 4]. In contrast, the later phase (several days to months) is associated with progressive expansion of the infarct area, release of additional cytokines, growth factors and PAI-1, further myocyte loss and, ultimately, global LV dilatation and dysfunction [3, 4]. In parallel, associated healing replaces the infarct with a robust collagen scar. Collagen deposition starts at one week and lasts up to months following MI [3, 4]. During the later phase stress-induced hormonal and biochemical factors such as acidic and basic growth factors, cytokines (TNF-α, IL-6, TGFβ) and angiotensin II are released [3, 4]. These dynamic quantitative and qualitative differences in stress-released factors, collagen deposition, fibroblast proliferation and phenotype formation early versus late post-MI result in time-dependent differences in the fibrotic microenvironment in the heart [3, 4].

Results of a recent study indicate that bone marrow-derived stem cells transplanted into infarcted rat heart with infarction demonstrate significantly attenuated mRNA expression of collagen types I and III, TIMP-1 and TGFβ1 at 7 and 28 days, suggesting that bone marrow stem cells may inhibit cardiac remodeling and fibrosis [42]. Moreover, Kudo et al. [5] have demonstrated that MSCs transplanted in the mouse heart decrease MI size and fibrosis. The molecular mechanisms involved in this process are unknown. Apoptosis in the heart is inhibited by antioxidants, angiotensin II inhibitors and expression of the antiapoptotic protein Bcl-2 [43–45]. Recent studies suggest that adult stem cell transplantation inhibits apoptosis of host myocardium [46]. Thus, our observation that transplantation of ES cells result in cardiac remodeling and regeneration is associated with improvement in cardiac function. Our unpublished data also suggest that local TIMP-1 levels were increased in the infarcted mouse heart following ES cells transplantation.

It has been reported that CM from Akt-MSCs inhibits apoptosis in cardiomyocytes [32, 33]. Furthermore, genes coding for VEGF, FGF2, HGF, IGF-1 and TB4 were upregulated, and are thus potential mediators of antiapoptotic effects observed with CM from Akt-MSCs [33]. Importantly, our recently published data suggest that antiapoptotic factors released from ES cells inhibit apoptosis and fibrosis in the infarcted heart [47].

Oxidative Stress, Apoptosis, Fibrosis, miRNA and Stem Cells

Oxidative stress appears to be the principle mediator of cardiac myocyte dysfunction in various pathologic conditions, causing both apoptosis and necrosis that leads to fibrosis and cardiac remodeling [2, 43, 44, 48]. We and others have reported significant amount of apoptosis and fibrosis in the models of oxidative stress such as

ischemia-reperfusion, infarcted myocardium and doxorubicin-induced cardiomyopathy and heart failure [2, 43, 44, 49, 50]. Activation of the signaling cascades PI3K/Akt, ERK1/2, TIMP-1 and MMPs have been implicated in cardiac remodeling (apoptosis and fibrosis) induced by a wide variety of stimuli [2, 43, 44, 49, 50]. Use of antioxidant drugs trolox, probucol, carvedilol and other agents such as bradykinin, cardiotrophin-1, insulin, insulin growth factor-1 and urocortin that reduce ischemia-reperfusion injury in animal models is associated with a decrease in apoptosis and fibrosis and an upregulation of the PI3K/Akt, ERK1/2 and TIMP-1 pathways, respectively [2, 43, 44, 49–51]. Moreover, we have recently published that transplanted ES cells inhibit myocardial apoptosis and fibrosis, in vivo [52], as well as factors released from ES cells inhibit H_2O_2-induced H9c2 cell apoptosis in the cell culture [53, 54]. Next, the measured levels of antioxidants using commercially available total antioxidants capacity (TAC) kit (Biovision) in ES cell-conditioned medium were significantly high (~100-fold) compared with the growth medium. These data suggest that inhibition of apoptosis in our ES cell models may be mediated through increased antioxidant levels present in the ES condition medium along with TIMP-1 as reported previously [47, 53].

Additionally, miRNAs are small noncoding RNAs of 20–24 nucleotides and play a major role in the gene regulation during a variety of cell processes including apoptosis, hypertrophy, fibrosis and cardiac differentiation [55–60]. It has been recently reported that miR-21 plays an important role in the enhanced survival of cardiac fibroblast [61]. Stress signals trigger miR-21 that inhibits SPRY1 and increases ERK-MAPK that leads to enhanced fibroblast survival and increased fibrosis, remodeling and cardiac dysfunction in the transgenic mouse model of cardiac failure [61]. As stated above, we demonstrated the presence of apoptosis and fibrosis that leads to cardiac remodeling in the oxidative stress model of infarcted heart and this cardiac remodeling was inhibited with ES cell transplantation that releases antioxidants. However, there are no reports that explore the role of miR-21 pathway in fibrosis and remodeling in the infarcted mouse heart as well as the effects of transplanted ES cells. We postulate that cardiac fibrosis in the infarcted heart is triggered by oxidative stress mediated through the miR-21 pathway associated with enh-anced fibroblast survival that contribute in fibrosis and remodeling with decreased cardiac function. We also predict that antioxidants, antifi-brotic and antiapoptotic factors released from ES cells will inhibit miR-21 and associated ERK-MAPK fibroblast cell survival with decreased fibrosis and remodeling and improved cardiac function.

Recent studies suggest the use of miRNAs and antiapoptotic genes Akt/Bcl2 in cell prolifera-tion, differentiation, hypertrophy and apoptosis [32, 43, 55, 56]. Another study suggests that miR-1 but not miR-133 overexpression in ES cells enhances early cardiac progenitor marker Nkx2.5 [48]. Similarly, miR-1 overexpression in C2C12 myoblasts promotes myogenesis, whereas miR-133 enhances proliferation [56].

Transplanted ES Cells and Teratoma Formation

Mammalian ES cells can form complex teratomas when engrafted into an immune-deficient host is a well-recognized characteristic of ES cells [62, 63]. Following transplantation of ES cells, the formed teratoma include highly organized and well-differentiated cell types representative of all three germ layers including keratinized cells, hair follicles, muscle cells, cardiomyocytes, epithe-lial cells, neural ganglia and pigmented cells [7, 62–64]. Therefore, the hampering of the clinical use of ES cells due to teratoma formation is consid-ered a major potential limitation in its therapeutic use; however, human ES cells with careful atten-tion has already been reached in the clinical trial approved by food and drug administration (FDA).

It has been hypothesized that following trans-plantation, undifferentiated ES cells will be exposed to various combinations of cytokine/growth factor signals in their own local micro-environment of tissue where they would be transplanted. Examined in the liver toxicity model of CCl4, transplanted undifferentiated ES cells (1×10^5 cells) successfully differentiated into hepatic cells, suggesting that local liver-spe-cific cytokines/growth factors may have directed ES cells differentiation into liver-specific cell types, however; no evidence of teratoma forma-tion was observed [9, 65, 66]. Moreover, we and others have shown that transplantation of up to 300,000 undifferentiated ES cells into the infarcted mouse heart by direct injection is safe and effective for cardiac regeneration as no tera-toma was detected for a period of 12 weeks [21]. Similarly, other studies performed have trans-planted undifferentiated ES cells and have not observed teratoma formation in the heart [24, 25, 67]. A detailed study on teratoma formation was conducted by Nussbaum et al. in the heart follow-ing transplantation of varying doses of ES cells (68 suggested that transplantation of fewer than 100,000 undifferentiated ES cells into the mouse heart does not cause teratoma). This study cor-roborated with our published data. Interestingly, they suggested teratomas formation if more than 100,000 ES cells are injected into normal or infarcted mouse hearts [68]. The exact discrepan-cies in these data are not clearly understood, however, a couple of points in this regard are detailed as below. Nussbaum et al. injected 100,000 ES cells in a single intramyocardial injection compared with 30,000 cells injected at three different sites in the mouse heart [9, 68]. It has been predicted that a large number of ES cells injected at a given specific site will lead to the formation of ES cell clumps, which may have generated teratoma formation; however, further studies are needed for better clarification. Recently, BMP2-primed ES cells (30 million) transplanted in infarcted sheep heart shows no evidence of teratoma formation [23].

In contrast, there are studies that suggest that teratoma formation do occur following ES cell transplantation [68, 69]. However, before we reach any clear conclusion on the issue of teratoma formation following transplantation in the heart, we must consider the number of ES cells used for transplantation, priming the ES cells with growth factors and to have better understanding on the microenvironment where ES cells are exposed, see our review for details [70].

Conclusions

Growing progress in cardiac cell therapy is exciting; however, there is still need to identify an appropriate cell type required for complete cardiac regeneration. Moreover, factors released from both ES and adult stem cells demonstrated to be an additional key player in the inhibition of apoptosis and fibrosis which ultimately contributes to improved cardiac function. Clinical trials in the patients using adult stem cells have failed at large; however, modest improvements were evident. Various investigators are modulating existing ES or adult stem cells via priming with growth factors, transfecting stem cells with anti-apoptotic genes to enhance cardiac repair and regeneration. Recently, identified induced pluripotent stem cells from patients and animals have gained another attraction to examine their potential as a future cell type of choice to regenerate injured myocardium. Next, many clinical trials using MSCs and CSCs are ongoing with improved strategies; however, their outcome is still awaiting in the near future.

References

1. Boersma E, Mercado N, Poldermans D, et al. Acute myocardial infarction. Lancet. 2003;361:847–58.
2. Anversa P, Olivetti G, Leri A, et al. Myocyte cell death and ventricular remodeling. Curr Opin Nephrol Hypertens. 1997;6:169–76.
3. Jugdutt BI. Ventricular remodeling after infarction and the extracellular collagen matrix: when is enough enough? Circulation. 2003;108:1395–403.
4. Jugdutt BI, Menon V, Kumar D, et al. Vascular remodeling during healing after myocardial infarction in the dog model: effects of reperfusion, amlodipine and enalapril. J Am Coll Cardiol. 2002;39:1538–45.
5. Kudo M, Wang Y, Wani MA, et al. Implantation of bone marrow stem cells reduces the infarction and fibrosis in ischemic mouse heart. J Mol Cell Cardiol. 2003;35:1113–9.
6. Kumar D, Kamp TJ, LeWinter MM. Embryonic stem cells: differentiation into cardiomyocytes and potential for heart repair and regeneration. Coron Artery Dis. 2005;16:111–6.
7. Singla DK, Sobel BE. Enhancement by growth factors of cardiac myocyte differentiation from embryonic stem cells: a promising foundation for cardiac regeneration. Biochem Biophys Res Commun. 2005;335:637–42.
8. Singla DK, Sun B. Transforming growth factor-beta2 enhances differentiation of cardiac myocytes from embryonic stem cells. Biochem Biophys Res Commun. 2005;332:135–41.
9. Singla DK, Hacker TA, Ma L, et al. Transplantation of embryonic stem cells into the infarcted mouse heart: formation of multiple cell types. J Mol Cell Cardiol. 2006;40:195–200.
10. Puceat M. TGFbeta in the differentiation of embryonic stem cells. Cardiovasc Res. 2006;74:256–61.
11. Kawai T, Takahashi T, Esaki M, et al. Efficient cardiomyogenic differentiation of embryonic stem cell by fibroblast growth factor 2 and bone morphogenetic protein 2. Circ J. 2004;68:691–702.
12. Balsam LB, Wagers AJ, Christensen JL, et al. Haematopoietic stem cells adopt mature haematopoietic fates in ischaemic myocardium. Nature. 2004;428:668–73.
13. Behfar A, Zingman LV, Hodgson DM, et al. Stem cell differentiation requires a paracrine pathway in the heart. FASEB J. 2002;16:1558–66.
14. Beltrami AP, Urbanek K, Kajstura J, et al. Evidence that human cardiac myocytes divide after myocardial infarction. N Engl J Med. 2001;344:1750–7.
15. Haider HK, Ashraf M. Bone marrow stem cell transplantation for cardiac repair. Am J Physiol Heart Circ Physiol. 2005;288:H2557–67.
16. Beltrami AP, Barlucchi L, Torella D, et al. Adult cardiac stem cells are multipotent and support myocardial regeneration. Cell. 2003;114:763–76.
17. Urbanek K, Rota M, Cascapera S, et al. Cardiac stem cells possess growth factor-receptor systems that after activation regenerate the infarcted myocardium, improving ventricular function and long-term survival. Circ Res. 2005;97:663–73.
18. Urbanek K, Torella D, Sheikh F, et al. Myocardial regeneration by activation of multipotent cardiac stem cells in ischemic heart failure. Proc Natl Acad Sci USA. 2005;102:8692–7.
19. Urbanek K, Cesselli D, Rota M, et al. Stem cell niches in the adult mouse heart. Proc Natl Acad Sci USA. 2006;103:9226–31.
20. Urbanek K, Quaini F, Tasca G, et al. Intense myocyte formation from cardiac stem cells in human cardiac hypertrophy. Proc Natl Acad Sci USA. 2003;100:10440–5.
21. Hodgson DM, Behfar A, Zingman LV, et al. Stable benefit of embryonic stem cell therapy in myocardial infarction. Am J Physiol Heart Circ Physiol. 2004;287:H471–9.
22. Spinale FG. Matrix metalloproteinases: regulation and dysregulation in the failing heart. Circ Res. 2002;90:520–30.

23. Menard C, Hagege AA, Agbulut O, et al. Transplantation of cardiac-committed mouse embryonic stem cells to infarcted sheep myocardium: a preclinical study. Lancet. 2005;366:1005–12.

24. Kofidis T, de Bruin JL, Yamane T, et al. Insulin-like growth factor promotes engraftment, differentiation, and functional improvement after transfer of embryonic stem cells for myocardial restoration. Stem Cells. 2004;22:1239–45.

25. Kofidis T, de Bruin JL, Yamane T, et al. Stimulation of paracrine pathways with growth factors enhances embryonic stem cell engraftment and host-specific differentiation in the heart after ischemic myocardial injury. Circulation. 2005;111:2486–93.

26. Emgard M, Hallin U, Karlsson J, et al. Both apoptosis and necrosis occur early after intracerebral grafting of ventral mesencephalic tissue: a role for protease activation. J Neurochem. 2003;86:1223–32.

27. Guerette B, Skuk D, Celestin F, et al. Prevention by anti-LFA-1 of acute myoblast death following transplantation. J Immunol. 1997;159:2522–31.

28. Nakano M, Matsumoto I, Sawada T, et al. Caspase-3 inhibitor prevents apoptosis of human islets immediately after isolation and improves islet graft function. Pancreas. 2004;29:104–9.

29. Schierle GS, Hansson O, Leist M, et al. Caspase inhibition reduces apoptosis and increases survival of nigral transplants. Nat Med. 1999;5:97–100.

30. Muller-Ehmsen J, Whittaker P, Kloner RA, et al. Survival and development of neonatal rat cardiomyocytes transplanted into adult myocardium. J Mol Cell Cardiol. 2002;34:107–16.

31. Zhang M, Methot D, Poppa V, et al. Cardiomyocyte grafting for cardiac repair: graft cell death and antideath strategies. J Mol Cell Cardiol. 2001;33:907–21.

32. Gnecchi M, He H, Liang OD, et al. Paracrine action accounts for marked protection of ischemic heart by Akt-modified mesenchymal stem cells. Nat Med. 2005;11:367–8.

33. Gnecchi M, He H, Noiseux N, et al. Evidence supporting paracrine hypothesis for Akt-modified mesenchymal stem cell-mediated cardiac protection and functional improvement. FASEB J. 2006;20:661–9.

34. Anversa P, Kajstura J, Olivetti G. Myocyte death in heart failure. Curr Opin Cardiol. 1996;11:245–51.

35. Anversa P, Kajstura J. Myocyte cell death in the diseased heart. Circ Res. 1998;82:1231–3.

36. Anversa P, Leri A, Kajstura J, et al. Myocyte growth and cardiac repair. J Mol Cell Cardiol. 2002;34:91–105.

37. Jugdutt BI. Remodeling of the myocardium and potential targets in the collagen degradation and synthesis pathways. Curr Drug Targets Cardiovasc Haematol Disord. 2003;3:1–30.

38. Askari AT, Brennan ML, Zhou X, et al. Myeloperoxidase and plasminogen activator inhibitor 1 play a central role in ventricular remodeling after myocardial infarction. J Exp Med. 2003;197:615–24.

39. Creemers E, Cleutjens J, Smits J, et al. Disruption of the plasminogen gene in mice abolishes wound healing after myocardial infarction. Am J Pathol. 2000; 156:1865–73.

40. Creemers EE, Cleutjens JP, Smits JF, et al. Matrix metalloproteinase inhibition after myocardial infarction: a new approach to prevent heart failure? Circ Res. 2001;89:201–10.

41. Takeshita K, Hayashi M, Iino S, et al. Increased expression of plasminogen activator inhibitor-1 in cardiomyocytes contributes to cardiac fibrosis after myocardial infarction. Am J Pathol. 2004;164:449–56.

42. Xu X, Xu Z, Xu Y, et al. Selective down-regulation of extracellular matrix gene expression by bone marrow derived stem cell transplantation into infarcted myocardium. Circ J. 2005;69:1275–83.

43. Kumar D, Lou H, Singal PK. Oxidative stress and apoptosis in heart dysfunction. Herz. 2002;27:662–8.

44. Kumar D, Jugdutt BI. Apoptosis and oxidants in the heart. J Lab Clin Med. 2003;142:288–97.

45. Limana F, Urbanek K, Chimenti S, et al. bcl-2 overexpression promotes myocyte proliferation. Proc Natl Acad Sci USA. 2002;99:6257–62.

46. Kocher AA, Schuster MD, Szabolcs MJ, et al. Neovascularization of ischemic myocardium by human bone-marrow-derived angioblasts prevents cardiomyocyte apoptosis, reduces remodeling and improves cardiac function. Nat Med. 2001;7:430–6.

47. Fatma S, Selby DE, Singla RD, et al. Factors released from embryonic stem cells stimulate c-kit-FLK-1(+ve) progenitor cells and enhance neovascularization. Antioxid Redox Signal. 2010;13:1857–65.

48. Ivey KN, Muth A, Arnold J, et al. MicroRNA regulation of cell lineages in mouse and human embryonic stem cells. Cell Stem Cell. 2008;2:219–29.

49. Kumar D, Kirshenbaum L, Li T, et al. Apoptosis in isolated adult cardiomyocytes exposed to adriamycin. Ann NY Acad Sci. 1999;874:156–68.

50. Kumar D, Kirshenbaum LA, Li T, et al. Apoptosis in adriamycin cardiomyopathy and its modulation by probucol. Antioxid Redox Signal. 2001;3:135–45.

51. Hausenloy DJ, Yellon DM. Survival kinases in ischemic preconditioning and postconditioning. Cardiovasc Res. 2006;70:240–53.

52. Singla DK, Lyons GE, Kamp TJ. Transplanted embryonic stem cells following mouse myocardial infarction inhibit apoptosis and cardiac remodeling. Am J Physiol Heart Circ Physiol. 2007;293:H1308–14.

53. Singla DK, McDonald DE. Factors released from embryonic stem cells inhibit apoptosis of H9c2 cells. Am J Physiol Heart Circ Physiol. 2007;293: H1590–5.

54. Singla DK, Singla RD, McDonald DE. Factors released from embryonic stem cells inhibit apoptosis in H9c2 cells through P1-3kinase/Akt but not ERK pathway. Am J Physiol Heart Circ Physiol. 2008;295: H907–13.

55. Care A, Catalucci D, Felicetti F, et al. MicroRNA-133 controls cardiac hypertrophy. Nat Med. 2007;13: 613–8.

56. Chen JF, Mandel EM, Thomson JM, et al. The role of microRNA-1 and microRNA-133 in skeletal muscle proliferation and differentiation. Nat Genet. 2006;38: 228–33.

57. Kwon C, Han Z, Olson EN, et al. MicroRNA1 influences cardiac differentiation in *Drosophila* and regulates Notch signaling. Proc Natl Acad Sci USA. 2005;102:18986–91.

58. van Rooij E, Sutherland LB, Liu N, et al. A signature pattern of stress-responsive microRNAs that can evoke cardiac hypertrophy and heart failure. Proc Natl Acad Sci USA. 2006;103:18255–60.

59. van Rooij E, Olson EN. MicroRNAs: powerful new regulators of heart disease and provocative therapeutic targets. J Clin Invest. 2007;117:2369–76.

60. van Rooij E, Olson EN. MicroRNAs put their signatures on the heart. Physiol Genomics. 2007;31: 365–6.

61. Thum T, Gross C, Fiedler J, et al. MicroRNA-21 contributes to myocardial disease by stimulating MAP kinase signalling in fibroblasts. Nature. 2008;456: 980–4.

62. Reubinoff BE, Pera MF, Fong CY, et al. Embryonic stem cell lines from human blastocysts: somatic differentiation in vitro. Nat Biotechnol. 2000;18: 399–404.

63. Thomson JA, Itskovitz-Eldor J, Shapiro SS, et al. Embryonic stem cell lines derived from human blastocysts. Science. 1998;282:1145–7.

64. Gertow K, Wolbank S, Rozell B, et al. Organized development from human embryonic stem cells after injection into immunodeficient mice. Stem Cells Dev. 2004;13:421–35.

65. Kuai XL, Cong XQ, Du ZW, et al. Treatment of surgically induced acute liver failure by transplantation of HNF4-overexpressing embryonic stem cells. Chin J Dig Dis. 2006;7:109–16.

66. Moriya K, Yoshikawa M, Saito K, et al. Embryonic stem cells develop into hepatocytes after intrasplenic transplantation in CCl4-treated mice. World J Gastroenterol. 2007;13:866–73.

67. Min JY, Yang Y, Converso KL, et al. Transplantation of embryonic stem cells improves cardiac function in postinfarcted rats. J Appl Physiol. 2002;92:288–96.

68. Nussbaum J, Minami E, Laflamme MA, et al. Transplantation of undifferentiated murine embryonic stem cells in the heart: teratoma formation and immune response. FASEB J. 2007;21:1345–57.

69. Swijnenburg RJ, Tanaka M, Vogel H, et al. Embryonic stem cell immunogenicity increases upon differentiation after transplantation into ischemic myocardium. Circulation. 2005;112:I166–72.

70. Singla DK. Embryonic stem cells in cardiac repair and regeneration. Antioxid Redox Signal. 2009;11: 1857–63.

Part II

Cardiac Hypertrophy and Heart Failure

Macroscopic and Microscopic Aspects of Cardiac Dysfunction in Congestive Heart Failure

Henk E.D.J. ter Keurs

Abstract

The macroscopic hallmarks of congestive heart failure (CHF) are slowed cardiac contraction and relaxation as well as loss of the inotropic effect of increased heart rate. Over time these abnormalities may progress causing ultimate pump failure and life-threatening arrhythmias. At the microscopic level, the calcium ion (Ca^{2+}) plays a crucial role in normal cardiac contraction. However, Ca^{2+} trafficking may go astray in CHF and jeopardize the exquisite mechanism of systole and diastole, triggering arrhythmias. Several factors, including gene mutations, acute ischemia, and unfavourable cardiac remodelling, modify Ca^{2+} transport at various loci in cardiac myocytes and may weaken the cells. The interplay between weakened and strong segments in non-uniform cardiac muscle may further lead to mechano-electric feedback mediating an early diastolic Ca transient caused by the rapid force decrease during the relaxation phase. These rapid force changes in non-uniform muscle may cause arrhythmogenic Ca^{2+} waves to propagate by activation of neighbouring SR by diffusing Ca^{2+} ions.

Keywords

Congestive heart failure • Systole • Diastole • Tachycardia-induced inotropism • Arrhythmias

Introduction

Function of Normal Myocardium

H.E.D.J. ter Keurs (✉)
Department of Physiology and Biophysics,
University of Calgary, Calgary, Alberta, Canada
e-mail: terkeurs@ucalgary.ca

This chapter will summarize macroscopic and microscopic cardiac dysfunctions against the background of a description of the principles of the normally functioning heart. The normal heart

N.S. Dhalla, M. Nagano, B. Ostadal (eds.), *Molecular Defects in Cardiovascular Disease*,
DOI 10.1007/978-1-4419-7130-2_8, © Springer Science+Business Media, LLC 2011

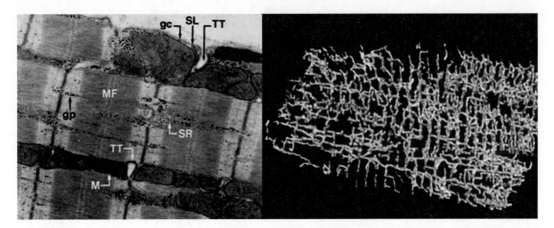

Fig. 1 Space is at a premium in the cardiac myocyte which is densely packed with myofibrils (MF) accompanied by sarcoplasmic reticulum (SR), which are connected by dyads to transverse tubules (TT) and are powered by the mitochondria (Mit). The *right-hand panel* (Modified from [1]) shows that the transverse tubules form a dense mesh in the cardiac cell with both transverse and longitudinal components

contracts at regular intervals driven by the electrical impulses of the sinus node. When the energy demand of the body increases, the macroscopic response of the heart consists of increased haemodynamic energy delivery to the circulation at an increased but still regular heart rate [2]. It is well known that force of the heart beat is adjusted to the requirements of the circulation by several mechanisms (1) stretch underlying Starling's law of the heart; (2) the "Anrep"-effect of stretch on the concentration of calcium (Ca^{2+}) ions in the cytosol and hence in the storage organelle of the myocyte: the sarcoplasmic reticulum (SR); (3) the positive inotropic effects of increased heart rate; (4) the effects of nor-adrenaline on Ca^{2+} transport in the myocyte as well as the responsiveness of the contractile apparatus to Ca^{2+} ions; (5) the effects of both hormonal systems and mechanical loading conditions on growth of cardiac cells; (6) the effects of modification of the composition of cardiac cells that accompany growth in a manner that is specific for the stimulus that induces growth. The first four mechanisms are quite fast and generate a new steady in less than a minute or even instantaneously such as the Starling effect. The effects of growth are remarkably rapid as well but a new steady state still requires several months to achieve a steady state.

In order to achieve a forceful heart beat as well as rapid complete relaxation in-between heart beats, Ca^{2+} ions should rapidly appear and disappear rapidly stays and at the right time in the cardiac myocyte. For the purpose of the current discussion, we will defend the simplest scenario that allows a heart to contract and put the maximal amount of energy into the circulation during systole while it completely relaxes and receives venous blood during diastole as a superbly compliant structure. How this might work is a useful introduction into the mainstay of the discussion what might happen when Ca^{2+} trafficking goes astray in congestive heart failure (CHF).

Figure 1 shows that a cardiac myocyte is completely packed with myofibrils enveloped in a network of Ca^{2+} storing intracellular tubules (the sarcoplasmic reticulum or SR) and mitochondria which accompany virtually every sarcomere in the myofibril. The cell membrane conveys electrical information in the form of the action potential in a fraction of a millisecond to the latter trio of organelles by tubules, which invaginate the surface perpendicular to the cell axis at every Z-disk.

The transverse tubules form a network that extends cell membrane and extracellular space throughout the core of the cell and reduces the

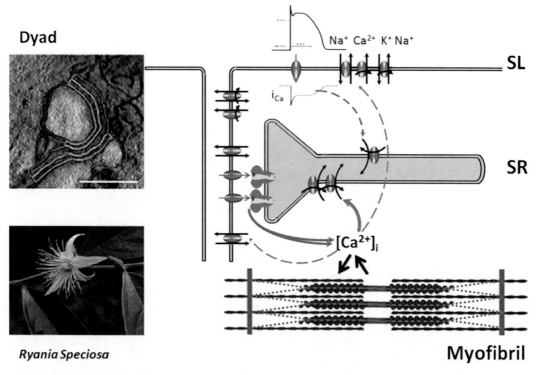

Dyad

Ryania Speciosa

Myofibril

Fig. 2 Magnification of a dyad, the contact site of SR, and TT[4]. The diagram illustrates the sequence of Ca^{2+} events starting with the action potential. The Ca^{2+} channels of the SR dominate the scene because of the magnitude of its Ca^{2+} fluxes (indicated by *arrows*; *red* for Ca^{2+} release; *green* for Ca^{2+} removal; and *black* indicating the interaction with the contractile proteins). The plant *Ryania speciosa* (*inset*) defends itself against insects by the production of the alkaloid ryanodine which binds specifically to the SR-Ca^{2+} channel. The dominant ligand for Ca^{2+} in the cardiac myocyte is the troponin-C molecule on the actin filament

distance between extracellular events and the centre of the sarcomere to less than a micrometer. The transverse tubules comprise ~60% of the total cell membrane area [3]. Calcium transport, as in the model illustrated in Fig. 2, allows the heart to cycle between diastole and systole by shuttling Ca^{2+} ions between the extracellular milieu and the interior of the myocytes and even more importantly by shuttling Ca^{2+} ions between the SR and the cytosol.

An asset of cardiac muscle, that allows rapid activation and relaxation of cardiac muscle, is that when the transverse tubules pass the SR a specialized structure, the dyad or triad, is formed by the terminal cisternae of the SR which embrace the transverse tubular membrane [4, 5] (Fig. 2). Ca^{2+} channels and Na^+/Ca^{2+} exchange proteins (NCX) occupy the transverse tubular

membranes co-localizing with the Ca^{2+} channels of the SR [named after ryanodine, the insecticidal alkaloid produced by the plant *Ryania speciosa* (Fig. 2)]. At the interface between the terminal cisternae transverse tubular proteins, especially L-type Ca^{2+} channels make close contact with Ca^{2+} channels of the SR. Some of the terminal cisternae remain free.

Figure 2 shows the relationship between the membrane action potential, which invades the myocyte along its transverse tubules and Ca^{2+} release by the SR. In short, a large Na^+ current carried by several Na^+ channel isoforms [6] rapidly depolarizes the cell to +30 mV in a millisecond. The i_{Na} raises the [Na^+] in the dyadic cleft and reverses the gradient for Na^+–Ca^{2+} exchange; the increased [Na^+] dissipates in a few milliseconds. The depolarization also opens (again in a millisecond) the membrane L-type Ca^{2+} channels. Rapid partial repolarization to 0 mV by the transient outward K^+ current (i_{to}) drives a maximal Ca^{2+} current spike through the Ca^{2+} channels [7] into the clefts of the dyads and triads between the transverse tubules and the terminal cisternae of the SR [8, 9]. The Ca^{2+} ions in the clefts bind to regulatory sites on the cytosolic domains of L-type Ca^{2+} channel itself and rapidly –but partially – inactivate the channels terminating the Ca^{2+} current spike and leaving a tonic Ca^{2+} current until the cells repolarize to −40 mV. Second, binding of Ca^{2+} to the Ca-binding domains (CBDs) of NCX rapidly activates [10–12] the exchanger and allows Ca^{2+} entry through "reverse mode" transport by NCX adding to Ca^{2+} entry into the cleft [10]. Lastly, Ca^{2+} binds to the ryanodine receptors, which triggers a large and rapid flux of Ca^{2+} ions through these channels from the SR into the cytosol. The magnitude of the Ca^{2+} flux depends on the degree of filling of the SR with Ca^{2+} ions and the interval between the action potentials because the ryanodine receptors need to recover (~0.3 s) before they are ready for the next release.

The released Ca^{2+} diffuses over a very short distance (~1 μm) into the cytosol of the adjacent myofibril and starts two simultaneous events. The mechanically important event is that Ca^{2+} binds to the protein troponin-C on the actin filaments in sarcomeres of the myofibril. Binding of Ca^{2+} to troponin-C starts a chain reaction which results in the movement of the inhibitory protein tropomyosin away from the binding sites for myosin cross-bridges, thus enabling the cross-bridges to convert chemical energy of ATP into force development and sliding of the filaments and thus sarcomere shortening. This process is amazingly close to synchronous in the hundred million billion sarcomeres of the normal left ventricle and allows rapid pressure development and brisk ejection of blood [13].

The event that is important to relaxation is that released Ca^{2+} also reaches the Ca^{2+} pumps [the sarco-endoplasmic Ca^{2+} pump proteins (SERCA2)] of the SR that envelops the same myofibril. SERCA2 responds to a slight rise in the concentration of Ca^{2+} by rapidly sequestering Ca^{2+} back into the SR. A more modest amount (~30%) of the released Ca^{2+} is simultaneously extruded from the cell by ion-exchange proteins that borrow the energy from the gradient of Na^+ ions across the cell membrane. This Na/Ca exchanger (NCX) is also important because 3–4 Na^+ ions enter the cell during transport of a single Ca^{2+} ion. By consequence the cell tends to become more positive during extrusion of Ca^{2+}. During the normal action potential this Ca^{2+} extrusion by NCX only slows the repolarization somewhat, but we will see the consequences of this depolarization when spontaneous Ca^{2+} release occurs later in this chapter.

We know that the transverse tubules carry more than half of the NCX molecules of the membrane and also a substantial fraction of the L-type Ca^{2+} channels. Ca^{2+} ions enter through both proteins during the action potential and thus add to the Ca^{2+} load of the SR. The presence of these transport molecules in the transverse tubular membrane contributes to the heart rate-dependent increase in force owing to an increase of the amount of Ca^{2+} that enters the cell per unit time. Hence, increasing the heart rate increases the Ca^{2+} load of the SR and thereby increases Ca^{2+} release following the action potential. In terms of macroscopic behaviour of the heart, this phenomenon is known as the inotropic effect of increased heart rate.

An interesting puzzle is whether the Ca^{2+} transport shows any activity during diastole. The answer to this puzzle is complex. It has long been known that ion channels may open spontaneously, although this is at rest (of the channel) a rare event. It is not unexpected that when a L-type Ca^{2+} channel opens in the transverse tubule, the resulting Ca^{2+} influx may trigger Ca^{2+} release by ryanodine receptors or clusters thereof in the terminal cisternae: these events are now known as Ca^{2+} sparklets triggering Ca^{2+} sparks [14, 15]. Furthermore, the ryanodine receptors respond to Ca^{2+}; so some may respond to Ca^{2+} release by neighbouring terminal cisternae by Ca^{2+} release. This phenomenon is noticeable in the form of Ca^{2+} waves in cardiac myocytes.

The puzzle regarding spontaneous activity of the Ca^{2+} system during diastole, thus reduces to the question: do Ca^{2+} sparks and Ca^{2+} waves occur

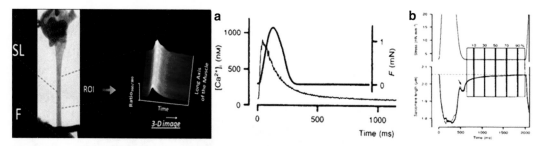

Fig. 3 Trabeculae, endocardially running fascicles of myocardium, respond to an action potential by uniform calcium release, uniform sarcomere length changes followed by quiescence during the diastolic interval

during diastole in normal myocardium? Again, we propose a simple scenario: the incidence of these events in normal cardiac fascicles is vanishingly small. We do so on the basis of many years of work with isolated cardiac fascicles or trabeculae that can be found on the endocardial side of the ventricle. We have used trabeculae from many species, including ferret, cat, pig, and rabbit, but the main source over the years has been the rat right ventricle. Their behaviour is strikingly similar. It has been shown by Loiselle et al. [16] that these muscles are virtually identical to the fascicles that comprise the wall of the heart. The attraction of using these thin (usually <100 μm) muscles is that one can study the contractile process at the level of the sarcomeres, by using light-diffraction techniques, while loading the specimen with Ca^{2+}-sensitive fluorescent dyes permits continuous measurement of the cytosolic $[Ca^{2+}]$. Figure 3 reveals that the action potential-induced $[Ca^{2+}]$ transient is uniform and shows a rapid rise and a simple monotonic decline throughout the muscle without variations in time or space during diastole.

The action potential brings the muscle from a compliant passive structure to the impressive force of ~0.5 kg cm^{-2}. In these experiments, the sarcomeres shorten during contraction because they are able to stretch the connections of the muscle with the equipment. After relaxation, sarcomere length remains constant without perceptible fluctuations [17] and the microscopic image of the muscle is crystal clear and completely quiescent [18]. Studies using confocal microscopy after loading of the muscle with the ester of the Ca^{2+} probe Fluo 4(-AM) confirm that the cells neither show Ca^{2+}

sparks nor Ca^{2+} waves. These observations support the notion that cells in intact normal myocardium are completely quiescent during diastole. The consequence of the resulting low $[Ca^{2+}]$ in the cytosol is that the passive force in the structure is completely supported by the titin molecules inside the myocytes (see Fig. 2) and the collagen meshwork surrounding myocytes and collagen bundles alongside the fascicles [19–21]. Some studies have suggested that a small amount of spontaneous contractile activity can be found in normal cells or normal muscle, but in our hands spontaneous activity was usually caused by the experimenter, for example by raising the $[Ca^{2+}]$ in the medium surrounding the muscle.

Interaction Between $[Ca^{2+}]$ and Force Development

The release of Ca^{2+} by the SR amounts to ~40 μM per heart beat and brings the free $[Ca^{2+}]_i$ from ~0.1 to ~1 μM. The most important cellular ligand for Ca^{2+} is troponin-C (75 μM in the cell), which has one binding site for Ca^{2+} ions at this range of $[Ca^{2+}]_i$, but probably binds Ca^{2+} ions by one or more cooperative mechanisms. Three cooperative mechanisms are currently actively studied: (1) troponin-C bound to Ca^{2+} enhances binding of Ca^{2+} ions by the neighbouring troponin-C, (2) cross-bridge attachment enhances binding of Ca^{2+} ions to adjacent troponin-C, and (3) force exerted by the cross-bridges on the actin filament deforms actin and the troponin complex riding on actin and allosterically enhances binding of

Fig. 4 Model of activation of the contractile proteins. The released Ca²⁺ ions bind to the regulatory protein on actin in the myofibril and allow force development. Force development itself retards the dissociation of Ca²⁺ from the troponin-C–Ca complex, thereby enhancing the sensitivity of cardiac muscle to Ca²⁺

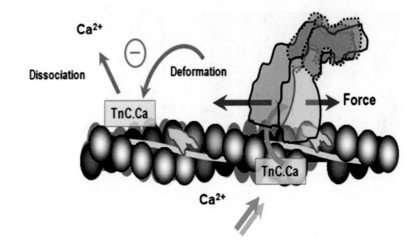

Ca²⁺ ions to troponin-C on the filament by slowing the rate at which the Ca²⁺ ion leaves the troponin-C–Ca complex (the off-rate of Ca²⁺). These feedback mechanisms are of outstanding importance in the heart because they permit a highly effective coupling between the Ca²⁺ release process and the mechanical response of the sarcomere to the released Ca²⁺ ions (Fig. 4).

In fact, we have shown [22] that the feedback of cross-bridge force to Ca²⁺ binding predicts fundamental properties known for cardiac muscle. The molecular mechanism that couples actin deformation to the troponin-C–Ca²⁺ off-rate is unknown, but in view of the realistic reproduction of the steady-state force–[Ca²⁺] relationships and force–sarcomere length relationships at varied activation levels for $[Ca^{2+}]_i$, the mechanism merits further investigation. This interaction between force and Ca²⁺ predicts that the muscle behaves during the heart beat as if it were in a steady state and shows only little effect of shortening against a load, thereby explaining that the end systolic force sarcomere length relationship is fixed as has been observed experimentally [23]. Hence, this interaction between force and Ca²⁺ binding to troponin-C explains the well-known end systolic pressure volume relationship of the left ventricle as well as Starling's law of the heart [22]. The combination of these predictions of the postulated force-Ca-troponin-C feedback makes it a useful working model for cardiac muscle and should stimulate further

studies of the dynamics of the interaction between troponin-C and Ca²⁺.

The time course of $[Ca^{2+}]_i$ and force during contraction is predicted by this model and is similar to those in experiments on trabeculae. We will see that an important consequence of this behaviour is that a force-decrease accelerates dissociation of Ca²⁺ from Ca²⁺–troponin-C. This phenomenon is experimentally well known [24, 25]; therefore, we propose that the latter mechanism plays an important role in non-uniform muscle and may be arrhythmogenic.

Congestive Heart Failure

Too Little Ca²⁺: Slower Release and Slower Removal

Myocardial infarction (MI) leads to ventricular dilatation and dysfunction and ultimately to CHF. There is considerable evidence that failure of Ca²⁺ transport in myocytes is a central cause of contractile dysfunction in CHF. Left ventricular myocardial infarction (MI) causes remodelling of infarct area into a scar as well as remodelling of and viable myocardium to enable it to generate the increased workload. With time though, a substantial infarct may be followed by CHF; characterized by reduced force of the heart beat as well as slower onset of contraction and slower relaxation. One of the hall marks of CHF has been shown to be that muscle strips from LV of human hearts in CHF develop less force than those from normal LV, especially at increased heart rate [26]. The same is found in the experimental studies of CHF. The important consequence of the loss of inotropism of an increased heart rate is that the heart loses a powerful feedback mechanism which normally allows it to respond to and increased haemodynamic load. Hence, the heart will rely more on other feedback mechanisms, such as increased filling pressure and increased β-adrenergic drive which may enhance further patho-physiological remodelling. The fundamental question, therefore, is: what are the causes of the reduced force output?

Several hypotheses have been put forward to account for the observed reduction of contractile force in CHF. We will focus here on the abnormalities that pertain to abnormal Ca^{2+} transport. The trigger for Ca^{2+} release by the SR is probably reduced as a result of the loss of transient outward K^+ current (which is known to occur in CHF [27, 28]), because the action potential decays in that scenario abnormally slowly from the Na^+ equilibrium potential, which reduces the driving force for Ca^{2+} current through the L-type Ca^{2+} channels. Because Ca^{2+} release is steeply dependent on i_{L-Ca} [29], the reduced Ca^{2+} influx triggers a smaller Ca^{2+} release through the SR-Ca^{2+} channels [30]. Furthermore, the reduced early Ca^{2+} entry through the L-type Ca^{2+} channels will delay the activation of the Na/Ca exchanger so that the contribution of Ca^{2+} entry through early reverse mode Na/Ca exchange will decrease further lowering the trigger for SR-Ca^{2+} release [31]. Both mechanisms would lead to a reduction of force at increased heart rate, which is the hallmark of CHF.

Reduced SR-Ca^{2+} pump activity described in both human CHF and experimental models of CHF is accompanied by increased expression and activity of the Na^+/Ca^{2+} exchanger [32]. Such changes could be responsible for slower relaxation of muscles in CHF, reduced SR-Ca^{2+} load and force, particularly at increased heart rate.

Both dysregulation of SR-Ca^{2+} channels and inadequate coupling between T-tubular L-type Ca^{2+} channels and the corresponding SR-Ca^{2+} channels have been proposed. Both could lead to

reduced force in CHF; however, such changes would be frequency independent.

The action potential duration (APD) of myocytes from hearts in CHF is increased as it is in LVH. Such APD prolongation is expected to permit an increased Ca^{2+} influx [33], providing an increased SR-Ca^{2+} load [34] and would counter the effects of changes in SERCA2 and NCX on force in CHF. On the other hand, there is mounting evidence that maintenance of structurally intact transverse tubules is at fault in CHF: the tubules are not rigorously connected to the surface membrane anymore and their regular structure is lost [35]. We know that the transverse tubules carry more than half of the NCX molecules of the membrane and also a substantial fraction of the L-type Ca^{2+} channels. Ca^{2+} ions enter through both proteins during the action potential and thus contribute to the Ca^{2+} load of the SR. Loss of this source of Ca^{2+} would contribute to reduced inotropism of increased heart rate in CHF. Furthermore, regions of the cell that lose their tight coupling to the action potential owing to loss of the transverse tubular proximity will now rely more on Ca^{2+} diffusion and propagated Ca^{2+} release and the rate of development of force will decrease. The loss of the proximity of NCX predicts a shift of Ca^{2+} removal toward SERCA2. Therefore, relaxation in CHF muscle is slowed even more.

Ca^{2+} at the Wrong Time: Diastolic Ca^{2+} Sparks, Ca^{2+} Waves, and Contractions

Multiple populations of Ca^{2+} sparks have been identified in normal rat trabeculae, as well as in guinea pig myocytes. Myocytes from SHR rats with LVH, cells exhibit an increased global Ca^{2+} transient as well as a redistribution of Ca^{2+} sparks to those with larger amplitudes without any changes in ryanodine receptors proteins. "Big" sparks in hypertrophied cells occurred without an alteration in trigger Ca^{2+} or overall SR content [36]. On the other hand, Ca^{2+} sparks appeared lower and slower in human myocytes from failing hearts. Gomez et al. showed in models ranging from LVH to CHF no changes of sparks when compared to control and suggested that

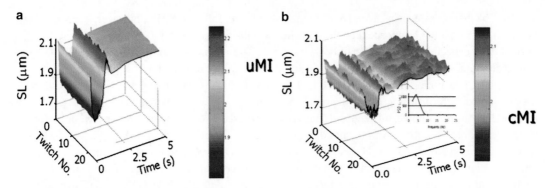

Fig. 5 Hypertrophy of rat cardiac muscle such as after a myocardial infarction does not yet affect quiescence of the Ca^{2+} transport system (uMI in *panel* a). However, development of frank CHF by the animal is associated with dramatic spontaneous diastolic Ca^{2+} release leading to spontaneous diastolic sarcomere contractions and loss of active force (cMI in *panel* b)

abnormalities in EC coupling in these CHF cells may be due to the changes in the spatial organization of the dyad. Some ryanodine receptors in transverse tubuli are coupled to L-type Ca^{2+} channels but other ryanodine receptors maybe "orphaned" [37]. That is, ryanodine receptors are still able to function but are "physically" isolated from Ca^{2+} influx channels, predicting reduced global cellular Ca^{2+} transients [38].

Lakatta's group observed that light-scatter by papillary muscles of normal rat fluctuated spontaneously. These fluctuations appeared related to spontaneous random sarcomere contractions in cells. Spontaneous light intensity fluctuations appeared to be coupled to asynchronous Ca^{2+} oscillations and caused increased force of the muscle during diastole as well as reduced active force development [39]. These findings differ quantitatively from the behaviour of sarcomeres in non-failing trabeculae, which are typically quiescent during diastole at physiological $[Ca^{2+}]_o$. Figure 5a illustrates both the quiescence during diastole and reproducible shortening during the twitch (Figs. 3 and 5a) as well as rapid uniform lengthening during relaxation [40].

Figure 5 shows dramatically that this uniform behaviour is lost in trabeculae from the heart of animals with CHF, where spontaneous sarcomere motion occurs at low $[Ca^{2+}]$ and increased steeply with further increase of $[Ca^{2+}]_o$. This increase

was sevenfold larger in the muscles from CHF compared to controls. Microscopic inspection of these muscles confirmed that the spontaneous sarcomere length variations were in fact caused by Ca^{2+} waves causing contractions that propagate within individual cells. The spontaneous diastolic activity caused the shortening of sarcomeres following an action potential to become highly variable and reduced force of the twitch by as much as 30% [18]. Spontaneous diastolic activity also increased following stimulation at a high rate and during catecholamine stimulation in cardiac muscle from CHF and contributing to the inability of failing cardiac muscle to increase its force in response to increased heart rate and sympathetic stimulation.

The spontaneous diastolic contractile activity in CHF appears to be due to a greater sensitivity of SR-Ca^{2+} channels to the SR-Ca^{2+} load. Fabiato described in the early 1970s that the SR starts to release its Ca^{2+} when the amount of Ca^{2+} in the SR exceeds a threshold level [41, 42]. Indeed, reduction of the SR-Ca^{2+} load in muscles from animals with CHF – for example by a small amount of ryanodine – eliminated the spontaneous contractions and restored force development. The failure of membrane L-type Ca^{2+} channel blockers to do the same reinforces the notion that the malfunction underlying spontaneous activity in CHF resides in the SR-Ca^{2+} channel. It is not yet known what the molecular mechanism of this abnormality is, although several mechanisms have been proposed including channel oxidation or nitrosylation [40].

Excessive phosphorylation of the channel owing to the high β_1-adrenergic drive of the heart in chronic CHF has been postulated as a cause of spontaneous Ca^{2+} leak from the SR. Intuitively this is an attractive proposition because β-blockers, especially Carvedilol, form the backbone of treatment of CHF, CHF in dog and human heart is thought to be accompanied by increased phosphorylation of ryanodine receptors by protein-kinase-A (PKA) causing the protein FK506-binding protein (FKBP)12.6 to dissociate from ryanodine receptors, which increases the open probability of ryanodine receptors [41]. However, the question whether ryanodine receptors are excessively phosphorylated in CHF is debated and the effect of increased phosphorylation of ryanodine receptors on dissociation of FKBP12.6 from ryanodine receptors is controversial [42–46].

The behaviour of the SR-Ca^{2+} channels has been explored in detail since the discovery that mutations of the SR-Ca^{2+} channel protein are involved in malignant arrhythmias. Interestingly, recent work has shown that variants of the cardiac ryanodine receptor may associate (the A allele of the rs3766871 variant) with the incidence of lethal cardiac arrhythmias in acquired CHF or (the A allele of the rs790896 variant) may act as a protective factor against sudden cardiac death [47].

Ca^{2+} Coming from the "Wrong" Source: Troponin-C

Non-uniform muscle. Arrhythmias are a main contributor to mortality in CHF patients. Electrical non-uniformity plays a major role in the re-entry mechanism of arrhythmia and has been well investigated [48]. Much less is known about arrhythmogenicity of non-uniform segmental wall motion, with areas of hypokinesis, akinesis, and dyskinesis, which are well-known signs of ischemic heart disease and CHF [49, 50]. Differences in the motion pattern around the LV may result from changes in the intrinsic force-generating

capacity of the myocytes in the fascicles, which may cause reduced systolic shortening or even lead to segment lengthening during contraction of surrounding healthier tissue. For example, acute ischemia causes acute loss of force-generating capacity of the cardiac cell by impairment of excitation–contraction coupling and may lead to non-uniform systolic strain distribution in the LV wall. We have also seen in the above that spontaneous random diastolic Ca^{2+} release weakens the segment in which this occurs and therefore leads to weak segments contracting in series with more normal strong segments. Although non-uniform excitation contraction coupling has been linked to a variety of arrhythmogenic heart diseases [51], the role of non-uniform contraction in arrhythmogenesis has received far less attention.

Arrhythmogenic Ca^{2+} Waves in Non-uniform Muscle

Several studies have shown that contraction of non-uniform myocardium itself causes the generation of Ca^{2+} waves. The increased free $[Ca^{2+}]$ during these waves activates NCX-mediated Ca^{2+} extrusion and Ca^{2+}-sensitive non-selective channels in the sarcolemma and therefore induces delayed after-depolarizations (DADs) that trigger action potentials[53]. This arrhythmogenic phenomenon in non-uniform myocardium has been coined reverse excitation contraction coupling [52–55]. Reverse excitation contraction coupling may be clinically relevant as it has been shown that when patients receive resynchronization pacing which can improve the mechanical uniformity, both the incidence of sudden death and the degree of heart failure are reduced [56].

The behaviour of weak and strong segments of myocardium [57] is predicted by a force balance owing to their force–length relationship and force–velocity relationships. The strong segments stretch the weaker segments of myocardium during systole and release the weaker segment rapidly during relaxation. *Intriguingly*, we found that the force decline during relaxation is accompanied by a Ca^{2+} surge which triggers Ca^{2+} waves starting from the border between the segments.

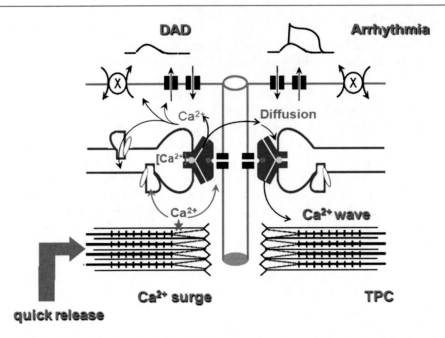

Fig. 6 A model for Ca²⁺-mediated arrhythmias: Rapid reduction of force (e.g. quick release of a weak segment by relaxation of the strong segment) induces a surge of Ca²⁺ ions coming off troponin-C. The SR is sufficiently recovered to respond by local Ca²⁺ release. Ca²⁺ diffuses along the cell and triggers further Ca²⁺ release in the form of Ca²⁺ waves. The rise of [Ca²⁺] owing to these events leads to NCX-mediated Ca²⁺ extrusion. This process depolarizes the cell (DAD) and may initiate a new action potential

These Ca²⁺ waves always start during force relaxation of a contraction and propagate into both the strong and the weak segments. The local [Ca²⁺]$_i$ surge occurs always at the same moment during relaxation. We have proposed that this cause is probably Ca²⁺ that dissociates from troponin-C. It is important to repeat here that troponin-C–Ca is a huge reservoir of Ca²⁺ ions during contraction. This Ca²⁺ is normally transported back to the SR and extruded from the cell, but during non-uniform contractions this reservoir can release so much Ca²⁺ that it triggers SR-Ca²⁺ release in the absence of an action potential. This phenomenon appeared to be highly arrhythmogenic; on the other hand the arrhythmias disappeared when the muscle uniformity was restored [55].

We proposed in the above that the molecular mechanism underlying force dependence of Ca²⁺ binding to troponin-C is probably that cross-bridge force exerted on the actin filament deforms the troponin-C molecule, thus retarding the dissociation of Ca²⁺ from troponin-C (Fig. 3) [57].

This mechanism predicts that the observed Ca²⁺ surge starts upon rapid relaxation of the strong segments which rapidly unloads the weak segments [13, 58]. The initial Ca²⁺ surge following rapid force relaxation can be explained by force feedback to Ca²⁺ binding by TnC, because the rapid force decline is expected to accelerate Ca²⁺ dissociation form TnC. This Ca²⁺ surge occurs when the SR-Ca²⁺ channels have recovered sufficiently from the last action potential-driven Ca²⁺ release so that they can respond to the Ca²⁺ surge by renewed Ca²⁺ release, which then propagates mediated by diffusion of Ca²⁺ along the length of the myofibrils as illustrated in Fig. 6. The transient increase of [Ca²⁺]$_i$ during this process leads to a depolarization owing to NCX-mediated Ca²⁺ removal called a DAD, because it occurs during diastole. When the DAD exceeds the threshold for action potential generation recurrence of this process may induce the spontaneous series of action potentials that comprises a triggered arrhythmia.

Discussion and Outlook

Cardiac fascicles, made non-uniform so that a segment becomes weaker than the adjacent muscle segments, show three patterns of response in or near the weakened segment (1) a local Ca^{2+} surge late during relaxation; (2) the surge triggers propagated Ca^{2+} waves; (3) the Ca^{2+} wave may trigger arrhythmia. SR-loading facilitates the generation of Ca^{2+} waves. Figure 6 clearly shows that these arrhythmias are completely reversible and disappear when uniformity in the muscle is restored. The requirements for the initiation of arrhythmogenic Ca^{2+} waves are that the region from where the Ca^{2+} waves start has a Ca^{2+}-loaded SR and exhibits active contraction, albeit weaker than that of the adjacent muscle. These requirements are met in the border of the weak segment if the paradigm to weaken the segment lowers intracellular $[Ca^{2+}]$ or SR-Ca^{2+} load, or reduces cross-bridge activity. The same requirements are met inside the weak segment following the exposure of the muscle to $[Ca^{2+}]_o$ levels which reduce contractile force in proportion to an increase of spontaneous Ca^{2+} release by the overloaded SR, as in failing heart. The mechanism of propagation of the Ca^{2+} waves needs further study in order to fully explain the high propagation velocity of the waves and test the hypothesis of Ca^{2+} diffusion coupled by Ca^{2+} diffusion, which permits a high propagation velocity if the Ca^{2+} ligands in the cell are partially occupied.

Conclusions

We have seen that several factors, including gene mutations, acute ischemia, and unfavourable cardiac remodelling, modify Ca^{2+} transport at various loci in cardiac myocytes and may weaken the cells in CHF especially at increased heart rate. In this scenario, the interplay between weaker and stronger segments in non-uniform cardiac muscle may cause arrhythmogenic Ca^{2+} waves to propagate by activation of neighbouring SR by diffusing Ca^{2+} ions. Facing the problem of treatment and prevention of arrhythmias it is re-assuring that the development of drugs that stabilize the Ca^{2+}-handling system has started [59].

Acknowledgements This work was supported by grants HL-58860-O6A2 and HL-66140 from the National Heart and Lung Institute of the NIH, by the Canadian Institutes for Health Research, and the Heart and Stroke Foundation of Alberta, the North West Territories, and Nunavut. H.E.D.J. ter Keurs is Senior Investigator of the Alberta Heritage Foundation for Medical Research.

References

1. Jayasinghe ID, Cannell MB, Soeller C (2009) Organization of ryanodine receptors, transverse tubules and sodium calcium exchanger in rat myocytes. Biophys. J 97:2664–2673.
2. Endoh M. Force-frequency relationship in intact mammalian ventricular myocardium: physiological and pathophysiological relevance. Eur J Pharmacol. 2004;500:73–86.
3. Pasek M, Simurda J, Christe G, et al. Modelling the cardiac transverse-axial tubular system. Prog Biophys Mol Biol. 2008;96:226–43.
4. Maio A, Karko K, Snopko RM, et al. T-tubule formation in cardiacmyocytes: two possible mechanisms? J Muscle Res Cell Motil. 2007;28:231–41.
5. Hayashi T, Martone ME, Yu ZY, et al. Three-dimensional electron microscopy reveals new details of membrane systems for Ca^{2+} signaling in the heart. J Cell Sci. 2009;122:1005–13.
6. Maier SK, Westenbroek RE, Schenkman KA, et al. An unexpected role for brain-type sodium channels in coupling of cell surface depolarization to contraction in the heart. Proc Natl Acad Sci USA. 2002;99:4073–8.
7. Polakova E, Zahradnikova Jr A, Pavelkova J, et al. Local calcium release activation by DHPR calcium channel openings in rat cardiac myocytes. J Physiol. 2008;586:3839–54.
8. Renken C, Hsieh CE, Marko M, et al. Structure of frozen-hydrated triad junctions: a case study in motif searching inside tomograms. J Struct Biol. 2009;165:53–63.
9. ter Keurs HEDJ, Boyden PA. Calcium and arrhythmogenesis. Physiol Rev. 2007;87:457–506.
10. Neco P, Rose B, Huynh N, et al. Sodium-calcium exchange is essential for effective triggering of calcium release in mouse heart. Biophys J. 2010;99:755–64.
11. Hilge M, Aelen J, Perrakis A, et al. Structural basis for Ca^{2+} regulation in the Na^+/Ca^{2+} exchanger. Ann NY Acad Sci. 2007;1099:7–15.
12. Hilge M, Aelen J, Foarce A, et al. Ca^{2+} regulation in the Na^+/Ca^{2+} exchanger features a dual electrostatic switch mechanism. Proc Natl Acad Sci USA. 2009;106:14333–8.

13. Hunter PJ, McCulloch AD, ter Keurs HEDJ. Modelling the mechanical properties of cardiac muscle. Prog Biophys Mol Biol. 1998;69:289–331.

14. Cheng HP, Lederer WJ. Calcium sparks. Physiol Rev. 2008;88:1491–545.

15. Wang SQ, Song LS, Lakatta EG, et al. Ca^{2+} signalling between single L-type Ca^{2+} channels and ryanodine receptors in heart cells. Nature. 2001;410:592–6.

16. Goo S, Joshi P, Sands G, et al. Trabeculae carneae as models of the ventricular walls: implications for the delivery of oxygen. J Gen Physiol. 2009;134:339–50.

17. Stuyvers BD, Miura M, ter Keurs HE. Dynamics of viscoelastic properties of rat cardiac sarcomeres during the diastolic interval: involvement of Ca^{2+}. J Physiol. 1997;502:661–77.

18. Obayashi M, Xiao BL, Stuyvers BD, et al. Spontaneous diastolic contractions and phosphorylation of the cardiac ryanodine receptor at serine-2808 in congestive heart failure in rat. Cardiovasc Res. 2006;69:140–51.

19. Granzier HL, Labeit S. The giant protein titin: a major player in myocardial mechanics, signaling, and disease. Circ Res. 2004;94:284–95.

20. Baudino TA, Carver W, Giles W, et al. Cardiac fibroblasts: friend or foe? Am J Physiol Heart Circ Physiol. 2006;291:H1015–26.

21. Hanley PJ, Young AA, LeGrice IJ, et al. 3-Dimensional configuration of perimysial collagen fibres in rat cardiac muscle at resting and extended sarcomere lengths. J Physiol. 1999;517:831–7.

22. ter Keurs HEDJ, Shinozaki T, Zhang YM, et al. Sarcomere mechanics in uniform and non-uniform cardiac muscle: A link between pump function and arrhythmias. Prog Biophys Mol Biol. 2008;97:312–31.

23. Suga H, Yamada O, Goto Y, et al. Peak isovolumic pressure-volume relation of puppy left ventricle. Am J Physiol. 1986;250:167–72.

24. Housmans PR, Lee NKM, Blinks JR. Active shortening retards the decline of the intracellular calcium transient in mammalian heart muscle. Science. 1983;221:159–61.

25. Kurihara S, Komukai K. Tension-dependent changes of the intracellular Ca^{2+} transients in ferret ventricular muscles. J Physiol. 1995;489:617–25.

26. Mulieri LA, Hasenfuss G, Leavitt B, et al. Altered myocardial force-frequency relation in human heart failure. Circulation. 1992;85:1743–50.

27. Beuckelmann DJ, Nabauer M, Erdmann E. Alterations of $^{K+}$ currents in isolated human ventricular myocytes from patients with terminal heart failure. Circ Res. 1993;73:379–85.

28. Nabauer M, Kaab S. Potassium channel down-regulation in heart failure. Cardiovasc Res. 1998;37:324–34.

29. Polakova E, Zahradnikova Jr A, Pavelkova J, et al. Local calcium release activation by DHPR calcium channel openings in rat cardiac myocytes. J Physiol. 2008;586:3839–54.

30. Cooper PJ, Soeller C, Cannell MB. Excitation-contraction coupling in human heart failure examined by action potential clamp in rat cardiac myocytes. J Mol Cell Cardiol. 2010;49:911–7.

31. Thomas MJ, Sjaastad I, Andersen K, et al. Localization and function of the Na^+/Ca^{2+}-exchanger in normal and detubulated rat cardiomyocytes. J Mol Cell Cardiol. 2003;35:1325–37.

32. Hobai IA, O'Rourke B. Enhanced Ca^{2+}-activated Na^+-Ca^{2+} exchange activity in canine pacing-induced heart failure. Circ Res. 2000;87:690–8.

33. Tomaselli GF, Marban E. Electrophysiological remodeling in hypertrophy and heart failure. Cardiovasc Res. 1999;42:270–83.

34. Sah R, Ramirez RJ, Kaprielan R, et al. Alterations in action potential profile enhances excitation-contraction coupling in rat cardiac myocytes. J Physiol. 2001;533:201–14.

35. Brette F, Orchard C. Resurgence of cardiac T-tubule research. Physiology (Bethesda). 2007;22:167–73.

36. Izu LT, Mauban JR, Balke CW, et al. Large currents generate cardiac Ca^{2+} sparks. Biophys J. 2001;80:88–102.

37. Gomez AM, Guatimosim S, Dilly KW, et al. Heart failure after myocardial infarction: altered excitation-contraction coupling. Circulation. 2001;104:688–93.

38. Sobie EA, Guatimosim S, Gomez-Viquez L, et al. The Ca^{2+} leak paradox and rogue ryanodine receptors: SR Ca^{2+} efflux theory and practice. Prog Biophys Mol Biol. 2006;90:172–85.

39. Lakatta EG. Functional implications of spontaneous sarcoplasmic reticulum Ca^{2+} release in the heart. Cardiovasc Res. 1992;26:193–214.

40. Davidoff AW, Boyden PA, Schwartz K, et al. Congestive heart failure after myocardial infarction in the rat: cardiac force and spontaneous sarcomere activity. Ann NY Acad Sci. 2004;1015:84–95.

41. Fabiato A, Fabiato F. Excitation-contraction coupling of isolated cardiac fibers with disrupted or closed sarcolemma. Circ Res. 1972;31:293–307.

42. Fabiato A. Calcium-induced release of calcium from the cardiac sarcoplasmic reticulum. Am J Physiol Cell Physiol. 1983;245:C1–14.

43. Marx SO, Reiken S, Hisamatsu Y, et al. PKA phosphorylation dissociates FKBP12.6 from the calcium release channel (ryanodine receptor): defective regulation in failing hearts. Cell. 2000;101:365–76.

44. Jiang DW, Xiao BL, Wang RW, et al. RyR2 mutations linked to ventricular tachycardia increase store overload induced Ca^{2+} release (SOICR) activity and luminal Ca^{2+} activation without altering FKBP12.6-RyR2 interaction. Biophys J. 2005;88:189A.

45. Xiao BL, Jiang MT, Zhao MC, et al. Characterization of a novel protein kinase a phosphorylation site, serine-2030, reveals no hyperphosphorylation of the cardiac ryanodine receptor in heart failure. Biophys J. 2005;88:188A.

46. Xiao JM, Tian XX, Jones PP, Bolstad J, Kong HH, Wang RW, et al. Removal of FKBP12.6 does not alter the conductance and activation of the cardiac ryanodine receptor or the susceptibility to stress-induced ventricular arrhythmias. J Biol Chem. 2007;282:34828–38.

47. Ran Y, Chen J, Li N, et al. Common RyR2 variants associate with ventricular arrhythmias and sudden

cardiac death in chronic heart failure. Clin Sci (Lond). 2010;119(5):215–23.

48. Kleber AG, Rudy Y. Basic mechanisms of cardiac impulse propagation and associated arrhythmias. Physiol Rev. 2004;84:431–88.

49. Young AA, Dokos S, Powell KA, et al. Regional heterogeneity of function in nonischemic dilated cardiomyopathy. Cardivasc Res. 2001;49:308–18.

50. Siogas K, Pappas S, Graekas G, et al. Segmental wall motion abnormalities alter vulnerability to ventricular ectopic beats associated with acute increases in aortic pressure in patients with underlying coronary artery disease. Heart. 1998;79:268–73.

51. Janse MJ. Electrophysiological changes in heart failure and their relationship to arrhythmogenesis. Cardiovasc Res. 2004;61:208–17.

52. ter Keurs HEDJ, Shinozaki T, Zhang YM, et al. Sarcomere mechanics in uniform and nonuniform cardiac muscle: a link between pump function and arrhythmias. Ann NY Acad Sci. 2008;1123:79–95.

53. ter Keurs HEDJ, Zhang YM, Miura M. Damage induced arrhythmias: reversal of excitation-contraction coupling. Cardiovasc Res. 1998;40:444–55.

54. Miura M, Wakayama Y, Endoh H, et al. Spatial nonuniformity of excitation-contraction coupling can enhance arrhythmogenic-delayed afterdepolarizations in rat cardiac muscle. Cardiovasc Res. 2008; 80:55–61.

55. Wakayama Y, Miura M, Stuyvers BD, et al. Spatial nonuniformity of excitation-contraction coupling causes arrhythmogenic Ca^{2+} waves in rat cardiac muscle. Circ Res. 2005;96:1266–73.

56. Cleland JGF, Daubert JC, Erdmann E, et al. Longer-term effects of cardiac resynchronization therapy on mortality in heart failure [the CArdiac REsynchronization-Heart Failure (CARE-HF) trial extension phase]. Eur op Heart J. 2006;27: 1928–32.

57. ter Keurs HEDJ, Wakayama Y, Sugai Y, et al. Role of sarcomere mechanics and Ca^{2+} overload in Ca^{2+} waves and arrhythmias in rat cardiac muscle. Ann NY Acad Sci. 2006;1080:248–67.

58. Wakayama Y, Sugai Y, Kagaya Y, et al. Stretch and quick release of cardiac trabeculae accelerates Ca^{2+} waves and triggered propagated contractions. Am J Physiol Circ Physiol. 2001;281:H2133–42.

59. Wehrens XH, Lehnart SE, Reiken SR, et al. Protection from cardiac arrhythmia through ryanodine receptor-stabilizing protein calstabin2. Science. 2004; 304:292–6.

Cardiac Dysfunction and Metabolism: Unravelling the Molecular Cross-Talk

Vijay Sharma and John H. McNeill

Abstract

The interactions between cardiac metabolism and function at the molecular level are complex, but can be understood in terms of several broad concepts. First, function and metabolism are linked by acute mechanisms involving coupling of ATP demand to ATP synthesis, AMPK activation and various covalent and allosteric modifications of key enzymes, and by transcriptional mechanisms. Second, altered metabolic fluxes are not primary causes of cardiac injury; injury is caused by the cytoplasmic accumulation of toxic metabolic intermediates. These intermediates accumulate when there is a mismatch between the supply and utilization of metabolic fuels, and this can be produced either by excessive supply or reduced metabolic flux of a fuel. Third, changes in metabolism can be adaptive (as occurs in physiological hypertrophy), maladaptive in parallel with cardiac dysfunction (as occurs in pathological hypertrophy), or maladaptive as an antecedent and cause of cardiac dysfunction (as occurs in pathological hypertrophy). Finally, from an evolutionary perspective, disease results when the metabolic and functional phenotype is inappropriate for the environment; this can result from a phenotypically inappropriate response (e.g. pathological hypertrophy), or from a constraint that prevents the heart from adapting appropriately (e.g. reduced metabolic reserve). This book chapter reviews the latest evidence that is emerging about the operation of interactions between metabolism and function at the metabolic level in terms of these key concepts.

J.H. McNeill (✉)
Division of Pharmacology and Toxicology,
Faculty of Pharmaceutical Sciences,
The University of British Columbia,
Vancouver, Canada
e-mail: jmcneill@interchange.ubc.ca

N.S. Dhalla, M. Nagano, B. Ostadal (eds.), *Molecular Defects in Cardiovascular Disease*,
DOI 10.1007/978-1-4419-7130-2_9, © Springer Science+Business Media, LLC 2011

Keywords

Diabetes • Cardiac metabolism • Cardiac hypertrophy • Mitochondrial respiration • Myocardial energetic • Diabetic cardiomyopathy • Foetal gene program • Fibrosis • Oxidative stress • Sarcomere • β-Oxidation • Circadian clock • BMal • Ceramide • NFAT pathway • Exercise training • Insulin • Sirtuins • Resveratrol • Cardiac risk factors • Apoptosis

Introduction

There has been increasing interest in recent years in the interrelationship between heart function and metabolism, and the extent to which alterations in cardiac metabolism are causes or consequences of cardiac dysfunction. It has been shown that, in the advanced stages of disease, the hypertrophied and failing heart increases its reliance on glycolysis and glucose oxidation, although fatty acid oxidation remains the predominant fuel [1–3]. This change occurs in parallel with the development of pathological hypertrophy and heart failure. Conversely, in the diabetic heart, a shift of metabolism occurs which precedes the onset of heart failure. Transport of glucose into the cardiomyocyte is dependent on the Glut-4 transporter whose translocation, translation, and transcription are all decreased by diabetes [4]. The diabetic heart is, therefore, less able to use glucose as an energy source, and relies more heavily on alternative substrates such as fatty acids and ketones [5]. The cross-talk between cardiac function and metabolism is complex, and the challenge now facing researchers is not only to identify the pathways involved, but also to determine the contribution these pathways make to the development of heart failure.

Regulation of Cardiac Metabolism

The heart requires a constant supply of adenosine triphosphate (ATP) for muscular contraction and the maintenance of ionic homeostasis [6]. Under aerobic conditions most of this ATP (>95%) is generated by mitochondrial oxidative phosphorylation. Oxidation of energy substrates is coupled to the reduction of nicotinamide adenine dinucleotide (NADH) and flavoproteins. ATP and its metabolic intermediates are continuously channelled between the mitochondria, the myofibrils, the sarcoplasmic reticulum and the sarcolemma. This exquisite coupling system between oxidative phosphorylation and myofibril contraction allows ATP demand to be precisely and instantly met over a wide range of workloads (see ref. [7] for review). Further communication is required to ensure that the supply of energy substrates responds to changes in ATP demand. This role is fulfilled by AMP-activated protein kinase (AMPK), which is activated by an increase in the AMP/ATP ratio (a signal of ATP depletion) and acts to deactivate ATP-consuming pathways and activate ATP-producing pathways [8].

The heart is an omnivorous organ which has the ability to use any energy substrate provided to it (lipids, carbohydrates, ketone bodies, and amino acids); however, the normal heart derives most of its ATP from the metabolism of fatty acids and carbohydrates [9]. Although fatty acid oxidation produces more ATP, glucose oxidation is more efficient in terms of oxygen consumption. For optimal cardiac efficiency, the normal heart maintains a balance of 60–80% fatty acid oxidation and 20–40% pyruvate oxidation; the heart derives approximately equal amounts of pyruvate from glycolysis and lactate metabolism [10, 11]. Ketone utilization is concentration-dependent; in situations where blood ketone levels rise (starvation and diabetes), ketones become a major cardiac fuel [12, 13].

The metabolism of glucose and fatty acids by the heart is summarized in Fig. 1. Glucose-6-phosphate, the glycolytic substrate, is obtained from endogenous glycogen stores and from exogenous glucose taken up by the Glut-1 and Glut-4

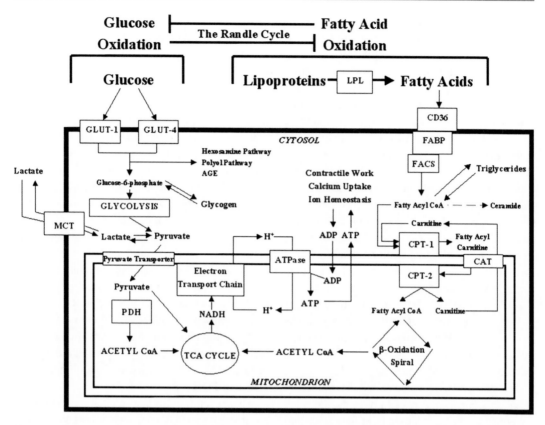

Fig. 1 Summary of fatty acid and glucose metabolism. Glucose is taken up by Glut-1 and Glut-4 transporters and is converted by glycolysis to pyruvate. Pyruvate then enters the mitochondria to be oxidized, producing acetyl CoA. Fatty acids are liberated from lipoproteins by LPL, and are taken up by CD36 and FABP. LCAS converts the fatty acid to a CoA ester which is then taken up by the carnitine shuttle system to the mitochondria. The fatty acyl CoA undergoes β-oxidation, removing two carbons per turn of the cycle and generating acetyl CoA. Acetyl CoA, generated by either pathway, enters the TCA cycle to generate reducing equivalents (NADH). These pass electrons to the electron transport chain which creates an electrochemical proton gradient to drive ATP synthesis. ATP synthesis is exquisitely coupled to the systems which create the ATP demand (*LPL* lipoprotein lipase, *CD36* fatty acid translocase, *FABP* fatty acid-binding protein, *FACS* fatty acyl CoA synthase, *CPT* carnitine palmitoyltransferase, *CAT* carnitine acyl transferase, *CoA* coenzyme A, *TCA cycle* tricarboxylic acid cycle, *AGE* advanced glycosylation end-product, *PDH* pyruvate dehydrogenase, *MCT* monocarboxylate transporter, *PDH* pyruvate dehydrogenase, *NADH* reduced nicotinamide adenine dinucleotide, *ATP* adenosine triphosphate, *ADP* adenosine monophosphate)

glucose transporters. Glucose uptake is regulated by Glut-4 and is responsible for the majority of glucose uptake [11, 14, 15]. Glycolysis comprises a series of reactions which convert glucose-6-phosphate to pyruvate. In the normal aerobic heart, the major fate of pyruvate is decarboxylation to acetyl CoA, catalyzed by the pyruvate dehydrogenase complex (PDH) in the mitochondria [16]. Lactate is metabolized to pyruvate, but pyruvate is also metabolized to lactate. Under aerobic conditions, the normal heart is a net consumer of lactate; the heart only becomes a net producer of lactate when the glycolytic flux exceeds the rate of pyruvate oxidation [11].

Fatty acids are released from chylomicrons and VLDL by lipoprotein lipase (LPL) on the luminal surface and are then taken up into the cardiomyocyte by fatty acid transporters such as CD36 [17]. Upon entry to the cytoplasm, fatty acids are bound by fatty acid-binding protein (FABP) until they are esterified to fatty acyl CoA by fatty acyl CoA synthetase (FACS). Fatty acyl CoA has two major fates: it can enter the mitochondria to be oxidized, or it can be esterified to triglyceride and store [18, 19]. A small proportion of palmitoyl CoAs is also converted to ceramides [19].

Whereas short and medium-chain acyl CoAs can pass freely into the mitochondria to be oxidized, long-chain acyl CoAs cannot cross the mitochondrial membrane and must be transported. This function is carried out by a carnitine-dependent shuttle system, consisting of carnitine palmitoyltransferase 1 (CPT-1), carnitine palmitoyltransferase 2 (CPT-2), and carnitine acyltransferase (CAT). Acyl CoA enters the β-oxidation spiral, a series of four reactions which cleaves two carbons (one acetyl CoA molecule) from the acyl CoA molecule per cycle and generates NADH and $FADH_2$. There are specific enzymes for long-, medium-, and short-chain acyl CoAs [20]. Acetyl CoA enters the TCA cycle to generate additional reducing equivalents which drive oxidative phosphorylation.

The rate of fatty acid oxidation is determined by the plasma concentration of fatty acids, the work performed by the heart, the entry of fatty acids into the cytoplasm, the entry of fatty acids into the mitochondrion, and the activity of the enzymes involved in the β-oxidation spiral [14, 21]. High rates of fatty acid oxidation increase the ratios of $NADH/NAD^+$ and acetyl CoA/free CoA, both of which feedback and inhibit glucose oxidation by decreasing flux through PDH [14]. High rates of fatty acid oxidation also increase citrate production. Citrate inhibits glycolysis by inhibiting the key glycolytic enzyme phosphofructokinase (PFK). This is known as the Randle cycle. Conversely, high rates of glycolysis and glucose oxidation can feed back to inhibit fatty acid oxidation. At the level of CPT-1, fatty acid oxidation is controlled by malonyl CoA, a potent inhibitor which binds CPT-1 on the cytosolic side [22]; tonic inhibition of CPT-1 by malonyl CoA is always present, but a rise in malonyl CoA levels inhibits fatty acid oxidation while a fall relieves inhibition [23, 24]. Metabolism in the heart is summarized in Fig. 1.

Regulation of the expression of the enzymes, transporters, and kinases that comprise the metabolic machinery enables the heart to adapt more permanently when the stimulus to do so is sustained. The mitochondria contain DNA which codes for 13 electron transport chain subunits (for complexes 1, III, IV, and V), but all other components of the metabolic machinery are coded for in the nuclear DNA [25]. There are several important inter-related nuclear transcriptional regulators of metabolism genes. The first are the peroxisome proliferator-activated receptors (PPARs). PPARs form heterodimers with retinoid X receptors (RXR). Formation of an active PPAR/RXR complex requires binding of (1) 9-cis-retinoic acid to the RXR and (2) long-chain fatty acids or an exogenous PPAR ligand to the PPAR. Upon activation, the complex translocates to the nucleus and binds to PPAR response elements (PPREs) within the promoter regions of its target genes. In the heart, the major isoform is PPAR-α, and its target genes encompass the full pathway of fatty acid metabolism from fatty acid uptake to the β-oxidation spiral, as well as pyruvate dehydrogenase kinase-4 (PDK-4), the major inhibitory kinase of PDH [26].

The second important regulator is PPAR-γ coactivator-1α (PGC-1α). PGC-1α regulates the capacity of the cell to generate ATP so that, when ATP demand increases, the reserve of the metabolic machinery can meet the demand [27, 28]. The major role of PGC-1α in cardiac muscle is to increase mitochondrial biogenesis and mitochondrial oxidative phosphorylation capacity. PGC-1α binds and enhances the action of other transcription factors including PPAR-α, myocyte-enhancer factor 2A (MEF-2A), and orphan nuclear receptor oestrogen-related receptor α ($ERR^{-\alpha}$) [29, 30].

Cardiac Hypertrophy

Cardiac hypertrophy refers to an increase in cardiomyocyte size (accompanied by increased protein synthesis and reorganization of sarcomeric structure) without cardiomyocyte multiplication, and is the major mechanism by which growth of the heart occurs after birth [31, 32]. Its importance to the study of heart failure is illustrated by its close association with heart failure and its known causes (most notably hypertension and ischaemic heart disease) and by the fact that its presence is a predictor of heart failure progression and confers a worse prognosis.

There are two forms of cardiac hypertrophy:

1. Physiological hypertrophy is a reversible adaptation which increases cardiac output to meet increased metabolic demands. It occurs postnatally and in response to pregnancy or exercise. At the molecular level, the expression of sarcomeric proteins is increased.

2. Pathological hypertrophy is a response to pathological stress signals such as neurohormonal activation, sustained increases in pressure (either due to backpressure from a downstream constriction, or from systemic hypertension), inflammation, or injury. Myocardial vascularization is impaired and fibrosis occurs. At the molecular level, the most notable change is a shift in gene expression from the adult to the foetal pattern, referred to as the "foetal gene program". Foetal genes are considered markers of pathological hypertrophy. Increased parallelism of muscle fibres which reduces their collective ability to generate force [33].

The induction of cardiac hypertrophy is associated with a number of changes in metabolism. A shift in substrate preference from fatty acids to glucose is seen in both physiological and pathological hypertrophy. Acceleration of glycolysis is an additional change which occurs only in pathological hypertrophy [1, 33–35]. Although up-regulation of glycolytic enzymes has been reported in this setting [36, 37], acceleration of glycolysis cannot be fully explained by changes in gene or protein expression, and is predominantly due to changes in the acute regulation of glycolytic flux which are incompletely understood. AMPK has been implicated as a mediator of accelerated glycolysis. AMPK is activated in pathological hypertrophy. Inhibition of AMPK ameliorates accelerated glycolysis but does not prevent it, indicating that other pathways must also be involved [38, 39]. By contrast, the decrease in fatty acid oxidation is predominantly due to decreased expression of fatty acid oxidative enzymes and fatty acid uptake/transport proteins [1, 33–35, 40]. However, low levels of myocardial carnitine, a cofactor required for fatty

acid uptake into mitochondria by the carnitine shuttle system, have also been implicated [40].

PPAR-α has been reported to be down-regulated in cardiac hypertrophy, which partly explains the decrease in fatty acid oxidation that occurs [41], and the polymorphism PPARA IVS7 2498 is associated with left ventricular hypertrophy in humans [42]. Activation of PPAR-γ can prevent cardiac hypertrophy induced by angiotensin-II or endothelin-1 [43, 44]. PPAR-γ agonists can attenuate the cardiac hypertrophic response to pressure overload [44, 45]. The mechanism involves binding of PPAR-γ to NFATc4 which prevents NFATc4 translocation to the nucleus and, therefore, inhibits the calcineurin/NFAT pathway [46, 47]. Despite these findings, the role of PPAR-γ in cardiac hypertrophy is less clear than that of PPAR-α, partly because its expression levels probably vary between the cell types present. Also, clinical trials of PPAR-γ agonists in cardiovascular disease (carried out to investigate the benefits of their insulin-sensitizing properties) have produced conflicting results; most notably, the DREAM trial identified a small but significant increase in the occurrence of congestive heart failure with rosiglitazone treatment [48]. Concern about the adverse cardiovascular effects of rosiglitazone recently led to its withdrawal from the European market.

Nuclear factor-κB is simultaneously involved in switching the substrate preference of the heart from fatty acids to glucose and in the activation of the foetal gene program. Five family members of NF-κB exist of which the p105/p50 is most crucial for this role. The same pathway can also be activated by unloading of the heart; in this situation, it has been found that loss of p105/p50 attenuates down-regulation of PPAR-α genes and the switch to glucose preference, but does not affect activation of the foetal gene program [49]. The NF-κB pathway can also be activated in response to oxidative stress induced by a range of stimuli, including cytokines and hyperglycemia. Activation of fibrotic and hypertrophic responses by this pathway has been extensively studied, but thorough evaluation of the metabolic consequences is awaited [50–54].

Ligand binding of PPARs requires the recruitment of coactivators such as PGC-1α and heterodimerization with the RXR. PGC-1α is enriched in metabolically active tissues, and is responsible for regulating the capacity of the cell for oxidative phosphorylation, regulating genes involved in oxidative phosphorylation, fatty acid oxidation, and mitochondrial biogenesis [28, 55–57]. PGC-1α expression in the heart increases after birth and during starvation, and in both cases this is associated with an increase in fatty acid oxidation [28].

It is unclear whether either physiological or pathological hypertrophy is always associated with significant alterations in the levels of PGC-1α or its target genes. Studies have produced conflicting results; no change [58–61], an increase [62–65], and a decrease [66] in PGC-1α levels and/or its known gene targets have been reported. However, recent studies have established a molecular link between PGC-1α signalling and the hypertrophic response in the cyclin-dependent kinase-7 (Cdk7)/cyclin H/ménage-a-trois-1 (MAT1) heterotrimer. PGC-1α coactivators require MAT1 for their operation. MAT1, in turn, is activated in response to hypertrophic growth signals from the Gq, calcineurin-, and biomechanical stress-dependent pathways [67]. Cardiac-specific ablation of MAT1 does not alter the normal growth of the heart but leads to the development of fatal heart failure. This is associated with selective repression of energy metabolism genes, including known PGC-1α targets [67]. To our knowledge, studies looking at MAT1 overexpression have not been carried out.

There is clearer evidence that progression to heart failure is associated with a dramatic impairment of mitochondrial function which has been observed in a wide range of animal models [68–73] and in humans [74, 75]. Down-regulation of PGC-1α and its target genes in heart failure, as well as of other transcription factors involved in mitochondrial biogenesis (mtTFA, NRFs), has also been reported in numerous animal models of heart failure [59, 69, 76–78] and in humans [79]. These data indicate that while down-regulation of PGC-1α is not a consistently observed feature of physiological or pathological hypertrophy in the absence of heart failure, it is a key feature of progression to heart failure.

Studies of cardiac-specific PGC-1α overexpression and knockout have revealed important insights into the interrelation between cardiac metabolism and function. The response of the heart to targeted PGC-1α overexpression depends on the developmental stage [57]:

1. When induced during neonatal life, overexpression causes marked mitochondrial proliferation with a detrimental effect on cardiac function.
2. When induced during adult life, overexpression causes modest mitochondrial proliferation with accumulation of aggregates of abnormal mitochondria. Wall thinning and chamber dilation occurs, associated with cardiac dysfunction.
3. Constitutive PGC-1α overexpression causes marked proliferation of large mitochondria leading to a severe dilated cardiomyopathy with systolic dysfunction and massive oedema. The cardiomyopathy is fatal and the mice die within 6 weeks of birth.

Cardiac-specific knockout of PGC-1α produces cardiac dysfunction and a diminished capacity to increase work when hearts are exposed to physiological stimuli. Fatty acid oxidation and overall oxidative capacity are reduced, associated with down-regulation of mitochondrial genes. Intriguingly, mitochondrial volume is unaltered, suggesting that other transcription factors can compensate for the role of PGC-1α in mitochondrial biogenesis, but not for its role in cardiac metabolism [80, 81].

Responses to exercise training in mice, a model of physiological hypertrophy, have been assessed following combined cardiomyocyte-specific knockout of the IGF-1 receptor and the insulin receptor (CIGF1RKO mice) and knockout of the insulin receptor alone (CIRKO mice). The hypertrophic response to exercise includes increases in PGC-1α and glycogen content in this model, and this response was preserved following isolated loss of insulin signalling but prevented by the combined loss of insulin receptor and IGF-1 signalling. In the latter situation, glycogen content and PGC-1α were not increased, meaning that the capacity of the heart to increase its capacity for oxidative phosphorylation was blunted, and AMPK was activated presumably in response to the energetic stress imposed by the exercise regime [82].

PGC-1α is subject to deacetylation and activation by sirtuin-1 (SIRT-1). Sirtuins have been implicated as mediators of lifespan expansion [83]. SIRT-1 has been implicated in a range of metabolic responses including regulation of oxidative metabolism (which is likely to be via its effects on PGC-1α), insulin signalling, and tolerance to oxidative stress [84–86]. SIRT-1 is activated by the plant-derived polyphenol resveratrol which has been shown to exhibit a range of cardioprotective effects [87–90].

Diabetic Cardiomyopathy

Diabetic cardiomyopathy is a disease process in which diabetes produces a direct and continuous myocardial insult even in the absence of ischemic, hypertensive, or valvular disease. It can act synergistically with hypertension or ischemia to damage heart muscle, but can also cause heart failure in its own right. The clinical course of diabetic cardiomyopathy is long, and can be divided into three stages [91]. In the early stage, the cardiomyopathy presents with mild asymptomatic diastolic dysfunction which is associated with ultrastructural changes in tissue architecture, impaired calcium handling, oxidative stress, and changes in cardiac metabolism. As the disease progresses, evidence of left ventricular hypertrophy appears which is associated with more severe diastolic dysfunction and mild systolic dysfunction. Cardiomyocyte apoptosis and necrosis, myocardial fibrosis, mild autonomic neuropathy, and activation of the renin–angiotensin system appear at this stage. Finally, combined systolic and diastolic dysfunctions occur which are associated with cardiac microvascular disease, severe autonomic neuropathy, and systemic sympathetic nervous system activation. This late stage is frequently associated with hypertension and the onset of ischemia [91]. The mechanisms underlying the process are poorly understood, but an overall picture is emerging. The sustained diabetic cardiac insult appears to be produced by two

major factors: hyperglycemia, a major mediator of many diabetic complications, and a shift in energy substrate selection by the heart [4]. This disease process impairs both passive and active mechanical properties of the myocardium; the compliance of the heart wall decreases (due to increased cross-linking of collagen, cardiac hypertrophy, and fibrosis [4, 92]), and contractility also decreases.

Cardiac metabolism in the diabetic heart differs from that in the non-diabetic hypertrophied and failing heart. Despite the fact that fatty acid oxidation increases dramatically in the diabetic heart, the delivery of free fatty acids into the cardiomyocyte exceeds its capacity to metabolize and store them. Intermediate products of fatty acid metabolism, particularly long-chain acyl-coenzyme As (Acyl CoAs), therefore accumulate in the cytoplasm [5]. Long-chain acyl CoAs are converted into ceramides, toxic substances which induce reactive oxygen species (ROS) and cardiomyocyte apoptosis [19].

Hyperglycemia, coupled with the marked decrease in glucose oxidation, increases the formation of ROS by several mechanisms [93]. Prolonged exposure of proteins to hyperglycemia induces a series of chemical reactions which eventually lead to the irreversible formation of advanced glycation end-products (AGEs) which act on their own receptors (RAGE) to increase the synthesis of diacylglycerol [94, 95]. Increased de novo synthesis of diacylglycerol, either by increased flux of glucose through the aldose reductase/polyol pathway or by RAGE activation, leads to the activation of protein kinase C (PKC) isoforms and stress-signalling pathways [96, 97]. Activation of these pathways increases mitochondrial ROS production, stimulates apoptosis, and increases the transcription of pro-inflammatory and pro-fibrotic genes [93]. In addition, flux of glucose through the hexosamine biosynthetic pathway (HBP) leads to O-linked-*N*-acetylglucosamination and activation of transcription factors which also regulate pro-inflammatory and pro-fibrotic genes [98].

At the level of mitochondria, the generation of ROS in response to hyperglycemia and hyperlipidemia produces mitochondrial damage.

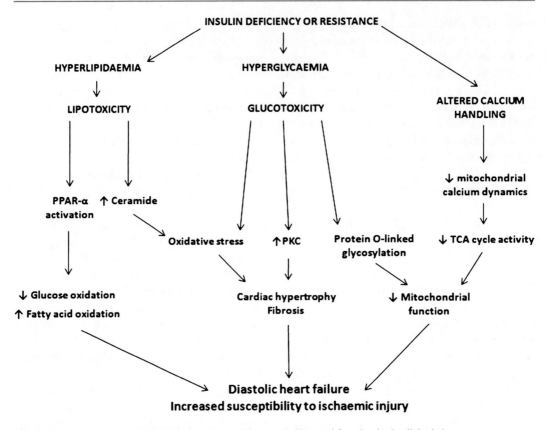

Fig. 2 Summary of the molecular links between cardiac metabolism and function in the diabetic heart

Despite simultaneous activation of the mitochondrial biogenesis program, mitochondrial efficiency decreases [99]. It has been observed that progression to heart failure is associated with decreased expression of uncoupling proteins (UCPs), particularly UCP2 and UCP3. These proteins regulate the mitochondrial membrane potential. The significance of this function in the heart is incompletely understood, but it is known that UCP2 and UCP3 can decrease superoxide radical generation by complex I of the respiratory chain [100], and there is some evidence that these proteins also protect against exogenous ROS [101]. However, UCPs decrease coupling between TCA cycle flux and ATP synthesis. Down-regulation of UCPs would be expected to increase TCA cycle/ATP synthesis coupling (a beneficial effect) but also to increase oxidative stress (a harmful effect). It is, therefore, unclear whether down-regulation of

UCPs is an adaptive or a maladaptive response (see ref. [102] for review).

The molecular links between metabolism and function in the diabetic heart are summarized in Fig. 2. Recent studies have shed considerable light on the underlying molecular basis of diabetic cardiomyopathy. Transcriptional regulators of cardiac metabolism have emerged as key mediators of the pathogenesis. The first of these are the PPARs of which PPAR-α is a major isoform in the heart. PPAR-α is a transcription factor which is bound and activated by free fatty acids and acts as a "lipostat", inducing genes involved in every step of fatty acid metabolism [103]. PPAR-α up-regulates enzymes at every step of the fatty acid oxidation pathway as well as inhibitors of glucose oxidation such as PDK-4, but it is the transcriptional control of mitochondrial long-chain acyl CoA uptake which has the greatest impact on the overall fatty acid oxidation rate [104]. When PPAR-α is overexpressed in the heart, a phenotype similar to that seen in diabetic cardiomyopathy is induced, with cardiac dysfunction and hypertrophy, reduced glucose oxidation, and increased sensitivity to ischemic injury. Furthermore, when PPAR-α is overexpressed in diabetic hearts, the phenotype produced by diabetes is worsened [5]. Deletion of PPAR-α is sufficient to protect diabetic hearts against the development of diabetic cardiomyopathy [5, 105]. PPAR-α activation is, therefore, essential to the pathogenesis of diabetic cardiomyopathy. The phenotype of PPAR-α overexpression is exacerbated by feeding the mice a high-fat diet and rescued in both cases by CD-36 deficiency, suggesting that PPAR-α induces cardiomyopathy by creating a mismatch between fatty acid uptake and oxidation that leads to fatty acid accumulation in the cytoplasm and lipotoxicity [106]. Intriguingly, however, CD36 deficiency does not prevent cardiac hypertrophy, presumably because this deficiency can be a cause of hypertrophy. Indeed, as discussed below, it appears that cardiac hypertrophy can be associated with over or under-activation of PPAR-α. Consistent with this idea, overexpression of the fatty acid transport protein FATP1 creates a similar phenotype to both diabetic cardiomyopathy and PPAR-α overexpression [107]. Cardiac-specific overexpression of PDK-4 produces a phenotype of reduced glucose oxidation and increased fatty acid oxidation, but no overt cardiomyopathy [108]. This indicates that it is the cytoplasmic accumulation of lipids rather than the rate of fatty acid oxidation per se that is the primary cause of cardiomyopathy.

An important potential link between function and metabolism is the transduction of signals from the sympathetic nervous system. We have previously shown that the β-blocker metoprolol inhibits fatty acid oxidation in the diabetic heart, an effect which is partly mediated by an acute mechanism (possibly involving covalent modification of CPT-1) and partly by a transcriptional mechanism [109, 110]. The latter involves repression of the PGC-1α/PPAR-α complex at the CPT-1 promoter by the contractile responsive element upstream stimulatory factor-2 (USF-2). As USF-2 is usually up-regulated in response to an increase in contractile function, this raises the intriguing possibility that fatty acid oxidation is transcriptionally repressed by an improvement in cardiac function. It is unclear whether USF-2 has wider effects on PPAR-α or PGC-1α targets. Binding of USF-2 decreased PGC-1α acetylation, probably by blocking the acetylation site, and would therefore be expected to increase PGC-1α activity overall. This would be a logical response to increased contractile function, and requires further investigation.

Elevation of glucose-derived intermediates is also an important mechanism of diabetic cardiomyopathy [111, 112]. Hyperglycemia, coupled with a marked decrease in glucose oxidation, increases glycogen formation and also increases flux of glucose through alternative metabolic pathways. Activation of PKC isoforms and the induction of oxidative stress are important consequences of this diversion. Hyperglycemia-induced activation of PKCβ2 has been shown to contribute to diabetic nephropathy by increasing the expression of TGFβ and CTGF [23]. The same effect occurs in the diabetic heart in both mice and rats, and can be prevented by insulin treatment [30].

Gene expression can also be altered in the heart by glucose, an effect mediated by the aldose reductase (AR)/polyol and HBPs. Aldose reductase catalyses the conversion of glucose to sorbitol, which is subsequently converted into fructose by sorbitol dehydrogenase (SDH) using NAD^+ [29, 113]. Excess glucose enters the polyol pathway, stimulating AR but not SDH; the result being an accumulation of sorbitol [113]. Increased flux through the polyol pathway has several consequences: the $NADH/NAD^+$ ratio is increased, leading to inhibition of glycolysis, and the consumption of NADPH increases. Reduction in the availability of NADPH compromises the ability of myocytes to regenerate reduced glutathione [93], potentially interfering with the heart's ability to cope with oxidative stress.

The HBP converts glucose-6-phosphate to hexosamine-6-phosphate which, in turn, is converted into uridine-5'-diphosphate-N-acetylglucosamine (UDP-GlcNAc). Approximately 5% of the glucose which enters cardiac myocytes is metabolized by this route. In the kidney, increased flux through this pathway in vitro leads to enhanced expression of tissue growth factor-β1 and fibronectin [114, 115] which is prevented by inhibitors of the rate-limiting step catalyzed by glutamine:fructose-6-phosphate-aminotransferase (GFAT) [116]. UDP-GlcNAc serves as an important substrate for protein glycosylation which is thought to play a role in decreased expression of several key components of the mitochondrial oxidative phosphorylation complexes as well as increased expression of pro-inflammatory proteins [93]. An important mechanism of this effect is the glycosylation of key transcription factors such as sp-1, leading to an increase in their binding affinity for DNA [98]. Significantly, the expression of GFAT has been shown to be increased by palmitate in human myotubes, indicating that palmitate can increase HBP flux through changes in protein expression. Whether this effect also occurs in the heart is unknown.

An Evolutionary Perspective on Heart Failure and Cardiac Metabolism

The application of evolutionary biology to the study of human disease has given rise to the concept that disease can result from adaptations conferred by the genome which are inappropriate for the environment in which humans live and can also be applied to the function of cells, tissues, organs, and systems responding to their local environments within the human body. An important concept in ecology and genetics is that of the reaction norm, which describes the pattern of phenotypes that a single genotype can produce across a range of environments. The pattern provides a map of the adaptations that are possible which could be considered as "a map of plasticity". In the heart, reaction norms include metabolic plasticity and the ability to undergo growth and remodelling. Function is compromised when the reaction norms move beyond what is adaptive to what is maladaptive.

The application of this evolutionary perspective to heart failure has been reviewed recently [117]. When the myocardium starts to fail, the reaction norms aim to restore both normal cardiac output and normal energy economy. The adaptations which permit this include reexpression of the foetal phenotype, which slows V_{max}, cardiac hypertrophy which restores wall stress, and a decrease in heat production per gram of tension, achieved by metabolic plasticity [117]. Once heart failure progresses, these processes become maladaptive because a slowing of V_{max} contributes to decreased contractile function and remodelling of the heart impairs its mechanical function.

Environmental constraint of reaction norms can affect heart function. To respond to increases in demand, the heart needs the ability not only to adapt its energy production, but to have ready access to metabolic fuels. To this end, the importance of the endogenous cardiac fuel stores of glycogen and TAG is being increasingly recognized. These stores have been referred to as the "metabolic reserve" of the heart, and a disturbance in this reserve limits the heart's metabolic plasticity and results in dysfunction when the heart is stressed [118].

Restoration of the environment to which the phenotype is adapted can be cardioprotective because it eliminates the mismatch responsible for the disease. The best example of this is provided by the cardioprotective effects of moderate calorie restriction. The mechanisms of the cardioprotective effect have been shown to involve attenuation of oxidative stress, mitochondrial dysfunction, inflammation, apoptosis, and autophagy in the heart (see ref. [119] for review). Moderate calorie restriction also reduces cardiac risk factors as whole [119]. The thrifty gene hypothesis suggests that the emergence of many cardiac risk factors is due to a mismatch between the high-energy intake/low activity environment of the modern human and a genotype which evolved on the background of a low-energy intake/high activity environment. Moderate calorie restriction, therefore, goes some way to restoring a low-energy intake environment, conferring a second level of cardioprotection by reducing cardiac risk factors in the whole body.

Molecular Time

One of most important adaptations for a cell, tissue, organ system or organism is the ability to anticipate and prepare for predictable cyclical changes in the environment. Sheer stress on the heart wall is a relevant example. It peaks during the awake phase due to increased physical activity. Exercise training is also typically undertaken during this period, whereas sustained pressure increases are maintained throughout the waking and sleeping phases. Physiological hypertrophy may therefore represent a response to sheer stress stimulation during the waking phase, whereas pathological hypertrophy represents a response to inappropriate stimulation during the sleep phase (see ref. [120] for review).

If the appearance of a stimulus follows a circadian pattern, then the reaction norm can be employed by linking the phenotype not just to the environmental signal, but to an internal timekeeping mechanism which can anticipate the appearance of that signal. It has been discovered that all cells in the body possess such a mechanism, a molecular clock, which is summarized in Fig. 3. The molecular clock is intricately interwoven with a range of metabolic loops, including redox status and an NAD^+-dependent loop involving SIRT-1 [120]. CLOCK function may be regulated by AMPK. AMPK activates casein kinase 1 which in turn leads to phosphorylation of period proteins, targeting them for degradation. This has the effect of decreasing the period length of the cycle and inducing a phase shift. Chronic activation of AMPK would be expected to induce a

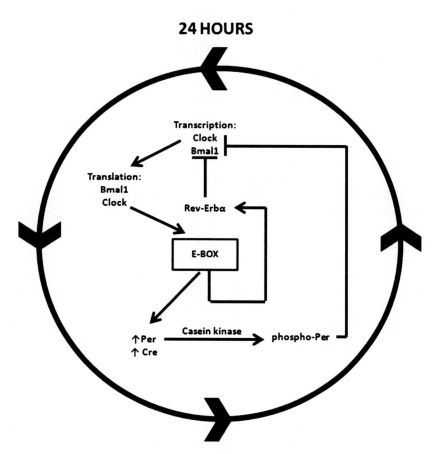

Fig. 3 The molecular circadian clock in the cardiomyocyte. The clock forms an auto-regulatory loop which cycles every 24 h

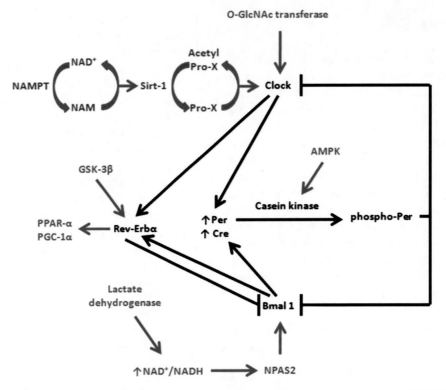

Fig. 4 Interactions between the molecular circadian clock (represented in *black*) and metabolism (represented in *blue*) in the cardiomyocyte. ProX is an undefined protein.

AMPK AMP-activated protein kinase, *NAMPT* nicotinamide phosphoribosyltransferase, *NPAS* neuronal PAS domain protein, *GSK* glycogen synthase kinase

phase advance in the circadian pattern of clock genes [121, 122]. Such a phase advance has been reported to occur in the diabetic heart. These interactions are summarized in Fig. 4.

The disposition of glucose and fatty acids differs between the awake and sleep phases. During the awake phase, glucosyl units are channelled towards complete oxidation both from exogenous uptake via glut-4 and glycogenolysis. During the sleep phase, exogenous fatty acids are channelled into synthetic pathways for phospholipids, DAG, and TAG and oxidation of fatty acids is reduced. Therefore, the susceptibility of the heart to cytoplasmic accumulation of fatty acids and depression of cardiac function is greatest during the sleep phase (see ref. [123] for review). This circadian periodicity is regulated at the molecular level by the clock transcriptional system. Metabolic genes which are clock output genes include those which code for PDK-4, UCP-3,

diacylglycerol acyltransferase 2 (an enzyme in the TAG synthesis pathway), and adiponutrin (a TAG lipase) [124–126]. PDK-4 activity can be increased by combined administration of fatty acids and a cAMP analogue in isolated cardiomyocytes, suggesting that circadian variation in adrenergic tone and fatty acid disposition act together to alter the expression of PDK-4 [127]. That this effect may be mediated by increased cytoplasmic accumulation of fatty acid intermediates is suggested by the observation that ceramide can induce a similar effect [128].

Cardiac-specific expression of a dominant negative CLOCK mutant produces a loss of *pdk4* and *ucp3* oscillations, chronic elevation of adiponectin expression, chronic repression of *dgat2*, and an inability to increase TAG synthesis in response to fasting; this is associated with chronic induction of genes which favour dephosphorylation, inhibition of PI3 kinase-mediated insulin signalling, and inhibition of key steps in β-adrenergic signalling: the inhibitory subunit of cAMP-dependent protein kinase and the catalytic subunit of protein phosphatase-1 [123, 129].

Conclusions

The interactions between cardiac metabolism and function at the molecular level can be understood in terms of several broad concepts. First, altered metabolic fluxes are not primary causes of cardiac injury; injury is caused by the cytoplasmic accumulation of toxic metabolic intermediates. These intermediates accumulate when there is a mismatch between the supply and utilization of metabolic fuels, and this can be produced either by excessive supply or reduced metabolic flux of a fuel. Second, changes in metabolism can be adaptive (as occurs in physiological hypertrophy), maladaptive in parallel with cardiac dysfunction (as occurs in pathological hypertrophy), or maladaptive as an antecedent and cause of cardiac dysfunction (as occurs in pathological hypertrophy). Finally, from an evolutionary perspective, disease results when the phenotype is inappropriate for the environment; this can result from an inappropriate response (e.g. pathological hypertrophy), or from an environmental constraint (e.g. reduced metabolic reserve). The story of the interaction of metabolism and function is one of the exquisite balance and plasticity. Disturbance in the balance or misdirection of the plasticity results in disease.

Acknowledgements Studies quoted from our laboratory were supported by the Canadian Institutes of Health Research (CIHR).

References

1. Allard MF, Schonekess BO, Henning SL, English DR, Lopaschuk GD. Contribution of oxidative metabolism and glycolysis to ATP production in hypertrophied hearts. Am J Physiol Heart Circ Physiol. 1994;267:H742–50.
2. Zhang J, Duncker DJ, Ya X, et al. Effect of left ventricular hypertrophy secondary to chronic pressure overload on transmural myocardial 2-deoxyglucose uptake. A 31P NMR spectroscopic study. Circulation. 1995;92:1274–83.
3. Apstein CS. Glucose-insulin-potassium for acute myocardial infarction: remarkable results from a new prospective, randomized trial. Circulation. 1998;98:2223–6.
4. Chatham JC, Forder JR, McNeill JH. The heart in diabetes. Norwell, MA: Kluwer; 1996.
5. Severson DL. Diabetic cardiomyopathy: recent evidence from mouse models of type 1 and type 2 diabetes. Can J Physiol Pharmacol. 2004;82:813–23.
6. Brown GC. Control of respiration and ATP synthesis in mammalian mitochondria and cells. Biochem J. 1992;284:1–13.
7. Saks VA, Kuznetsov AV, Vendelin M, et al. Functional coupling as a basic mechanism of feedback regulation of cardiac energy metabolism. Mol Cell Biochem. 2004;256–257:185–99.
8. Carling D. The AMP-activated protein kinase cascade – a unifying system for energy control. Trends Biochem Sci. 2004;29:18–24.
9. Keul J, Doll E, Keppler D, et al. Variations of arterial substrate level under the influence of physical work. Int Z Angew Physiol. 1966;22:356–85.
10. Lopaschuk GD. Optimizing cardiac energy metabolism: how can fatty acid and carbohydrate metabolism be manipulated? Coron Artery Dis. 2001;12 Suppl 1:S8–11.
11. Stanley WC, Recchia FA, Lopaschuk GD. Myocardial substrate metabolism in the normal and failing heart. Physiol Rev. 2005;85:1093–129.
12. Avogaro A, Nosadini R, Doria A, et al. Myocardial metabolism in insulin-deficient diabetic humans without coronary artery disease. Am J Physiol Endocrinol Metab. 1990;258:E606–18.
13. Hall JL, Stanley WC, Lopaschuk GD, et al. Impaired pyruvate oxidation but normal glucose uptake in diabetic pig heart during dobutamine-induced work. Am J Physiol Heart Circ Physiol. 1996;271: H2320–9.
14. Stanley WC, Lopaschuk GD, Hall JL, et al. Regulation of myocardial carbohydrate metabolism under normal and ischaemic conditions. Potential for pharmacological interventions. Cardiovasc Res. 1997;33:243–57.
15. Young LH, Coven DL, Russell III RR. Cellular and molecular regulation of cardiac glucose transport. J Nucl Cardiol. 2000;7:267–76.
16. Randle PJ. Fuel selection in animals. Biochem Soc Trans. 1986;14:799–806.
17. Augustus AS, Kako Y, Yagyu H, et al. Routes of FA delivery to cardiac muscle: modulation of lipoprotein lipolysis alters uptake of TG-derived FA. Am J Physiol Endocrinol Metab. 2003;284:E331–9.
18. Lopaschuk GD, Belke DD, Gamble J, et al. Regulation of fatty acid oxidation in the mammalian heart in health and disease. Biochim Biophys Acta. 1994;1213:263–76.
19. Bielawska AE, Shapiro JP, Jiang L, et al. Ceramide is involved in triggering of cardiomyocyte apoptosis

induced by ischemia and reperfusion. Am J Pathol. 1997;151:1257–63.

20. Bing RJ, Siegel A, Ungar I, et al. Metabolism of the human heart. II. Studies on fat, ketone and amino acid metabolism. Am J Med. 1954;16:504–15.

21. Opie L. The heart: physiology, from cell to circulation. Philadelphia, PA: Lippincot-Raven; 1998.

22. Kerner J, Hoppel C. Fatty acid import into mitochondria. Biochim Biophys Acta. 2000;1486:1–17.

23. McGarry JD, Brown NF. The mitochondrial carnitine palmitoyltransferase system. From concept to molecular analysis. Eur J Biochem. 1997;244:1–14.

24. McGarry JD, Mills SE, Long CS, et al. Observations on the affinity for carnitine, and malonyl-CoA sensitivity, of carnitine palmitoyltransferase I in animal and human tissues. Demonstration of the presence of malonyl-CoA in non-hepatic tissues of the rat. Biochem J. 1983;214:21–8.

25. Scarpulla RC. Nuclear activators and coactivators in mammalian mitochondrial biogenesis. Biochim Biophys Acta. 2002;1576:1–14.

26. Francis GA, Annicotte JS, Auwerx J. PPAR-alpha effects on the heart and other vascular tissues. Am J Physiol Heart Circ Physiol. 2003;285:H1–9.

27. Arany Z, He H, Lin J, et al. Transcriptional coactivator PGC-1 alpha controls the energy state and contractile function of cardiac muscle. Cell Metab. 2005;1:259–71.

28. Lehman JJ, Barger PM, Kovacs A, et al. Peroxisome proliferator-activated receptor gamma coactivator-1 promotes cardiac mitochondrial biogenesis. J Clin Invest. 2000;106:847–56.

29. Huss JM, Torra IP, Staels B, et al. Estrogen-related receptor alpha directs peroxisome proliferator-activated receptor alpha signaling in the transcriptional control of energy metabolism in cardiac and skeletal muscle. Mol Cell Biol. 2004;24:9079–91.

30. Huss JM, Kelly DP. Nuclear receptor signaling and cardiac energetics. Circ Res. 2004;95:568–78.

31. Rohini A, Agrawal N, Koyani CN, et al. Molecular targets and regulators of cardiac hypertrophy. Pharmacol Res. 2010;61:269–80.

32. Dorn 2nd GW, Robbins J, Sugden PH. Phenotyping hypertrophy: eschew obfuscation. Circ Res. 2003;92:1171–5.

33. Labarthe F, Khairallah M, Bouchard B, et al. Fatty acid oxidation and its impact on response of spontaneously hypertensive rat hearts to an adrenergic stress: benefits of a medium-chain fatty acid. Am J Physiol Heart Circ Physiol. 2005;288:H1425–36.

34. Nascimben L, Ingwall JS, Lorell BH, et al. Mechanisms for increased glycolysis in the hypertrophied rat heart. Hypertension. 2004;44:662–7.

35. Vincent G, Khairallah M, Bouchard B, et al. Metabolic phenotyping of the diseased rat heart using 13C-substrates and ex vivo perfusion in the working mode. Mol Cell Biochem. 2003;242:89–99.

36. Bishop SP, Altschuld RA. Increased glycolytic metabolism in cardiac hypertrophy and congestive failure. Am J Physiol. 1970;218:153–9.

37. Overturf M, Sybers H, Schaper J, et al. Hypertension and atherosclerosis in cholesterol-fed rabbits. II. One-kidney, one clip Goldblatt hypertension treated with nifedipine. Atherosclerosis. 1987;66:63–76.

38. Allard MF, Parsons HL, Saeedi R, et al. AMPK and metabolic adaptation by the heart to pressure overload. Am J Physiol Heart Circ Physiol. 2007;292:H140–8.

39. Saeedi R, Saran VV, Wu SS, et al. AMP-activated protein kinase influences metabolic remodeling in H9c2 cells hypertrophied by arginine vasopressin. Am J Physiol Heart Circ Physiol. 2009;296:H1822–32.

40. Sambandam N, Lopaschuk GD, Brownsey RW, et al. Energy metabolism in the hypertrophied heart. Heart Fail Rev. 2002;7:161–73.

41. Barger PM, Brandt JM, Leone TC, et al. Deactivation of peroxisome proliferator-activated receptor-alpha during cardiac hypertrophic growth. J Clin Invest. 2000;105:1723–30.

42. Jamshidi Y, Montgomery HE, Hense HW, et al. Peroxisome proliferator-activated receptor alpha gene regulates left ventricular growth in response to exercise and hypertension. Circulation. 2002;105:950–5.

43. Sakai S, Miyauchi T, Irukayama-Tomobe Y, et al. Peroxisome proliferator-activated receptor-gamma activators inhibit endothelin-1-related cardiac hypertrophy in rats. Clin Sci (Lond). 2002;103 Suppl 48:16S–20.

44. Asakawa M, Takano H, Nagai T, et al. Peroxisome proliferator-activated receptor gamma plays a critical role in inhibition of cardiac hypertrophy in vitro and in vivo. Circulation. 2002;105:1240–6.

45. Sivarajah A, McDonald MC, Thiemermann C. The cardioprotective effects of preconditioning with endotoxin, but not ischemia, are abolished by a peroxisome proliferator-activated receptor-gamma antagonist. J Pharmacol Exp Ther. 2005;313:896–901.

46. Molkentin JD, Lu JR, Antos CL, et al. A calcineurin-dependent transcriptional pathway for cardiac hypertrophy. Cell. 1998;93:215–28.

47. Bao Y, Li R, Jiang J, et al. Activation of peroxisome proliferator-activated receptor gamma inhibits endothelin-1-induced cardiac hypertrophy via the calcineurin/NFAT signaling pathway. Mol Cell Biochem. 2008;317:189–96.

48. Gerstein HC, Yusuf S, Bosch J, et al. Effect of rosiglitazone on the frequency of diabetes in patients with impaired glucose tolerance or impaired fasting glucose: a randomised controlled trial. Lancet. 2006;368:1096–105.

49. Razeghi P, Wang ME, Youker KA, et al. Lack of NF-kappaB1 (p105/p50) attenuates unloading-induced downregulation of PPARalpha and PPARalpha-regulated gene expression in rodent heart. Cardiovasc Res. 2007;74:133–9.

50. Eisner V, Criollo A, Quiroga C, et al. Hyperosmotic stress-dependent NFkappaB activation is regulated

by reactive oxygen species and IGF-1 in cultured cardiomyocytes. FEBS Lett. 2006;580:4495–500.

51. Monnier L, Mas E, Ginet C, et al. Activation of oxidative stress by acute glucose fluctuations compared with sustained chronic hyperglycemia in patients with type 2 diabetes. JAMA. 2006;295:1681–7.

52. Houstis N, Rosen ED, Lander ES. Reactive oxygen species have a causal role in multiple forms of insulin resistance. Nature. 2006;440:944–8.

53. Yamamoto K, Ohki R, Lee RT, et al. Peroxisome proliferator-activated receptor gamma activators inhibit cardiac hypertrophy in cardiac myocytes. Circulation. 2001;104:1670–5.

54. Sheng L, Ye P, Liu YX, et al. Peroxisome proliferator-activated receptor beta/delta activation improves angiotensin II-induced cardiac hypertrophy in vitro. Clin Exp Hypertens. 2008;30:109–19.

55. Finck BN, Bernal-Mizrachi C, Han DH, et al. A potential link between muscle peroxisome proliferator-activated receptor-alpha signaling and obesity-related diabetes. Cell Metab. 2005;1:133–44.

56. Lin J, Wu H, Tarr PT, et al. Transcriptional coactivator PGC-1 alpha drives the formation of slow-twitch muscle fibres. Nature. 2002;418:797–801.

57. Russell LK, Mansfield CM, Lehman JJ, et al. Cardiac-specific induction of the transcriptional coactivator peroxisome proliferator-activated receptor gamma coactivator-1alpha promotes mitochondrial biogenesis and reversible cardiomyopathy in a developmental stage-dependent manner. Circ Res. 2004;94:525–33.

58. Kayar SR, Conley KE, Claassen H, et al. Capillarity and mitochondrial distribution in rat myocardium following exercise training. J Exp Biol. 1986;120: 189–99.

59. Kemi OJ, Hoydal MA, Haram PM, et al. Exercise training restores aerobic capacity and energy transfer systems in heart failure treated with losartan. Cardiovasc Res. 2007;76:91–9.

60. Murakami T, Shimomura Y, Fujitsuka N, et al. Differential adaptation to endurance training between heart and gastrocnemius muscle mitochondria in rats. Biochem Mol Biol Int. 1995;36:285–90.

61. Terblanche SE, Gohil K, Packer L, et al. The effects of endurance training and exhaustive exercise on mitochondrial enzymes in tissues of the rat (Rattus norvegicus). Comp Biochem Physiol A Mol Integr Physiol. 2001;128:889–96.

62. Coleman R, Weiss A, Finkelbrand S, et al. Age and exercise-related changes in myocardial mitochondria in mice. Acta Histochem. 1988;83:81–90.

63. Iemitsu M, Miyauchi T, Maeda S, et al. Cardiac hypertrophy by hypertension and exercise training exhibits different gene expression of enzymes in energy metabolism. Hypertens Res. 2003;26: 829–37.

64. Kuo WW, Chu CY, Wu CH, et al. The profile of cardiac cytochrome c oxidase (COX) expression in an accelerated cardiac-hypertrophy model. J Biomed Sci. 2005;12:601–10.

65. Stuewe SR, Gwirtz PA, Agarwal N, et al. Exercise training enhances glycolytic and oxidative enzymes in canine ventricular myocardium. J Mol Cell Cardiol. 2000;32:903–13.

66. Wagner RA, Tabibiazar R, Powers J, et al. Genome-wide expression profiling of a cardiac pressure overload model identifies major metabolic and signaling pathway responses. J Mol Cell Cardiol. 2004;37: 1159–70.

67. Sano M, Izumi Y, Helenius K, et al. Menage-a-trois 1 is critical for the transcriptional function of PPARgamma coactivator 1. Cell Metab. 2007;5: 129–42.

68. De Sousa E, Veksler V, Bigard X, et al. Heart failure affects mitochondrial but not myofibrillar intrinsic properties of skeletal muscle. Circulation. 2000;102: 1847–53.

69. Garnier A, Fortin D, Delomenie C, et al. Depressed mitochondrial transcription factors and oxidative capacity in rat failing cardiac and skeletal muscles. J Physiol. 2003;551:491–501.

70. Javadov S, Huang C, Kirshenbaum L, et al. NHE-1 inhibition improves impaired mitochondrial permeability transition and respiratory function during postinfarction remodelling in the rat. J Mol Cell Cardiol. 2005;38:135–43.

71. Jullig M, Hickey AJ, Chai CC, et al. Is the failing heart out of fuel or a worn engine running rich? A study of mitochondria in old spontaneously hypertensive rats. Proteomics. 2008;8:2556–72.

72. Marin-Garcia J, Goldenthal MJ, Moe GW. Abnormal cardiac and skeletal muscle mitochondrial function in pacing-induced cardiac failure. Cardiovasc Res. 2001;52:103–10.

73. Sharov VG, Goussev A, Lesch M, et al. Abnormal mitochondrial function in myocardium of dogs with chronic heart failure. J Mol Cell Cardiol. 1998; 30:1757–62.

74. Mettauer B, Zoll J, Garnier A, et al. Heart failure: a model of cardiac and skeletal muscle energetic failure. Pflugers Arch. 2006;452:653–66.

75. Sharov VG, Todor AV, Silverman N, et al. Abnormal mitochondrial respiration in failed human myocardium. J Mol Cell Cardiol. 2000;32:2361–7.

76. Sun CK, Chang LT, Sheu JJ, et al. Losartan preserves integrity of cardiac gap junctions and PGC-1 alpha gene expression and prevents cellular apoptosis in remote area of left ventricular myocardium following acute myocardial infarction. Int Heart J. 2007;48: 533–46.

77. Watson PA, Reusch JE, McCune SA, et al. Restoration of CREB function is linked to completion and stabilization of adaptive cardiac hypertrophy in response to exercise. Am J Physiol Heart Circ Physiol. 2007;293:H246–59.

78. Witt H, Schubert C, Jaekel J, et al. Sex-specific pathways in early cardiac response to pressure overload in mice. J Mol Med. 2008;86:1013–24.

79. Sebastiani M, Giordano C, Nediani C, et al. Induction of mitochondrial biogenesis is a maladaptive

mechanism in mitochondrial cardiomyopathies. J Am Coll Cardiol. 2007;50:1362–9.

80. Lehman JJ, Boudina S, Banke NH, et al. The transcriptional coactivator PGC-1alpha is essential for maximal and efficient cardiac mitochondrial fatty acid oxidation and lipid homeostasis. Am J Physiol Heart Circ Physiol. 2008;295:H185–96.

81. Leone TC, Lehman JJ, Finck BN, et al. PGC-1alpha deficiency causes multi-system energy metabolic derangements: muscle dysfunction, abnormal weight control and hepatic steatosis. PLoS Biol. 2005;3: e101.

82. Kim J, Wende AR, Sena S, et al. Insulin-like growth factor I receptor signaling is required for exercise-induced cardiac hypertrophy. Mol Endocrinol. 2008; 22:2531–43.

83. Guarente L, Picard F. Calorie restriction – the SIR2 connection. Cell. 2005;120:473–82.

84. Shinmura K, Tamaki K, Bolli R. Impact of 6-mo caloric restriction on myocardial ischemic tolerance: possible involvement of nitric oxide-dependent increase in nuclear Sirt1. Am J Physiol Heart Circ Physiol. 2008;295:H2348–55.

85. Alcendor RR, Gao S, Zhai P, et al. Sirt1 regulates aging and resistance to oxidative stress in the heart. Circ Res. 2007;100:1512–21.

86. Rodgers JT, Lerin C, Gerhart-Hines Z, et al. Metabolic adaptations through the PGC-1 alpha and SIRT1 pathways. FEBS Lett. 2008;582:46–53.

87. Seya K, Kanemaru K, Sugimoto C, et al. Opposite effects of two resveratrol (trans-3,5,4′-trihydroxystilbene) tetramers, vitisin A and hopeaphenol, on apoptosis of myocytes isolated from adult rat heart. J Pharmacol Exp Ther. 2009;328:90–8.

88. Ray PS, Maulik G, Cordis GA, et al. The red wine antioxidant resveratrol protects isolated rat hearts from ischemia reperfusion injury. Free Radic Biol Med. 1999;27:160–9.

89. Juric D, Wojciechowski P, Das DK, et al. Prevention of concentric hypertrophy and diastolic impairment in aortic-banded rats treated with resveratrol. Am J Physiol Heart Circ Physiol. 2007;292:H2138–43.

90. Bertelli AA, Giovannini L, Giannessi D, et al. Antiplatelet activity of synthetic and natural resveratrol in red wine. Int J Tissue React. 1995;17:1–3.

91. Fang ZY, Prins JB, Marwick TH. Diabetic cardiomyopathy: evidence, mechanisms, and therapeutic implications. Endocr Rev. 2004;25:543–67.

92. Ulrich P, Cerami A. Protein glycation, diabetes, and aging. Recent Prog Horm Res. 2001;56:1–21.

93. Wold LE, Ceylan-Isik AF, Ren J. Oxidative stress and stress signaling: menace of diabetic cardiomyopathy. Acta Pharmacol Sin. 2005;26:908–17.

94. Brownlee M. Biochemistry and molecular cell biology of diabetic complications. Nature. 2001;414:813–20.

95. Brownlee M, Cerami A, Vlassara H. Advanced glycosylation end products in tissue and the biochemical basis of diabetic complications. N Engl J Med. 1988;318:1315–21.

96. Koya D, King GL. Protein kinase C activation and the development of diabetic complications. Diabetes. 1998;47:859–66.

97. Keogh RJ, Dunlop ME, Larkins RG. Effect of inhibition of aldose reductase on glucose flux, diacylglycerol formation, protein kinase C, and phospholipase A2 activation. Metabolism. 1997;46:41–7.

98. Jiang T, Che Q, Lin Y, et al. Aldose reductase regulates TGF-beta1-induced production of fibronectin and type IV collagen in cultured rat mesangial cells. Nephrology (Carlton). 2006;11:105–12.

99. Sack MN. Type 2 diabetes, mitochondrial biology and the heart. J Mol Cell Cardiol. 2009;46:842–9.

100. Liu SS. Generating, partitioning, targeting and functioning of superoxide in mitochondria. Biosci Rep. 1997;17:259–72.

101. Teshima Y, Akao M, Jones SP, et al. Uncoupling protein-2 overexpression inhibits mitochondrial death pathway in cardiomyocytes. Circ Res. 2003;93: 192–200.

102. Laskowski KR, Russell 3rd RR. Uncoupling proteins in heart failure. Curr Heart Fail Rep. 2008;5:75–9.

103. Djouadi F, Brandt JM, Weinheimer CJ, et al. The role of the peroxisome proliferator-activated receptor alpha (PPAR alpha) in the control of cardiac lipid metabolism. Prostaglandins Leukot Essent Fatty Acids. 1999;60:339–43.

104. Brandt JM, Djouadi F, Kelly DP. Fatty acids activate transcription of the muscle carnitine palmitoyltransferase I gene in cardiac myocytes via the peroxisome proliferator-activated receptor alpha. J Biol Chem. 1998;273:23786–92.

105. Finck BN, Lehman JJ, Leone TC, et al. The cardiac phenotype induced by PPARalpha overexpression mimics that caused by diabetes mellitus. J Clin Invest. 2002;109:121–30.

106. Yang J, Sambandam N, Han X, et al. CD36 deficiency rescues lipotoxic cardiomyopathy. Circ Res. 2007;100:1208–17.

107. Chiu HC, Kovacs A, Blanton RM, et al. Transgenic expression of fatty acid transport protein 1 in the heart causes lipotoxic cardiomyopathy. Circ Res. 2005;96:225–33.

108. Zhao G, Jeoung NH, Burgess SC, et al. Overexpression of pyruvate dehydrogenase kinase 4 in heart perturbs metabolism and exacerbates calcineurin-induced cardiomyopathy. Am J Physiol Heart Circ Physiol. 2008;294:H936–43.

109. Sharma V, Dhillon P, Wambolt R, et al. Metoprolol improves cardiac function and modulates cardiac metabolism in the streptozotocin (STZ) diabetic rat. Am J Physiol Heart Circ Physiol. 2008;294: H1609–20.

110. Sharma V, Dhillon P, Parsons H, et al. Metoprolol represses PGC1alpha-mediated carnitine palmitoyltransferase-1B expression in the diabetic heart. Eur J Pharmacol. 2009;607:156–66.

111. Young ME, McNulty P, Taegtmeyer H. Adaptation and maladaptation of the heart in diabetes: Part II:

potential mechanisms. Circulation. 2002;105: 1861–70.

112. Taegtmeyer H, McNulty P, Young ME. Adaptation and maladaptation of the heart in diabetes: Part I: general concepts. Circulation. 2002;105:1727–33.

113. Narayanan S. Aldose reductase and its inhibition in the control of diabetic complications. Ann Clin Lab Sci. 1993;23:148–58.

114. Weigert C, Brodbeck K, Lehmann R, et al. Overexpression of glutamine:fructose-6-phosphate-amidotransferase induces transforming growth factor-beta1 synthesis in NIH-3T3 fibroblasts. FEBS Lett. 2001;488:95–9.

115. Burt DJ, Gruden G, Thomas SM, et al. P38 mitogen-activated protein kinase mediates hexosamine-induced TGFbeta1 mRNA expression in human mesangial cells. Diabetologia. 2003;46:531–7.

116. Kolm-Litty V, Sauer U, Nerlich A, et al. High glucose-induced transforming growth factor beta1 production is mediated by the hexosamine pathway in porcine glomerular mesangial cells. J Clin Invest. 1998; 101:160–9.

117. Swynghedauw B, Delcayre C, Samuel JL, et al. Molecular mechanisms in evolutionary cardiology failure. Ann NY Acad Sci. 2010;1188:58–67.

118. Kassiotis C, Rajabi M, Taegtmeyer H. Metabolic reserve of the heart: the forgotten link between contraction and coronary flow. Prog Cardiovasc Dis. 2008;51:74–88.

119. Marzetti E, Wohlgemuth SE, Anton SD, et al. Cellular mechanisms of cardioprotection by calorie restriction: state of the science and future perspectives. Clin Geriatr Med. 2009;25:715–32.

120. Durgan DJ, Young ME. The cardiomyocyte circadian clock: emerging roles in health and disease. Circ Res. 2010;106:647–58.

121. Meng QJ, Logunova L, Maywood ES, et al. Setting clock speed in mammals: the CK1 epsilon tau mutation in mice accelerates circadian pacemakers by selectively destabilizing PERIOD proteins. Neuron. 2008;58:78–88.

122. Um JH, Yang S, Yamazaki S, et al. Activation of 5′-AMP-activated kinase with diabetes drug metformin induces casein kinase Iepsilon (CKIepsilon)-dependent degradation of clock protein mPer2. J Biol Chem. 2007;282:20794–8.

123. Bray MS, Young ME. Diurnal variations in myocardial metabolism. Cardiovasc Res. 2008;79:228–37.

124. Durgan DJ, Hotze MA, Tomlin TM, et al. The intrinsic circadian clock within the cardiomyocyte. Am J Physiol Heart Circ Physiol. 2005;289:H1530–41.

125. Young ME, Razeghi P, Cedars AM, et al. Intrinsic diurnal variations in cardiac metabolism and contractile function. Circ Res. 2001;89:1199–208.

126. Stavinoha MA, Rayspellicy JW, Hart-Sailors ML, et al. Diurnal variations in the responsiveness of cardiac and skeletal muscle to fatty acids. Am J Physiol Endocrinol Metab. 2004;287:E878–87.

127. Priestman DA, Orfali KA, Sugden MC. Pyruvate inhibition of pyruvate dehydrogenase kinase. Effects of progressive starvation and hyperthyroidism in vivo, and of dibutyryl cyclic AMP and fatty acids in cultured cardiac myocytes. FEBS Lett. 1996;393: 174–8.

128. Park TS, Hu Y, Noh HL, et al. Ceramide is a cardiotoxin in lipotoxic cardiomyopathy. J Lipid Res. 2008;49:2101–12.

129. Bray MS, Shaw CA, Moore MW, et al. Disruption of the circadian clock within the cardiomyocyte influences myocardial contractile function, metabolism, and gene expression. Am J Physiol Heart Circ Physiol. 2008;294:H1036–47.

Metabolic Remodelling of the Hypertrophied Heart

Jiazhen M. Dai and Michael F. Allard

Abstract

The heart develops hypertrophy in response to persistent elevation in cardiac workload. Depending on the nature of the stimulus, cardiac hypertrophy can be categorized as pathologic or physiologic, each of which is accompanied by distinctly different phenotypic alterations including alterations in energy metabolism. These unique metabolic phenotypes may, in part, explain the differing functional outcomes of pathologically and physiologically hypertrophied hearts, especially notable following an ischemic stress. Thus, the mechanisms underlying remodelling in pathologic and physiologic cardiac hypertrophy have been the focus of many studies. A number of molecules including AMP-activated protein kinase, peroxisome proliferator-activated receptor-α, peroxisome proliferator-activated receptor gamma coactivator 1, protein kinase C, phosphoinositide-3 kinase/protein kinase B, and reactive oxygen species have been implicated as participating in the process of metabolic remodelling in cardiac hypertrophy.

Keywords

Physiologic cardiac hypertrophy • Pathologic cardiac hypertrophy • Fatty acid oxidation • Glucose oxidation • Glycolysis • Ischemia-reperfusion • AMP-activated protein kinase

Introduction

Prolonged increases in haemodynamic workload lead to development of cardiac hypertrophy. In addition to increased mass, the heart demonstrates phenotypic plasticity by developing a number of quantitative and qualitative alterations that collectively are referred to as remodelling [1]. This hypertrophic remodelling response is

M.F. Allard (✉)
Department of Pathology and Laboratory Medicine/James Hogg Research Centre, University of British Columbia, Vancouver, British Columbia, Canada
e-mail: mike.allard@pathology.ubc.ca

N.S. Dhalla, M. Nagano, B. Ostadal (eds.), *Molecular Defects in Cardiovascular Disease*, DOI 10.1007/978-1-4419-7130-2_10, © Springer Science+Business Media, LLC 2011

accompanied by changes in interstitial and vascular compartments of the heart [1] as well as by changes in cardiac myocytes, including alterations in energy metabolism [2–4]. Stimuli leading to cardiac hypertrophy may be pathologic, as occurs with pressure or volume overload caused by hypertension or valvular heart disease, or physiologic, as occurs with endurance exercise training [5]. Pathologic and physiologic stimuli lead to distinct hypertrophic phenotypes in the heart [6].

In the case of pathologic cardiac hypertrophy, the hypertrophy initially normalizes myocardial wall stress and oxygen consumption [7] and allows the heart to maintain cardiac output in the presence of increased haemodynamic workload [8], but over the long term, it is associated with the development of heart failure and increased risk for sudden death [9]. Pathologically hypertrophied hearts also have a reduced ability to cope with a subsequent acute metabolic stress, such as occurs during ischemia-reperfusion [10, 11]. Therefore, pathologic cardiac hypertrophy may be considered maladaptive under these conditions. This finding is significant because cardiac hypertrophy and coronary artery disease are both highly prevalent conditions that commonly co-exist [12]. Conversely, physiologic cardiac hypertrophy, which is accompanied by improved cardiac performance, is not associated with detrimental long-term outcomes [5, 13]. In fact, physiological cardiac hypertrophy may be viewed as a true adaptive response because the ability of the exercise adapted heart to cope with a subsequent acute metabolic stress is enhanced [2].

In addition to functional differences, pathologically and physiologically hypertrophied hearts demonstrate distinctive differences in other phenotypic characteristics including energy metabolism [6]. In this chapter, we will review current findings on remodelling of energy metabolism in pathologic and physiologic cardiac hypertrophy focusing on the underlying cellular signalling mechanisms that potentially contribute to the changes observed.

Myocardial Energy Metabolism

Fatty Acid Oxidation

The heart derives its energy primarily from catabolism of exogenous long-chain fatty acids, such as palmitate and oleate, and from endogenous triglycerides (Fig. 1) [14, 15]. Membrane-bound and cytosolic fatty acid-binding proteins (FABPpm and FABPc) as well as fatty acid translocase (FAT/CD36) facilitate the uptake and transport of long-chain fatty acids into the myocardium from fatty acids bound to albumin or present in lipoproteins [16]. These long-chain fatty acids are esterified with coenzyme A by fatty-acyl-CoA synthetase to prevent efflux and to enable further catabolism. Intracellular free fatty acids can either be incorporated into triacylglycerols or transported into the mitochondrial matrix for oxidation by the β-oxidation spiral and the tricarboxylic acid cycle [17]. A complex process involving three carnitine-dependent enzymes, carnitine palmitoyl transferase 1 (CPT1), carnitine acyl translocase (CT) and carnitine palmitoyl transferase 2 (CPT2), transports the long-chain fatty acid derivatives across the mitochondrial membrane to the site of oxidation in the mitochondrial matrix [17]. The rate of transport into mitochondria and oxidation of long-chain fatty acids is controlled largely by CPT1.

Glycolysis and Glucose Oxidation

In addition to fatty acids, carbohydrates such as exogenous glucose and its endogenous storage form, glycogen, as well as lactate are also used by the heart to produce energy (Fig. 1) [14, 18]. Myocardial glucose uptake is facilitated by the glucose transporters, GLUT1 and GLUT4 [14, 19]. Basal glucose uptake is largely accounted for by the presence of GLUT1 in the sarcolemma of cardiac myocytes [19]. Stimulation of glucose uptake by insulin or during metabolic stress,

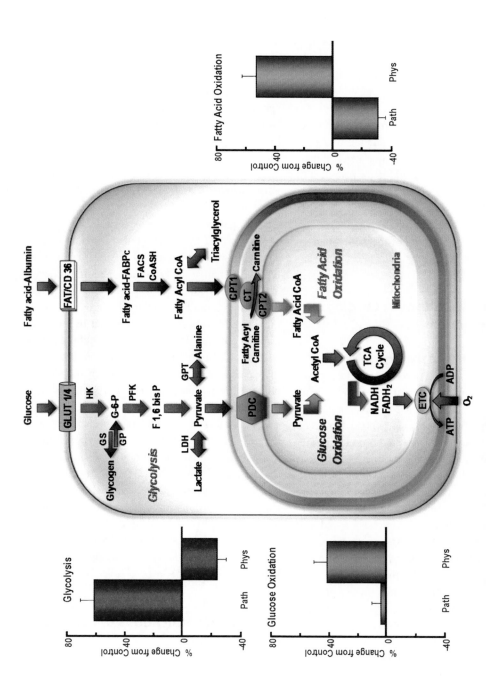

Fig. 1 Substrate utilization in myocardium. *Glut1/4* glucose transporters 1 and 4, *HK* hexokinase, *G-6-P* glucose-6-phosphate; *GS* glycogen synthase, *GP* glycogen phosphory-lase, *PFK* phosphofructokinase, *F 1,6 bis P* fructose 1,6 bisphosphate, *LDH* lactate dehydrogenase, *GPT* glutamatepyruvate transaminase; *PDC* pyruvate dehydrogenase complex, *FAT/CD36* fatty acid transporters, *FABPc* cytosolic fatty acid-binding protein, *FACS* fatty-acyl-CoA synthetase, *CoASH* coenzyme A, *CPT1* carnitine palmitoyl transferase-1, *CT* carnitine acyl translocase, *CPT1* carnitine palmitoyl transferase-2, *TCA cycle* tricarboxylic acid cycle, *ETC* electron transport chain. Path, pathological cardiac hypertrophy. Inserted *bar graphs* illustrating the dramatic variation in glycolysis, glucose oxidation, and fatty acid oxidation between Pathologic (Path) and Physiologic (Phys) cardiac hypertrophy

caused by increased work or ischemia, is primarily due to translocation of glucose transporters, especially GLUT4, from intracellular sites to the sarcolemma [19]. Once in the intracellular compartment, glucose is rapidly phosphorylated and can then be incorporated into glycogen or catabolized directly to pyruvate by glycolysis [14, 19]. Pyruvate can be oxidized to CO_2 in mitochondria or nonoxidatively catabolized to lactate and alanine [14, 19]. The extent of glucose transport via glucose transporters and flux through the reactions catalyzed by hexokinase and 6-phosphofructo-1-kinase (PFK1) are major determinants of glycolytic rates in the heart [19]. The extent of oxidation of pyruvate, which may be derived from glucose, glycogen, or lactate via the lactate dehydrogenase (LDH) reaction, is determined principally by the activation state of the mitochondrial pyruvate dehydrogenase complex (PDC) [19].

Metabolic Alterations in Cardiac Hypertrophy

Pathologic Cardiac Hypertrophy

Oxidation of long-chain fatty acids is low in hypertrophied hearts studied in vivo or as isolated preparations (Fig. 1) [3, 4, 20, 21]. However, oxidation of octanoate, a medium-chain fatty acid that does not require carnitine for transport into the mitochondria, is not reduced [20], indicating that the capacity of mitochondrial β-oxidation is not impaired in pathologically hypertrophied hearts. In contrast to reduced long-chain fatty acid oxidation, glycolysis is accelerated in hypertrophied hearts (Fig. 1) before, during, and after ischemia [4, 22, 23]. Despite the acceleration of glycolysis, glucose oxidation is not correspondingly increased and may, in fact, be lower than in non-hypertrophied hearts (Fig. 1) [3, 4, 23, 24]. As a result of these changes in catabolism of glucose, non-oxidative glycolysis (i.e., the proportion of glucose passing through glycolysis that is not oxidized) is higher in pathologically hypertrophied hearts than in non-hypertrophied hearts (Fig. 2) [25]. This pattern of energy substrate utilization that

develops in pathologic cardiac hypertrophy resembles that in foetal hearts [26], an alteration that has been said to reflect the recurrence of a foetal metabolic profile or phenotype [8]. It is worth noting that the substrate utilization profile described here is observed in hearts hypertrophied by pressure overload [4, 27], in volume overload [28], and in hearts hypertrophied in the setting of genetically induced hypertension in spontaneously hypertensive rats (SHRs) [3] as well as in patients with hypertrophied-failing hearts [29].

Physiologic Cardiac Hypertrophy

As with pathologic stimuli, exercise training that causes cardiac hypertrophy also leads to significant alterations in myocardial substrate utilization with changes in both fatty acid and glucose catabolism [2]. In contrast to pathologic cardiac hypertrophy, oxidation of long-chain fatty acids is increased in hearts hypertrophied by exercise training compared with non-hypertrophied hearts (Fig. 1) [2]. Furthermore, glucose oxidation is increased while glycolytic rates are reduced in physiologic cardiac hypertrophy (Fig. 1) [2]. As a consequence of these changes, the fraction of glucose oxidized is higher in exercised-induced hypertrophied hearts than in non-hypertrophied hearts (Fig. 2) [2]. These dramatic differences in the pattern of substrate utilization (or metabolic phenotype) between pathologic and physiologic cardiac hypertrophy indicates that the alterations in metabolic flux induced by prolonged changes in haemodynamic are substantially influenced by the nature of the stimulus leading to cardiac hypertrophy.

Functional Implications of Cardiac Hypertrophy

Coincident with the different patterns of metabolic remodelling discussed above, the functional outcome also differs between pathologically and physiologically hypertrophied hearts, especially after an ischemic stress. Specifically, functional

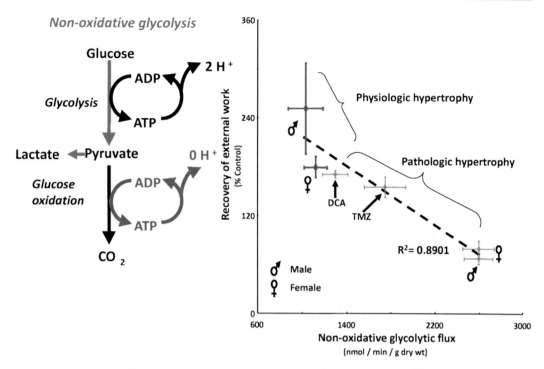

Fig. 2 Non-oxidative glycolysis (*green arrows*) and its relationship to recovery of function after ischemia in rodent models of cardiac hypertrophy. *DCA* dichloroace-tate, *TMZ* trimetazidine. Note the difference in proton (H⁺) production between oxidative and non-oxidative glycolysis

recovery is lower in pathologic cardiac hypertrophy [10, 11, 30] but higher in physiologic cardiac hypertrophy [2] as compared with corresponding non-hypertrophied hearts. The well-recognized connection between myocardial energy metabolism and function of the heart [8] raises the distinct possibility that alterations in substrate utilization are, at least partly, responsible for the different functional outcomes after ischemia observed between the two forms of cardiac hypertrophy.

Alterations in glucose catabolism may be a key determinant of functional outcome of hypertrophied hearts following an ischemic insult. This view is supported by the finding that an inverse relationship exists between the extent of non-oxidative glycolysis (i.e., glucose passing through glycolysis that is not oxidized to CO_2 in mitochondria) and recovery of function after ischemia in pathologically and physiologically hypertrophied hearts (Fig. 2) [2, 11, 31]. Of additional relevance in this regard are observations that reduction of

non-oxidative glycolysis (by stimulating glucose oxidation or by reducing glycolysis) substantially improves function, including contractile efficiency of non-ischemic and ischemic-reperfused hypertrophied hearts [11, 31, 32]. As in non-hypertrophied hearts, this beneficial effect presumably occurs, at least in part, by decreasing myocardial H⁺ production [19, 33]. Such a reduction favours recovery of intracellular pH, which could limit Ca^{2+} overload by way of successive trans-sarcolemmal H⁺/Na⁺ and Na⁺/Ca^{2+} exchange, and thus reduces the energetic cost associated with the maintenance of ion homeostasis [19]. This would, in turn, lead to improved post-ischemic contractile function and efficiency [19]. In pathologically hypertrophied hearts, production of proton (H⁺), which adversely affects contractile efficiency [34] is accelerated, because glycolysis is accelerated but glucose oxidation is not (i.e., non-oxidative glycolysis is high) [33]. Accelerated glycolysis may, however, be beneficial in conditions such as hypertrophied hearts exposed to hypoxia or very mild ischemia because glycolytic ATP production is increased with minimal glycolytic metabolite accumulation [30]. On the other hand, accelerated glycolysis contributes to a poor outcome in the setting of severe ischemia because it causes an enhanced accumulation of H^+ and other potentially harmful metabolites such as lactate and $NADH_2$ associated with glycolysis [32]. Therefore, the increase in fractional oxidation of glucose with a decline in non-oxidative glycolysis and the concomitant reduction in H^+ production from glucose catabolism might partly explain the improved post-ischemic function of the physiologically hypertrophied heart [2].

Differential remodelling of fatty acid metabolism may also play a role in the differing outcomes of pathologic and physiologic cardiac hypertrophy. Reduced rates of fatty acid oxidation in pathologic cardiac hypertrophy, which in turn leads to accumulation of free fatty acids and their derivatives [19], may be an important contributing factor. Several mechanisms have been proposed to account for this detrimental effect, including cytoplasmic and mitochondrial accumulation of toxic intermediates, such as ceramide, which is a by-product of fatty acid metabolism [35], and direct detrimental effects of fatty acids on mitochondrial membranes and proteins [36]. Therefore, reduced fatty acid oxidation may contribute to the poor post-ischemic outcome of the pathologically hypertrophied heart by allowing accumulation of cytoplasmic fatty acids. In contrast, higher rates of fatty acid oxidation in physiologically hypertrophied hearts are associated with an improved outcome after ischemia. This raises the possibility that enhanced rates of fatty acid oxidation protect these hearts from the noxious effects of fatty acids after ischemia, possibly by preventing the accumulation of fatty acids and activated fatty acids, limiting their toxic effects. In addition, despite higher rates of fatty acid oxidation, fractional glucose oxidation is greater in physiologically hypertrophied hearts, a somewhat paradoxical finding when the well-recognized negative effect of fatty acid oxidation on rates of glucose oxidation is considered [37]. This observation suggests that the inhibitory effect of high levels of fatty acid oxidation on glucose metabolism is circumvented in these hearts, a possibility that requires study in the future.

Cellular Mechanisms of Metabolic Remodelling

Fatty Acid Oxidation

Flux through metabolic pathways in the heart is controlled and regulated at several steps, rather than at a single rate-limiting step [16]. Each step is itself controlled by multiple factors, including allosteric modulation, phosphorylation and dephosphorylation, changes in subcellular distribution and/or alterations in gene expression [19]. In pathologic cardiac hypertrophy, reduced expression of oxidative enzymes [38] and fatty acid uptake/transport proteins [16] as well as low levels of myocardial carnitine [20, 28], a co-factor required for long-chain fatty acid transport into mitochondria, have been proposed to be responsible for the switch away from fatty acid oxidation. Of significance is the fact that down-regulation of corresponding fatty acid oxidation proteins typically only occurs in hypertrophied hearts with the onset of failure [38], a key observation because alterations of substrate utilization have already occurred in the non-failing hypertrophied heart indicating other non-transcriptional-translational factors are involved. The hypertrophied hearts of SHRs are an exception in that FAT/CD36 is markedly reduced or not detectable in myocardium at messenger RNA (mRNA) and protein levels, even in the absence of failure [39].

In physiologically hypertrophied hearts, the overall protein content of FABPpm and FAT/CD36 is similar to that in non-hypertrophied hearts [2], indicating that the capacity of fatty acid uptake is not changed. However, the possibility exists that increased sarcolemmal distribution of FAT/CD36 from intracellular sources may occur to raise the rate of cellular fatty acid uptake [40] and thus, contribute to the enhanced rate of fatty acid oxidation. Furthermore, elevated expression of FABPc, which also facilitates the transport of fatty acid to the outer mitochondrial membrane [41], may participate in increased delivery of cytoplasmic fatty acid to mitochondria in hearts of rats undergoing exercise training [42]. This possibility is supported by an enhanced expression of the mitochondrial fatty acid transport protein, mitochondrial CPT1 (mCPT1), in hearts of trained rats [43]. With increased fatty acid uptake into the mitochondria, expression and activity of mitochondrial enzymes and proteins involved in oxidative catabolism of fatty acid may be up-regulated. Unfortunately, attempts at identifying definitive candidates have not yet been unequivocally successful. Rats undergoing treadmill running show no change in cardiac protein content of long-chain acyl-CoA dehydrogenase (LCAD) and medium-chain acyl-CoA dehydrogenase (MCAD), which are enzymes catalyzing the first step of fatty acid oxidation in the β-oxidation spiral [2]. Similarly, the expression of mCPT-1 as well as the activities of citrate synthase and complexes I and IV of the respiratory chain in rats with swimming-induced cardiac hypertrophy are comparable to those in sedentary control rats [39]. In contrast, Rimbaud et al. reported elevated mRNA expression of mCPT-1 and MCAD in hearts of rats exposed to treadmill running [43]. The differing observations among these studies may be a reflection of variations in key methodological factors, such as animal strain and training protocols.

Glucose Oxidation

The metabolic profile of glucose use in pathologic cardiac hypertrophy is not fully accounted for by changes in expression of key metabolic enzymes and proteins [25]. Alterations in myocardial content of GLUT1 and GLUT4 have not been consistently observed in pathologically hypertrophied hearts [24, 43, 44]. However, distribution of glucose transport proteins has been observed in pathologically hypertrophied hearts that may contribute to the alterations in glucose use observed [44]. Expression and activity of a number of glycolytic enzymes, including hexokinase II, muscle-specific PFK1 (M-PFK1), glyceraldehyde-3-phosphate dehy-

drogenase (GAPDH) and pyruvate dehydrogenase kinase (PDK) isozyme 4, were found by some to be enhanced in pathologic cardiac hypertrophy [39]. Others, however, found that changes in expression of relevant enzymes and proteins did not adequately account for the changes observed [25], while isoenzymes of LDH were seen to shift toward more anaerobic foetal forms in pathologic cardiac hypertrophy [27]. Notably, the low rates of fractional oxidation of glucose, resulting from imbalance between glycolysis and mitochondrial pyruvate oxidation, cannot be explained by a reduction in expression or activity of either PDC or citrate synthase [27].

In physiologic cardiac hypertrophy, there is also no unequivocal evidence that alterations in glycolysis or glucose oxidation are related to changes in expression of relevant enzymes or proteins [2, 13]. For instance, despite an elevated rate of glucose uptake [45], no change in the protein content of GLUT4 was found in hearts of rats undergoing exercise training [2]. Similarly, the protein expression of glycolytic enzymes such as M-PFK1, GAPDH, LDH and enolase were not changed [2, 39], although activities of LDH and other glycolytic enzymes including hexokinase and pyruvate kinase were elevated in physiological cardiac hypertrophy [13]. There was also no difference in the level of PDC protein subunits and PDK between control and physiologically hypertrophied rats hearts [2, 43]. In addition, cardiac glycogen content has been found to be increased in mice following exercise training [46]. Whether this translates into elevation of catabolism of glucose derived from glycogen and its contribution to the enhanced glucose oxidation rate requires further study.

Taken together, remodelling of fatty acid and glucose metabolism in pathologically and physiologically hypertrophied hearts is not fully or adequately explained by changes in expression of relevant proteins and enzymes. Changes in subcellular localization, allosteric factors and covalent modulation [19], as well as organization of energy transfer networks coupling ATP producing pathways to sites of ATP demand may play important roles [47]. A number of signalling molecules with possible involvement in metabolic remodelling of hypertrophied hearts that act by transcriptional and/or non-transcriptional mechanisms are currently under investigation and a selected number are discussed below.

Potential Signalling Molecules in Hypertrophic Metabolic Remodelling

AMP-Activated Protein Kinase

AMP-activated protein kinase (AMPK), which is highly expressed in the heart [48], is a highly conserved family of protein kinases with a major role in the control and regulation of energy metabolism [49]. Activity of AMPK is subject to allosteric regulation by the level of AMP and ATP [49], and it can also be altered by phosphorylation via upstream kinases such as LKB1 and calcium/calmodulin-dependent protein kinase kinase (CaMKK) [50]. LKB1 is highly expressed in the heart and is considered to be the major upstream kinase that phosphorylates AMPK in response to elevations in AMP/ATP ratio [51]. Activation of AMPK by agents acting through Gq-linked G-protein coupled receptors and a calcium-dependent pathway involving CaMKKβ [52] occur in the absence of changes in energy status. CaMKKβ protein is expressed in the heart and the level of expression does not change with cardiac hypertrophy [53].

Metabolic and Other Actions of AMPK

Activation of AMPK stimulates fatty acid oxidation by increasing fatty acid uptake and mitochondrial oxidation [17, 48]. Fatty acid uptake is increased because AMPK activation leads to translocation of fatty acid transport proteins to the sarcolemma [54] and increased recruitment of lipoprotein lipase to the capillary endothelium [55]. By phosphorylating and inhibiting acetyl CoA carboxylase, AMPK activation causes a reduction in malonyl-CoA, a key allosteric inhibitor of CPT-1 [56]. AMPK activation increases glucose uptake in the heart by causing sarcolemmal translocation of glucose transport proteins [57]. AMPK phosphory-

lates and activates 6-phosphofructo-2-kinase to produce more fructose-2,6-bisphosphate ($F26P_2$) [58]. $F26P_2$ is a critical activator of PFK-1, a major determinant of glycolytic rates [59], leading to stimulation of glycolysis. In addition to these metabolic actions, AMPK is also known to participate in the control and regulation of protein synthesis, where it is viewed by some as a negative regulator of hypertrophy, as well as in control of gene expression and mitochondrial biogenesis [60–62].

AMPK in Pathologic and Physiologic Cardiac Hypertrophy

AMPK is activated and glycolysis is accelerated in pathologically hypertrophied rat hearts with [44] or without [53] changes in cellular energy state indicating both energy state-dependent and energy state-independent pathways are involved in activation of AMPK. We found that pharmacologic or molecular reduction of AMPK activity partially abrogates accelerated glycolytic rates in hypertrophied H9c2 cells, a line of cells derived from embryonic rat ventricle [63]. These results provide strong support for the concept that AMPK is involved in alterations in glucose use in pathologic cardiac hypertrophy, and is at least partly responsible for the acceleration of glycolysis in pathologically hypertrophied heart muscle cells. Activation of AMPK does not lead to stimulation of fatty acid oxidation because oxidation of fatty acids is impaired by other mechanisms in pathologic cardiac hypertrophy.

The role of AMPK in metabolic remodelling of physiologic cardiac hypertrophy is not yet fully understood [64]. In skeletal muscle, AMPK activation leads to increased uptake and oxidation of glucose and fatty acid as well as expression of metabolically relevant proteins and enzymes [61]. Furthermore, activation of AMPK results in increase in expression of PPARγ coactivator-1α (PGC-1α), a regulator of mitochondrial biogenesis and coactivator of peroxisome proliferator-activated receptor-α (PPARα), a key regulator of lipid metabolism [49, 65]. Specifically, activation of AMPK leads to phosphorylation and "activation" of the transcription factor PPARα [66], as well as increased expression of

PPARα and the coactivator PPARγ coactivator-1 (PGC-1α) [65]. PPARα and PGC-1α are well recognized for their roles in causing mitochondrial biogenesis and increasing expression of metabolic proteins in mitochondria, especially those related to oxidation of fatty acids [67]. Thus, it is conceivable, but not yet proven, that AMPK is involved in the regulation of metabolic remodelling in physiologic cardiac hypertrophy.

Peroxisome Proliferator-Activated Receptor-α

As a member of the family of nuclear receptors, PPARα is the primary transcriptional regulator of genes encoding enzymes and proteins that are involved in mitochondrial fatty acid oxidation [67, 68]. In pathologic cardiac hypertrophy, the expression of PPARα is low as compared to that in non-hypertrophied hearts [68–70]. This alteration in PPARα expression is accompanied by reduction in expression of genes encoding mCPT1, PDK4, MCAD and mitochondrial uncoupling proteins [70]. As mentioned, activity and expression of metabolic proteins is not typically altered significantly until heart failure occurs [69]. Down-regulation of PPARα in agonist-induced hypertrophy of isolated cardiac myocytes has been shown to be due to post-transcriptional deactivation by the mitogen-activated protein kinase, ERK1/2 [68]. In physiologic cardiac hypertrophy, on the other hand, mRNA expression of PPARα is increased coincidentally with up-regulation of mCPT1 and MCAD [43], suggesting possible involvement of PPARα-related signalling in the enhanced rates of fatty acid oxidation in exercise adapted hearts.

Peroxisome Proliferator-Activated Receptor Gamma Coactivator 1 (PGC-1)

As a coactivator of PPARα, PGC-1 interacts with PPARα to regulate lipid metabolism [69]. Thus, in addition to down-regulation of PPARα, reduced expression of PGC-1α may contribute to the reduced expression of enzymes involved in mitochondrial transport and oxidation of fatty acid in pathologic cardiac hypertrophy [69]. Conversely, in physiologic cardiac hypertrophy, PGC-1α is activated with a concurrent increase in fatty acid oxidation capacity [71]. Through its interaction with another nuclear receptor, nuclear respiratory factor 1, PGC-1 also promotes mitochondrial biogenesis [69], which may in turn contribute to the enhanced oxidative potential of the physiologically hypertrophied heart.

Protein Kinase C

Protein kinase C (PKC) is a family of serine/threonine protein kinases, which can be classified into three groups based on the upstream second messengers involved. The classical PKC (α, β1, β2 and γ) requires diacylglycerol (DAG) and Ca^{2+} for activation, while the novel PKC (δ, ε, θ and η) requires only DAG, but not Ca^{2+}, for activity. The atypical PKC (ζ and λ) does not require stimulation by DAG or Ca^{2+} [72]. PKC is recognized for its involvement in the regulation of substrate utilization in the heart, and a change in PKC content alters cardiac metabolism and contractility [73, 74]. In left ventricular hypertrophy induced by pressure overload, PKC activity is elevated with increased expression of isozymes including PKC-β1, PKC-β2 and PKC-ε in membrane and nuclear-cytoskeletal fractions [75]. Although activation of PKC has been implicated in the pathogenesis of cardiac hypertrophy and heart failure [72, 76], little is currently known about its specific role in metabolic remodelling of cardiac hypertrophy.

Phosphoinositide-3 Kinase/Protein Kinase B

Signalling via the phosphoinositide-3 kinase (PI3K)/protein kinase B (Akt) cascade is involved in cardiac growth in response to physiological and pathological stimuli [76, 77]. Physiological stimuli, such as exercise and growth factors like insulin derived growth factor-1 (IGF-1), lead to stimulation of class 1a PI3K, which contains the catalytic p110α subunit. Use of genetically modified mice, including those with overexpression of constitutively active PI3Kα or dominant negative p110α, showed the critical importance of this pathway to the development of physiological cardiac hypertrophy but not pathological cardiac hypertrophy [78]. Pathologic stimuli, including trophic factors such as angiotensin, endothelin and norepinephrine, also stimulate the PI3K pathway by acting through G-protein coupled receptors [76, 77]. In contrast to physiological stimuli, these pathological stimuli lead to activation of a different PI3K isoform, specifically class 1b PI3K which contains the catalytic p110γ subunit; an isoform shown to be involved in the development of pathologic cardiac hypertrophy but not normal physiologic growth of the heart [79].

Akt is a serine/threonine kinase downstream of PI3K that is involved in the regulation of cellular growth and metabolism of the heart [76]. There are three Akt isoforms, namely Akt1, Akt2 and Akt3, with Akt1 and Akt2 being highly expressed in the heart [76]. In studies using genetically modified mice with overexpression of activated forms of Akt, it was discovered that short term activation of Akt or Akt activation resulting in mild-moderate increases in cardiac mass led to a physiological cardiac hypertrophy phenotype, while longer term activation of Akt and Akt activation leading severe increases in mass resulted in a phenotype typical of pathologic cardiac hypertrophy [77, 80, 81]. A blunting of cardiac hypertrophy in response to exercise training and an exaggeration of cardiac hypertrophy in response to pressure overload was observed in mice with ablation of Akt1 [82], indicating Akt1 can have a positive or negative role in the development of hypertrophy depending upon the nature of stimulus. In contrast to Akt1, Akt2 plays less of a role in cardiac growth, and is instead involved in insulin-stimulated cardiac glucose uptake and metabolism [83]. Notably, pathologically hypertrophied hearts demonstrate reduced responsiveness to insulin, whose signal is also mediated via the PI3K/Akt pathway [24]. The specific defects responsible are not yet known, however.

Two signalling molecules distal to Akt play important roles in the hypertrophic response.

These include the mammalian target of Rapamycin (mTOR), a key regulator of protein synthesis, and glycogen synthase kinase-3, which is also involved in the regulation of protein synthesis as well as the control of transcription factors involved in cardiac hypertrophic growth [84]. It is important to recognize that both these molecules may also be regulated by G-protein coupled receptor mechanisms independent of Akt [84].

PI3K/Akt signalling can thus be involved in both physiologic and pathologic forms of cardiac hypertrophy. The key factors and the mechanisms by which they act to determine whether activation of this pathway participates in development of pathologic or physiologic cardiac hypertrophy are not yet known with certainty. Additionally, specific details of the role of this signalling cascade in the development of the unique metabolic phenotypes of physiologically and pathologically hypertrophied hearts remained to be fully characterized.

Hypoxia Inducible Factor-1α

Hypoxia inducible factor-1α (HIF1α) is a factor induced by hypoxic stimuli that is involved in transcriptional regulation of enzymes and proteins in glycolysis [85–87]. It can also be induced by mechanical stress under normoxic conditions mediated by a series of upstream signalling events involving activation of stretch-activated channels and PI3K/Akt signalling [85]. HIF1α has been found to be up-regulated in hypertrophic cardiomyopathy and cardiac hypertrophy induced by pressure overload [45, 88]. Given that overexpression of HIF1α elevates myocardial expression of glycolytic genes [45, 87], it is tempting to speculate that the increased HIF1α observed in pathological cardiac hypertrophy may participate in metabolic remodelling by altering expression of key metabolic enzymes and proteins. Of note, swimming-induced cardiac hypertrophy was not accompanied by an elevation of HIFα [89], indicating that HIFα may be involved in remodelling of pathologic cardiac hypertrophy but not physiologic cardiac hypertrophy.

Reactive Oxygen Species

Reactive oxygen species (ROS) are highly reactive molecules containing oxygen, which includes hydrogen peroxide, hydroxyl radical and superoxide anion. During mitochondrial oxidative phosphorylation, ROS such as superoxide anions (O_2^-) are generated as natural by-products of ATP production [90]. When produced at low levels, ROS may serve as signalling molecules involved in regulation of apoptosis, cell proliferation and cell differentiation [91]. However, when ROS production is higher and/or exceeds the capacity of the cellular antioxidant scavenging system, the resultant increase in oxidative stress will cause damage to key cellular components including mitochondria [92]. Notably, ROS have been implicated as signalling molecules in the pathogenesis of cardiac hypertrophy [93]. In SHRs, there is good evidence that hypertrophic growth is mediated by ROS-induced inhibition of AMPK/LKB1 signalling, which allows enhanced activation of mTOR and p70S6K; a process that was ameliorated by use of the antioxidant agent, resveratrol [94]. Levels of ROS are elevated in cardiac myocytes hypertrophied in response to α-adrenergic stimuli and pressure overload [93, 95]. This increase in ROS may be mediated, at least in part, by monoamine oxidase-A (MAO-A), which is also up-regulated in pathologically hypertrophied hearts [96]. Bound to the outer mitochondrial membrane, MAO oxidatively deaminates biogenic amines and produces hydrogen peroxide [97]. Therefore, enhanced MAO-A activity would be expected to raise the ROS level by increased production of hydrogen peroxide. Oxidant signalling has also been linked to stimulation of glucose uptake and glycolysis [98] and might, therefore, contribute to the development of the metabolic phenotype of pathologic cardiac hypertrophy. Another source of ROS in this setting is nicotinamide adenine dinucleotide phosphate-oxidase, whose expression rises in pressure overload cardiac hypertrophy [99]. The role and specific details of the possible contribution of ROS to hypertrophic remodelling is an area of great interest that remains to be fully characterized.

Conclusions

The specific nature of the stimulus leading to cardiac hypertrophy influences the heart's metabolic response to long-term changes in haemodynamic workload. As a result, the altered pattern of substrate utilization (or metabolic phenotype) differs dramatically between pathologic and physiologic cardiac hypertrophy with directionally opposite changes in energy substrate utilization. The metabolic remodelling in pathologic and physiologic cardiac hypertrophy also affects heart function, particularly the hypertrophied heart's ability to withstand stresses during ischemia-reperfusion. Therefore, understanding the mechanisms underlying metabolic remodelling in both types of cardiac hypertrophy will provide valuable insights into the development of therapeutic targets to improve cardiac function of patients with pathologically hypertrophied hearts. Various subcellular signalling molecules, such as AMPK, PPARα, PGC-1, PKC, HIF1α, PI3K/Akt and ROS have been implicated in the pathogenesis of cardiac hypertrophy. However, their role and the signalling mechanism(s) linking these molecules to metabolic remodelling in both pathologic and physiologic cardiac hypertrophy remain to be fully characterized and clearly warrant further study.

Acknowledgements This work was supported by CIHR. We thank Mr. Rich Wambolt and all the current and former members of the Allard laboratory who have contributed to the studies summarized here.

References

1. Swynghedauw B. Phenotypic plasticity of adult myocardium: molecular mechanisms. J Exp Biol. 2006; 209:2320–7.
2. Burelle Y, Wambolt RB, Grist M, et al. Regular exercise is associated with a protective metabolic phenotype in the rat heart. Am J Physiol Heart Circ Physiol. 2004;287:H1055–63.
3. Vincent G, Khairallah M, Bouchard B, et al. Metabolic phenotyping of the diseased rat heart using 13C-substrates and ex vivo perfusion in the working mode. Mol Cell Biochem. 2003;242:89–99.
4. Allard MF, Schonekess BO, Henning SL, et al. Contribution of oxidative metabolism and glycolysis

to ATP production in hypertrophied hearts. Am J Physiol Heart Circ Physiol. 1994;267:H742–50.

5. Richey PA, Brown SP. Pathological versus physiological left ventricular hypertrophy: a review. J Sports Sci. 1998;16:129–41.

6. Allard MF. Energy substrate metabolism in cardiac hypertrophy. Curr Hypertens Rep. 2004;6:430–5.

7. Grossman W, Jones D, McLaurin LP. Wall stress and patterns of hypertrophy in the human left ventricle. J Clin Invest. 1975;56:56–64.

8. Taegtmeyer H. Genetics of energetics: transcriptional responses in cardiac metabolism. Ann Biomed Eng. 2000;28:871–6.

9. Frohlich ED, Apstein C, Chobanian AV, et al. The heart in hypertension. N Engl J Med. 1992;327: 998–1008.

10. Gaasch WH, Zile MR, Hoshino PK, et al. Tolerance of the hypertrophic heart to ischemia. Studies in compensated and failing dog hearts with pressure overload hypertrophy. Circulation. 1990;81:1644–53.

11. Wambolt RB, Lopaschuk GD, Brownsey RW, et al. Dichloroacetate improves postischemic function of hypertrophied rat hearts. J Am Coll Cardiol. 2000; 36:1378–85.

12. Kannel WB. Risk stratification in hypertension: new insights from the Framingham study. Am J Hypertens. 2000;13:3S–10.

13. Moore RL, Palmer BM. Exercise training and cellular adaptations of normal and diseased hearts. Exerc Sport Sci Rev. 1999;27:285–315.

14. Neely JR, Morgan HE. Relationship between carbohydrate and lipid metabolism and the energy balance of heart muscle. Annu Rev Physiol. 1974;36:413–57.

15. Saddik M, Lopaschuk GD. Myocardial triglyceride turnover and contribution to energy substrate utilization in isolated working rat hearts. J Biol Chem. 1991;266:8162–70.

16. van der Vusse GJ, van Bilsen M, Glatz JF. Cardiac fatty acid uptake and transport in health and disease. Cardiovasc Res. 2000;45:279–93.

17. Lopaschuk GD, Belke DD, Gamble J, et al. Regulation of fatty acid oxidation in the mammalian heart in health and disease. Biochim Biophys Acta. 1994;1213:263–76.

18. Henning SL, Wambolt RB, Schonekess BO, et al. Contribution of glycogen to aerobic myocardial glucose utilization. Circulation. 1996;93:1549–55.

19. Stanley WC, Lopaschuk GD, Hall JL, et al. Regulation of myocardial carbohydrate metabolism under normal and ischaemic conditions. Cardiovasc Res. 1997;33: 243–57.

20. el Alaoui-Talibi Z, Landormy S, Loireau A, et al. Fatty acid oxidation and mechanical performance of volume-overloaded rat hearts. Am J Physiol Heart Circ Physiol. 1992;262:H1068–74.

21. Hajri T, Ibrahimi A, Coburn CT, et al. Defective fatty acid uptake in the spontaneously hypertensive rat is a primary determinant of altered glucose metabolism, hyperinsulinemia, and myocardial hypertrophy. J Biol Chem. 2001;276:23661–6.

22. Schonekess BO, Brindley PG, Lopaschuk GD. Calcium regulation of glycolysis, glucose oxidation, and fatty acid oxidation in the aerobic and ischemic heart. Can J Physiol Pharmacol. 1995;73:1632–40.

23. Wambolt RB, Henning SL, English DR, et al. Regression of cardiac hypertrophy normalizes glucose metabolism and left ventricular function during reperfusion. J Mol Cell Cardiol. 1997;29:939–48.

24. Allard MF, Wambolt RB, Longnus SL, et al. Hypertrophied rat hearts are less responsive to the metabolic and functional effects of insulin. Am J Physiol Endocrinol Metab. 2000;279:E487–93.

25. Saeedi R, Wambolt RB, Parsons H, et al. Gender and post-ischemic recovery of hypertrophied rat hearts. BMC Cardiovasc Disord. 2006;6:8.

26. Lopaschuk GD, Spafford MA, Marsh DR. Glycolysis is predominant source of myocardial ATP production immediately after birth. Am J Physiol Heart Circ Physiol. 1991;261:H1698–705.

27. Sambandam N, Lopaschuk GD, Brownsey RW, et al. Energy metabolism in the hypertrophied heart. Heart Fail Rev. 2002;7:161–73.

28. El Alaoui-Talibi Z, Guendouz A, Moravec M, et al. Control of oxidative metabolism in volume-overloaded rat hearts: effect of propionyl-L-carnitine. Am J Physiol Heart Circ Physiol. 1997;272:H1615–24.

29. de las Fuentes L, Herrero P, Peterson LR, et al. Myocardial fatty acid metabolism: independent predictor of left ventricular mass in hypertensive heart disease. Hypertension. 2003;41:83–7.

30. Anderson PG, Allard MF, Thomas GD, et al. Increased ischemic injury but decreased hypoxic injury in hypertrophied rat hearts. Circ Res. 1990;67:948–59.

31. Saeedi R, Grist M, Wambolt RB, et al. Trimetazidine normalizes post-ischemic function of hypertrophied rat hearts. J Pharmacol Exp Ther. 2005;314:446–54.

32. Allard MF, Emanuel PG, Russell JA, et al. Preischemic glycogen reduction or glycolytic inhibition improves postischemic recovery of hypertrophied rat hearts. Am J Physiol Heart Circ Physiol. 1994;267:H66–74.

33. Lopaschuk GD, Wambolt RB, Barr RL. An imbalance between glycolysis and glucose oxidation is a possible explanation for the detrimental effects of high levels of fatty acids during aerobic reperfusion of ischemic hearts. J Pharmacol Exp Ther. 1993;264:135–44.

34. Hata K, Takasago T, Saeki A, et al. Stunned myocardium after rapid correction of acidosis. Increased oxygen cost of contractility and the role of the $Na^{(+)}$-H^+ exchange system. Circ Res. 1994;74:794–805.

35. Ford DA. Alterations in myocardial lipid metabolism during myocardial ischemia and reperfusion. Prog Lipid Res. 2002;41:6–26.

36. Korge P, Honda HM, Weiss JN. Effects of fatty acids in isolated mitochondria: implications for ischemic injury and cardioprotection. Am J Physiol Heart Circ Physiol. 2003;285:H259–69.

37. Randle PJ, Garland PB, Hales CN, et al. The glucose fatty-acid cycle. Its role in insulin sensitivity and the metabolic disturbances of diabetes mellitus. Lancet. 1963;1:785–9.

38. Sack MN, Rader TA, Park S, et al. Fatty acid oxidation enzyme gene expression is downregulated in the failing heart. Circulation. 1996;94:2837–42.
39. Iemitsu M, Miyauchi T, Maeda S, et al. Cardiac hypertrophy by hypertension and exercise training exhibits different gene expression of enzymes in energy metabolism. Hypertens Res. 2003;26:829–37.
40. Luiken JJ, Arumugam Y, Dyck DJ, et al. Increased rates of fatty acid uptake and plasmalemmal fatty acid transporters in obese Zucker rats. J Biol Chem. 2001;276:40567–73.
41. van der Vusse GJ, van Bilsen M, Glatz JF, et al. Critical steps in cellular fatty acid uptake and utilization. Mol Cell Biochem. 2002;239:9–15.
42. Zonderland ML, Bar PR, Reijneveld JC, et al. Different metabolic adaptation of heart and skeletal muscles to moderate-intensity treadmill training in the rat. Eur J Appl Physiol Occup Physiol. 1999;79:391–6.
43. Rimbaud S, Sanchez H, Garnier A, et al. Stimulus specific changes of energy metabolism in hypertrophied heart. J Mol Cell Cardiol. 2009;46:952–9.
44. Tian R, Musi N, D'Agostino J, et al. Increased adenosine monophosphate-activated protein kinase activity in rat hearts with pressure-overload hypertrophy. Circulation. 2001;104:1664–9.
45. Krishnan J, Suter M, Windak R, et al. Activation of a HIF1alpha-PPARgamma axis underlies the integration of glycolytic and lipid anabolic pathways in pathologic cardiac hypertrophy. Cell Metab. 2009;9:512–24.
46. Kim J, Wende AR, Sena S, et al. Insulin-like growth factor I receptor signaling is required for exercise-induced cardiac hypertrophy. Mol Endocrinol. 2008;22:2531–43.
47. De Sousa E, Veksler V, Minajeva A, et al. Subcellular creatine kinase alterations. Implications in heart failure. Circ Res. 1999;85:68–76.
48. Kudo N, Barr AJ, Barr RL, et al. High rates of fatty acid oxidation during reperfusion of ischemic hearts are associated with a decrease in malonyl-CoA levels due to an increase in 5'-AMP-activated protein kinase inhibition of acetyl-CoA carboxylase. J Biol Chem. 1995;270:17513–20.
49. Hardie DG, Sakamoto K. AMPK: a key sensor of fuel and energy status in skeletal muscle. Physiology (Bethesda). 2006;21:48–60.
50. Carling D, Sanders MJ, Woods A. The regulation of AMP-activated protein kinase by upstream kinases. Int J Obes (Lond). 2008;32 Suppl 4:S55–9.
51. Sakamoto K, McCarthy A, Smith D, et al. Deficiency of LKB1 in skeletal muscle prevents AMPK activation and glucose uptake during contraction. EMBO J. 2005;24:1810–20.
52. Woods A, Dickerson K, Heath R, et al. Ca^{2+}/calmodulin-dependent protein kinase kinase-beta acts upstream of AMP-activated protein kinase in mammalian cells. Cell Metab. 2005;2:21–33.
53. Allard MF, Parsons HL, Saeedi R, et al. AMPK and metabolic adaptation by the heart to pressure overload. Am J Physiol Heart Circ Physiol. 2007;292:H140–8.
54. Chabowski A, Momken I, Coort S, et al. Prolonged AMPK activation increases the expression of fatty acid transporters in cardiac myocytes and perfused hearts. Mol Cell Biochem. 2006;288:201–12.
55. An D, Pulinilkunnil T, Qi D, et al. The metabolic "switch" AMPK regulates cardiac heparin-releasable lipoprotein lipase. Am J Physiol Endocrinol Metab. 2005;288:E246–53.
56. McGarry JD. Malonyl-CoA and carnitine palmitoyltransferase I: an expanding partnership. Biochem Soc Trans. 1995;23:481–5.
57. Russell III RR, Bergeron R, Shulman GI, et al. Translocation of myocardial GLUT-4 and increased glucose uptake through activation of AMPK by AICAR. Am J Physiol Heart Circ Physiol. 1999;277:H643–9.
58. Marsin A-S, Bertrand L, Rider MH, et al. Phosphorylation and activation of heart PFK-2 by AMPK has a role in the stimulation of glycolysis during ischemia. Curr Biol. 2000;10:1247–55.
59. Narabayashi H, Lawson JW, Uyeda K. Regulation of phosphofructokinase in perfused rat heart. Requirement for fructose 2,6-bisphosphate and a covalent modification. J Biol Chem. 1985;260:9750–8.
60. Winder WW, Holmes BF, Rubink DS, et al. Activation of AMP-activated protein kinase increases mitochondrial enzymes in skeletal muscle. J Appl Physiol. 2000;88:2219–26.
61. Holmes BF, Kurth-Kraczek EJ, Winder WW. Chronic activation of 5'-AMP-activated protein kinase increases GLUT-4, hexokinase, and glycogen in muscle. J Appl Physiol. 1999;87:1990–5.
62. Jorgensen SB, Richter EA, Wojtaszewski JF. Role of AMPK in skeletal muscle metabolic regulation and adaptation in relation to exercise. J Physiol. 2006;574:17–31.
63. Saeedi R, Saran VV, Wu SSY, et al. AMP-activated protein kinase influences metabolic remodeling in H9c2 cells hypertrophied by arginine vasopressin. Am J Physiol Heart Circ Physiol. 2009;296:H1822–32.
64. Musi N, Hirshman MF, Arad M, et al. Functional role of AMP-activated protein kinase in the heart during exercise. FEBS Lett. 2005;579:2045–50.
65. Terada S, Goto M, Kato M, et al. Effects of low-intensity prolonged exercise on PGC-1 mRNA expression in rat epitrochlearis muscle. Biochem Biophys Res Commun. 2002;296:350–4.
66. Burns KA, Vanden Heuvel JP. Modulation of PPAR activity via phosphorylation. Biochim Biophys Acta. 2007;1771:952–60.
67. Finck BN. The PPAR regulatory system in cardiac physiology and disease. Cardiovasc Res. 2007;73:269–77.
68. Barger PM, Brandt JM, Leone TC, et al. Deactivation of peroxisome proliferator-activated receptor-alpha during cardiac hypertrophic growth. J Clin Invest. 2000;105:1723–30.
69. Lehman JJ, Kelly DP. Gene regulatory mechanisms governing energy metabolism during cardiac hypertrophic growth. Heart Fail Rev. 2002;7:175–85.

70. Akki A, Smith K, Seymour AM. Compensated cardiac hypertrophy is characterised by a decline in palmitate oxidation. Mol Cell Biochem. 2008;311: 215–24.

71. O'Neill BT, Kim J, Wende AR, et al. A conserved role for phosphatidylinositol 3-kinase but not Akt signaling in mitochondrial adaptations that accompany physiological cardiac hypertrophy. Cell Metab. 2007;6:294–306.

72. Malhotra R, D'Souza KM, Staron ML, et al. Gαq-mediated activation of GRK2 by mechanical stretch in cardiac myocytes. J Biol Chem. 2010;285:13748–60.

73. Mayr M, Chung Y-L, Mayr U, et al. Loss of PKC-{delta} alters cardiac metabolism. Am J Physiol Heart Circ Physiol. 2004;287:H937–45.

74. Liu Q, Chen X, MacDonnell SM, et al. Protein kinase C{alpha}, but not PKC{beta} or PKC{gamma}, regulates contractility and heart failure susceptibility: implications for ruboxistaurin as a novel therapeutic approach. Circ Res. 2009;105:194–200.

75. Gu X, Bishop SP. Increased protein kinase C and isozyme redistribution in pressure-overload cardiac hypertrophy in the rat. Circ Res. 1994;75:926–31.

76. Dorn II GW, Force T. Protein kinase cascades in the regulation of cardiac hypertrophy. J Clin Invest. 2005;115:527–37.

77. Shiojima I, Sato K, Izumiya Y, et al. Disruption of coordinated cardiac hypertrophy and angiogenesis contributes to the transition to heart failure. J Clin Invest. 2005;115:2108–18.

78. McMullen JR, Shioi T, Zhang L, et al. Phosphoinositide 3-kinase(p110alpha) plays a critical role for the induction of physiological, but not pathological, cardiac hypertrophy. Proc Natl Acad Sci USA. 2003;100: 12355–60.

79. Patrucco E, Notte A, Barberis L, et al. PI3Kgamma modulates the cardiac response to chronic pressure overload by distinct kinase-dependent and -independent effects. Cell. 2004;118:375–87.

80. Condorelli G, Drusco A, Stassi G, et al. Akt induces enhanced myocardial contractility and cell size in vivo in transgenic mice. Proc Natl Acad Sci USA. 2002;99:12333–8.

81. Matsui T, Li L, Wu JC, et al. Phenotypic spectrum caused by transgenic overexpression of activated Akt in the heart. J Biol Chem. 2002;277:22896–901.

82. DeBosch B, Treskov I, Lupu TS, et al. Akt1 is required for physiological cardiac growth. Circulation. 2006;113:2097–104.

83. DeBosch B, Sambandam N, Weinheimer C, et al. Akt2 regulates cardiac metabolism and cardiomyocyte survival. J Biol Chem. 2006;281:32841–51.

84. Proud CG. Ras, PI3-kinase and mTOR signaling in cardiac hypertrophy. Cardiovasc Res. 2004;63: 403–13.

85. Kim CH, Cho YS, Chun YS, et al. Early expression of myocardial HIF-1alpha in response to mechanical stresses: regulation by stretch-activated channels and the phosphatidylinositol 3-kinase signaling pathway. Circ Res. 2002;90:E25–33.

86. Semenza GL, Roth PH, Fang HM, et al. Transcriptional regulation of genes encoding glycolytic enzymes by hypoxia-inducible factor 1. J Biol Chem. 1994;269: 23757–63.

87. Xue W, Cai L, Tan Y, et al. Cardiac-specific overexpression of HIF-1{alpha} prevents deterioration of glycolytic pathway and cardiac remodeling in streptozotocin-induced diabetic mice. Am J Pathol. 2010;177: 97–105.

88. Shyu KG, Liou JY, Wang BW. Carvedilol prevents cardiac hypertrophy and overexpression of hypoxia-inducible factor-1alpha and vascular endothelial growth factor in pressure-overloaded rat heart. J Biomed Sci. 2005;12:409–20.

89. Luo J, McMullen JR, Sobkiw CL, et al. Class IA phosphoinositide 3-kinase regulates heart size and physiological cardiac hypertrophy. Mol Cell Biol. 2005;25:9491–502.

90. Ritchie RH, Delbridge LM. Cardiac hypertrophy, substrate utilization and metabolic remodelling: cause or effect? Clin Exp Pharmacol Physiol. 2006;33: 159–66.

91. Sauer H, Wartenberg M. Reactive oxygen species as signaling molecules in cardiovascular differentiation of embryonic stem cells and tumor-induced angiogenesis. Antioxid Redox Signal. 2005;7:1423–34.

92. Tsutsui H, Kinugawa S, Matsushima S. Mitochondrial oxidative stress and dysfunction in myocardial remodelling. Cardiovasc Res. 2009;81:449–56.

93. Akki A, Zhang M, Murdoch C, et al. NADPH oxidase signaling and cardiac myocyte function. J Mol Cell Cardiol. 2009;47:15–22.

94. Dolinsky VW, Chan AYM, Robillard Frayne I, et al. Resveratrol prevents the prohypertrophic effects of oxidative stress on LKB1. Circulation. 2009;119: 1643–52.

95. Nakamura K, Fushimi K, Kouchi H, et al. Inhibitory effects of antioxidants on neonatal rat cardiac myocyte hypertrophy induced by tumor necrosis factor-alpha and angiotensin II. Circulation. 1998;98: 794–9.

96. Kong SW, Bodyak N, Yue P, et al. Genetic expression profiles during physiological and pathological cardiac hypertrophy and heart failure in rats. Physiol Genomics. 2005;21:34–42.

97. Mialet-Perez J, Bianchi P, Kunduzova O, et al. New insights on receptor-dependent and monoamine oxidase-dependent effects of serotonin in the heart. J Neural Transm. 2007;114:823–7.

98. Fischer Y, Thomas J, Kamp J, et al. 5-Hydroxytryptamine stimulates glucose transport in cardiomyocytes via a monoamine oxidase-dependent reaction. Biochem J. 1995;311:575–83.

99. Li JM, Gall NP, Grieve DJ, et al. Activation of NADPH oxidase during progression of cardiac hypertrophy to failure. Hypertension. 2002;40:477–84.

Mechanisms for the Regulation of Phospholipase C Gene Expression in Cardiac Hypertrophy

Paramjit S. Tappia

Abstract

Phospholipase C (PLC) is considered to mediate the cardiomyocyte hypertrophic response to norepinephrine. However, a paucity of information exists regarding the regulation of specific PLC isozyme gene and protein expression as well as activities in normal and hypertrophied myocardium. In this chapter, the role of PLC isozymes in cardiac hypertrophy as well as some of the mechanisms that are involved in the regulation of PLC isozyme gene expression, protein abundance and activities are discussed. On the basis of the available literature, it is suggested that specific PLC isozymes could be involved in the cardiomyocyte response to different hypertrophic stimuli and that modification of the transcriptional regulation of PLC isozymes could also prevent the progression of cardiac hypertrophy and its transition to heart failure.

Keywords

Phospholipase C • Adult cardiomyocytes • Signal transduction • Regulation of gene expression • Cardiac hypertrophy

Introduction

Phospholipase C Isozymes in the Heart

Although the signal transduction processes following agonist–receptor interaction have not been completely elucidated for most agonists,

P.S. Tappia (✉)
Asper Clinical Research Institute, St. Boniface Hospital Research and Department of Human Nutritional Sciences, University of Manitoba, Winnipeg, Canada
e-mail: ptappia@sbrc.ca

phospholipid signal transduction pathways are emerging as important mediators of the cardiomyocyte response to external stimuli [1–3]. The cardiac sarcolemma (SL) membrane associated phospholipase C (PLC) isozymes play a key role in early activation of intracellular signal transduction pathways known to regulate a variety of cell functions [4–7]. Extracellular signals such as neurotransmitters, hormones and growth factors, evoke intracellular responses by activating PLC [7–17]. In fact, a number of different agonists including norepinephrine (NE), Angiotensin II (Ang II) and endothelin-1 (ET-1), by binding to their specific receptors stimulate G-protein (Gq subfamily) for subsequent activation of PLC [7]. PLC isozymes are also present in the cytosolic compartment of the cardiomyocyte and the physiological concentrations of PIP_2 dissolved in the cytosol are negligible [13]; thus, in vivo, cytosolic PLC isozymes must migrate to the membrane where their lipid substrate resides [13].

The activation of PLC results in the hydrolysis of phosphatidylinositol 4,5 bisphosphate (PIP_2) to produce DAG and IP_3. The functional significance of IP_3 in the heart has been up for debate [18, 19]. The IP_3 receptors (IP_3R) are ubiquitous intracellular Ca^{2+} release channels [20]. However, relative to ryanodine receptor (RyR), which is the main source of Ca^{2+} in excitation–contraction coupling (ECC), low levels of IP_3R are present in the cardiomyocyte [21]. The IP_3R may contribute to altered ECC and arrhythmogenesis in atria [22, 23]. The type 2 IP_3R, which is the predominant subtype in cardiomyocytes, is located mainly in the nuclear envelope in ventricular cardiomyocytes, but its role in the heart is poorly understood. ET-1 elicits local nuclear envelope Ca^{2+} release via type 2 IP_3R [20]. It was suggested that the local Ca^{2+} release results in the activation (derepression) of transcription, thus providing a mechanism of how PLC-derived IP_3 may be involved in altered gene expression in hypertrophy; so-called excitation–transcription coupling [20]. Interestingly, overexpression of IP_3 5-phosphatase has been shown to result in reduced IP_3 responses to α_1-AR agonists acutely, but with longer stimulation, an overall increase in PLC activity was observed, which was associated with a selective increase in expression of PLC β_1 that served to normalize IP_3 content in neonatal rat cardiomyocytes [19]. It was suggested that the level of IP_3 selectively regulates the expression of PLC β_1. Furthermore, it was also demonstrated that hearts from type 2 IP_3R knock-out mice showed heightened PLC β_1 expression. Accordingly, it was concluded that IP_3 and type 2 IP_3R regulate PLC β_1 and thereby maintain levels of IP_3 [19], providing further functional significance for IP_3 in the heart. On the other hand, DAG acts in conjunction with phosphatidylserine and in some cases Ca^{2+} to activate different PKC

isoforms containing a cysteine-rich C-1 domain [24]. PKC family members displaying responsiveness to DAG modulate contractile properties and promote cell growth and survival [25–29]. It is interesting to note that PLC-derived DAG would produce a physiological response that is mediated by PKC depending on the fatty acid species in the DAG molecule [30, 31]. In this regard, polyunsaturated fatty acid containing DAG is considered as a more potent activator of PKC [30, 31]. The PLC family consists of six subfamilies: PLC β, γ, δ, ε, ζ and η [7, 32–36], and PLC β, δ, γ and ε isozymes appear to be the predominant forms expressed in the heart [37–39]. Although these isozymes display differences in structure and activating mechanisms, Ca^{2+} is required for their activity, but their Ca^{2+} sensitivity varies [7, 32, 40]. However the distinct role of each of the PLC isozymes in cardiomyocyte hypertrophy and the extent of their overlap has yet to be completely defined.

Regulation of PLC Gene Expression, Protein Levels and Activities in Cardiac Hypertrophy

We have previously reported that the NE-induced increases in atrial natriuretic factor (ANF, a marker for cardiac hypertrophy) gene expression as well as protein synthesis that can be attenuated by U73122, an inhibitor of PLC activities, as well as by an α_1-adrenoceptor (α_1-AR) blocker, prazosin [8] in isolated adult left ventricular (LV) cardiomyocytes. The role of PLC in the development of different types of cardiac hypertrophy, in vivo, has also been documented. For example, the development of cardiac hypertrophy in stroke prone spontaneously hypertensive rats has been reported to involve PLC signalling pathway [41, 42]. Furthermore, the development of cardiac hypertrophy in cardiomyopathic hamster (BIO 14.6) was found to be associated with an increase in PLC activity [43]. In addition, we have previously reported an increase in PLC isozyme gene and protein expression as well as activities in the hypertrophied rat heart due to volume overload induced by an arteriovenous shunt [44, 45]. Of note, it was demonstrated that increases in PLC β_1 and γ_1 were associated with the hypertrophic stage in this model [35]. It should be noted that the receptor of most growth factors are transmembrane tyrosine kinases and transduce their signal via PLC γ [7, 10]. In fact, Ang II may also mediate some of its cardiac effects by activation of PLC γ_1 [46].

The status of PLC β_1 levels in cardiac hypertrophy due to pressure overload induced by ligation of the descending thoracic aorta in the guinea pig has also been examined [47]. In this study, quantitative immunoblotting revealed that PLC β_1 and Gαq protein levels were unchanged during hypertrophy. However, translocation of PKC isozymes from cytosol to membranous fractions was elevated. These investigators suggested that PKC translocation occurred without changes in Gαq and PLC-β protein abundance and that it might be due to increases in Gαq and PLC β_1 activity rather than upregulation of expression [47]; however, PLC β_1 activity was not determined in this study. Several studies have shown that antagonism of the α_1-AR, Ang II type 1 receptor and ET-1 type A receptor types results in mitigation of cardiac hypertrophy and its progression to heart failure [48–56]. An upregulation of PLC β_3 protein expression as well as activity has been reported in the development of cardiac hypertrophy in 2K1C hypertensive rats [57]; furthermore these investigators observed an increase in the protein levels of PLC β_3 in neonatal rat cardiomyocytes in response to Ang II that could be inhibited with losartan, an AT$_1$ receptor blocker [57]. Interestingly, we have previously demonstrated that treatment with losartan immediately after the induction of volume overload hypertrophy (due to arteriovenous shunt) resulted in an attenuation of PLC isozyme gene expression, which was found to be correlated to regression of cardiac hypertrophy [45]. It is possible that losartan could also have attenuated PLC isozyme activities.

The development of hypertrophy in cultured rat neonatal cardiomyocytes induced by ET-1 has been reported to be due to the activation of PLC β isozymes [58]. Furthermore, the expression pattern of the PLC β isozyme subfamily has also been investigated in neonatal rat cardiomyocytes after stimulation with different hypertrophic stimuli [59]. In this study, under control conditions and after stimulation with NE, cardiomyocytes expressed similar amounts of PLC β_3 mRNA. However, in the presence of foetal calf serum, additional expression of PLC β_1 was induced. Growth hormone and insulin-like growth factor-I (IGF-I) both induced a substantial increase in PLC β_3 mRNA expression. In addition, the response to growth factor could not be abolished by the IGF-I receptor blocker IGF-I analogue indicating an IGF-I-independent action of growth hormone. Furthermore, it was shown that the upregulation of PLC β_3 by IGF-I was abolished by preincubation of cardiomyocytes with the IGF-I receptor antagonist IGF-I analogue, the tyrosine kinase inhibitor genistein, the extracellular signal-related kinase (ERK) inhibitor PD 98059, the phosphatidylinositol-3 (PI-3)-kinase inhibitor wortmannin and the p70 S6 kinase inhibitor rapamycin. Induction of the immediate early genes c-myc, c-fos and c-jun by IGF-I was abolished by preincubation with antisense oligos against PLC β_3. These investigators concluded that the expression of PLC β isozymes in cardiomyocytes is differentially regulated by different hypertrophic stimuli [59]. Moreover, the upregulation of PLC β_3 by IGF-I is dependent on the activity of tyrosine kinase, ERK, PI3 kinase and p70 S6 kinase and PLC β_3 expression seems to be required for the induction of immediate early genes by IGF-I. Accordingly, the involvement of the PLC β subfamily in signal transduction of receptors other than G-protein-coupled receptors such as IGF-I receptors was suggested. While PLC β isozymes, β_1 and β_3 have been extensively characterized in cardiac tissue, recently PLC β_4 mRNA expression levels > PLC β_{1-3} have been reported in human LV tissue [60]. Furthermore, these investigators demonstrated that PLC β_4 mRNA levels are increased in response to Angiotensin II in mouse HL-1 cardiomyocytes, suggesting that this isoform may also have a role to play in the development of cardiac hypertrophy.

Fas receptor activation, a classical death signal causing apoptosis via activation of the caspase cascade [61], has been recognized as a novel pathway mediating cardiomyocyte hypertrophy in vitro and in vivo [62]. These investigators demonstrated that Fas activation by Fas ligand induced a hypertrophic response in cultured neonatal rat cardiomyocytes. Furthermore, in *lpr* mice lacking functional Fas, a rapid-onset of left ventricular (LV) dilatation and failure, absence of compensatory hypertrophy and increased mortality, due to pressure overload, was also demonstrated indicating that hypertrophy was dependent on Fas activity [62]. In addition, in the same cell type, Fas activation has been shown to induce NFAT nuclear translocation [63]. These investigators also demonstrated that the hypertrophy was abolished by U73122 (PLC inhibitor) and xestospongin C (an IP_3 receptor blocker), demonstrating Fas-mediated hypertrophy is dependent on the PLC-IP_3 pathway. Mechanical stress induced by cell stretching in neonatal cardiomyocytes has also been reported to increase PLC activity [64]. However, in these studies [63, 64] no attempt was made to identify the PLC isozymes responsible for such responses. It is important to note that while some studies have reported changes in the expression levels of PLC β isozymes in the hypertrophic response in neonatal cardiomyocytes [57, 59], the signalling function i.e., PLC activities is determined by the interaction with Gαq and thus increases in the myocardial PLC isozyme mRNA levels alone, does not necessarily signify a role of PLC isozymes in cardiac hypertrophy.

Stimulation of signalling pathways via Gαq and rac1 provokes cardiac hypertrophy in cultured cardiomyocytes and transgenic mouse models [65–68]. Furthermore, Ang II type 1 receptor (a Gαq-coupled receptor), overexpression has been reported to induce cardiac hypertrophy [69]. The first transgenic murine cardiac hypertrophy model to support a Gαq mechanism of hypertrophy was over expression of the wild-type Gαq in the heart using the α-MHC promoter [65]. Indeed, a fourfold overexpression of Gαq resulted in increased heart weight and cardiomyocyte size along with marked increases in ANF, α-skeletal actin and β-myosin heavy chain expression. In view of the fact that an essential downstream effector for Gαq is PLC β [7], these observations would appear to implicate the activation of PLC β isozymes in cardiac hypertrophy. Gαq expression in vivo constitutively elevates cardiac PLC β activity [70, 71]. The transgenic mouse line (αq*52) in which cardiac-specific expression of hemagglutinin (HA) epitope-tagged constitutively active mutant of the Gαq subunit (HAαq*) leads to activation of PLC β, the immediate downstream target of HAαq*, with subsequent development of cardiac hypertrophy and dilation. However, in a second, independent line in the same genetic background (αq*44h) with lower expression of HAαq* protein that ultimately results in the same phenotype of dilated cardiomyopathy, no correlation with PLC activity was seen [72].

G-proteins are subject to direct regulation by RGS (regulators of G protein signalling) proteins, which shorten the duration of the cellular response to external signals and generally cause a reduction in hormone sensitivity [73]. Although the primary mode of action of RGS proteins is to accelerate termination of the signal by decreasing the lifetime of active, GTP-bound Gα subunits, some RGS proteins can also inhibit signal generation by antagonizing Gα-mediated effector activation [74]. In this regard, recently it has been reported that endogenous ventricular RGS2 expression is selectively reduced in two different models of cardiac hypertrophy (transgenic Gαq expression and pressure overload), which was linked to elevated PLC β activity [75]. These investigators suggested that endogenous RGS2 exerts a functionally important inhibitory restraint on Gq/11-mediated PLC β activation and hypertrophy and concluded that loss of cardiac fine-tuning of PLC β signalling by RGS2 down-regulation could potentially play a pathophysiological role in the development of Gq/11-mediated cardiac hypertrophy.

The cardiac-targeted overexpression of $α_{1A}$-AR results in a small increase in the NE-stimulated, but not basal, PLC activity. However, no morphological, histological or echocardiographic evidence of LV hypertrophy was observed [76]. In addition, apart from an increase in ANF mRNA, expression of other hypertrophy-associated genes was unchanged.

On the other hand, cardiac-specific expression of α_{1B}-AR in mice results in the activation of PLC as evidenced by an increase in myocardial DAG content [77]. Furthermore, a phenotype consistent with cardiac hypertrophy developed in the adult transgenic mice with increase heart/body weight ratios, cardiomyocyte cross-sectional areas and ventricular ANF mRNA levels [77]. Thus, it would appear that the α_{1B}-AR is primarily implicated in hypertrophy.

We have earlier reported that NE-mediated cardiac hypertrophy may occur due to stimulation of α_1-AR and PLC activity [8]. We have also examined the signal transduction mechanisms involved in the regulation of PLC isozyme gene expression in adult cardiomyocytes in response to NE [9]. In this study, it was revealed that the NE-induced increases in PLC β_1, β_3, γ_1, and δ_1 isozyme mRNA and protein levels were attenuated in cardiomyocytes pretreated with either prazosin, an α_1-AR blocker or U73122, an inhibitor of PLC activities. The effects of prazosin and U73122 were associated with inhibition of PLC activity. The inhibition of NE-stimulated PLC protein and gene expression by bisindolylmaleimide-1, a PKC inhibitor, and PD98059, an ERK1/2 inhibitor, indicated that PKC-MAPK signalling may be involved in this signal transduction pathway. Furthermore, significant increases in mRNA levels and protein contents for all PLC isozymes were found in cardiomyocytes treated with phorbol 12-myristate 13-acetate, a PKC activator. Taken together, it was suggested that PLC isozymes may regulate their own gene expression through a PKC and ERK1/2-dependent pathway (Fig. 1). It should be noted that U73122 has been reported to exert non-specific actions in different cell types [78–82]; however, these were observed at concentrations that are between 100- and 10,000-fold greater than the concentration used in our studies [8, 9]. It is pointed out that the NE-induced IP_3 generation in neonatal rat cardiomyocytes has been reported to be primarily due to α_1-AR-mediated activation of PLC β_1 [83]. PLC β_1 exists as two splice variants, PLC β_{1a} and PLC β_{1b}, which differ only in their C-terminal sequences of 64 and 31 amino acids, respectively. While PLC β_{1a} is localized in the cytoplasm, PLC

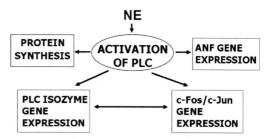

Fig. 1 Possible role of PLC activation in the progression of cardiac hypertrophy. *PLC* phospholipase C, *ANF* atrial natriuretic factor. Reproduced from Clin Lipidol. 2009;4:79–90 with permission of Future Medicine Ltd

β_{1b} targets to the SL and is enriched in caveolae [84], where α_1-AR signalling is also localized [85]. Furthermore, in cardiomyocytes, responses initiated by α_1-AR activation involve only PLC β_{1b}, thus the selective targeting of this splice variant to the SL membrane provides a potential target to reduce hypertrophy [85]. Indeed, recently it has been shown that the overexpression of one splice variant of PLC β_1, specifically PLC β_{1b}, in neonatal rat cardiomyocytes causes increased cell size, elevated protein/DNA ratio, and heightened expression of the hypertrophy-related marker gene, atrial natriuretic peptide [86]. The other splice variant, PLC β_{1a}, had no effect. Expression of a 32-amino acid C-terminal PLC β_{1b} peptide, which competes with PLC β_{1b} for sarcolemmal association, prevented PLC activation and eliminated hypertrophic responses initiated by Gq or Gq-coupled α_1-adrenergic receptors. In contrast, a PLC β_{1a} C-terminal peptide altered neither PLC activity nor cellular hypertrophy. It was concluded that hypertrophic responses initiated by Gq are mediated specifically by PLC β_{1b}. This study provided further evidence that preventing PLC β_{1b} association with the sarcolemma may provide a useful therapeutic target to limit hypertrophy.

An increased expression of the protooncogene, *c-fos* is associated with the initiation of cardiac hypertrophy [87]. Similarly, it has been reported that the stretching of isolated neonatal cardiomyocytes or exposure to NE also elevates *c-fos* mRNA levels and produces cellular hypertrophy [88–90]. Although the pathway that mediates the NE-induction of *c-fos* in other cell types has been shown to involve PKC, the identity of the specific PLC isozymes that may be part of this signalling pathway is not known. In addition, since ERK1/2 is considered to play a major role in the upregulation of the mRNA and protein levels of the immediate early gene *c-jun* [90], it is possible that this transcription factor may play a role in the regulation of PLC isozyme mRNA levels in response to α_1-AR stimulation in adult cardiomyocytes. Although it is well known that both *c-fos* and *c-jun* regulate the expression of a number of genes in the heart [91–94], our studies [95] using *c-fos* and *c-jun* siRNA have indicated that these transcription factors might also regulate the expression of specific PLC isozymes. It should be noted that under our experimental conditions, NE treatment of adult rat cardiomyocytes for 2 h did not induce any change in NFAT3, NFκB, MEF2C and MEF2D mRNA levels, suggesting that these transcription factors may not regulate the early increase in PLC isozyme gene expression in response to NE [96]. Furthermore, our studies revealed that specific PLC isozymes may be involved in the regulation of *c-fos* and *c-jun* gene expression in response to NE [96]. This raises the intriguing possibility of a reciprocal regulation of PLC isozyme and *c-fos* and *c-jun* gene expression in adult cardiomyocytes. In fact, PLC may play an important role in a cycle of events that may be involved in the progression of the cardiomyocyte hypertrophic response (Fig. 1).

While our observations have placed the activation of PLC isozymes as an important signalling event in hypertrophy of the adult heart [8, 9, 44, 97], a loss of PLC ε signalling in PLC ε knock-out mice has recently been suggested to sensitize the heart to development of hypertrophy in response to chronic isoproterenol treatment [39]. However, cardiac hypertrophy independent of PLC activation has also been reported [72, 98]. Nonetheless, from the aforementioned discussion it possible that specific PLC isozymes might play a contributory role in the signal transduction pathways activated in cardiac hypertrophy. It is worth pointing out that

we as well as others have reported that phosphatidic acid (PA), a product of phospholipase D (PLD) activities, can stimulate PLC isozyme activities [97, 99, 100]. We also believe that PA can induce an increase in PLC isozyme gene expression [101]. Interestingly, we have previously reported that PA may be a potential signal transducer for cardiac hypertrophy [97]. In fact, we have also previously reported that PA is a potent stimulator of PLC isozyme activities. Accordingly, it can be suggested that the generation of PA in cardiac hypertrophy may be involved in the perpetuation and amplification of the cardiomyocyte hypertrophic response that might involve increases in PLC isozyme gene and protein expression as well as their activities.

An upregulation during cardiac hypertrophy is not limited to PLC. In rat heart, abdominal aortic banding (constriction to 50% of original lumen) induced hypertrophy in the left ventricle (as shown by weight index and ANP expression) is accompanied increases in the mRNA expressions of both PLD1 and PLD2. Furthermore, a similar induction of PLD mRNA and protein expression was observed in hypertrophied human hearts of individuals (39- to 45-year-old) who had died from non-cardiac causes [102]. It is interesting to note that PLC-β stimulated by ET-1, may cross-talk with PLD [103]. Some of our earlier work [101] has shown that NE induces an increase in both PLD1 and PLD2 isozyme gene expression in adult rat cardiomyocytes. In addition, both prazosin, U73122 and Bis-1 inhibited the NE-induced increase in PLD1 isozyme gene expression. Activation of PKC with PMA resulted in an increase in the mRNA expression of PLD1 isozyme only, while blockade of ERK1/2 activity with PD98059 specifically prevented the NE-induced increase in PLD1 isozyme gene expression. These data demonstrate that the NE-induced increase in PLD1 gene expression occurs via a PKC-ERK1/2 dependent pathway whereas increase in PLD2 gene expression induced by NE occurs via PKC-ERK1/2 independent pathway. Thus, PLC activation may also play a significant role in the upregulation of PLD isozyme gene expression during cardiac hypertrophy. In fact, it could be suggested that upregulation of both PLC

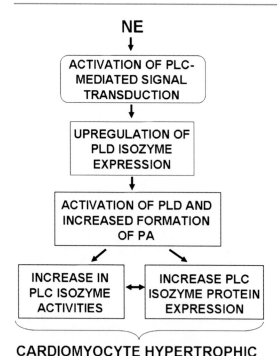

NE
↓
ACTIVATION OF PLC-
MEDIATED SIGNAL
TRANSDUCTION
↓
UPREGULATION OF
PLD ISOZYME
EXPRESSION
↓
ACTIVATION OF PLD AND
INCREASED FORMATION
OF PA

INCREASE IN
PLC ISOZYME
ACTIVITIES ⟷ INCREASE PLC
ISOZYME PROTEIN
EXPRESSION

CARDIOMYOCYTE HYPERTROPHIC
RESPONSE

Fig. 2 Possible mechanism of interaction between PLC and PLD in adult cardiomyocytes during cardiac hypertrophy. *PLC* phospholipase C, *PLD* phospholipase D, *PA* phosphatidic acid. Reproduced from Clin Lipidol. 2009;4:79–90 with permission of Future Medicine Ltd

Conclusions

In this chapter, we have presented information on the involvement of PLC-mediated signal transduction events in cardiac hypertrophy. We have also identified some of the signal transduction mechanisms involved in the molecular regulation of PLC as well as PLD isozymes. Although significant in roads have been made, much more remains to be done in understanding the role of PLC in cardiac hypertrophy. For example, the contribution of PLC with respect to other myocardial signalling systems involved in the hypertrophic response needs to be evaluated. While some information on the molecular regulation of PLC isozymes has been provided many aspects remain to be completely understood. The intriguing and exciting concept of PLC activities being involved in the regulation of self isozyme gene expression as well as PLC activation regulating the expressions levels of PLD raises the idea that PLC is a key component that may not only initiate cardiac hypertrophy, but may also be involved in the perpetuation of the hypertrophic response. In spite of this, the involvement of specific PLC isozymes as well as the extent of functional overlap in cardiac hypertrophy needs to be verified i.e., if overexpression of specific PLC isozymes in cardiomyocytes in vitro and in vivo results in hypertrophic phenotype. While some studies have shown prazosin in mitigating the progression of cardiac hypertrophy to heart failure [48, 49, 106–108] and losartan to attenuate cardiac hypertrophy, a direct inhibition of PLC (isozyme gene expression, protein contents and activities) and regression of cardiac hypertrophy needs to be demonstrated in vivo. It should be noted that the discussion in this article is not meant to de-emphasize the activation of different signal transduction pathways and their role in cardiac hypertrophy, but from the evidence provided it is proposed that specific PLC isozymes might constitute additional therapeutic targets for drug discovery for the treatment of cardiac hypertrophy and its progression to heart failure.

and PLC-induced PLD gene expression may constitute part of a signal transduction system for the augmentation/perpetuation of the hypertrophic response to NE (Fig. 2). However, it remains to be determined if the changes in PLD isozyme gene expression also translate to corresponding changes at the protein level as well as in activities. While a linkage between PLC and PLD might exist in the heart, a link between PLD and PLA$_2$ with PLC has been suggested and considered to be mediated via lipid products in TSA-201 cells [104]. In view of the above observations it is possible that a similar cross-talk linking these phospholipases together may also exist in cardiomyocytes, which not only regulates protein function, but also the expression of phospholipases. Support for this concept is provided, in part, by our previous report of a PLA$_2$-mediated activation of PLD in rat heart [105].

Acknowledgements The work reported in this article was supported by the Heart and Stroke Foundation of Manitoba. Infrastructural support was provided by the St. Boniface Hospital Research Foundation.

References

1. Opie LH. The heart: physiology, from cell to circulation. 3rd ed. New York: Lippincott-Raven; 1998.
2. Lamers JM, De Jonge HW, Panagia V, et al. Receptor-mediated signalling pathways acting through hydrolysis of membrane phospholipids in cardiomyocytes. Cardioscience. 1993;4:121–31.
3. Izumo S, Aoki H. Calcineurin – the missing link in cardiac hypertrophy. Nat Med. 1998;4:661–2.
4. Tappia PS, Singal T, Dent MR, et al. Phospholipid-mediated signaling in diseased myocardium. Future Lipidol. 2006;1:701–17.
5. Tappia PS, Dent MR, Dhalla NS. Oxidative stress and redox regulation of phospholipase D in myocardial disease. Free Radic Biol Med. 2006;41:349–61.
6. Tappia PS. Phospholipid-mediated signaling systems as novel targets for treatment of heart disease. Can J Physiol Pharmacol. 2007;85:25–41.
7. Rhee SG. Regulation of phosphoinositide-specific phospholipase C. Annu Rev Biochem. 2001;70:281–312.
8. Singal T, Dhalla NS, Tappia PS. Phospholipase C may be involved in norepinephrine-induced cardiac hypertrophy. Biochem Biophys Res Commun. 2004;320:1015–9.
9. Singal T, Dhalla NS, Tappia PS. Norepinephrine-induced changes in gene expression of phospholipase C in cardiomyocytes. J Mol Cell Cardiol. 2006;41:126–37.
10. Tappia PS, Padua RR, Panagia V, et al. Fibroblast growth factor-2 stimulates phospholipase C β in adult cardiomyocytes. Biochem Cell Biol. 1999;77:569–75.
11. Guo Y, Rebecchi M, Scariata S. Phospholipase C β_2 binds to and inhibits phospholipase C δ_1. J Biol Chem. 2005;280:1438–47.
12. Fukami K. Structure, regulation, and function of phospholipase C isozymes. J Biochem. 2002;131:293–9.
13. James SR, Downes CP. Structural and mechanistic features of phospholipases C: effectors of inositol phospholipid-mediated signal transduction. Cell Signal. 1997;9:329–36.
14. Lopez I, Mak EC, Ding J, et al. A novel bifunctional phospholipase C that is regulated by Gα12 and stimulates the Ras/mitogen-activated protein kinase pathway. J Biol Chem. 2001;276:2758–65.
15. Heredia Mdel P, Delgado C, Pereira L, et al. Neuropeptide Y rapidly enhances $[Ca^{2+}]_i$ transients and Ca^{2+} sparks in adult rat ventricular myocytes through Y1 receptor and PLC activation. J Mol Cell Cardiol. 2005;38:205–12.
16. Balogh J, Wihlborg AK, Isackson H, et al. Phospholipase C and cAMP-dependent positive inotropic effects of ATP in mouse cardiomyocytes via P2Y11-like receptors. J Mol Cell Cardiol. 2005;39:223–30.
17. Yin G, Yan C, Berk BC. Angiotensin II signaling pathways mediated by tyrosine kinases. Int J Biochem Cell Biol. 2003;35:780–3.
18. Kockskämper J, Zima AV, Roderick HL, et al. Emerging roles of inositol 1,4,5-trisphosphate signaling in cardiac myocytes. J Mol Cell Cardiol. 2008;45:128–47.
19. Vasilevski O, Grubb DR, Filtz TM, et al. Ins(1,4,5)P$_3$ regulates phospholipase C β1 expression in cardiomyocytes. J Mol Cell Cardiol. 2008;45:679–84.
20. Wu X, Zhang T, Bossuyt J, et al. Local InsP$_3$-dependent perinuclear Ca^{2+} signaling in cardiac myocyte excitation-transcription coupling. J Clin Invest. 2006;116:675–82.
21. Bers DM. Cardiac excitation-contraction coupling. Nature. 2002;415:198–205.
22. Mackenzie L, Bootman MD, Laine M, et al. The role of inositol 1,4,5-trisphosphate receptors in Ca^{2+} signaling and the generation of arrhythmias in rat atrial myocytes. J Physiol. 2004;555:395–409.
23. Zima AV, Blatter LA. Inositol 1,4,5-trisphosphate-dependent Ca^{2+} signaling in cat atrial excitation-contraction coupling and arrhythmias. J Physiol. 2004;555:607–15.
24. Newton AC, Johnson JE. Protein kinase C: a paradigm for regulation of protein function by two membrane-targeting modules. Biochim Biophys Acta. 1998;1376:155–72.
25. Malhotra A, Kang BP, Opawumi D, et al. Molecular biology of protein kinase C signaling in cardiac myocytes. Mol Cell Biochem. 2001;225:97–107.
26. Kamp TJ, Hell JW. Regulation of cardiac L-type calcium channels by protein kinase A and protein kinase C. Circ Res. 2000;87:1095–102.
27. Churchill E, Budas G, Vallentin A, et al. PKC isozymes in chronic cardiac disease: possible therapeutic targets? Annu Rev Pharmacol Toxicol. 2008;48:569–99.
28. Dorn 2nd GW, Force T. Protein kinase cascades in the regulation of cardiac hypertrophy. J Clin Invest. 2005;115:527–37.
29. Sabri A, Steinberg SF. Protein kinase C isoform-selective signals that lead to cardiac hypertrophy and the progression of heart failure. Mol Cell Biochem. 2003;251:97–101.
30. Hodgkin MN, Pettitt TR, Martin A, et al. Diacylglycerols and phosphatidates: which molecular species are intracellular messengers? Trends Biochem Sci. 1998;23:200–4.
31. Pettitt TR, Martin A, Horton T, et al. Diacylglycerol and phosphatidate generated by phospholipases C and D, respectively, have distinct fatty acid compositions and functions. Phospholipase D-derived diacylglycerol does not activate protein kinase C in porcine aortic endothelial cells. J Biol Chem. 1997;272:17354–9.
32. Rebecchi MJ, Pentyala SN. Structure, function, and control of phosphoinositide-specific phospholipase C. Physiol Rev. 2000;80:1291–335.
33. Song C, Hu CD, Masago M, et al. Regulation of a novel human phospholipase C, PLCε, through membrane targeting by Ras. J Biol Chem. 2001;276:2752–7.

34. Saunders CM, Larman MG, Parrington J, et al. PLC ζ: a sperm-specific trigger of Ca^{2+} oscillations in eggs and embryo development. Development. 2002;129: 3533–44.

35. Wing MR, Bourdon DM, Harden TK. PLC-ε: a shared effector protein in Ras-, Rho-, and G αβγ-mediated signaling. Mol Interv. 2003;3:273–80.

36. Hwang JI, Oh YS, Shin KJ, et al. Molecular cloning and characterization of a novel phospholipase C, PLC-η. Biochem J. 2005;389:181–6.

37. Tappia PS, Liu S-Y, Shatadal S, et al. Changes in sarcolemmal PLC isoenzymes in postinfarct congestive heart failure: partial correction by imidapril. Am J Physiol. 1999;277:H40–9.

38. Wolf RA. Association of phospholipase C-δ with a highly enriched preparation of canine sarcolemma. Am J Physiol. 1992;263:C1021–8.

39. Wang H, Oestreich EA, Maekawa N, et al. Phospholipase C ε modulates β-adrenergic receptor-dependent cardiac contraction and inhibits cardiac hypertrophy. Circ Res. 2005;97:1305–13.

40. Asemu G, Dhalla NS, Tappia PS. Inhibition of PLC improves postischemic recovery in isolated rat heart. Am J Physiol Heart Circ Physiol. 2004;287: H2598–605.

41. Kawaguchi H, Sano H, Iizuka K, et al. Phosphatidylinositol metabolism in hypertrophic rat heart. Circ Res. 1993;72:966–72.

42. Shoki M, Kawaguchi H, Okamoto H, et al. Phosphatidylinositol and inositolphosphatide metabolism in hypertrophied rat heart. Jpn Circ J. 1992;56: 142–7.

43. Sakata Y. Tissue factors contributing to cardiac hypertrophy in cardiomyopathic hamsters (BIO14.6): involvement of transforming growth factor-β1 and tissue renin-angiotensin system in the progression of cardiac hypertrophy. Hokkaido Igaku Zasshi. 1993;68:18–28.

44. Dent MR, Dhalla NS, Tappia PS. Phospholipase C gene expression, protein content and activities in cardiac hypertrophy and heart failure due to volume overload. Am J Physiol Heart Circ Physiol. 2004;282:H719–27.

45. Dent MR, Aroutiounova N, Dhalla NS, et al. Losartan attenuates phospholipase C isozyme gene expression in hypertrophied hearts due to volume overload. J Cell Mol Med. 2006;10:470–9.

46. Katan M. Families of phosphoinositide-specific phospholipase C: structure and function. Biochim Biophys Acta. 1998;1436:5–17.

47. Jalili T, Takeishi Y, Song G, et al. PKC translocation without changes in Gαq and PLC-β protein abundance in cardiac hypertrophy and failure. Am J Physiol. 1999;277:H2298–304.

48. Giles TD, Sander GE, Thomas MG, et al. α-adrenergic mechanisms in the pathophysiology of left ventricular heart failure-An analysis of their role in systolic and diastolic dysfunction. J Mol Cell Cardiol. 1986;18:33–43.

49. Prasad K, O'Neil CL, Bharadwaj B. Effect of prolonged prazosin treatment on hemodynamic and biochemical changes in the dog heart due to chronic pressure overload. Jpn Heart J. 1984;25:461–76.

50. Motz W, Klepzig M, Strauer BE. Regression of cardiac hypertrophy: experimental and clinical results. J Cardiovasc Pharmacol. 1987;10:S148–52.

51. Zakynthinos E, Pierrutsakos CH, Daniil Z, et al. Losartan controlled blood pressure and reduced left ventricular hypertrophy but did not alter arrhythmias in hypertensive men with preserved systolic function. Angiology. 2005;56:439–49.

52. Kanno Y, Kaneko K, Kaneko M, et al. Angiotensin receptor antagonist regresses left ventricular hypertrophy associated with diabetic nephropathy in dialysis patients. J Cardiovasc Pharmacol. 2004;43:380–6.

53. Ruzicka M, Yuan B, Leenen FH. Effects of enalapril versus losartan on regression of volume overload-induced cardiac hypertrophy in rats. Circulation. 2004;90:484–91.

54. Rothermund L, Vetter R, Dieterich M, et al. Endothelin-A receptor blockade prevents left ventricular hypertrophy and dysfunction in salt-sensitive experimental hypertension. Circulation. 2002;106: 2305–8.

55. Yamamoto K, Masuyama T, Sakata Y, et al. Prevention of diastolic heart failure by endothelin type A receptor antagonist through inhibition of ventricular structural remodeling in hypertensive heart. J Hypertens. 2002; 20:753–61.

56. Lund AK, Goens MB, Nunez BA, et al. Characterizing the role of endothelin-1 in the progression of cardiac hypertrophy in aryl hydrocarbon receptor (AhR) null mice. Toxicol Appl Pharmacol. 2006;212:127–35.

57. Bai H, Wu LL, Xing DQ, et al. Angiotensin II induced upregulation of Gαq/11, phospholipase C β$_3$ and extracellular signal-regulated kinase 1/2 via angiotensin II type 1 receptor. Chin Med J. 2004;117: 88–93.

58. Lamers JM, Eskildsen-Helmond YE, Resink AM, et al. Endothelin-1-induced phospholipase C-β and D and protein kinase C isoenzyme in signaling leading to hypertrophy in rat cardiomyocytes. J Cardiovasc Pharmacol. 1995;26:S100–3.

59. Schnabel P, Mies F, Nohr T, et al. Differential regulation of phospholipase C-β isozymes in cardiomyocyte hypertrophy. Biochem Biophys Res Commun. 2000;275:1–6.

60. Otaegui D, Querejeta R, Arrieta A, et al. Phospholipase C β4 isozyme is expressed in human, rat, and murine heart left ventricles and in HL-1 cardiomyocytes. Mol Cell Biochem. 2010;337:167–73.

61. Nagata S. Apoptosis by death factor. Cell. 1997;88: 355–65.

62. Badorff C, Ruetten H, Mueller S, et al. Fas receptor signaling inhibits glycogen synthase kinase 3 β and induces cardiac hypertrophy following pressure overload. J Clin Invest. 2002;109:373–81.

63. Barac YD, Zeevi-Levin N, Yaniv G, et al. The 1,4,5-inositol trisphosphate pathway is a key component in Fas-mediated hypertrophy in neonatal rat ventricular myocytes. Cardiovasc Res. 2005;68:75–86.

64. Ruwhof C, van Wamel JT, Noordzij LA, et al. Mechanical stress stimulates phospholipase C activity and intracellular calcium ion levels in neonatal cardiomyocytes. Cell Calcium. 2001;29:73–83.

65. D'Angelo DD, Sakata Y, Lorenz JN, et al. Transgenic Gαq overexpression induces cardiac contractile failure in mice. Proc Natl Acad Sci USA. 1997;94: 8121–6.

66. Sakata Y, Hoit BD, Liggett SB, et al. Decompensation of pressure-overload hypertrophy in Gαq-overexpressing mice. Circulation. 1998;97:1488–95.

67. Adams JW, Sakata Y, Davis MG, et al. Enhanced Gαq signaling: a common pathway mediates cardiac hypertrophy and apoptotic heart failure. Proc Natl Acad Sci USA. 1998;95:10140–5.

68. Sussman MA, Welch S, Walker A, et al. Altered focal adhesion regulation correlates with cardiomyopathy in mice expressing constitutively active rac1. J Clin Invest. 2000;105:875–86.

69. Paradis P, Dali-Youcef N, Paradis FW, et al. Overexpression of angiotensin II type I receptor in cardiomyocytes induces cardiac hypertrophy and remodeling. Proc Natl Acad Sci USA. 2000;97: 931–6.

70. Mende U, Kagen A, Cohen A, et al. Transient cardiac expression of constitutively active Gαq leads to hypertrophy and dilated cardiomyopathy by calcineurin-dependent and independent pathways. Proc Natl Acad Sci USA. 1998;95:13893–8.

71. Mende U, Kagen A, Meister M, et al. Signal transduction in atria and ventricles of mice with transient cardiac expression of activated G protein αq. Circ Res. 1999;85:1085–91.

72. Mende U, Semsarian C, Martins DC, et al. Dilated cardiomyopathy in two transgenic mouse lines expressing activated G protein αq: lack of correlation between phospholipase C activation and the phenotype. J Mol Cell Cardiol. 2001;33:1477–91.

73. Hollinger S, Hepler JR. Cellular regulation of RGS proteins: modulators and integrators of G protein signaling. Pharmacol Rev. 2002;54:527–59.

74. Anger T, Zhang W, Mende U. Differential contribution of GTPase activation and effector antagonism to the inhibitory effect of RGS proteins on Gq-mediated signaling in vivo. J Biol Chem. 2004;279:3906–15.

75. Zhang W, Anger T, Su J, et al. Selective loss of fine tuning of Gq/11 signaling by RGS2 protein exacerbates cardiomyocyte hypertrophy. J Biol Chem. 2006;281:5811–20.

76. Lin F, Owens WA, Chen S, et al. Targeted α$_{1B}$-adrenergic receptor overexpression induces enhanced cardiac contractility but not hypertrophy. Circ Res. 2001;89:343–50.

77. Milano CA, Dolber PC, Rockman HA, et al. Myocardial expression of a constitutively active 1β-adrenergic receptor in transgenic mice induces cardiac hypertrophy. Proc Natl Acad Sci USA. 1994;91:10109–13.

78. Heemskerk JWM, Farndale RW, Sage SO. Effects of U73122 and U73343 on human platelet calcium signalling and protein tyrosine phosphorylation. Biochim Biophys Acta. 1997;1355:81–8.

79. Jin W, Lo TM, Loh HH, et al. U73122 inhibits phospholipase C-dependent calcium mobilization in neuronal cells. Brain Res. 1994;642:237–43.

80. Mogami H, Mills CL, Gallagher DV. Phospholipase C inhibitor, U73122, releases intracellular Ca^{2+}, potentiates Ins(1,4,5)P-3-mediated Ca^{2+} release and directly activates inn channels in mouse pancreatic acinar cells. Biochem J. 1997;324:645–51.

81. Muto Y, Nagao T, Urushidani T. The putative phospholipase C inhibitor U73122 and its negative control, U73343, elicit unexpected effects on the rabbit parietal cell. J Pharmacol Exp Ther. 1997;282:1379–88.

82. Berven LA, Barritt GJ. Evidence obtained using single hepatocytes for inhibition by the phospholipase C inhibitor U73122 of store-operated Ca^{2+} inflow. Biochem Pharmacol. 1995;49:1373–9.

83. Arthur JF, Matkovich SJ, Mitchell CJ, et al. Evidence for selective coupling of α$_1$-adrenergic receptors to phospholipase C-β1 in rat neonatal cardiomyocytes. J Biol Chem. 2001;276:37341–6.

84. Grubb DR, Vasilevski O, Huynh H, et al. The extreme C-terminal region of phospholipase C β$_1$ determines subcellular localization and function; the "b" splice variant mediates α$_1$- adrenergic receptor responses in cardiomyocytes. FASEB J. 2008;22:2768–74.

85. Morris JB, Huynh H, Vasilevski O, et al. α$_1$-Adrenergic receptor signaling is localized to caveolae in neonatal rat cardiomyocytes. J Mol Cell Cardiol. 2006; 41:117–25.

86. Filtz TM, Grubb DR, McLeod-Dryden TJ, et al. Gq-initiated cardiomyocyte hypertrophy is mediated by phospholipase Cβ$_{1b}$. FASEB J. 2009;23:3564–70.

87. Barka T, van der Noen H, Shaw PA. Proto-oncogene fos (c-fos) expression in the heart. Oncogene. 1987;1:439–43.

88. Hannan RD, West AK. Adrenergic agents, but not tri-iodo-L-thyronine induce c-fos and c-myc expression in the rat heart. Basic Res Cardiol. 1991;86:154–64.

89. Iwaki K, Sukhatme VP, Shubeita HE, et al. α- and β-adrenergic stimulation induces distinct patterns of immediate early gene expression in neonatal rat myocardial cells. fos/jun expression is associated with sarcomere assembly; Egr-1 induction is primarily an α$_1$-mediated response. J Biol Chem. 1990;265: 13809–17.

90. Komuro I, Kaida T, Shibazaki Y, et al. Stretching cardiac myocytes stimulates protooncogene expression. J Biol Chem. 1990;265:3595–8.

91. Hefti MA, Harder BA, Eppenberger HM, et al. Signaling pathways in cardiac myocyte hypertrophy. J Mol Cell Cardiol. 1997;29:2873–92.

92. Chiu R, Boyle WJ, Meek J, et al. The c-Fos protein interacts with c-Jun/AP-1 to stimulate transcription of AP-1 responsive genes. Cell. 1988;54:541–52.

93. Lijnen P, Petrov V. Antagonism of the re1nin-angiotensin system, hypertrophy and gene expression in cardiac myocytes. Methods Fund Exp Clin Pharmacol. 1999;21:363–74.

94. Omura T, Yoshiyama M, Yoshida K, et al. Dominant negative mutant of c-Jun inhibits cardiomyocyte hypertrophy induced by endothelin 1 and phenylephrine. Hypertension. 2002;39:81–6.

95. Singal T, Dhalla NS, Tappia PS. Reciprocal regulation of transcription factors and PLC isozyme gene expression in adult cardiomyocytes. J Cell Mol Med. 2010;14:1824–35.

96. Singal T, Dhalla NS, Tappia PS. Regulation of c-Fos and c-Jun gene expression by phospholipase C activity in adult cardiomyocytes. Mol Cell Biochem. 2009;327:229–39.

97. Dhalla NS, Xu Y-J, Sheu S-S, et al. Phosphatidic acid: a potential signal transducer for cardiac hypertrophy. J Mol Cell Cardiol. 1997;29:2865–71.

98. Small K, Feng JF, Lorenz J, et al. Cardiac specific overexpression of transglutaminase II (Gh) results in a unique hypertrophy phenotype independent of phospholipase C activation. J Biol Chem. 1999;23:21291–6.

99. Tappia PS, Yu CH, Di Nardo P, et al. Depressed responsiveness of phospholipase C isoenzymes to phosphatidic acid in congestive heart failure. J Mol Cell Cardiol. 2001;33:431–40.

100. Henry RA, Boyce SY, Kurz T, et al. Stimulation and binding of myocardial phospholipase C by phosphatidic acid. Am J Physiol. 1995;269:C349–58.

101. Tappia PS, Singal T. Regulation of phospholipase C in cardiac hypertrophy. Clin Lipidol. 2009;4:79–90.

102. Peivandi AA, Huhn A, Lehr HA, et al. Upregulation of phospholipase D expression and activation in ventricular pressure-overload hypertrophy. J Pharmacol Sci. 2005;98:244–54.

103. Eskildsen-Helmond YE, Bezstarosti K, Dekkers DH, et al. Cross-talk between receptor-mediated phospholipase C-β and D via protein kinase C as intracellular signal possibly leading to hypertrophy in serum-free cultured cardiomyocytes. J Mol Cell Cardiol. 1997;29:2545–59.

104. Murthy SN, Chung PH, Lin L, et al. Activation of phospholipase Cε by free fatty acids and cross talk with phospholipase D and phospholipase A$_2$. Biochemistry. 2006;45:10987–97.

105. Liu SY, Tappia PS, Dai J, et al. Phospholipase A$_2$-mediated activation of phospholipase D in rat heart sarcolemma. J Mol Cell Cardiol. 1998;30:1203–14.

106. Strauer BE, Bayer F, Brecht HM, et al. The influence of sympathetic nervous activity on regression of cardiac hypertrophy. J Hypertens. 1985;3:S39–44.

107. Strauer BE. Progression and regression of heart hypertrophy in arterial hypertension: pathophysiology and clinical aspects. Z Kardiol. 1995;74:171–8.

108. Strauer BE. Regression of myocardial and coronary vascular hypertrophy in hypertensive heart disease. J Cardiovasc Pharmacol. 1988;12:S45–54.

Molecular Changes in Fatty Acid Oxidation in the Failing Heart

Jagdip S. Jaswal, Wendy Keung, Wei Wang,
John R. Ussher, and Gary D. Lopaschuk

Abstract

Heart failure is emerging as a leading cause of morbidity and mortality in developed countries and is accompanied by alterations in myocardial fatty acid metabolism. In contrast to the normal heart, where fatty acid and glucose metabolism are reciprocally regulated, this dynamic relationship is perturbed in the failing heart. These metabolic alterations negatively impact both cardiac efficiency and function. Depending on the severity/stage of heart failure, the contribution of overall myocardial oxidative metabolism (fatty acid β-oxidation and glucose oxidation) to adenosine triphosphate (ATP) production can be depressed. Nonetheless, the balance between fatty acid β-oxidation and glucose oxidation is amenable to pharmacological intervention at multiple levels of each metabolic pathway. The alterations in fatty acid β-oxidation and the associated metabolic phenotype of accompany heart failure are described here. Furthermore, as myocardial fatty acid β-oxidation has emerged as a novel therapeutic target to limit the decrements in ventricular function, the rationale for the use of pharmacological agents that optimize fatty acid β-oxidation to improve cardiac function in the setting of heart failure will be described.

Keywords

Heart failure • Cardiac efficiency • Fatty acid oxidation • Glucose oxidation • Mitochondria

Introduction

Myocardial energy substrate metabolism and contractile function are tightly coupled, and high rates of adenosine triphosphate (ATP) synthesis and hydrolysis are necessary to meet the energetic requirements of cardiac contraction. However,

G.D. Lopaschuk (✉)
Departments of Pediatrics and Pharmacology,
University of Alberta, Mazankowski Alberta Heart Institute,
Edmonton, Alberta, Canada
e-mail: gary.lopaschuk@ualberta.ca

N.S. Dhalla, M. Nagano, B. Ostadal (eds.), *Molecular Defects in Cardiovascular Disease*,
DOI 10.1007/978-1-4419-7130-2_12, © Springer Science+Business Media, LLC 2011

myocardial ATP stores are low relative to the amounts of ATP required to maintain cardiac contraction, ionic homeostasis, and basal metabolism. Consequently, the myocardial ATP pool undergoes complete turnover at least once every 10 s, and the heart cycles the equivalent of ~6 kg of ATP in a 24 h period [1–3]. To accommodate its energy demands, the heart possesses a high degree of metabolic plasticity, evident from its ability to utilize a variety of energy substrates, including fatty acids, carbohydrates (primarily glucose and lactate), as well as ketones to generate ATP. The contribution of each energy substrate to ATP generation is highly regulated, and there is interdependence/inter-regulation between the utilization of different substrates. In the adult heart, under physiological conditions, upwards of 95% of ATP production is attributable to mitochondrial oxidative phosphorylation, to which the contribution of fatty acid β-oxidation ranges from 40 to 80% [4–7], with the remaining balance being contributed by carbohydrate (glucose and lactate) and ketone body oxidation [6–9].

Cardiovascular pathologies can perturb the balance between the various pathways of energy substrate metabolism, and these alterations can contribute to the progression of myocardial disease and/or injury. Ischemic heart disease (e.g. angina, acute myocardial infarction) occurs when coronary flow, and hence oxygen supply, is insufficient to meet the oxygen requirements of the heart. The consequences of myocardial ischemia are dependent on the nature and severity of the ischemic episode and the elapsed time to subsequent reperfusion (i.e. the re-establishment of coronary flow to the previously ischemic areas of the myocardium), and can manifest as reversible or irreversible injury, the latter associated with cardiac myocyte death. Alterations in cardiac structure, deficits in cardiac mechanical function, and perturbations in energy substrate metabolism can accompany ischemic heart disease.

Improvements in medical therapy, refinements in revascularization procedures, and a decrease in the prevalence of cardiovascular risk factors including hypertension, hypercholesterolemia, and smoking have led to increased numbers of patients surviving the consequences of myocardial ischemia [10, 11]. However, stemming from these beneficial improvements in survival is an increase in the prevalence of heart failure. Heart failure is a complex clinical syndrome, characterized by the progressive inability of the heart to fill with, and eject adequate amounts of blood to meet the needs of the body [12]. The majority of heart failure arises from pre-existing ischemic heart disease, but can also be of non-ischemic/idiopathic origin [1, 3]. Heart failure has emerged as the leading cause of morbidity and mortality in developed countries [13]. In addition to being accompanied by well characterized neuro-hormonal alterations, including activation of the renin–angiotensin–aldosterone system (RAAS) and activation of the sympathetic nervous system [14, 15], heart failure is also accompanied by alterations in myocardial energy metabolism. The focus of this chapter will center on the alterations in energy substrate metabolism that occur in heart failure, since it is now clear that these metabolic changes contribute to the severity and outcomes of heart failure.

Classically, the treatment of heart failure has centered on the use of pharmacological agents that alter systemic and/or cardiac hemodynamics. As knowledge of the mechanisms regulating cardiac energy substrate metabolism increases and as alterations in energy substrate metabolism accompany heart failure, the modulation and optimization of energy metabolism represents a novel and promising therapeutic intervention in heart failure. One particular pathway of energy substrate metabolism that is altered in heart failure is fatty acid ß-oxidation. As such, overviews of: (1) cardiac fatty acid β-oxidation and its regulation, (2) the influence of fatty acid β-oxidation on cardiac efficiency and function, (3) the metabolic phenotype of the failing heart, and (4) the mechanistic rationale for the use of pharmacological agents that modify fatty acid β-oxidation to limit the deleterious consequences of heart failure will be described.

Oxidative Metabolism of Fatty Acids and Glucose

Under aerobic conditions, the majority (~95%) of myocardial ATP is produced via mitochondrial oxidative phosphorylation [1, 3]. Reducing equivalents (protons and electrons) are carried from energy substrates to the mitochondrial electron transport chain by the reduced forms of flavin adenine dinucleotide ($FADH_2$) and nicotinamide adenine dinucleotide (NADH), generated by dehydrogenase reactions participating in the fatty acid β-oxidation pathway, the oxidation of pyruvate (i.e. glucose oxidation), and the tricarboxylic acid (TCA) cycle. The contributions of fatty acid β-oxidation and carbohydrate oxidation to overall myocardial ATP production are determined by cardiac and systemic hemodynamic factors including chronotropic state and inotropic state, as well as preload and peripheral vascular resistance [1].

Fatty Acid β-Oxidation

Circulating free fatty acids (FFAs) bound to albumin are a significant source of non-esterified FFAs for cardiac ATP production [16–18]. Fatty acids can also originate from circulating chylomicrons and very low density lipoprotein (VLDL) [19, 20] via the action of lipoprotein lipase, or can be liberated from endogenous triacylglycerol stores. The uptake of fatty acids from the circulation is governed by the trans-sarcolemmal fatty acid concentration gradient. Following liberation from chylomicrons or VLDL, or dissociation from plasma albumin, fatty acids either directly enter cardiac myocytes by passive diffusion, or indirectly following binding to the plasma membrane isoform of fatty acid binding protein (FABPpm). Following dissociation from albumin, fatty acids can also enter cells by facilitated transport via fatty acid translocase proteins (FATPs) or FAT/CD36, or following binding to FABPpm and subsequent protein-mediated transport by FAT/CD36 [21–23].

Following uptake, fatty acids are activated via esterification to coenzyme A (CoA), an ATP-dependent process catalyzed by a family of fatty acyl-CoA synthases. In the cytosol, acyl-CoA molecules are bound to acyl-CoA binding protein (ACBP), and can be utilized for a number of processes including the synthesis of phospholipids and triacylglycerol, intracellular signal transduction, or mitochondrial fatty acid β-oxidation [1].

Impermeability of the inner mitochondrial membrane to fatty acyl-CoA molecules necessitates the use of carnitine as a shuttle mechanism to transfer fatty acid moieties into the mitochondrial matrix, and is facilitated by a complex of proteins [24]. Fatty acyl-CoA molecules are converted to their respective fatty acyl-carnitine moieties by carnitine-palmitoyl transferase I (CPT i), which itself is localized to the outer mitochondrial membrane [25, 26]. Carnitine translocase then shuttles fatty acyl-carnitine molecules into the mitochondrial matrix, where the action of carnitine-palmitoyl transferase II (CPT II) (localized to the inner leaflet of the inner mitochondrial membrane) regenerates a fatty acyl-CoA molecule [27–29]. In the mitochondrial matrix, fatty acyl-CoA molecules undergo fatty acid β-oxidation, which progressively shortens acyl-CoA molecules by 2 carbon units through the liberation of acetyl-CoA (which is further metabolized in the TCA cycle). Fatty acid β-oxidation also generates reducing equivalents (NADH and $FADH_2$) which serve as electron donors for the electron transport chain and ATP generation via oxidative phosphorylation. The process of fatty acid β-oxidation is mediated by the enzymes acyl-CoA dehydrogenase, enoyl-CoA hydratase, 3-L-hydroxyacyl-CoA dehydrogenase, and 3-ketoacyl-CoA thiolase (Fig. 1). The oxidative metabolism of poly- and monounsaturated fatty acids is more complex, as it requires additional enzymes including 2,4-dienoyl-CoA reductase and enoyl-CoA isomerase to generate a *trans* double bond, prior to fatty acid β-oxidation by the four major enzymes above [30].

Regulation of Fatty Acid β-Oxidation

The circulating concentrations of fatty acids, the activities of the enzymes of β-oxidation, as well as the intracellular levels of malonyl-CoA are all important factors regulating the rates of fatty acid β-oxidation [31, 32]. Circulating FFA concentrations increase following fasting and decrease in the postprandial state due to the antilipolytic effects of insulin [33–35]. An increase in catecholamine discharge (an important component of heart failure) stimulates lipolysis, and so increases

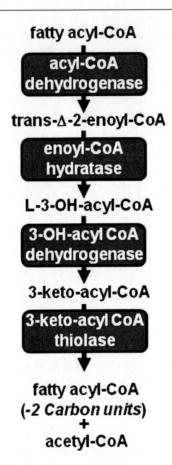

fatty acyl-CoA

acyl-CoA dehydrogenase

trans-Δ-2-enoyl-CoA

enoyl-CoA hydratase

L-3-OH-acyl-CoA

3-OH-acyl CoA dehydrogenase

3-keto-acyl-CoA

3-keto-acyl CoA thiolase

fatty acyl-CoA (-2 Carbon units) + acetyl-CoA

Fig. 1 Mitochondrial fatty acid β-oxidation. The enzymes involved in mitochondrial fatty acid β-oxidation. Mitochondrial fatty acid β-oxidation is mediated by the successive actions of the enzymes acyl-CoA dehydrogenase, enoyl-CoA hydratase, 3-L-hydroxyacyl-CoA dehydrogenase, and 3-ketoacyl-CoA thiolase. The end products of mitochondrial fatty acid β-oxidation are acetyl-CoA and an acyl-CoA molecule that is 2-carbon units shorter from when it entered the β-oxidation pathway. The newly generated acyl-CoA molecule can re-enter the β-oxidation pathway and be progressively shortened, liberating acetyl-CoA which is utilized in the tricarboxylic acid cycle

the circulating concentrations of FFAs, thereby increasing the availability of fatty acids to cardiac muscle. One of the consequences of increased fatty acid availability is an increase in the rates of myocardial fatty acid β-oxidation. The activities of the enzymes of mitochondrial fatty acid β-oxidation also regulate the overall rates of fatty acid metabolism [3, 36]. Acyl-CoA dehydrogenase is sensitive to the mitochondrial ratio of FAD/FADH$_2$, 3-L-hydroxyacyl-CoA dehydrogenase is sensitive

to the ratio of NAD$^+$/NADH, and 3-ketoacyl-CoA thiolase is sensitive to the CoA/acetyl-CoA ratio.

The intracellular content of malonyl-CoA also functions as a key regulator of myocardial fatty acid β-oxidation [37, 38]. Malonyl-CoA regulates fatty acid β-oxidation by inhibiting the activity of CPT I, the rate limiting enzyme of mitochondrial fatty acid uptake [39–41]. In the myocardium, intracellular malonyl-CoA content is determined by its rates of synthesis and degradation, as well as by cardiac energy demand [42]. Acetyl-CoA carboxylase (ACC) is responsible for malonyl-CoA synthesis, while malonyl-CoA decarboxylase (MCD) is responsible for malonyl-CoA degradation [37, 38]. Mitochondrial citrate can also influence cytosolic malonyl-CoA content. A proportion of citrate that is not oxidized by the TCA cycle can be translocated via the tricarboxylate transporter from the mitochondrial matrix to the cytosolic compartment. Once in the cytosol, citrate can allosterically activate ACC [43] or contribute to the formation of cytosolic acetyl-CoA via the ATP citrate lyase reaction [44, 45]. The activity of ACC and hence malonyl-CoA synthesis is also under covalent control. ACC is subject to phosphorylation/inhibition by 5′-AMP activated protein kinase (AMPK), which is central to? the regulation of both fatty acid and carbohydrate metabolism [46–54].

Glucose Metabolism

Glucose utilization by the heart is initiated via its cellular uptake, a complex process coupled to the rates of: (1) glucose delivery to the interstitial space, (2) glucose transport into the cell, and (3) glucose phosphorylation in the intracellular compartment [55]. As glucose is a hydrophilic molecule, it enters cells via a facilitative transport process, mediated by a family of glucose transporters (GLUTs), with GLUT1 and GLUT4 being particularly important in cardiac muscle [56–59]. The majority of GLUT4 is stored in intracellular compartments, whereas GLUT1 has a pronounced sarcolemmal localization [23]. The stimulation of myocardial glucose transport involves an increase in the recruitment of GLUT1 as well as GLUT4 from intracellular compartments to the sarcolemma [56]. Once glucose enters the cytosolic compartment, the enzymes hexokinase I and/or hexokinase II phosphorylate glucose, thereby generating glucose-6-phosphate (G-6-P). As glucose is phosphorylated nearly as rapidly as it is translocated into the cardiac myocyte, the intracellular concentration of free glucose is negligible, thereby maintaining a steep downward concentration gradient from the interstitial- to intracellular-space [60]. Glucose-6-phosphate (G-6-P) serves as substrate for either of two metabolic fates, storage as glycogen, or catabolism by glycolysis.

In the aerobic setting, the major end-product of glycolysis is pyruvate, the mitochondrial oxidation of which requires transport via a monocarboxylate carrier [61]. Although mitochondrial pyruvate can be subject to carboxylation yielding oxaloacetate, the majority is subjected to oxidative decarboxylation mediated by the pyruvate dehydrogenase (PDH) complex to generate acetyl-CoA [62–64]. The multienzyme PDH complex mediates the rate limiting reaction of glucose oxidation (i.e. pyruvate oxidation). The complex comprises PDH, PDH kinase (PDHK), and PDH phosphatase (PDHP), and is regulated by substrate/product ratios as well as by covalent modification [65–67]. PDH is inhibited by increased ratios of $NADH/NAD^+$ and/or acetyl-CoA/CoA, while flux through PDH increases in response to increased pyruvate generation from glycolysis [65, 68, 69]. Covalent modification via reversible phosphorylation also represents an important mechanism for the regulation of PDH, and hence glucose oxidation. In response to increases in acetyl-CoA and NADH, PDHK phosphorlyates and inhibits PDH [65, 68]; conversely, PDHP dephosphorylates and increases PDH activity and glucose oxidation.

Integrated Regulation of Fatty Acid β-Oxidation and Glucose Oxidation in the Heart

The relationship between fatty acids and glucose for oxidative metabolism (glucose/fatty acid cycle) was originally described by Randle et al. in 1963 [35]. The molecular mechanisms governing the glucose/fatty acid cycle are manifest at various points in the pathways involved in the breakdown of each substrate. Although both glucose uptake and glycolysis can be inhibited by elevated fatty acid ß-oxidation rates, the most prominent inhibitory effect is exerted at the level of the PDH complex and glucose oxidation [34, 35] due to increased acetyl-CoA and NADH production from fatty acid β-oxidation (Fig. 2). Inhibition of PDH uncouples the processes of glycolysis and glucose oxidation, and can lead to the production of intracellular acidosis subsequent to the hydrolysis of glycolytically derived ATP, a proton producing reaction [70, 71]. The effects of this uncoupling between glycolysis and glucose oxidation may influence cardiac ionic homeostasis and efficiency, especially when cardiac energetics are compromised in the setting of heart failure.

In contrast, increasing the contribution of glucose oxidation to acetyl-CoA production (which improves the coupling between glycolysis and glucose oxidation) can reciprocally decrease fatty acid ß-oxidation secondary to inhibition of 3-ketoacyl-CoA thiolase, the terminal enzyme of fatty acid β-oxidation (Fig. 2). Furthermore, NADH generated from glucose oxidation can decrease fatty acid β-oxidation by inhibiting both the acyl-CoA dehydrogenase and 3-hydroxyacyl-CoA dehydrogenase enzymes. Glucose-derived acetyl-CoA can also influence fatty acid β-oxidation via alterations in mitochondrial fatty acid uptake. An increase in glucose-derived acetyl-CoA via the actions of the enzymes carnitine acetyl-transferase [3, 72] and ACC can increase the generation of cytosolic malonyl-CoA, a potent endogenous inhibitor of CPT I and thus decrease mitochondrial fatty acid uptake and subsequent oxidation.

Cardiac Energy Substrate Metabolism and Cardiac Efficiency

Cardiac efficiency refers to the relationship between mechanical energy generated (i.e. cardiac work) and energy consumed (i.e. oxygen consumption – MVO_2) by the ventricle during

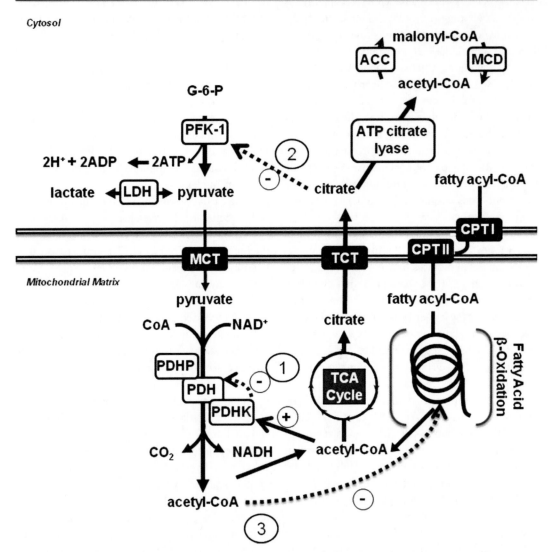

Fig. 2 The glucose/fatty acid cycle. The glucose/fatty acid cycle describes the reciprocal relationship between fatty acid and glucose metabolism. Acetyl-CoA and NADH produced from fatty acid β-oxidation can inhibit the pyruvate dehydrogenase (PDH) complex (1). Citrate derived from fatty acid β-oxidation-derived acetyl-CoA inhibits phosphofructokinase-1 (PFK-1), which in turn can lead to an inhibition of hexokinase by glucose-6-phosphate (G-6-P) (2). Increasing the contribution of glucose oxidation for the generation of acetyl-CoA decreases fatty acid β-oxidation via feedback inhibition of 3-ketoacyl-CoA thiolase. Furthermore, NADH derived from glucose oxidation can decrease fatty acid β-oxidation via feedback inhibition of both the acyl-CoA dehydrogenase and 3-hydroxyacyl-CoA dehydrogenase reactions (3). Mitochondrial citrate can also gain access to the cytosol and increase acetyl-CoA content (described in text). Acetyl-CoA itself can be translocated from the mitochondrial matrix to the cytosol via carnitine acetyl-transferase. In the cytosolic compartment acetyl-CoA can generate malonyl-CoA via the action of acetyl-CoA carboxylase (ACC), and malonyl-CoA can function as an endogenous inhibitor of carnitine-palmitoyl transferase I (CPT I), the rate limiting step of mitochondrial fatty acid uptake

contraction, and can be expressed as the work/MVO$_2$ ratio [73]. MVO$_2$ provides an adequate measure of energy input for contraction as cardiac muscle under aerobic conditions meets the majority (>95%) of its energetic requirements via the oxidation of fatty acids and carbohydrates [3]. Furthermore, as the rates of oxidative metabolism are tightly coupled to energy demand, there is a good correlation between MVO_2 and cardiac work [74, 75]. Alterations in fatty acid β-oxidation have the potential to markedly influence cardiac efficiency [76], and therefore could have important consequences on the failing heart (as will be discussed). As the majority of ATP utilized to drive cardiac contraction is generated by mitochondrial oxidative phosphorylation, cardiac efficiency itself can be influenced by both the efficiency of ATP generation and hydrolysis (i.e. the efficiency of converting chemical energy into mechanical energy). Cardiac efficiency can thus be decreased as a result of increased MVO_2 [77–79], decreased LV work [80, 81], or a combination of both [80, 81]. Interestingly, there are relatively few studies that have examined cardiac mechanical efficiency in the failing heart, and there appear to be discrepant results between these studies. Previous studies have demonstrated a preservation of cardiac efficiency secondary to decreases in oxygen consumption [82, 83]; while, in contrast, others have demonstrated decreased cardiac efficiency secondary to oxygen wasting effects in the failing heart [84, 85]. Targeting the balance between fatty acid β-oxidation and glucose oxidation (i.e. the glucose/fatty acid cycle) may represent a suitable therapeutic intervention in the failing heart to improve both cardiac efficiency and function.

Phosphorous/oxygen (P/O) ratios depend on the type of energy substrate utilized for the production of NADH and $FADH_2$, and describe the number of molecules of ATP that are produced relative to the number of oxygen atoms reduced in the process of oxidative phosphorylation [86]. Comparing fatty acids (e.g. palmitate) and glucose as energy substrates, the complete oxidation of 1 molecule of palmitate generates 105 molecules of ATP, while that of glucose generates 31 molecules of ATP. Clearly fatty acid β-oxidation generates the larger amount of ATP relative to glucose oxidation; however, this comes at an increased oxygen cost. As such, the P/O ratio of palmitate (2.28) is less than that of glucose (2.58), rendering glucose more efficient at generating ATP with respect to oxygen consumed. Therefore, for any level of cardiac work, an increased dependence on fatty acids relative to carbohydrates as an oxidative fuel (which occurs during the early stages of heart failure) can

decrease cardiac efficiency. Based exclusively on P/O ratios of oxidative metabolism, cardiac efficiency differs by a theoretical value of ~13% when using either palmitate or glucose as a sole energy substrate. However, reported differences in cardiac efficiency are much greater, approximating 25–40%, thereby suggesting additional mechanisms may influence cardiac efficiency by regulating the balance between fatty acid β-oxidation and glucose oxidation (see below).

The translocation of protons from the matrix space to the inter-membrane space by complexes I, III, and IV of the electron transport chain is required for the synthesis of ATP via oxidative phosphorylation [86, 87]. The ensuing movement of protons into the mitochondrial matrix via the F_1/F_0 ATP synthase provides the chemical energy necessary for ATP synthesis [87]. The translocation of protons from the inter-membrane space into the matrix space can be uncoupled from ATP synthesis, if protons do not utilize the F_1/F_0 ATP synthase. Uncoupling proteins (UCPs) provide an alternate route for the movement of protons down the electrochemical gradient from the inter-membrane space to the matrix, and so can decrease ATP synthesis. UCP2 and UCP3 are the predominant UCP isoforms present in ventricular muscle, and their expression is upregulated in response to elevated plasma FFA levels [88]. Furthermore, although equivocal [91], recent reports indicate that elevated expression of UCP3 is involved in fatty acid-induced uncoupling of oxidative phosphorylation [89, 90]. Interestingly, in the failing heart, a positive correlation between circulating fatty acid levels and the expression of UCP2 and UCP3 has been described [92]. This may contribute to the decreased efficiency of ATP generation associated with the use of fatty acids as an energy substrate, and uncouple oxidative phosphorylation decreasing overall ATP synthesis and cardiac efficiency [93]. Increased cardiac fatty acid utilization in the insulin resistant/diabetic state, which often accompanies heart failure (see below) is also associated with increased MVO_2, uncoupled respiration, decreased ATP synthesis rates, and decreased cardiac efficiency [77–81].

Although debatable [94], an additional postulated function of UCP3 is the export of fatty acid anions from the mitochondrial matrix. Such an action may induce ATP wasting secondary to the futile cycling of fatty acid metabolites. When fatty acyl-CoA supply exceeds the capacity of mitochondrial fatty acid β-oxidation [95], excess fatty acyl-CoA molecules can be hydrolyzed by a mitochondrial thioesterase (MTE), liberating free CoA, and generating fatty acid anions. As mitochondria cannot regenerate the fatty acyl-CoA moiety (a prerequisite for fatty acid β-oxidation), the fatty acid anion is proposed to be exported to the cytosolic compartment by the putative transport function of UCPs. Indeed recent reports demonstrate that interventions that increase fatty acid availability (e.g. high-fat diet, fasting, and diabetes), also increase the mRNA and protein expression of both UCP3 and MTE [96–98], as well as increasing MTE activity and mitochondrial export of palmitate [98]. These effects may rid the mitochondrial matrix of fatty acid anions and prevent the depletion of matrix CoA [99]. Fatty acids can also cycle between their activated acyl-CoA moieties and the myocardial triacylglycerol pool [16, 18], an effect that is estimated to account for 30% of total energy expenditure in isolated cardiac myocytes [100].

Futile cycling of fatty acid metabolites by the above routes may compromise cardiac efficiency, as the cycled fatty acid metabolite requires activation/esterification to CoA via FACS prior to subsequent metabolism. The FACS reaction consumes the equivalent of 2 ATP molecules, and as such may increase ATP wasting, thereby decreasing the efficiency of ATP utilization for contractile purposes.

Metabolic Phenotype in the Failing Heart

Heart failure can arise from a diverse set of pathologies that eventually result in alterations in cardiac contractile function and reflex neuro-endocrine activation (sympathetic nervous system, and the RAAS). Multiple cardiovascular disease states ranging from ischemic heart disease, hypertension,

as well as cardiomyopathies of genetic origin can progress ultimately to heart failure. In addition to clinical studies examining patients with heart failure, various experimental/animal models have been developed to produce heart failure including pressure-overload, volume-overload, rapid ventricular pacing, genetic modifications (transgenic animals), or myocardial infarction [101, 102]. Combined, these different clinical and experimental approaches have been used to help define the metabolic phenotype of the failing heart.

Multiple abnormalities in energy generating processes coincide with the progression of heart failure. In advanced stages of heart failure, myocardial ATP content decreases to ~30–40% of the values compared to those in the normal heart [103–106], and there are decreases in phosphocreatine content (see refs. [2, 107, 108] for reviews). Furthermore, the PCr/ATP ratio is decreased in heart failure and correlates well with New York Heart Association (NYHA) functional class [109]. These findings suggest defects in the ability to produce ATP in the failing heart and/or a decrease in cardiac efficiency in the failing heart. Heart failure is also accompanied by defects in myocardial oxygen consumption and mitochondrial electron transport chain activity in its advanced stages (see refs. [2, 3] for reviews). These alterations in ATP generating processes suggest that changes in energy substrate metabolism are important biochemical mediators of, and contributors to, the progression of heart failure.

Fatty Acid and Glucose Utilization in Heart Failure

Heart failure itself is heterogeneous in nature, and as such the accompanying changes in energy substrate metabolism are very complex. More specifically, the metabolic phenotype of the failing heart appears to be, at least partially, dependent on the stage/severity of the syndrome (Fig. 3a, b); however, the metabolic alterations during these various stages are equivocal. In ventricular

Fig. 3 (continued) the stage and severity of heart failure (b). These alterations in fatty acid β-oxidation and glucose oxidation contribute to decreasing the contribution of oxidative phosphorylation to overall ATP production in early/moderate and severe heart failure relative to the normal heart (b)

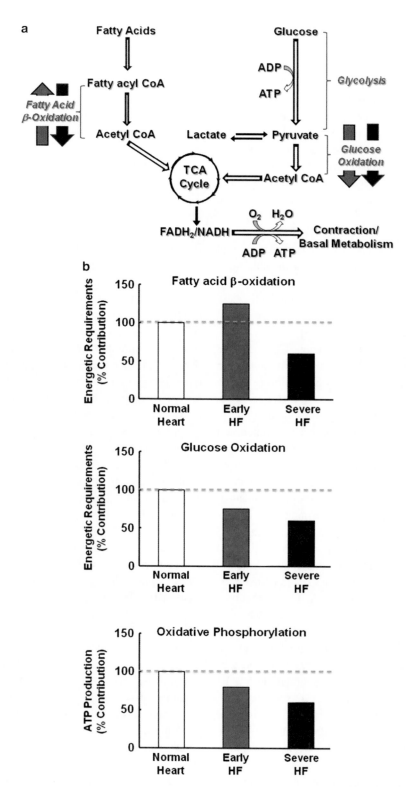

Fig. 3 As heart failure progresses, changes occur in myocardial energy substrate metabolism. In early/moderate heart failure (*filled grey arrows*), there may be an initial upregulation of fatty acid β-oxidation. As heart failure progresses to its more severe stages (*filled black arrows*), fatty acid β-oxidation is suppressed (**a**). In early/moderate heart failure glucose oxidation is suppressed (*filled grey arrows*). As heart failure progresses to its more severe stages, glucose oxidation is further suppressed (*filled black arrows*) (**a**). These contributions of fatty acid β-oxidation and glucose oxidation to overall cardiac energetics relative to the normal heart differ depending on

homogenates from hearts subjected to pressure overload with preserved ejection fraction, the rates of fatty acid β-oxidation are similar, whereas the rates of glycolysis are accelerated relative to homogenates obtained from normal hearts, [110]. Fatty acid β-oxidation rates are also similar in ventricular homogenates from hearts subjected to myocardial infarction and subsequent heart failure at a time point when there is a down-regulation in genes encoding enzymes involved in fatty acid uptake and β-oxidation [111]. These findings also extrapolate to the organ level, where fatty acid β-oxidation rates are not different in acute heart failure secondary to aortic banding in rats [112], or in the canine microembolization model, where glucose uptake and oxidation are also preserved relative to the normal heart [113].

Previous studies indicate that despite decreased fatty acid uptake (likely owing to decreased regional coronary blood flow), cardiac fatty acid β-oxidation rates are normal in patients with asymptomatic hypertrophic cardiomyopathy [114]. Furthermore, in NYHA functional class III patients, fatty acid utilization is increased secondary to enhanced lipolysis [115]. Increased fatty acid utilization is also accompanied by elevated plasma lactate concentrations, indicative of fatty acid-induced impairments of whole-body carbohydrate oxidation [115], owing possibly to the mechanisms operative in the glucose/fatty acid cycle. Of further interest, in clinically stable NYHA functional class II and III patients, cardiac fatty acid uptake [116, 117] and subsequent oxidation [116] were greater than that observed in healthy controls, while glucose uptake [117] and oxidation were lower [116]. These alterations in cardiac fatty acid and glucose utilization in NYHA functional class II-III patients may have negative consequences on cardiac efficiency. Thus, targeting the balance between fatty acid β-oxidation and glucose oxidation may represent a viable therapeutic approach in the failing heart.

Recent experimental studies indicate overall mitochondrial oxidative metabolism is depressed in severe end-stage heart failure. Decreased mitochondrial state 3 respiration and decreased fatty acid (i.e. oleate) and glucose oxidation [118, 119]

are manifest 20 weeks following pressure overload-induced heart failure. However, the ratio between fatty acid β-oxidation and glucose oxidation is not altered. These results contrast those in the canine model of severe heart failure induced by rapid ventricular pacing, where fatty acid β-oxidation rates are decreased, while glucose oxidation rates are increased [120–122]. The increase in carbohydrate oxidation appears to be paradoxical, as protein expression of PDH is decreased, while that of its negative regulator, PDHK4 is increased [120]. The mechanisms underlying the decrease in fatty acid β-oxidation in severe heart failure are less ambiguous, as decreased fatty acid β-oxidation is accompanied by decreased expression of retinoid X receptor (PPAR binding partner) and by decreased expression of medium-chain acyl-CoA dehydrogenase (MCAD) [121]. Of interest, the metabolic phenotype observed during pacing-induced heart failure is reversible, as the rates of fatty acid β-oxidation increase, while the rates of glucose oxidation decrease during a recovery phase following discontinuation of rapid ventricular pacing [122]. These effects may again point to the utility of targeting the balance between fatty acid β-oxidation and glucose oxidation as a therapeutic approach in the management of heart failure.

In the clinical setting, the rates of both fatty acid uptake and oxidation are decreased in patients with dilated cardiomyopathy (ejection fraction ~32%), while the rates of glucose uptake are increased [123]. There is also an inability to increase glucose uptake in response to pacing stress in such patients, which may contribute to deficits in mechanical efficiency [123]. These defects in fatty acid and glucose uptake may suggest a considerable degree of ineffective energy substrate utilization. Furthermore, energy substrate supply is a critical determinant of cardiac performance and efficiency in patients with heart failure. Acute reductions in circulating fatty acid levels in response to acipimox (an inhibitor of lipolysis) treatment are accompanied by large reductions in fatty acid uptake, and decreased cardiac efficiency [124]. These results indicate that circulating FFAs are an important energy substrate in the failing heart, and are in line with the previous suggestion that, "the heart functions best when it oxidizes two substrates simultaneously [125]." Alternatively, these findings also lend support to previous observations demonstrating that pharmacologically targeting the balance between fatty acid β-oxidation and glucose oxidation as opposed to limiting fatty acid availability may be a more viable therapeutic strategy to improve cardiac efficiency in these patients (see below).

Sympathetic Nervous Activity, Plasma FFAs, and Insulin Resistance in Heart Failure

Heart failure is characteristically attended by hyperactivity of the sympathetic neuro-humoral axis in an effort to preserve cardiac output (see refs. [14, 15] for reviews). For the purposes of this chapter, we will only deal with the neuronal limb of the sympathetic nervous system and its contribution to elevated plasma fatty acid levels during heart failure. However, it should be noted that the participation of the humoral limb and the RAAS is equally important [126, 127]. In heart failure increased sympathetic nervous system activity is associated with increased circulating norepinephrine levels, spillover of norepinephrine from activated sympathetic nerve fibers to the plasma, and increased central sympathetic outflow [128]. Norepinephrine spillover is a prominent effect, as circulating levels in untreated heart failure patients can approach those observed in healthy individuals following intense exercise [129].

Excessive levels of circulating norepinephrine can increase adipose tissue lipolysis, and concomitantly increase the delivery of circulating FFAs to the heart. Therefore, one would anticipate that these effects can negatively affect the balance between fatty acid β-oxidation and glucose oxidation, resulting in impaired cardiac efficiency. The activation of cardiac β_1- and β_2-adrenoceptors also elicits chronotropic and inotropic effects, which increases subsequent oxygen consumption rates. Interestingly, β_1-adrenoceptors are down-regulated and norepinephrie uptake decreased in the failing heart [130, 131]. Regardless, as heart failure patients have elevations of sympathetic nervous

system activity, the availability of circulating FFAs is increased. Furthermore, increases in cardiac energy demand brought about by increased cardiac work are associated with elevated fatty acid oxidation rates [132].

Sympathetic nervous system hyperactivity and excess catecholamine release also impair insulin sensitivity. Impaired insulin sensitivity contributes to increased circulation of FFA levels as well as the development of whole-body insulin resistance [133]. Clinical studies demonstrate that decreasing plasma FFA levels attenuates insulin resistance [134]. Insulin resistance is also highly prevalent in the pathogenesis of heart failure, evidenced by the observation that higher proinsulin levels (a surrogate marker for insulin resistance) can be observed in patients 20 years before the actual diagnosis of heart failure itself [135]. Furthermore, whole-body insulin resistance precedes the development of heart failure in humans [136, 137]. However, whether the myocardium itself is insulin resistant is a question of debate [138]. Studies utilizing ^{18}F-fluoro-2-deoxyglucose (FDG) positron emission tomography have shown that heart failure patients with type 2 diabetes do exhibit myocardial insulin resistance, as indicated by reductions in myocardial FDG uptake [139]. Also, there is a complete absence of insulin-stimulated myocardial glucose uptake following a hyperinsulinemic-euglycemic clamp in a canine model of rapid ventricular pacing-induced heart failure, indicative of profound myocardial insulin resistance [140, 141]. A consideration when interpreting metabolic changes in heart failure patients with accompanying insulin resistance/type 2 diabetes is that the metabolic phenotypes of each disease state can be in opposition. In both experimental and clinical studies, myocardial metabolism in insulin resistance is associated with enhanced fatty acid oxidation rates, depressed glucose oxidation rates, and depending on the severity of insulin resistance, either reduced or unchanged glycolysis rates [78, 79, 142–149]. In contrast, as the severity of HF increases, fatty acid oxidation rates decrease while glycolysis rates increase, with no real change in glucose oxidation as the heart adopts a fetal metabolic phenotype [1, 3].

Optimizing Energy Substrate Metabolism in the Failing Heart

Optimizing energy substrate metabolism, by targeting the glucose/fatty acid cycle to partially inhibit fatty acid β-oxidation, while increasing glucose oxidation (Fig. 4) may provide a means to increase the efficiency of ATP production and utilization in order to improve function in the failing heart. However, it is important to note that the severity and/or stage of heart failure may determine whether inhibition of fatty acid β-oxidation is a viable therapeutic approach, as in the most severe stages of heart failure, mitochondrial function is severely diminished. As such, there may be negative consequences associated with reducing oxidative capacity even further [3].

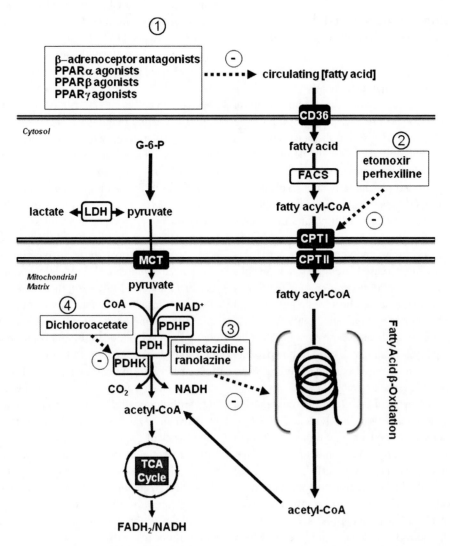

Fig. 4 Fatty acid oxidation can be targeted at different levels for treatment of heart failure. Circulating fatty acids can be decreased with the use of β-adrenoceptor antagonists, as well as various PPAR agonists (safety concerns regarding the use PPAR agonists in heart failure in outlined in text) (1). The mitochondrial uptake of long chain acyl-CoAs can be decreased with the use of carnitine palmitoyl tranferase-I (CPTI) inhibitors (2). Partial fatty acid oxidation inhibitors can inhibit the rates of myocardial fatty acid oxidation (3). Glucose oxidation can be increased with dichloroacetate, which inhibits pyruvate dehydrogenase kinase (PDHK) (4)

Targeting the Availability of Circulating FFAs

Owing to favorable effects on cardiac hemodynamics that result in oxygen-sparing and reductions in energy demand, β-adrenoceptor antagonists are mainstay therapy for the treatment of heart failure. In heart failure, treatment with β-adrenoceptor antagonists is associated with improved left ventricular performance, reversal of adverse left ventricular remodeling, reduced hospitalization, and ultimately enhanced patient survival [15]. Mechanisms underlying these protective effects in heart failure include: (1) upregulation of $β_1$-adrenoceptors, (2) inhibition of the cardiotoxic effects of excessive catecholamine discharge, (3) attenuation of pro-apoptotic, growth promoting, and vasoconstrictive pathways, (4) improvement in subendocardial coronary flow, (5) restoration of reflex control, and (6) improved myocardial performance due to reduced cardiac energy demand and oxygen consumption.

By reducing neuro-humoral hyperactivity, β-adrenoceptor antagonists contribute to decreasing catecholamine-induced lipolysis and therefore decrease circulating FFA availability and myocardial fatty acid extraction. Indeed, β-adrenoceptor antagonists lower plasma FFA concentrations [150, 151], an effect likely occurring secondary to decreased mobilization of fatty acids from adipose tissue [152]. Furthermore, several clinical studies suggest that the β-adrenoceptor antagonist, carvedilol, can decrease fatty acid uptake and oxidation [153, 154], while increasing LV function in the absence of increased oxygen utilization [155, 156], an effect indicative of shifting energy substrate utilization from fatty acid β-oxidation to carbohydrate oxidation. These effects may be attributed, at least in part to the ability of β-adrenoceptor antagonists to inhibit CPT I activity [157] and promote glucose oxidation [158]. These alterations in fatty and glucose metabolism have the potential to decrease the oxygen costs of ATP generation. Interestingly, metoprolol, does not alter circulating FFAs levels [159]. Nonetheless, β-adrenoceptor antagonists improve left ventricular function independent of alterations in cardiac oxygen consumption [155, 156], effects indicative of improved cardiac efficiency.

Members of the peroxisome proliferator activated receptor (PPAR) superfamily are involved in regulating fatty acid metabolism. There are three distinct PPAR isoforms (PPARα, PPARβ/δ, and PPARγ), and each has distinct effects on the cardiovascular system. PPARα is predominantly expressed in the heart, skeletal muscle, and liver; PPARβ/δ is expressed in a more ubiquitous manner, with high levels in both cardiac and skeletal muscle, whereas PPARγ is predominantly expressed in adipose tissue and exists at lower levels in cardiac and skeletal muscle [160].

Fibrates, are selective PPARα agonists, that decrease circulating FFAs, primarily by increasing hepatic expression of fatty acid oxidation enzymes [161], as well as increasing FACS expression [162]. The decrease in circulating FFA concentration and decreased cardiac fatty acid extraction may decrease myocardial fatty acid β-oxidation. These effects are evident in models of diet-induced obesity and insulin resistance, as mice subjected to diet-induced obesity and treatment with fenofibrate exhibit a significant increase in hepatic fatty acid oxidation rates [144]. Furthermore, this increase in extra-cardiac fatty acid oxidation is associated with a reduction in circulating triacylglycerol concentrations, likely contributing to the observed reduction in myocardial fatty acid β-oxidation and subsequent increase in glucose oxidation. Interestingly, fibrates can reduce infarct size in animal models [163] and improve the recovery of postischemic function [164]. These effects may suggest the possible utility of these compounds in optimizing energy metabolism in the failing heart.

PPARβ/δ is involved in regulating the expression of various genes involved in cardiac fatty acid metabolism including FACS, the muscle isoform of CPT I, long chain acyl-CoA dehydrogenase, and medium-chain acyl-CoA dehydrogenase [165–167]. Furthermore, the PPARβ/δ-mediated increases in the expression of genes involved in fatty acid metabolism are accompanied by the expected increases in the rates of myocardial fatty acid utilization, particularly increased rates of fatty acid β-oxidation [166, 168, 169]. Interestingly, PPARβ/δ is also involved in regulating the expression of genes involved in myocardial glucose metabolism, including GLUT4 and phosphofructokinase, and cardiac specific overexpression of PPARβ/δ increases the rates of myocardial glucose oxidation [170]. These effects may be beneficial by limiting the attenuation of oxidative metabolism in the failing heart while simultaneously favoring the predominant use of glucose as an oxidative fuel. However, these aspects remain to be investigated.

PPARγ is the molecular target of the thiazolidinedione (TZD) class of antidiabetic drugs. TZDs promote lipid sequestration in adipose tissue, thereby decreasing ectopic deposition and storage of excess lipid. Experimental studies have demonstrated a decrease in plasma triacylglycerol and FFA concentrations with TZD administration, while glucose [171] and lactate uptake [172] and oxidation [173] has been shown to increase. This increase in carbohydrate utilization, at the expense of fatty acid utilization may potentially improve cardiac efficiency. In contrast, cardiac specific overexpression of PPARγ is associated with the development of cardiomyopathy and disruption of mitochondrial architecture [174]. Furthermore clinical trials assessing the use of TZDs in diabetic heart failure patients have raised safety concerns. Specifically, increased fluid retention and vascular permeability have been implicated in worsening heart failure symptoms in diabetic patients [175]. The Prospective Pioglitazone Clinical Trial in Macrovascular Events (PROactive) study demonstrated an increased incidence of heart failure in patients treated with pioglitazone [176]. Recent meta-analysis of the risk of myocardial infarction and cardiovascular mortality suggests that rosiglitazone therapy causes an increased risk of myocardial infarction, although no increase in cardiovascular or all cause mortality was observed [177, 178]. Although TZDs appear to favorably alter fatty cardiac fatty acid and glucose oxidation, the use of these compounds to optimize energy metabolism in heart failure may be contraindicated due to safety concerns.

Targeting Mitochondrial Fatty Acid Uptake

CPT I is the rate limiting enzyme of mitochondrial fatty acid uptake and is an attractive target for inhibiting myocardial fatty acid β-oxidation. Several CPT I inhibitors have been developed, including etomoxir and perhexiline, both of which have been demonstrated to have oxygen-sparing and beneficial effects in the treatment of heart failure.

Etomoxir is an irreversible CPT I inhibitor [179]. The compound has been shown to improve myocardial function, concomitant with an increase in glucose oxidation after global ischemia [180–182] as well as in hearts from diabetic rodents [183, 184]. Thus etomoxir possesses anti-ischemic effects and may potentially be effective in the treatment of diabetic cardiomyopathy. Etomoxir treatment has also been shown to improve ventricular function in hearts subjected to pressure overload [185], which can progress to heart failure. Furthermore, etomoxir is also effective in treating heart failure by improving the rate of sarcoplasmic reticulum calcium uptake [186]. However, results of clinical trials with etomoxir have not been definitive. An open-label trial (80 mg daily for 3 months) showed improved LV ejection fraction, cardiac output at peak exercise, and clinical status in patients with NYHA class II heart failure [187]. In contrast, a double-blind multi-centered clinical trial had to be prematurely terminated due to unacceptable high liver transaminase levels in several etomoxir-treated patients [188]. Thus, whether this compound can be effectively utilized in the treatment of heart failure requires additional clinical studies.

Perhexiline was originally utilized as an anti-anginal agent in the 1970s. However, cases of hepatic toxicity and neuropathy related to phospholipid accumulation led to the decline of its use. It has recently been shown that perhexiline associated adverse effects can be reduced by titrating the plasma concentration between 150 and 600 ng/mL. Perhexiline has been demonstrated to be efficacious in the treatment of chronic heart failure, where it improves left ventricular ejection fraction and VO_2 max [189], as well as improving overall cardiac energetics [190]. These beneficial effects suggest that perhexiline-induced alterations in fatty acid utilization at the level of mitochondrial fatty acid uptake are therapeutically relevant in the treatment of heart failure.

Targeting Mitochondrial Fatty Acid β-Oxidation

Direct inhibition of the enzymes of mitochondrial fatty acid β-oxidation represents an additional approach to decrease fatty acid utilization in heart failure. A number of fatty acid β-oxidation inhibitors have been developed and have been proven effective in heart failure. Trimetazidine competitively inhibits long chain 3-ketoacyl-CoA thiolase (KAT) [191, 192], although this mechanism of action has been debated [193]. The inhibition of fatty acid β-oxidation is accompanied by an increase in glucose oxidation. This would be beneficial in heart failure as increased glucose oxidation relative to fatty acid β-oxidation can improve cardiac efficiency. Trimetazidine is effective in treating heart failure. Trimetazidine normalizes the PCr/ATP ratio in patients with ischemic cardiomyopathy [194] and improves NYHA functional class, LV end-diastoic volume, and ejection fraction in patients with heart failure and ischemic cardiomyopathy [194, 195]. Furthermore, in patients with idiopathic dilated cardiomyopathy, trimetazidine has been shown to improve LV ejection fraction. This improvement coincides with a decrease in myocardial fatty acid β-oxidation independent of alterations in MVO_2, implying an increase in carbohydrate oxidation [196]. Interestingly, improved ejection fraction is accompanied by a small decrease in fatty acid oxidation (~10%), suggesting that additional mechanisms may contribute to the observed benefit. Indeed, an increase in $β_1$-adrenoceptor occupancy with the use of trimetazidine has been observed [196], implicating that additional mechanisms contribute to its beneficial effects in the treatment of heart failure.

Ranolazine partially inhibits fatty acid β-oxidation, while increasing PDH activity [197, 198] and glucose oxidation [199, 200]. In addition to inhibiting fatty acid β-oxidation, ranolazine has also been shown to inhibit the electron transport chain in damaged and uncoupled mitochondria and is postulated to prevent ATP wasting from futile cycles [201]. Ranolazine also directly inhibits the late Na^+ current and prevents adverse increases in diastolic $(Ca^{2+})_i$ attributable to Na^+-dependent Ca^{2+} overload [202, 203]. Recently, it has been proposed that the inhibition of late Na^+ current is the mechanism responsible for the cardioprotective effects of ranolazine based on the apparent lower concentration (≤ 10 μM) [204] required for Na^+ current inhibition versus that required for partial fatty acid oxidation inhibition (100 μM) [193], as well as the observation that inhibition of fatty acid β-oxidation by the fatty acid β-oxidation inhibitor CVT-4325 does not improve postischemic function [205]. However, a number of studies have demonstrated improved cardiac function concomitant with increased glucose oxidation and decreased fatty acid oxidation at ranolazine concentrations ≤ 10 μM [197, 200]. Thus, it is possible that both late Na^+ current inhibition and partial inhibition of fatty acid β-oxidation contribute to the cardioprotective effects of ranolazine. In a canine model of heart failure, ranolazine can acutely increase ejection fraction, stroke volume, and mechanical efficiency without increasing oxygen consumption [206, 207], with 3 months of treatment attenuating the progression of LV remodeling and contractile dysfunction [208]. The beneficial effects of both trimetazidine and ranolazine in the failing heart suggest that altering the balance between fatty acid and glucose oxidation, such that it favors glucose oxidation, improves cardiac function.

Targeting the PDH Complex and Glucose Oxidation

Directly increasing myocardial glucose oxidation represents another approach to improve cardiac function. Dichloroacetate (DCA) stimulates the mitochondrial PDH complex via the inhibition of the activity of PDHK, and improved coupling between glycolysis and glucose oxidation contributes to the mechanism(s) by which DCA exerts its cardioprotective effects [209, 210]. Experimental studies indicate that DCA attenuates the transition from left ventricular hypertrophy to heart failure, a protective effect associated with improved myocardial energetics [211]. Clinical data pertaining to the use of DCA is scarce. However, in NYHA class III and IV heart failure patients, DCA infusion increased myocardial lactate uptake [212, 213], consistent with a stimulation of PDH activity. DCA also increased stroke volume, stroke work, and LV mechanical efficiency. Although rates of glucose or FFA uptake and oxidation were not measured, these results suggest that DCA increases pyruvate oxidation and mechanical efficiency by switching the heart towards the more efficient oxidative substrate. However, one should exercise caution in interpreting these results as this study lacks a vehicle-treated control group. Although limited to a small number of studies, preliminary data does suggest that DCA has beneficial effects against heart failure, which may be due to its effects on myocardial glucose oxidation and fatty acid β-oxidation.

Conclusions

Cardiac fatty β-oxidation is a highly regulated process that provides the bulk of myocardial ATP production. The balance between fatty acid β-oxidation and glucose oxidation is an important determinant of cardiac efficiency and cardiac function. Heart failure is characterized by a number of alterations in the oxidative metabolism of fatty acids and glucose that can depress contractile function. Shifting the balance between fatty acid β-oxidation and glucose oxidation by pharmacologically targeting: (1) the cellular uptake of energy substrates, (2) the transcriptional regulators of energy substrate metabolism, (3) mitochondrial fatty acid uptake, (4) mitochondrial fatty acid β-oxidation, and (5) glucose oxidation such that glucose oxidation is increased at the expense of

fatty acid β-oxidation can improve the efficiency of ATP generation utilization. These changes in fatty acid and glucose metabolism contribute it improving cardiac efficiency and function in the failing heart.

Acknowledgments This work was supported by a grant from the Canadian Institutes of Health Research to G.D.L. G.D.L. is an Alberta Heritage Foundation for Medical Research (AHFMR) Scientist. W.K. is supported by fellowship awards from the Heart and Stroke Foundation of Canada and AHFMR. W.W. is supported by a fellowship award from AHFMR. J.R.U. is supported by fellowship awards from AHFMR and the Canadian Institutes of Health Research.

References

1. Lopaschuk GD, Ussher JR, Folmes CD, et al. Myocardial fatty acid metabolism in health and disease. Physiol Rev. 2010;90:207–58.
2. Neubauer S. The failing heart – an engine out of fuel. N Engl J Med. 2007;356:1140–51.
3. Stanley WC, Recchia FA, Lopaschuk GD. Myocardial substrate metabolism in the normal and failing heart. Physiol Rev. 2005;85:1093–129.
4. Bing RJ, Siegel A, Ungar I, et al. Metabolism of the human heart. II. Studies on fat, ketone and amino acid metabolism. Am J Med. 1954;16:504–15.
5. Neely JM, Morgan HE. Relationship between carbohydrate metabolism and energy balance of heart muscle. Ann Rev Physiol. 1974;36:413–59.
6. Opie LH. Metabolism of the heart in health and disease. I. Am Heart J. 1968;76:685–98.
7. Opie LH. Metabolism of the heart in health and disease. II. Am Heart J. 1969;77:100–22.
8. Messer JV, Neill WA. The oxygen supply of the human heart. Am J Cardiol. 1962;9:384–94.
9. Messer JV, Wagman RJ, Levine HJ, et al. Patterns of human myocardial oxygen extraction during rest and exercise. J Clin Invest. 1962;41:725–42.
10. Ford ES, Ajani UA, Croft JB, et al. Explaining the decrease in U.S. deaths from coronary disease, 1980–2000. N Engl J Med. 2007;356:2388–98.
11. Ford ES, Capewell S. Coronary heart disease mortality among young adults in the U.S. from 1980 through 2002: concealed leveling of mortality rates. J Am Coll Cardiol. 2007;50:2128–32.
12. Hunt SA, Abraham WT, Chin MH, et al. Focused update incorporated into the ACC/AHA 2005 Guidelines for the Diagnosis and Management of Heart Failure in Adults A Report of the American College of Cardiology Foundation/American Heart Association Task Force on Practice Guidelines Developed in Collaboration With the International Society for Heart and Lung Transplantation. J Am Coll Cardiol. 2009;53:e1–90.

13. McMurray JJ, Pfeffer MA. Heart failure. Lancet. 2005;365:1877–89.

14. Opie LH, Knuuti J. The adrenergic-fatty acid load in heart failure. J Am Coll Cardiol. 2009;54:1637–46.

15. Triposkiadis F, Karayannis G, Giamouzis G, et al. The sympathetic nervous system in heart failure physiology, pathophysiology, and clinical implications. J Am Coll Cardiol. 2009;54:1747–62.

16. Saddik M, Lopaschuk GD. Myocardial triglyceride turnover and contribution to energy substrate utilization in isolated working rat hearts. J Biol Chem. 1991;266:8162–70.

17. Saddik M, Lopaschuk GD. The fate of arachidonic acid and linoleic acid in isolated working rat hearts containing normal or elevated levels of coenzyme A. Biochim Biophys Acta. 1991;1086:217–24.

18. Saddik M, Lopaschuk GD. Myocardial triglyceride turnover during reperfusion of solated rat hearts subjected to a transient period of global ischemia. J Biol Chem. 1992;267:3825–31.

19. Eaton RP. Synthesis of plasma triglycerides in endogenous hypertriglyceridemia. J Lipid Res. 1971;12: 491–7.

20. van der Vusse GJ, van Bilsen M, Glatz JF. Cardiac fatty acid uptake and transport in health and disease. Cardiovasc Res. 2000;45:279–93.

21. Bonen A, Campbell SE, Benton CR, et al. Regulation of fatty acid transport by fatty acid translocase/CD36. Proc Nutr Soc. 2004;63:245–9.

22. Koonen DP, Glatz JF, Bonen A, et al. Long-chain fatty acid uptake and FAT/CD36 translocation in heart and skeletal muscle. Biochim Biophys Acta. 2005;1736: 163–80.

23. Luiken JJ, Coort SL, Koonen DP, et al. Regulation of cardiac long-chain fatty acid and glucose uptake by translocation of substrate transporters. Pflugers Arch. 2004;448:1–15.

24. Murthy MS, Pande SV. Mechanism of carnitine acylcarnitine translocase-catalyzed import of acylcarnitines into mitochondria. J Biol Chem. 1984;259:9082–9.

25. Murthy MS, Pande SV. Some differences in the properties of carnitine palmitoyltransferase activities of the mitochondrial outer and inner membranes. Biochem J. 1987;248:727–33.

26. Murthy MS, Pande SV. Malonyl-CoA binding site and the overt carnitine palmitoyltransferase activity reside on the opposite sides of the outer mitochondrial membrane. Proc Natl Acad Sci USA. 1987;84:378–82.

27. Stanley WC, Chandler MP. Energy metabolism in the normal and failing heart: potential for therapeutic interventions. Heart Fail Rev. 2002;7:115–30.

28. Wolff AA, Rotmensch HH, Stanley WC, et al. Metabolic approaches to the treatment of ischemic heart disease: the clinicians' perspective. Heart Fail Rev. 2002;7:187–203.

29. McGarry JD, Brown NF. The mitochondrial carnitine palmitoyltransferase system. From concept to molecular analysis. Eur J Biochem. 1997;244:1–14.

30. Schulz H. Oxidation of fatty acids in eukaryotes. 5th ed. Amsterdam: Elsevier; 2007.

31. Dyck JR, Lopaschuk GD. Malonyl CoA control of fatty acid oxidation in the ischemic heart. J Mol Cell Cardiol. 2002;34:1099–109.

32. Kudo N, Barr AJ, Barr RL, et al. High rates of fatty acid oxidation during reperfusion of ischemic hearts are associated with a decrease in malonyl-CoA levels due to an increase in 5′-AMP-activated protein kinase inhibition of acetyl-CoA carboxylase. J Biol Chem. 1995;270:17513–20.

33. Frayn KN, Arner P, Yki-Jarvinen H. Fatty acid metabolism in adipose tissue, muscle and liver in health and disease. Essays Biochem. 2006;42:89–103.

34. Randle PJ. Regulatory interactions between lipids and carbohydrates: the glucose fatty acid cycle after 35 years. Diabetes Metab Rev. 1998;14:263–83.

35. Randle PJ, Garland PB, Hales CN, et al. The glucose fatty-acid cycle. Its role in insulin sensitivity and the metabolic disturbances of diabetes mellitus. Lancet. 1963;1:785–9.

36. Folmes CD, Lopaschuk GD. Role of malonyl-CoA in heart disease and the hypothalamic control of obesity. Cardiovasc Res. 2007;73:278–87.

37. Ussher JR, Lopaschuk GD. The malonyl CoA axis as a potential target for treating ischaemic heart disease. Cardiovasc Res. 2008;79:259–68.

38. Ussher JR, Lopaschuk GD. Targeting malonyl CoA inhibition of mitochondrial fatty acid uptake as an approach to treat cardiac ischemia/reperfusion. Basic Res Cardiol. 2009;104:203–10.

39. Paulson DJ, Ward KM, Shug AL. Malonyl CoA inhibition of carnitine palmityltransferase in rat heart mitochondria. FEBS Lett. 1984;176:381–4.

40. Saggerson ED. Carnitine acyltransferase activities in rat liver and heart measured with palmitoyl-CoA and octanoyl-CoA. Latency, effects of K⁺, bivalent metal ions and malonyl-CoA. Biochem J. 1982;202:397–405.

41. McGarry JD, Leatherman GF, Foster DW. Carnitine palmitoyltransferase I. The site of inhibition of hepatic fatty acid oxidation by malonyl-CoA. J Biol Chem. 1978;253:4128–36.

42. Reszko AE, Kasumov T, David F, et al. Regulation of malonyl-CoA concentration and turnover in the normal heart. J Biol Chem. 2004;279:34298–342301.

43. Munday MR. Regulation of mammalian acetyl-CoA carboxylase. Biochem Soc Trans. 2002;30:1059–64.

44. Comte B, Vincent G, Bouchard B, et al. A 13C mass isotopomer study of anaplerotic pyruvate carboxylation in perfused rat hearts. J Biol Chem. 1997;272: 26125–31.

45. Poirier M, Vincent G, Reszko AE, et al. Probing the link between citrate and malonyl-CoA in perfused rat hearts. Am J Physiol Heart Circ Physiol. 2002;283: H1379–86.

46. Carling D, Aguan K, Woods A, et al. Mammalian AMP-activated protein kinase is homologous to yeast and plant protein kinases involved in the regulation of carbon metabolism. J Biol Chem. 1994;269: 11442–8.

47. Dyck JR, Gao G, Widmer J, et al. Regulation of 5′-AMP-activated protein kinase activity by the

noncatalytic beta and gamma subunits. J Biol Chem. 1996;271:17798–8803.

48. Gao J, Waber L, Bennett MJ, et al. Cloning and mutational analysis of human malonyl-coenzyme A decarboxylase. J Lipid Res. 1999;40:178–82.

49. Hardie DG. Regulation of fatty acid synthesis via phosphorylation of acetyl-CoA carboxylase. Prog Lipid Res. 1989;28:117–46.

50. Hardie DG. Regulation of fatty acid and cholesterol metabolism by the AMP-activated protein kinase. Biochim Biophys Acta. 1992;1123:231–8.

51. Hardie DG. An emerging role for protein kinases: the response to nutritional and environmental stress. Cell Signal. 1994;6:813–21.

52. Hawley SA, Davison M, Woods A, et al. Characterization of the AMP-activated protein kinase kinase from rat liver and identification of threonine 172 as the major site at which it phosphorylates AMP-activated protein kinase. J Biol Chem. 1996;271:27879–87.

53. Stapleton D, Woollatt E, Mitchelhill KI, et al. AMP-activated protein kinase isoenzyme family: subunit structure and chromosomal location. FEBS Lett. 1997;409:452–6.

54. Weekes J, Hawley SA, Corton J, et al. Activation of rat liver AMP-activated protein kinase by kinase kinase in a purified, reconstituted system. Effects of AMP and AMP analogues. Eur J Biochem. 1994;219:751–7.

55. Wasserman DH, Ayala JE. Interaction of physiological mechanisms in control of muscle glucose uptake. Clin Exp Pharmacol Physiol. 2005;32:319–23.

56. Becker C, Sevilla L, Tomas E, et al. The endosomal compartment is an insulin-sensitive recruitment site for GLUT4 and GLUT1 glucose transporters in cardiac myocytes. Endocrinol. 2001;142:5267–76.

57. Fischer Y, Thomas J, Sevilla L, et al. Insulin-induced recruitment of glucose transporter 4 (GLUT4) and GLUT1 in isolated rat cardiac myocytes. Evidence of the existence of different intracellular GLUT4 vesicle populations. J Biol Chem. 1997;272:7085–92.

58. Schwenk RW, Luiken JJ, Bonen A, et al. Regulation of sarcolemmal glucose and fatty acid transporters in cardiac disease. Cardiovasc Res. 2008;79:249–58.

59. Wood IS, Trayhurn P. Glucose transporters (GLUT and SGLT): expanded families of sugar transport proteins. Br J Nutr. 2003;89:3–9.

60. Zierler K. Whole body glucose metabolism. Am J Physiol. 1999;276:E409–26.

61. Poole RC, Halestrap AP. Transport of lactate and other monocarboxylates across mammalian plasma membranes. Am J Physiol. 1993;264:C761–82.

62. Panchal AR, Comte B, Huang H, et al. Acute hibernation decreases myocardial pyruvate carboxylation and citrate release. Am J Physiol Heart Circ Physiol. 2001;281:H1613–20.

63. Panchal AR, Comte B, Huang H, et al. Partitioning of pyruvate between oxidation and anaplerosis in swine hearts. Am J Physiol Heart Circ Physiol. 2000; 279:H2390–8.

64. Pound KM, Sorokina N, Ballal K, et al. Substrate-enzyme competition attenuates upregulated anaplerotic flux through malic enzyme in hypertrophied rat heart and restores triacylglyceride content: attenuating upregulated anaplerosis in hypertrophy. Circ Res. 2009;104:805–12.

65. Sugden MC, Holness MJ. Recent advances in mechanisms regulating glucose oxidation at the level of the pyruvate dehydrogenase complex by PDKs. Am J Physiol Endocrinol Metab. 2003;284:E855–62.

66. Kolobova E, Tuganova A, Boulatnikov I, et al. Regulation of pyruvate dehydrogenase activity through phosphorylation at multiple sites. Biochem J. 2001; 358:69–77.

67. Korotchkina LG, Patel MS. Site specificity of four pyruvate dehydrogenase kinase isoenzymes toward the three phosphorylation sites of human pyruvate dehydrogenase. J Biol Chem. 2001;276:37223–9.

68. Holness MJ, Sugden MC. Regulation of pyruvate dehydrogenase complex activity by reversible phosphorylation. Biochem Soc Trans. 2003;31:1143–51.

69. Spriet LL, Heigenhauser GJ. Regulation of pyruvate dehydrogenase (PDH) activity in human skeletal muscle during exercise. Exerc Sport Sci Rev. 2002; 30:91–5.

70. Dennis SC, Gevers W, Opie LH. Protons in ischemia: where do they come from; where do they go to? J Mol Cell Cardiol. 1991;23:1077–86.

71. Roberts RA, Ghiasvand F, Parker D. Biochemistry of exercise-induced metabolic acidosis. Am J Physiol Regul Integr Comp Physiol. 2004;287:R502–16.

72. Lysiak W, Toth PP, Suelter CH, et al. Quantitation of the efflux of acylcarnitines from rat heart, brain, and liver mitochondria. J Biol Chem. 1986;261:13698–703.

73. Bing RJ, Hammond MM, Handelsman JC, et al. The measurement of coronary blood flow, oxygen consumption, and efficiency of the left ventricle in man. Am Heart J. 1949;38:1–24.

74. Suga H. Cardiac energetics: from E(max) to pressure-volume area. Clin Exp Pharmacol Physiol. 2003; 30:580–5.

75. Suga H. Ventricular energetics. Physiol Rev. 1990; 70:247–77.

76. Jaswal JS, Ussher JR, Lopaschuk GD. Myocardial fatty acid utilization as a determinant of cardiac efficiency and function. Future Lipidol. 2009;4:379–89.

77. Boudina S, Sena S, O'Neill BT, et al. Reduced mitochondrial oxidative capacity and increased mitochondrial uncoupling impair myocardial energetics in obesity. Circulation. 2005;112:2686–95.

78. Hafstad AD, Khalid AM, How OJ, et al. Glucose and insulin improve cardiac efficiency and postischemic functional recovery in perfused hearts from type 2 diabetic (db/db) mice. Am J Physiol Endocrinol Metab. 2007;292:E1288–94.

79. How OJ, Aasum E, Severson DL, et al. Increased myocardial oxygen consumption reduces cardiac efficiency in diabetic mice. Diabetes. 2006;55: 466–73.

80. Boudina S, Sena S, Theobald H, et al. Mitochondrial energetics in the heart in obesity-related diabetes: direct evidence for increased uncoupled respiration

and activation of uncoupling proteins. Diabetes. 2007;56:2457–66.

81. Mazumder PK, O'Neill BT, Roberts MW, et al. Impaired cardiac efficiency and increased fatty acid oxidation in insulin-resistant ob/ob mouse hearts. Diabetes. 2004;53:2366–74.

82. Huang Y, Hunyor SN, Jiang L, et al. Remodeling of the chronic severely failing ischemic sheep heart after coronary microembolization: functional, energetic, structural, and cellular responses. Am J Physiol Heart Circ Physiol. 2004;286:H2141–50.

83. Kameyama T, Chen Z, Bell SP, et al. Mechanoenergetic alterations during the transition from cardiac hypertrophy to failure in Dahl salt-sensitive rats. Circulation. 1998;98:2919–29.

84. Bengel FM, Permanetter B, Ungerer M, et al. Noninvasive estimation of myocardial efficiency using positron emission tomography and carbon-11 acetate – comparison between the normal and failing human heart. Eur J Nucl Med. 2000;27:319–26.

85. Morii I, Kihara Y, Inoko M, et al. Myocardial contractile efficiency and oxygen cost of contractility are preserved during transition from compensated hypertrophy to failure in rats with salt-sensitive hypertension. Hypertension. 1998;31:949–60.

86. Hinkle PC. P/O ratios of mitochondrial oxidative phosphorylation. Biochim Biophys Acta. 2005;1706:1–11.

87. Kadenbach B. Intrinsic and extrinsic uncoupling of oxidative phosphorylation. Biochim Biophys Acta. 2003;1604:77–94.

88. Murray AJ, Panagia M, Hauton D, et al. Plasma free fatty acids and peroxisome proliferator-activated receptor alpha in the control of myocardial uncoupling protein levels. Diabetes. 2005;54:3496–502.

89. Boehm EA, Jones BE, Radda GK, et al. Increased uncoupling proteins and decreased efficiency in palmitate-perfused hyperthyroid rat heart. Am J Physiol Heart Circ Physiol. 2001;280:H977–83.

90. Hidaka S, Kakuma T, Yoshimatsu H, et al. Streptozotocin treatment upregulates uncoupling protein 3 expression in the rat heart. Diabetes. 1999;48:430–5.

91. Bugger H, Boudina S, Hu XX, et al. Type 1 diabetic akita mouse hearts are insulin sensitive but manifest structurally abnormal mitochondria that remain coupled despite increased uncoupling protein 3. Diabetes. 2008;57:2924–32.

92. Murray AJ, Anderson RE, Watson GC, et al. Uncoupling proteins in human heart. Lancet. 2004; 364:1786–8.

93. Murray AJ, Cole MA, Lygate CA, et al. Increased mitochondrial uncoupling proteins, respiratory uncoupling and decreased efficiency in the chronically infarcted rat heart. J Mol Cell Cardiol. 2008; 44:694–700.

94. Seifert EL, Bezaire V, Estey C, et al. Essential role for uncoupling protein-3 in mitochondrial adaptation to fasting but not in fatty acid oxidation or fatty acid anion export. J Biol Chem. 2008;283:25124–31.

95. Hunt MC, Alexson SE. The role Acyl-CoA thioesterases play in mediating intracellular lipid metabolism. Prog Lipid Res. 2002;41:99–130.

96. Burgmaier M, Sen S, Philip F, Wilson CR, et al. Metabolic adaptation follows contractile dysfunction in the heart of obese zucker rats fed a high-fat "Western" diet. Obesity (Silver Spring). 2010;18:1895–901.

97. Stavinoha MA, RaySpellicy JW, Essop MF, et al. Evidence for mitochondrial thioesterase 1 as a peroxisome proliferator-activated receptor-alpha-regulated gene in cardiac and skeletal muscle. Am J Physiol Endocrinol Metab. 2004;287:E888–95.

98. King KL, Young ME, Kerner J, et al. Diabetes or peroxisome proliferator-activated receptor alpha agonist increases mitochondrial thioesterase I activity in heart. J Lipid Res. 2007;48:1511–7.

99. Himms-Hagen J, Harper ME. Physiological role of UCP3 may be export of fatty acids from mitochondria when fatty acid oxidation predominates: an hypothesis. Exp Biol Med (Maywood). 2001;226:78–84.

100. Myrmel T, Forsdahl K, Larsen TS. Triacylglycerol metabolism in hypoxic, glucose-deprived rat cardiomyocytes. J Mol Cell Cardiol. 1992;24:855–68.

101. Klocke R, Tian W, Kuhlmann MT, et al. Surgical animal models of heart failure related to coronary heart disease. Cardiovasc Res. 2007;74:29–38.

102. Monnet E, Chachques JC. Animal models of heart failure: what is new? Ann Thorac Surg. 2005; 79:1445–53.

103. Beer M, Seyfarth T, Sandstede J, et al. Absolute concentrations of high-energy phosphate metabolites in normal, hypertrophied, and failing human myocardium measured noninvasively with (31)P-SLOOP magnetic resonance spectroscopy. J Am Coll Cardiol. 2002;40:1267–74.

104. Conway MA, Allis J, Ouwerkerk R, et al. Detection of low phosphocreatine to ATP ratio in failing hypertrophied human myocardium by 31P magnetic resonance spectroscopy. Lancet. 1991;338:973–6.

105. Nascimben L, Friedrich J, Liao R, et al. Enalapril treatment increases cardiac performance and energy reserve via the creatine kinase reaction in myocardium of Syrian myopathic hamsters with advanced heart failure. Circulation. 1995;91:1824–33.

106. Tian R, Nascimben L, Kaddurah-Daouk R, et al. Depletion of energy reserve via the creatine kinase reaction during the evolution of heart failure in cardiomyopathic hamsters. J Mol Cell Cardiol. 1996; 28:755–65.

107. Ingwall JS. Energy metabolism in heart failure and remodelling. Cardiovasc Res. 2009;81:412–9.

108. Ingwall JS, Weiss RG. Is the failing heart energy starved? On using chemical energy to support cardiac function. Circ Res. 2004;95:135–45.

109. Neubauer S, Krahe T, Schindler R, et al. 31P magnetic resonance spectroscopy in dilated cardiomyopathy and coronary artery disease. Altered cardiac high-energy phosphate metabolism in heart failure. Circulation. 1992;86:1810–8.

110. Degens H, de Brouwer KF, Gilde AJ, et al. Cardiac fatty acid metabolism is preserved in the compensated hypertrophic rat heart. Basic Res Cardiol. 2006;101:17–26.

111. de Brouwer KF, Degens H, Aartsen WM, et al. Specific and sustained down-regulation of genes involved in fatty acid metabolism is not a hallmark of progression to cardiac failure in mice. J Mol Cell Cardiol. 2006;40:838–45.

112. O'Donnell JM, Fields AD, Sorokina N, et al. The absence of endogenous lipid oxidation in early stage heart failure exposes limits in lipid storage and turnover. J Mol Cell Cardiol. 2008;44:315–22.

113. Chandler MP, Kerner J, Huang H, et al. Moderate severity heart failure does not involve a downregulation of myocardial fatty acid oxidation. Am J Physiol Heart Circ Physiol. 2004;287:H1538–43.

114. Grover-McKay M, Schwaiger M, Krivokapich J, et al. Regional myocardial blood flow and metabolism at rest in mildly symptomatic patients with hypertrophic cardiomyopathy. J Am Coll Cardiol. 1989;13:317–24.

115. Lommi J, Kupari M, Yki-Jarvinen H. Free fatty acid kinetics and oxidation in congestive heart failure. Am J Cardiol. 1998;81:45–50.

116. Paolisso G, Gambardella A, Galzerano D, et al. Total-body and myocardial substrate oxidation in congestive heart failure. Metabolism. 1994;43:174–9.

117. Taylor M, Wallhaus TR, Degrado TR, et al. An evaluation of myocardial fatty acid and glucose uptake using PET with (18F)fluoro-6-thia-heptadecanoic acid and (18F)FDG in Patients with Congestive Heart Failure. J Nucl Med. 2001;42:55–62.

118. Bugger H, Schwarzer M, Chen D. Proteomic remodelling of mitochondrial oxidative pathways in pressure overload-induced heart failure. Cardiovasc Res. 2010;85(2):376–84.

119. Doenst T, Pytel G, Schrepper A, et al. Decreased rates of substrate oxidation ex vivo predict the onset of heart failure and contractile dysfunction in rats with pressure overload. Cardiovasc Res. 2010;86: 461–70.

120. Lei B, Lionetti V, Young ME, et al. Paradoxical downregulation of the glucose oxidation pathway despite enhanced flux in severe heart failure. J Mol Cell Cardiol. 2004;36:567–76.

121. Osorio JC, Stanley WC, Linke A, et al. Impaired myocardial fatty acid oxidation and reduced protein expression of retinoid X receptor-alpha in pacing-induced heart failure. Circulation. 2002;106:606–12.

122. Qanud K, Mamdani M, Pepe M, et al. Reverse changes in cardiac substrate oxidation in dogs recovering from heart failure. Am J Physiol Heart Circ Physiol. 2008;295:H2098–105.

123. Neglia D, De Caterina A, Marraccini P, et al. Impaired myocardial metabolic reserve and substrate selection flexibility during stress in patients with idiopathic dilated cardiomyopathy. Am J Physiol Heart Circ Physiol. 2007;293:H3270–8.

124. Tuunanen H, Engblom E, Naum A, et al. Free fatty acid depletion acutely decreases cardiac work and efficiency in cardiomyopathic heart failure. Circulation. 2006;114:2130–7.

125. Taegtmeyer H. Metabolism – the lost child of cardiology. J Am Coll Cardiol. 2000;36:1386–8.

126. Dzau VJ, Colucci WS, Hollenberg NK, et al. Relation of the renin-angiotensin-aldosterone system to clinical state in congestive heart failure. Circulation. 1981;63:645–51.

127. Re RN. Mechanisms of disease: local renin-angiotensin-aldosterone systems and the pathogenesis and treatment of cardiovascular disease. Nat Clin Pract Cardiovasc Med. 2004;1:42–7.

128. Pepper GS, Lee RW. Sympathetic activation in heart failure and its treatment with beta-blockade. Arch Intern Med. 1999;159:225–34.

129. Morris MJ, Cox HS, Lambert GW, et al. Region-specific neuropeptide Y overflows at rest and during sympathetic activation in humans. Hypertension. 1997;29:137–43.

130. Bohm M, La Rosee K, Schwinger RH, et al. Evidence for reduction of norepinephrine uptake sites in the failing human heart. J Am Coll Cardiol. 1995;25: 146–53.

131. Engelhardt S, Bohm M, Erdmann E, et al. Analysis of beta-adrenergic receptor mRNA levels in human ventricular biopsy specimens by quantitative polymerase chain reactions: progressive reduction of beta 1-adrenergic receptor mRNA in heart failure. J Am Coll Cardiol. 1996;27:146–54.

132. Neely JR, Whitmer M, Mochizuki S. Effects of mechanical activity and hormones on myocardial glucose and fatty acid utilization. Circ Res. 1976; 38(5 Suppl 1):I22–30.

133. Nonogaki K. New insights into sympathetic regulation of glucose and fat metabolism. Diabetologia. 2000;43:533–49.

134. Marangou AG, Alford FP, Ward G, et al. Hormonal effects of norepinephrine on acute glucose disposal in humans: a minimal model analysis. Metabolism. 1988;37:885–91.

135. Arnlov J, Lind L, Zethelius B, et al. Several factors associated with the insulin resistance syndrome are predictors of left ventricular systolic dysfunction in a male population after 20 years of follow-up. Am Heart J. 2001;142:720–4.

136. Petersen KF, Dufour S, Savage DB, et al. The role of skeletal muscle insulin resistance in the pathogenesis of the metabolic syndrome. Proc Natl Acad Sci USA. 2007;104:12587–94.

137. Shulman GI, Rothman DL, Jue T, et al. Quantitation of muscle glycogen synthesis in normal subjects and subjects with non-insulin-dependent diabetes by 13C nuclear magnetic resonance spectroscopy. N Engl J Med. 1990;322:223–8.

138. Doehner W, von Haehling S, Anker SD. Insulin resistance in chronic heart failure. J Am Coll Cardiol. 2008;52:239. author reply 239–240.

139. Dutka DP, Pitt M, Pagano D, et al. Myocardial glucose transport and utilization in patients with type 2 diabetes mellitus, left ventricular dysfunction, and coronary artery disease. J Am Coll Cardiol. 2006;48:2225–31.

140. Nikolaidis LA, Elahi D, Hentosz T, et al. Recombinant glucagon-like peptide-1 increases myocardial glucose uptake and improves left ventricular performance in conscious dogs with pacing-induced dilated cardiomyopathy. Circulation. 2004;110:955–61.

141. Nikolaidis LA, Elahi D, Shen YT, et al. Active metabolite of GLP-1 mediates myocardial glucose uptake and improves left ventricular performance in conscious dogs with dilated cardiomyopathy. Am J Physiol Heart Circ Physiol. 2005;289:H2401–8.

142. Aasum E, Belke DD, Severson DL, et al. Cardiac function and metabolism in Type 2 diabetic mice after treatment with BM 17.0744, a novel PPAR-alpha activator. Am J Physiol Heart Circ Physiol. 2002;283:H949–57.

143. Aasum E, Hafstad AD, Severson DL, et al. Age-dependent changes in metabolism, contractile function, and ischemic sensitivity in hearts from db/db mice. Diabetes. 2003;52:434–41.

144. Aasum E, Khalid AM, Gudbrandsen OA, et al. Fenofibrate modulates cardiac and hepatic metabolism and increases ischemic tolerance in diet-induced obese mice. J Mol Cell Cardiol. 2008;44:201–9.

145. Buchanan J, Mazumder PK, Hu P, et al. Reduced cardiac efficiency and altered substrate metabolism precedes the onset of hyperglycemia and contractile dysfunction in two mouse models of insulin resistance and obesity. Endocrinology. 2005;146:5341–9.

146. Hafstad AD, Solevag GH, Severson DL, et al. Perfused hearts from Type 2 diabetic (db/db) mice show metabolic responsiveness to insulin. Am J Physiol Heart Circ Physiol. 2006;290:H1763–9.

147. How OJ, Aasum E, Kunnathu S, et al. Influence of substrate supply on cardiac efficiency, as measured by pressure-volume analysis in ex vivo mouse hearts. Am J Physiol Heart Circ Physiol. 2005;288:H2979–85.

148. Peterson LR, Herrero P, Schechtman KB, et al. Effect of obesity and insulin resistance on myocardial substrate metabolism and efficiency in young women. Circulation. 2004;109:2191–6.

149. Ussher JR, Koves TR, Jaswal JS, et al. Insulin-stimulated cardiac glucose oxidation is increased in high-fat diet-induced obese mice lacking malonyl CoA decarboxylase. Diabetes. 2009;58:1766–75.

150. Brisse B, Tetsch P, Jacobs W, et al. Beta-adrenoceptor blockade in stress due to oral surgery. Br J Clin Pharmacol. 1982;13 Suppl 2:421S–7.

151. Newman RJ. Comparison of the antilipolytic effect of metoprolol, acebutolol, and propranolol in man. Br Med J. 1977;2:601–3.

152. Fellander G, Eleborg L, Bolinder J, et al. Microdialysis of adipose tissue during surgery: effect of local alpha- and beta-adrenoceptor blockade on blood flow and lipolysis. J Clin Endocrinol Metab. 1996;81:2919–24.

153. Igarashi N, Nozawa T, Fujii N, et al. Influence of beta-adrenoceptor blockade on the myocardial accumulation of fatty acid tracer and its intracellular metabolism in the heart after ischemia-reperfusion injury. Circ J. 2006;70:1509–14.

154. Wallhaus TR, Taylor M, DeGrado TR, et al. Myocardial free fatty acid and glucose use after carvedilol treatment in patients with congestive heart failure. Circulation. 2001;103:2441–6.

155. Eichhorn EJ, Bedotto JB, Malloy CR, et al. Effect of beta-adrenergic blockade on myocardial function and energetics in congestive heart failure. Improvements in hemodynamic, contractile, and diastolic performance with bucindolol. Circulation. 1990;82:473–83.

156. Eichhorn EJ, Heesch CM, Barnett JH, et al. Effect of metoprolol on myocardial function and energetics in patients with nonischemic dilated cardiomyopathy: a randomized, double-blind, placebo-controlled study. J Am Coll Cardiol. 1994;24:1310–20.

157. Panchal AR, Stanley WC, Kerner J, et al. Beta-receptor blockade decreases carnitine palmitoyl transferase I activity in dogs with heart failure. J Card Fail. 1998;4:121–6.

158. Podbregar M, Voga G. Effect of selective and nonselective beta-blockers on resting energy production rate and total body substrate utilization in chronic heart failure. J Card Fail. 2002;8:369–78.

159. Al-Hesayen A, Azevedo ER, Floras JS, et al. Selective versus nonselective beta-adrenergic receptor blockade in chronic heart failure: differential effects on myocardial energy substrate utilization. Eur J Heart Fail. 2005;7:618–23.

160. Madrazo JA, Kelly DP. The PPAR trio: regulators of myocardial energy metabolism in health and disease. J Mol Cell Cardiol. 2008;44:968–75.

161. Cook WS, Yeldandi AV, Rao MS, et al. Less extrahepatic induction of fatty acid beta-oxidation enzymes by PPAR alpha. Biochem Biophys Res Commun. 2000;278:250–7.

162. Schoonjans K, Staels B, Grimaldi P, et al. Acyl-CoA synthetase mRNA expression is controlled by fibric-acid derivatives, feeding and liver proliferation. Eur J Biochem. 1993;216:615–22.

163. Wayman NS, Hattori Y, McDonald MC, et al. Ligands of the peroxisome proliferator-activated receptors (PPAR-gamma and PPAR-alpha) reduce myocardial infarct size. FASEB J. 2002;16:1027–40.

164. Prasad MR, Clement R, Otani H, et al. Improved myocardial performance induced by clofibrate during reperfusion after acute myocardial infarction. Can J Physiol Pharmacol. 1988;66:1518–23.

165. Cheng L, Ding G, Qin Q, et al. Cardiomyocyte-restricted peroxisome proliferator-activated receptor-delta deletion perturbs myocardial fatty acid oxidation and leads to cardiomyopathy. Nat Med. 2004;10:1245–50.

166. Gilde AJ, van der Lee KA, Willemsen PH, et al. Peroxisome proliferator-activated receptor (PPAR) alpha and PPARbeta/delta, but not PPARgamma,

modulate the expression of genes involved in cardiac lipid metabolism. Circ Res. 2003;92:518–24.

167. Hondares E, Pineda-Torra I, Iglesias R, et al. PPARdelta, but not PPARalpha, activates PGC-1alpha gene transcription in muscle. Biochem Biophys Res Commun. 2007;354:1021–7.

168. Pellieux C, Montessuit C, Papageorgiou I, et al. Angiotensin II downregulates the fatty acid oxidation pathway in adult rat cardiomyocytes via release of tumour necrosis factor-alpha. Cardiovasc Res. 2009;82:341–50.

169. Planavila A, Laguna JC, Vazquez-Carrera M. Nuclear factor-kappaB activation leads to down-regulation of fatty acid oxidation during cardiac hypertrophy. J Biol Chem. 2005;280:17464–71.

170. Burkart EM, Sambandam N, Han X, et al. Nuclear receptors PPARbeta/delta and PPARalpha direct distinct metabolic regulatory programs in the mouse heart. J Clin Invest. 2007;117:3930–9.

171. Sidell RJ, Cole MA, Draper NJ, et al. Thiazolidinedione treatment normalizes insulin resistance and ischemic injury in the zucker Fatty rat heart. Diabetes. 2002;51:1110–7.

172. Zhu P, Lu L, Xu Y, et al. Troglitazone improves recovery of left ventricular function after regional ischemia in pigs. Circulation. 2000;101:1165–71.

173. Yue TL, Bao W, Gu JL, et al. Rosiglitazone treatment in Zucker diabetic Fatty rats is associated with ameliorated cardiac insulin resistance and protection from ischemia/reperfusion-induced myocardial injury. Diabetes. 2005;54:554–62.

174. Okere IC, Chandler MP, McElfresh TA, et al. Carnitine palmitoyl transferase-I inhibition is not associated with cardiac hypertrophy in rats fed a high-fat diet. Clin Exp Pharmacol Physiol. 2007; 34:113–9.

175. Lindenfeld J, Masoudi FA. Fluid retention with thiazolidinediones: does the mechanism influence the outcome? J Am Coll Cardiol. 2007;49:1705–7.

176. Dormandy JA, Charbonnel B, Eckland DJ, et al. Secondary prevention of macrovascular events in patients with type 2 diabetes in the PROactive Study (PROspective pioglitAzone Clinical Trial In macro-Vascular Events): a randomised controlled trial. Lancet. 2005;366:1279–89.

177. Nissen SE, Wolski K. Effect of rosiglitazone on the risk of myocardial infarction and death from cardiovascular causes. N Engl J Med. 2007;356:2457–71.

178. Nissen SE, Wolski K. Rosiglitazone revisited: an updated meta-analysis of risk for myocardial infarction and cardiovascular mortality. Arch Intern Med. 2010; in press

179. Reaven GM, Chang H, Hoffman BB. Additive hypoglycemic effects of drugs that modify free-fatty acid metabolism by different mechanisms in rats with streptozocin-induced diabetes. Diabetes. 1988;37:28–32.

180. Lopaschuk GD, McNeil GF, McVeigh JJ. Glucose oxidation is stimulated in reperfused ischemic hearts with the carnitine palmitoyltransferase 1 inhibitor, Etomoxir. Mol Cell Biochem. 1989;88:175–9.

181. Lopaschuk GD, Spafford MA, Davies NJ, et al. Glucose and palmitate oxidation in isolated working rat hearts reperfused after a period of transient global ischemia. Circ Res. 1990;66:546–53.

182. Lopaschuk GD, Wall SR, Olley PM, et al. Etomoxir, a carnitine palmitoyltransferase I inhibitor, protects hearts from fatty acid-induced ischemic injury independent of changes in long chain acylcarnitine. Circ Res. 1988;63:1036–43.

183. Schmitz FJ, Rosen P, Reinauer H. Improvement of myocardial function and metabolism in diabetic rats by the carnitine palmitoyl transferase inhibitor Etomoxir. Horm Metab Res. 1995;27:515–22.

184. Wall SR, Lopaschuk GD. Glucose oxidation rates in fatty acid-perfused isolated working hearts from diabetic rats. Biochim Biophys Acta. 1989;1006:97–103.

185. Turcani M, Rupp H. Etomoxir improves left ventricular performance of pressure-overloaded rat heart. Circulation. 1997;96:3681–6.

186. Rupp H, Vetter R. Sarcoplasmic reticulum function and carnitine palmitoyltransferase-1 inhibition during progression of heart failure. Br J Pharmacol. 2000;131:1748–56.

187. Schmidt-Schweda S, Holubarsch C. First clinical trial with etomoxir in patients with chronic congestive heart failure. Clin Sci (Lond). 2000;99:27–35.

188. Holubarsch CJ, Rohrbach M, Karrasch M, et al. A double-blind randomized multicentre clinical trial to evaluate the efficacy and safety of two doses of etomoxir in comparison with placebo in patients with moderate congestive heart failure: the ERGO (etomoxir for the recovery of glucose oxidation) study. Clin Sci (Lond). 2007;113:205–12.

189. Lee L, Campbell R, Scheuermann-Freestone M, et al. Metabolic modulation with perhexiline in chronic heart failure: a randomized, controlled trial of short-term use of a novel treatment. Circulation. 2005;112:3280–8.

190. Abozguia K, Elliott P, McKenna W, et al. Metabolic modulator perhexiline corrects energy deficiency and improves exercise capacity in symptomatic hypertrophic cardiomyopathy. Circulation. 2010;122:1562–9.

191. Kantor PF, Lucien A, Kozak R, et al. The antianginal drug trimetazidine shifts cardiac energy metabolism from fatty acid oxidation to glucose oxidation by inhibiting mitochondrial long-chain 3-ketoacyl coenzyme A thiolase. Circ Res. 2000;86:580–8.

192. Lopaschuk GD, Barr R, Thomas PD, et al. Beneficial effects of trimetazidine in ex vivo working ischemic hearts are due to a stimulation of glucose oxidation secondary to inhibition of long-chain 3-ketoacyl coenzyme a thiolase. Circ Res. 2003;93:e33–7.

193. MacInnes A, Fairman DA, Binding P, et al. The antianginal agent trimetazidine does not exert its functional benefit via inhibition of mitochondrial long-chain 3-ketoacyl coenzyme A thiolase. Circ Res. 2003;93:e26–32.

194. Fragasso G, Perseghin G, De Cobelli F, et al. Effects of metabolic modulation by trimetazidine on left ventricular function and phosphocreatine/adenosine triphosphate ratio in patients with heart failure. Eur Heart J. 2006;27:942–8.

195. Fragasso G, Palloshi A, Puccetti P, et al. A randomized clinical trial of trimetazidine, a partial free fatty acid oxidation inhibitor, in patients with heart failure. J Am Coll Cardiol. 2006;48:992–8.

196. Tuunanen H, Engblom E, Naum A, et al. Trimetazidine, a metabolic modulator, has cardiac and extracardiac benefits in idiopathic dilated cardiomyopathy. Circulation. 2008;118:1250–8.

197. Clarke B, Spedding M, Patmore L, et al. Protective effects of ranolazine in guinea-pig hearts during low-flow ischaemia and their association with increases in active pyruvate dehydrogenase. Br J Pharmacol. 1993;109:748–50.

198. Clarke B, Wyatt KM, McCormack JG. Ranolazine increases active pyruvate dehydrogenase in perfused normoxic rat hearts: evidence for an indirect mechanism. J Mol Cell Cardiol. 1996;28:341–50.

199. McCormack JG, Baracos VE, Barr R, et al. Effects of ranolazine on oxidative substrate preference in epitrochlearis muscle. J Appl Physiol. 1996;81:905–10.

200. McCormack JG, Barr RL, Wolff AA, et al. Ranolazine stimulates glucose oxidation in normoxic, ischemic, and reperfused ischemic rat hearts. Circulation. 1996;93:135–42.

201. Wyatt KM, Skene C, Veitch K, Hue L, et al. The antianginal agent ranolazine is a weak inhibitor of the respiratory complex I, but with greater potency in broken or uncoupled than in coupled mitochondria. Biochem Pharmacol. 1995;50:1599–606.

202. Fraser H, Belardinelli L, Wang L, et al. Ranolazine decreases diastolic calcium accumulation caused by ATX-II or ischemia in rat hearts. J Mol Cell Cardiol. 2006;41:1031–8.

203. Sossalla S, Wagner S, Rasenack EC, et al. Ranolazine improves diastolic dysfunction in isolated myocardium from failing human hearts – role of late sodium current and intracellular ion accumulation. J Mol Cell Cardiol. 2008;45:32–43.

204. Belardinelli L, Shryock JC, Fraser H. Inhibition of the late sodium current as a potential cardioprotective principle: effects of the late sodium current inhibitor ranolazine. Heart. 2006;92 Suppl 4:iv6–14.

205. Wang P, Fraser H, Lloyd SG, et al. A comparison between ranolazine and CVT-4325, a novel inhibitor of fatty acid oxidation, on cardiac metabolism and left ventricular function in rat isolated perfused heart during ischemia and reperfusion. J Pharmacol Exp Ther. 2007;321:213–20.

206. Chandler MP, Stanley WC, Morita H, et al. Short-term treatment with ranolazine improves mechanical efficiency in dogs with chronic heart failure. Circ Res. 2002;91:278–80.

207. Sabbah HN, Chandler MP, Mishima T, et al. Ranolazine, a partial fatty acid oxidation (pFOX) inhibitor, improves left ventricular function in dogs with chronic heart failure. J Card Fail. 2002;8:416–22.

208. Rastogi S, Sharov VG, Mishra S, et al. Ranolazine combined with enalapril or metoprolol prevents progressive LV dysfunction and remodeling in dogs with moderate heart failure. Am J Physiol Heart Circ Physiol. 2008;295:H2149–55.

209. Liu B, Clanachan AS, Schulz R, et al. Cardiac efficiency is improved after ischemia by altering both the source and fate of protons. Circ Res. 1996;79:940–8.

210. Liu Q, Docherty JC, Rendell JC, et al. High levels of fatty acids delay the recovery of intracellular pH and cardiac efficiency in post-ischemic hearts by inhibiting glucose oxidation. J Am Coll Cardiol. 2002;39:718–25.

211. Kato T, Niizuma S, Inuzuka Y, et al. Analysis of metabolic remodeling in compensated left ventricular hypertrophy and heart failure. Circ Heart Fail. 2010;3:420–30.

212. Bersin RM, Stacpoole PW. Dichloroacetate as metabolic therapy for myocardial ischemia and failure. Am Heart J. 1997;134:841–55.

213. Bersin RM, Wolfe C, Kwasman M, et al. Improved hemodynamic function and mechanical efficiency in congestive heart failure with sodium dichloroacetate. J Am Coll Cardiol. 1994;23:1617–24.

Cardiolipin Metabolism in Experimental and Human Heart Failure

Grant M. Hatch

Abstract

Heart failure accounts for approximately 5% of all medical admissions and is the single most common cause of hospital admissions in individuals aged 65 years and over. The biochemical mechanisms for the development of heart failure are beginning to emerge. Cardiolipin is a major mitochondrial membrane phospholipid required for the activity of key mitochondrial enzymes involved in cellular energy production. Loss of cardiolipin results in the inability of mitochondria to sustain oxidative phosphorylation. Cardiolipin metabolism is altered leading to reduction in tetralinoleoyl-cardiolipin levels in experimental animal models of heart failure and in humans. This loss in tetralinoleoyl-cardiolipin results in reduced mitochondrial function which may contribute to the development of heart failure. Thus, cardiolipin biosynthetic and remodeling enzymes may represent targets for pharmacotherapeutic modulation in both left ventricular- as well as right ventricular-mediated heart failure.

Keywords

Cardiolipin • Heart failure • Mitochondria • Phospholipid • Biosynthesis • Remodeling • Tafazzin • Huntington disease • Persistent pulmonary hypertension • Hypertensive heart failure–prone rat • Genetic disease • Yeast artificial chromosome mouse • Barth syndrome

G.M. Hatch (✉)
Department of Pharmacology and Therapeutics, Biochemistry and Medical Genetics, Internal Medicine, Faculty of Medicine, Center for Research and Treatment of Atherosclerosis, Manitoba Institute of Child Health, University of Manitoba, Winnipeg, Canada
e-mail: hatchgm@ms.umanitoba.ca

Introduction

Heart failure in humans occurs in 1–2% of the adult population and 6–10% of adults over 65 years of age (reviewed in ref. [1, 2]). The lifetime risk of developing heart failure is roughly one in five for a 40 year old and the prevalence is increasing. Heart failure accounts for approximately 5%

N.S. Dhalla, M. Nagano, B. Ostadal (eds.), *Molecular Defects in Cardiovascular Disease*,
DOI 10.1007/978-1-4419-7130-2_13, © Springer Science+Business Media, LLC 2011

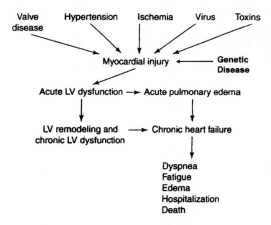

Fig. 1 The cause and functional consequences of left ventricular heart failure

of all medical admissions and is the single most common cause of admissions in people aged over 65 years. Although there are a number of different conditions that lead to left ventricular heart failure (see Fig. 1), the fundamental problem of heart failure is a decrease in the force of contraction of the myocardium for any given fiber length. The heart tries to compensate for the resulting decrease in stroke volume by increasing its end diastolic volume and by a reflex increase in contractility. This is called the compensated phase of heart failure. Eventually these compensatory mechanisms prove to be inadequate and heart failure occurs. Long term adjustments can be in the form of myocardial hypertrophy and eventually dilatation. The failing heart, due to an increase in its diameter, has to do much more work to generate an equivalent amount of wall tension compared to the normal heart (Laplace's law). This phase is called the decompensated phase. Increased venous pressure during heart failure causes an increase in capillary pressure leading to edema. Decreased cardiac output causes a reduction in renal blood flow which activates the renin-angiotensin-aldosterone axis; this causes water and salt retention and an increase in blood volume. This mechanism, while attempting to increase cardiac filling pressure and maintain output, causes a further increase in capillary pressure. Decreased blood pressure during failure causes a reflex increase in sympathetic activity,

arteriolar constriction, and increased cardiac afterload. Although done in an attempt to maintain blood flow to the brain and other organs, arteriolar constriction (increased afterload) further compromises stroke volume. Prolonged increase in preload and the elevated levels of catecholamines and angiotensin causes structural remodeling of the heart (hypertrophy and dilatation), which although initially is beneficial, later becomes detrimental for heart function resulting in increased diastolic stiffness and increased incidence of arrhythmia. The first line drug for treatment of heart failure is an angiotensin converting enzyme inhibitor. A diuretic is used if there is either pulmonary or systemic edema. In patients of ischemic heart disease a beta blocker is given in gradually increasing dose. Digoxin may be added if the above are not enough. A comprehensive review of the pharmacological treatment of heart failure and the most recent clinical trials for the drugs used in the treatment of heart failure was recently published [2].

Phospholipids are important structural and functional components of the cell membrane [3]. It is well documented that alteration in the composition of phospholipids within the heart are linked to sustained differences in myocardial electrical activity [4]. The major polyglycerophospholipid in mammalian tissues is bis-(1,2-diacyl-*sn*-glycero-3-phospho)-1′,3′-*sn*-glycerol or cardiolipin [5]. Cardiolipin (CL) comprises approximately 15–20% of the entire phospholipid phosphorus mass of the heart [5, 6]. CL is required for the activity of a number of key mitochondrial enzymes involved in cellular energy metabolism [7, 8]. In fact, it has been suggested that CL is the "glue" that holds the mitochondrial respiratory complex together [9]. Thus, maintenance of the appropriate content and fatty acid composition of CL in mitochondria is essential for proper heart function. Barth Syndrome is a X-linked genetic disorder and is the only disease in which the specific biochemical defect is a reduction in CL and accumulation of monolysocardiolipin (MLCL) (reviewed in ref. [10]). A reduced ability to remodel CL from MLCL is the molecular mechanism responsible for Barth Syndrome. Barth Syndrome patients rapidly develop cardiomyopathy shortly after birth and this is a main cause of death in these patients.

During the development of heart failure the heart becomes hypertrophied and mitochondrial energy production is unable to meet the requirements of the hypertrophied heart [11–13]. Alterations in CL have been observed in human and experimental models of heart failure and correlate closely with the loss of mitochondrial respiratory enzyme activity and disease progression [14]. The mechanisms responsible for this alteration in CL during the development of heart failure are beginning to emerge. The purpose of this chapter is to review recent studies on CL metabolism in human and experimental human heart failure and outline other potentially useful animal models.

Role of Cardiolipin in General Mitochondrial Function

CL is required for mitochondrial respiratory chain function and optimum oxygen consumption in mitochondria [15, 16]. For example, in rat heart subjected to ischemia and reperfusion, the reduction in complex III activity was coupled with a reduction in CL [17]. Under experimental conditions in which CL is removed or digested away from mitochondrial respiratory chain proteins by phospholipases, denaturation and complete loss of activity is observed [18]. CL interaction with these proteins is specific since substitution with other phospholipids does not fully reconstitute activity. CL may play a role in the regulation of mitochondrial mediated apoptosis. For example, oxidative damage to the CL molecule, via a CL-specific peroxidase activity of CL bound cytochrome c, is associated with cytochrome c release and apoptosis [19–21]. Ischemia leads to oxidative damage and subsequent phospholipase A_2 activation with hydrolysis of CL [22]. Moreover, CL itself is required for caspase-8 cleavage of Bid at the mitochondrial outer membrane [23].

In Barth Syndrome (BTHS) there is a reduction in tetralinoleoyl (L_4-CL) species of CL [reviewed in 10, 24, 25]. The decrease in CL is caused by a mutation in the BTHS gene transacylase tafazzin (TAZ). The TAZ gene product tafazzin remodels newly synthesized CL with linoleic acid and in patients with BTHS the ability to remodel CL is thus reduced. The severity of BTHS does not correlate between genotype and phenotype to date, suggesting that there may be other unknown factors that modulate disease severity. A characteristic feature of BTHS is the presentation of cardiomyopathy leading to weakness and fatigue. In a few cases, sudden, fatal ventricular tachycardia was shown to occur even during a period of seemingly good health. The skeletal and cardiomyocyte fatigue of BTHS leads to delayed motor development, and may even be a presenting factor. Myocyte fatigue is attributed to the mitochondrial deficiencies and these deficiencies in the respiratory chain lead to a decrease in oxidative phosphorylation. Other signs commonly associated with BTHS are neutropenia, 3-methylglucaconic aciduria, short stature, failure to thrive, and decreased plasma cholesterol.

Biosynthesis and Remodeling of Cardiac Cardiolipin

Mammalian cardiac CL is synthesized de novo via the cytidine-5′-diphosphate-1,2-diacylglycerol (CDP-DG) pathway (see Fig. 2) [6]. In the first step of this pathway, phosphatidic acid (PA) and CTP are converted to CDP-DG by CTP:PA cytidylyltransferase or CDP-DG synthetase (CDS). In the second and third steps of the pathway CDP-DG condenses with sn-glycerol-3-phosphate to form phophatidylglycerolphosphate (PGP) and then phosphatidylglycerol (PG), catalyzed by (PGP) synthase (PGPS) and PGP phosphatase, respectively. PGP does not normally accumulate in tissues due to the high enzymatic activity of the cardiac PGP phosphatase [26]. In the last step of the CL biosynthetic pathway, PG is converted to CL by condensation with CDP-DG catalyzed by cardiac CL synthase (CLS) [6]. Once synthesized de novo, CL is remodeled via deacylation by

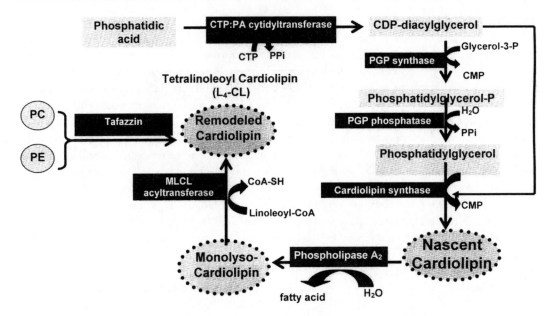

Fig. 2 Mitochondrial cardiolipin biosynthesis and remodeling pathways. See text for explanation. *PC* phosphatidyl-choline, *PE* phosphatidylethanolamine, *PGP* phosphatidylglycerolphosphate, *MLCL* monolysocardiolipin

phospholipase A followed by reacylation through acyl-Coenzyme A lysocardiolipin acyltransferase-1 in the endoplasmic reticulum or by MLCL AT-1 or the CL transacylase TAZ in mitochondria (reviewed in refs. [7, 10]).

Models of Experimental Heart Failure

There are several animal models of chronic heart failure, each with their own advantages and disadvantages (reviewed in ref. [27]). In this chapter, the discussion will be limited to experimental models of heart failure in which alteration of CL enzymes have been directly observed and in which the mechanism for the CL alteration has been addressed. The well known spontaneous hypertensive rat (SHR) has essentially normal cardiac function for up to one year and 57% of these animals develop clinically measureable heart failure at 18–24 months of age. In SHRs cardiac CL and phosphatidylethanolamine plasmalogen levels were significantly increased and phosphatidylcholine and phosphatidylethanolamine decreased compared to controls [28].

The mechanism for these changes is unknown. Although a good model to mimic the hypertension-induced heart failure in humans, the main disadvantage of the SHR model is the long duration of development of the disease, nearly 2 years [27]. In contrast, the hypertensive heart failure–prone (SHHF) rat carries the corpulent gene, which encodes an insufficient leptin receptor, and develops cardiomyopathy between 10 and 16 months. These rats develop myocardial hypertrophy, myocyte enlargement, myocardial fibrosis and neurohumoral activation similar to human congestive heart failure [29]. In addition, the SHHF rat model is ideal since it has other similarities to the actual human condition in that the heart failure develops in association with hypertension, hyperinsulinemia, and diabetes.

Cardiolipin Metabolism Is Altered in Heart Failure in SHHF Rats and in Humans

During the development of heart failure in SHHF rats the major cardiac CL species (tetralinoleoyl-CL or L_4-CL) was decreased whereas other minor

CL species were significantly increased [30]. In addition, these authors showed that left ventricular tissue, which makes up 50% of the heart by weight, had twice the amount of CL than right ventricular or septal tissue. The mechanism for these changes in CL mass and these regional differences in CL content was unknown. Recently we showed that mitochondrial CDS activity and CDS-1 mRNA were increased in SHHF rats and explants from humans in heart failure [31]. In contrast, CDS-2 mRNA was unaltered. Moreover, PGPS activity, but not mRNA, increased in SHHFs whereas CLS activity and mRNA decreased in SHHFs, but its mRNA was not significantly altered in humans. The CL remodeling enzymes, monolysocardiolipin acyltransferase (MLCL AT) and tafazzin, showed variable changes during heart failure. MLCL AT activity increased but tafazzin mRNA was decreased in SHHF rats and in explants of humans with heart failure. In contrast, the gene expression of acyl-Coenzyme A: lysocardiolipin acyltransferase-1, the endoplasmic reticulum MLCL AT, remained unaltered in SHHF rats. These results provided the first mechanisms whereby both CL biosynthesis and remodeling are altered during the development of heart failure. The increases in CDS, PGPS, and MLCL AT activities suggested compensatory mechanisms during the development of heart failure. In addition, the human data implied that similar trends in CL metabolism appear to occur in human heart failure. The above changes in mRNA expression and activities of CL biosynthetic and remodeling enzymes were not observed in age-matched control Sprague-Dawley rats indicating that these changes were specific to heart failure and not observed during nonpathological aging.

Novel Animal Models to Study CL Metabolism in Heart Failure

Persistent pulmonary hypertension of the newborn (PPHN) is characterized by high pulmonary vascular resistance due to the failure of normal pulmonary vascular relaxation at or shortly after birth (reviewed in refs. [32, 33]). The incidence

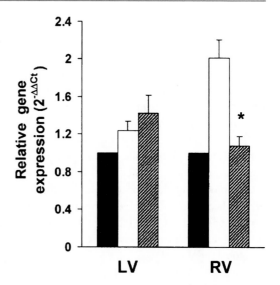

Fig. 3 Expression of cardiac tafazzin in PPHN piglets. New born piglets (<24 h old) were exposed to normoxic (21% oxygen) or hypoxic (10% oxygen) environment for 3 days then left ventricle (LV) and right ventricle (RV) isolated, total RNA prepared, and mRNA expression of tafazzin determined. *Closed bars*, newborn; *Open bars*, 3-day-old normoxic; *Hatched bars*, 3-day-old hypoxic. Data are expressed relative to constitutive expression of β-actin and represent the mean±SEM of three hearts. *$p<0.05$, 3-day-old control versus 3-day-old normoxic piglets

of PPHN is up to 6 per 1,000 live births with a resulting 10–30% mortality rate. Right-to-left shunting of blood across the ductus arterious and foramen ovale in PPHN causes the disturbances in cardiac performance by compromising the systemic and pulmonary circulation with right heart after-loading. In healthy term infants, PPHN is caused by perinatal hypoxia, inflammation, or direct lung injury. These patients develop a rapid right heart failure within a week. Exposure of newborn animals to hypoxia is a widely accepted model of PPHN and mimics the pathophysiological and histological features of human PPHN [34]. The newborn piglet develops PPHN within 1–3 days of exposure to hypoxia. In preliminary studies, we exposed new born piglets (<24 h old) to normoxic (21% oxygen) or hypoxic (10% oxygen) environment for 3 days and have examined mRNA expression of CL metabolism enzymes. Tafazzin mRNA expression was dramatically decreased in the right ventricle (RV) of hypoxic piglets (see Fig. 3). Non-functional mutations in the tafazzin gene lead to decreased

L_4-CL content [reviewed in 10], destabilization of mitochondrial supercomplexes [35], mitochondrial dysfunction and energy production [36]. Impairment of the mitochondrial energy-producing ability was involved in the development of right ventricular heart failure in monocrotaline-induced pulmonary hypertensive rats [37]. The decrease in tafazzin mRNA expression in RV of PPHN animals could lead to a reduction in L_4-CL formation with subsequent reduction in mitochondrial energy-producing ability leading to development of RV heart failure. Moreover, defects in the expression of other CL metabolism enzymes may further exacerbate cardiac dysfunction during the development of PPHN.

Huntington's disease (HD) is a neurodegenerative genetic disorder and is the most common genetic cause of repetitive abnormal movements called chorea (reviewed in ref. [38]). The prevalence of HD is 7 in 100,000 in the Caucasian population. Physical symptoms begin at any age, although the mean is 35–44 years of age. The second leading cause of death in HD is heart failure, over 30% of patients [39]. HD is caused by an expansion of a CAG trinucleotide sequence that encodes a polyglutamine tract in the huntingtin (Htt) protein [38]. Transgenic expression of an 83 residue polyglutamine repeat within the Htt protein in mice resulted in the development of heart failure within 5 months [40]. The cytotoxicity induced by Htt proteins is mediated, in part, by an alteration in normal mitochondrial dynamics. It is well documented that mitochondrial fusion protein expression is altered in heart failure [41]. Recently we demonstrated that expression of the mitochondrial fusion protein, mitofusion-2, may be involved in the regulation of CL de novo biosynthesis in human cells [42]. The effects of mutant Htt on cardiac function have been studied only in one animal model of HD that expresses an N-terminal fragment of mutant Htt, the R6/2 mouse [43]. In these mice cardiac performance was reduced, possibly due to an intrinsic defect of the cardiac tissue and its contractile function. R6/2 mice had reduced myocardial cross-sectional area and ventricular dilation. Mitochondria were smaller and rounder and markers of oxidative stress (protein nitration)

were increased. R6/2 mice are a drastic model of HD, become very sick by 10 weeks of age and are less accurate in terms of the neuropathology [44]. The yeast artificial chromosome mouse model of HD (YAC128) expresses the human HD gene containing 128 CAG repeats and develops motor abnormalities and age-dependent brain atrophy in a much slower disease course with symptoms developing between 4 and 9 months and may more accurately replicate that of the human condition [44]. In preliminary studies we have observed a significant 20% reduction in mRNA expression of tafazzin in hearts of YAC128 mice between 6.7 and 7.4 months of age. The decrease in tafazzin mRNA expression in hearts of HD animals could lead to a reduction in L_4-CL formation and subsequent reduction in mitochondrial energy-producing ability. In addition, the potential alterations in CL metabolism may point to an underlying pathology of the development of heart failure in HD.

Conclusions

In summary, alteration in CL level and CL metabolic genes occur in the SHHF model of heart failure, in explants from human heart failure patients, in a PPHN model of right heart failure, and in hearts of HD animals. Thus, it is clear that CL alterations indeed occur in the heart during the development of heart failure. What is less clear is whether these alterations in CL metabolic genes correspond directly to alterations in functional mitochondrial enzymatic activity (mitochondrial respiratory chain complex activities) and alterations in the level and the molecular species composition of CL in the PPHN and HD models of heart failure. The alterations in expression of tafazzin in PHHN piglets and YAC128 mice highlight the importance of these models in developing our understanding of CL metabolism in heart failure. In addition, it is also unclear if alterations in CL gene expression are associated with a functional deficit in PHHN and in HD. Moreover, will introduction or reduction of specific CL genes into experimental heart failure models restore mitochondrial and hence cardiac function? The above questions will form the future basis for studies on CL metabolism in experimental and human heart failure.

Acknowledgments The author wishes to acknowledge the contribution of Dr. Harjot Saini-Chohan for Figs. 2 and 3, Dr. Shyamala Dakshinamurti for PPHN piglet hearts and Dr. Simonetta Sipione for YAC128 mouse hearts. This work was supported by a grant from the Heart and Stroke Foundation of Manitoba, the Barth Syndrome Foundation of Canada, and the Huntington Foundation of Canada. G.M.H. is a Canada Research Chair in Molecular Cardiolipin Metabolism.

References

1. McMurray JJ, Pfeffer MA. Heart failure. Lancet. 2005;365:1877–89.
2. Saini-Chohan H, Hatch GM. Biological actions and metabolism of currently used pharmaceutical agents for the treatment of congestive heart failure. Curr Drug Metabol. 2009;10:206–19.
3. White DA. The phospholipid composition of mammalian tissues. In: Ansell GB, Hawthorne JN, Dawson RMC, editors. Form and function of phospholipids. Amsterdam: Elsevier; 1982. p. 441–82.
4. Reig J, Domingo E, Segura R, et al. Rat myocardial tissue lipids and their effect on ventricular electrical activity: influence on dietary lipids. Cardiovasc Res. 1993;27:364–70.
5. Hostetler KY. Polyglycerophospholipids: phosphatidylglycerol, di phosphatidylglyceroland bis (monoacylglycero)phosphate. In: Hawthorne JN, Ansell GB, editors. Phospholipids. Amsterdam: Elsevier; 1982. p. 215–61.
6. Hatch GM. Cardiolipin biosynthesis in the isolated rat heart. Biochem J. 1994;297:201–8.
7. Hatch GM. Cell biology of cardiac mitochondrial phospholipids. Biochem Cell Biol. 2004;82:99–112.
8. Hoch FL. Cardiolipins and biomembrane functions. Biochim Biophys Acta. 1992;1113:71–133.
9. Zhang M, Mileykovskaya E, Dowhan W. Gluing the respiratory chain together. Cardiolipin is required for supercomplex formation in the inner mitochondrial membrane. J Biol Chem. 2002;277:43553–6.
10. Hauff KD, Hatch GM. Cardiolipin metabolism and Barth Syndrome. Prog Lipid Res. 2006;45:91–101.
11. Ventura-Clapier R, Garnier A, Veksler V. Energy metabolism in heart failure. J Physiol. 2004;555:1–13.
12. Ingwall JS, Weiss RG. Is the failing heart energy starved? On using chemical energy to support cardiac function. Circ Res. 2004;95:135–45.
13. Neubauer S. The failing heart – an engine out of fuel. N Engl J Med. 2007;356:1140–51.
14. Sparagna GC, Chicco AJ, Murphy RC, et al. Loss of cardiac tetralinoleoyl cardiolipin in human and experimental heart failure. J Lipid Res. 2007;48:1559–70.
15. Ohtsuka T, Nishijima M, Suzuki K, et al. Mitochondrial dysfunction of a cultured Chinese hamster ovary cell mutant deficient in cardiolipin. J Biol Chem. 1993;268:22914–9.
16. Yamaoka S, Urade R, Kito M. Cardiolipin molecular species in rat heart mitochondria are sensitive to essential fatty acid-deficient dietary lipids. J Nutr. 1990;120:415–21.
17. Petrosillo G, Ruggiero FM, DiVenosa N, et al. Decreased complex III activity in mitochondria isolated from rat heart subjected to ischemia and reperfusion: role of reactive oxygen species and cardiolipin. FASEB J. 2003;17:714–6.
18. Hatch GM. Cardiolipin: biosynthesis, remodeling and trafficking in the heart and mammalian cells. Intl J Molec Med. 1998;1:33–41.
19. Nomura K, Imai H, Koumora T, et al. Mitochondrial phospholipid hydroperoxide glutathione peroxidase inhibits the release of cytochrome c from mitochondria by suppressing the peroxidation of cardiolipin in hypoglycaemia-induced apoptosis. Biochem J. 2000;351:83–93.
20. Orrenius S, Zhivotovsky B. Cardiolipin oxidation sets cytochrome c free. Nat Chem Biol. 2005;1:223–32.
21. Kagan VE, Tyurin V, Jiang J, et al. Cytochrome c acts as a cardiolipin oxygenase required for release of proapoptotic factors. Nat Chem Biol. 2005;1:223–32.
22. Muralikrishna Adibhatla R, Hatcher J. Phospholipase A2, reactive oxygen species, and lipid peroxidation in cerebral ischemia. Free Radic Biol Med. 2006;40:376–87.
23. Gonzalvez F, Schug ZT, Houtkooper RH, et al. Cardiolipin provides an essential activating platform for caspase-8 on mitochondria. J Cell Biol. 2008;183:681–96.
24. Schlame M. Cardiolipin synthesis for the assembly of bacterial and mitochondrial membranes. J Lipid Res. 2008;49:1607–20.
25. Houtkooper RH, Vaz F. Cardiolipin, the heart of mitochondrial metabolism. Cell Mol Life Sci. 2008;65:2493–506.
26. Cheng P, Hatch GM. Inhibition of cardiolipin biosynthesis in the hypoxic rat heart. Lipids. 1995;30:513–9.
27. Muders F, Elsner D. Animal models of chronic heart failure. Pharmacol Res. 2000;41:605–12.
28. Chi Y, Gupta RK. Alterations in heart and kidney membrane phospholipids in hypertension as observed by 31P nuclear magnetic resonance. Lipids. 1998;33:1023–30.
29. Carraway JW, Park S, McCune SA, et al. Comparison of irbesartan with captopril effects on cardiac hypertrophy and gene expression in heart failure-prone male SHHF/Mcc-fa(cp) rats. J Cardiovas Pharmacol. 1999;33:451–60.
30. Sparagna GC, Chicco AJ, Murphy RC, et al. Loss of cardiac tetralinoleoyl cardiolipin in human and experimental heart failure. J Lipid Res. 2007;48:1559–70.
31. Saini-Chohan HK, Holmes MG, Chicco AJ, et al. Cardiolipin biosynthesis and remodeling enzymes are

altered during development of heart failure. J Lipid Res. 2009;50:1600–9.

32. Therese P. Persistent pulmonary hypertension of the newborn. Paediatr Respir Rev. 2006;7 Suppl 1:S175–6.

33. Vosatka RJ. Persistent pulmonary hypertension of the newborn. N Eng J Med. 2002;346:864.

34. Berkenbosch JW, Baribeau J, Perreault T. Decreased synthesis and vasodilation to nitric oxide in piglets with hypoxia-induced pulmonary hypertension. Am J Physiol Lung Cell Mol Physiol. 2000;278: L276–83.

35. McKenzie M, Lazarou M, Thorburn DR, et al. Mitochondrial respiratory chain supercomplexes are destabilized in Barth Syndrome patients. J Mol Biol. 2006;361:462–9.

36. Ma L, Vaz FM, Gu L, et al. The human TAZ gene complements mitochondrial dysfunction in the yeast taz1Delta mutant. Implications for Barth syndrome. J Biol Chem. 2004;279:44394–9.

37. Daicho T, Yagi T, Abe Y, et al. Possible involvement of mitochondrial energy-producing ability in the development of right ventricular failure in monocrotaline-induced pulmonary hypertensive rats. J Pharmacol Sci. 2009;111:33–43.

38. Walker FO. Huntington's Disease. Lancet. 2007;369: 218–28.

39. Chiu E, Alexander L. Causes of death in Huntington's disease. Med J Aust. 1982;1:153.

40. Pattison JS, Sanbe A, Maloyan A, et al. Cardiomyocyte expression of a polyglutamine preamyloid oligomer causes heart failure. Circulation. 2008;117:2743–51.

41. Chen L, Gong Q, Stice J, et al. Mitochondrial OPA1, apoptosis, and heart failure. Cardiovasc Res. 2009; 84:91–9.

42. Xu FY, McBride H, Aceham D, et al. The dynamics of cardiolipin synthesis post mitochondrial fusion. Biochim Biophys Acta (Biomembranes). 2010; 1798:1577–85.

43. Mihm MJ, Amann DM, Schanbacher BL, et al. Cardiac dysfunction in the R6/2 mouse model of Huntington's disease. Neurobiol Dis. 2007;25:297–308.

44. Slow EJ, van Raamsdonk J, Rogers D, et al. Selective striatal neuronal loss in a YAC128 mouse model of Huntington disease. Hum Mol Genetics. 2003; 12:1555–67.

Mechanisms Underlying Development of Cardiomyocyte Hypertrophy via Na–H Exchange Stimulation

Morris Karmazyn

Abstract

Na–H exchange (NHE) is the principal mechanism by which the cardiac cell extrudes protons following the development of intracellular acidosis. Although ten isoforms of NHE have now been identified, cardiac cells possess primarily the ubiquitous NHE-1 subtype. There is now strong evidence that NHE-1 contributes to chronic maladaptive myocardial responses to injury including myocardial remodelling and the antiporter likely contributes to the development of heart failure. Experimental studies using both in vitro approaches as well as animal models of heart failure have consistently demonstrated salutary effects of NHE-1 inhibitors in attenuating hypertrophy in response to various stimuli as well as inhibiting heart failure in a large number of animal models. The beneficial effects of NHE-1 inhibitors reflect direct antiremodelling/antihypertrophic effects on the heart which occur via a number of intracellular processes including diminution of intracellular sodium accumulation, prevention of mitochondrial remodelling and reduction in the calcium-dependent activation of the hypertrophic calcineurin pathway. Taken together, NHE-1 inhibition represents a potentially effective therapeutic approach for the treatment of heart failure.

Keywords

Na–H exchange isoform 1 • Hypertrophy • Myocardial remodelling • Heart failure • Intracellular Na^+ concentrations • Calcineurin • NFAT • Mitochondria

Introduction

NHE is an important regulator of intracellular pH (pHi) in most cells including cardiomyocytes. To date, ten NHE isoforms have been identified (NHE-1 to NHE-10) [1–3]. NHE-1 is the ubiquitous isoform whereas newer isoforms (NHE-6 to

M. Karmazyn (✉)
Department of Physiology and Pharmacology,
The University of Western Ontario,
London, Ontario, Canada
e-mail: morris.karmazyn@schulich.uwo.ca

N.S. Dhalla, M. Nagano, B. Ostadal (eds.), *Molecular Defects in Cardiovascular Disease*,
DOI 10.1007/978-1-4419-7130-2_14, © Springer Science+Business Media, LLC 2011

NHE-9) function to maintain acidic pH values in Golgi and post-Golgi compartments due to their localization within these organelles [4]. NHE-10 is restricted to osteoclasts [3]. However, in terms of the heart, NHE-1 is the primary and most relevant NHE isoform serving as a target for therapeutic intervention. NHE-1 contains 815 amino acids and can be separated into two distinct functional domains: a 500-amino acid transmembrane domain, made up of 12 transmembrane spanning segments (responsible for proton extrusion) and a 315-amino acid hydrophilic cytoplasmic carboxy-terminal domain which contains regulatory sites [5–8]. The major determinant of NHE-1 activity under normal physiological conditions is intracellular pHi [9, 10]. Within the normal physiological pHi range, NHE-1 activity is negligible, but as pHi decreases, the exchanger becomes rapidly activated through a putative proton sensor located in the intracellular loop consisting of specific amino acid residues [11, 12]. A large number of autocrine/paracrine regulators increase NHE-1 activity by increasing the sensitivity of the proton sensor to pHi via phosphorylation [7, 8, 13] including endothelin-1, [14, 15] angiotensin II [16, 17] and α1-adrenergic agonists [18, 19] likely via mitogen-activated protein kinase (MAPK) [20–22].

Role of Hormonal, Paracrine and Autocrine Factors in Regulation of NHE-1 Activity: Potential Relevance to Pathology

As noted above, it is critical to note that NHE-1 activity is regulated by hormones, paracrine/autocrine regulators as well as mechanical stimuli such as stretch possibly through an identical mechanism involving phosphoinositide hydrolysis. This results in the subsequent activation of kinases which then stimulate NHE-1 activity via phosphorylation reactions through PKC or MAPKs [21–23]. In addition, it has been shown that 90-kDa ribosomal S6 kinase (RSK) is an important regulator of NHE-1 activity in ventricular myocytes in response to diverse factors including ischemia and reperfusion as well as

phenylephrine administration [24, 25]. Inhibition of phosphorylation-dependent NHE-1 activation in ventricular myocytes occurs through increased dephosphorylation by the catalytic subunit of type 2A protein phosphatase which is colocalized with NHE-1 in the intercalated disc region of ventricular myocytes [26].

Various factors involved in phosphorylation-dependent reactions which are prohypertrophic and which contribute to myocardial remodelling, including endothelin [14, 27, 28], angiotensin II [16, 29, 30], α1-adrenergic agonists [18, 19, 31] as well as growth factors [11] can all stimulate NHE-1 activity. Although these factors are indeed important for regulation of NHE-1 activity, it should be recalled that intracellular acidosis is the primary stimulus for NHE-1 activation and the regulation of NHE-1 activity by hormonal, autocrine and paracrine factors represents an ability of these agents to "fine-tune" activity of the exchanger. This is illustrated primarily by the ability of these factors to shift the pHi/NHE-1 activity relationship to the right, thus lowering the pHi threshold for NHE-1 activation. Taken together, it is evident that NHE-1 activity is stimulated by a multiplicity of signals, intracellular acidosis being the primary one among these. Under conditions of cardiac pathology involving ischemia plus the concomitant upregulation of many biochemical activators of NHE-1, one can envisage that the antiporter receives substantial input for its activation in disease states.

Theoretical Considerations for NHE-1 Involvement in Myocardial Remodelling

Myocardial hypertrophy, remodelling and heart failure represent many complex events but in general involve initiating factors such as an increase in mechanical load and upregulation of a large number of hormonal, paracrine and autocrine factors which contribute to the process through receptor-mediated changes in intracellular signalling [32]. One of the major reasons for considering NHE-1 as a potentially important contributor to the heart failure process is based on the fact that, already alluded to above, the antiporter represents a key downstream factor activated by many such factors including α_1-adrenoceptor agonists [18, 19, 31], angiotensin II [16, 29, 30] and endothelin-1 [14, 27, 28]. Indeed, in cardiac cells, NHE inhibitors block hypertrophic responses to various stimuli. Stretch-induced stimulation in protein synthesis in neonatal cardiac myocytes as well as stretch-induced alkalinization in feline papillary muscles can be blocked by NHE inhibitors [33, 34] as can norepinephrine-induced protein synthesis in cultured rat cardiomyocytes [35]. These studies reveal a commonality in terms of responses to a wide array of hypertrophic factors. Indeed, it is likely that NHE-1 activation represents a common response to mechanical stretch and a key player in the hypertrophic process [36]. Thus, cellular deformation under pathological conditions could lead to a cascade of events resulting in cell hypertrophy and eventual myocardial remodelling. It has been proposed that this occurs as a consequence of the activation of both angiotensin II AT_1 as well as the endothelin-1 ET_A receptors which then activate intracellular signal transduction pathways leading to increased NHE-1 activity and cell growth [36, 37]. This may occur in an autocrine or paracrine fashion in which stretch stimulates the local release of these peptides which then act on their respective receptor.

Experimental Evidence for NHE Involvement in Myocyte Hypertrophy and Heart Failure

Various lines of evidence support the concept of NHE-1 as a contributing factor to heart failure. In terms of NHE-1 activity, this was shown to be increased in experimental heart failure [38] as well as in hearts from patients with end-stage heart failure [39]. Moreover, an increasing number of studies have been reported supporting the concept that inhibition of NHE-1 is conducive to attenuation of the remodelling process and heart failure. Such findings have been observed in both

in vitro and in vivo models of hypertrophy and heart failure. In early studies, the nonspecific NHE inhibitor amiloride, a potassium-sparing diuretic, was shown to block norepinephrine-induced protein synthesis in cultured neonatal rat ventricular myocytes [35], although similar effects have been reported with HOE 694, a much more selective NHE-1 inhibitor [40]. Moreover, selective NHE-1 inhibition has been shown to suppress the hypertrophic effect of isoproterenol in rats [41]. Glucose-induced cardiac hypertrophy can also be attenuated by NHE-1 inhibition suggesting that targeting the NHE-1 system could represent an attractive therapeutic approach in diabetic cardiomyopathy [42]. NHE-1 inhibition also attenuates the direct hypertrophic effect of aldosterone in cultured myocytes through a mechanism involving reduced intracellular sodium levels [43] and reduces aldosterone-induced cardiac fibrosis [44].

In vivo studies using clinically relevant animal models have further advanced the concept of NHE-1-mediated hypertrophy and heart failure and have provided very strong evidence for the antiporter's involvement in these processes. Early studies have shown that orally administered amiloride, a nonspecific NHE inhibitor, reduces fibre diameter in rat coronary ligation [45] and murine dilated cardiomyopathy models [46]. Dietary administration of the NHE-1 specific inhibitor cariporide completely abrogated the increased length of surviving myocytes after 1 week of coronary artery occlusion and ameliorated contractile dysfunction in the absence of afterload reduction, thereby implicating a direct effect of the drug on myocardial remodelling [47]. Furthermore, more severe hypertrophy and heart failure observed at 3-month postinfarction follow-up are reduced by approximately 50% in animals treated with the NHE-1 inhibitor cariporide [48]. Of clinical importance, NHE-1 inhibition with the NHE-1 specific inhibitor EMD87580 (EMD) has been shown to reverse established heart failure and hypertrophy when drug administration is delayed by up to 4 weeks following induction of myocardial infarction [49]. It is critical to mention that in all these cases the effects of NHE-1 inhibition were observed in the absence of afterload reduction or reduction in infarct size. The salutary effect of NHE-1 inhibition in terms of both hypertrophy and left ventricular function can also be seen in a pacing model of heart failure in rabbits [50] as well as in hypertension-induced cardiac defects [51]. NHE-1 inhibition has also been shown by our group to be beneficial in reducing right ventricular hypertrophy secondary to pulmonary artery injury produced by monocrotaline. In this study, dietary cariporide was very effective in reducing the degree of right ventricular hypertrophy and its hemodynamic consequences but essentially leaving the pulmonary artery remodelling unaffected, thereby implicating a direct effect on the myocardium [52].

NHE-1 inhibition may also be involved in the antihypertrophic effects of other agents. For example, a recent report from Cingolani's group identified a beneficial effect of the phosphodiesterase 5A inhibitor sildenafil in rats subjected to 6 weeks coronary artery ligation as shown by improved left ventricular function and reduced hypertrophy, effects which were associated with reduced NHE-1 activity [53]. Moreover, sildenafil was found to exert a direct NHE-1 inhibitory property in myocytes subjected to intracellular acidosis produced by ammonium chloride pulsing [53].

Antiremodelling Effects of NHE-1 Inhibition in Genetic Models of Hypertrophy and Heart Failure

Further evidence for direct antiremodelling effect of NHE-1 inhibition stems from studies involving various genetic models of cardiac hypertrophy. It has been shown that hypertrophied cardiac tissue from the spontaneously hypertensive rat (SHR) exhibits increased NHE-1 activity [54, 55] which may contribute to the hypertrophic process in these animals. Indeed, cariporide has been shown to cause a regression of left ventricular hypertrophy similar to that seen with the vasodilators enalapril and nifedipine, but with no decrease in blood pressure in the SHR [56].

Mice with cardiac-specific overexpression of the β_1-adrenergic receptors show cardiac hypertrophy, fibrosis and development of heart failure, as well as an increased expression of NHE-1 [57]. Despite continued presence of β_1-adrenergic signalling, cariporide completely normalized NHE-1 expression and improved left ventricular function probably via selectively inhibited pathological hypertrophy while not affecting normal cardiac growth [57]. Protection by NHE-1 inhibition has also been demonstrated in the UM-X7.1 hamster which shows genetically determined phases of necrosis, hypertrophy and heart failure and which is used as a model of human hereditary cardiomyopathy [58]. In these animals, NHE-1 expression and activity is increased and accompanied by increased intracellular Na^+ and Ca^{2+} levels during the development of cardiac necrosis and hypertrophy, all of which were prevented by treating animals with EMD [58].

Although the genetic models described above are associated with increased protein expression and activity of NHE-1, other models of hypertrophy exist in which enhanced NHE-1 activity is not accompanied by an increase of NHE-1 expression. Thus, mice with global deletion of the atrial natriuretic peptide receptor (GC-A$^{-/-}$ mice) exhibit hypertension and marked cardiac hypertrophy which is associated with enhanced NHE-1 activity, subsequent alkalinization and increased intracellular Ca^{2+} concentrations [59]. These effects were prevented by treating the animals with cariporide which was associated with regression of cardiac hypertrophy and fibrosis, despite persistent arterial hypertension [59]. The salutary effects were associated with normalization of CaMKII and Akt pathways without affecting calcineurin and ERK1/2 MAPK, despite increased activation of all four signalling pathways in the hearts of GC-A$^{-/-}$ mice [59].

In a related but somewhat different model, mice with cardiomyocyte restricted deletion of GC-A (CM GC-A KO), demonstrate increased expression of NHE-1 and increased sensitivity to the hypertrophic effect of angiotensin II as well as the peptide's ability to increase intracellular Ca^{2+} concentrations [60]. These effects were significantly attenuated by cariporide suggesting that the increased sensitivity to angiotensin II was related, at least in part to NHE-1 activity [60]. Although, the exact mechanism through which GC-A could inhibit NHE-1 activity is still not clear, there is evidence that this inhibitory effect could also be mediated via a cGMP signalling pathway [59]. Indeed, studies from two different groups showed that increased cGMP levels inhibit NHE-1 activity in pressure overloaded cardiac hypertrophy [61], and postinfarction remodelling [53]. In a genetic model of type 2 diabetes with no obesity and hypertension but with cardiac hypertrophy (Goto–Kakizaki rat), activity of NHE-1 was found to be increased without changes in expression [62]. As in the other genetic models of hypertrophy, cariporide reduced the increased NHE-1 activity, decreased intracellular Ca^{2+} concentrations and attenuated the hypertrophic phenotype [62].

Possible Role of Gender in Influencing NHE-1 Dependent Responses

Although the influence of gender on the incidence of heart disease in general and heart failure specifically is well established, virtually nothing is known about the role which gender plays in NHE-1 dependent responses in the heart and the potential influence of gender on the beneficial effects of NHE-1 inhibitors. According to American Heart Association statistics, the remaining lifetime risk of developing heart failure in heart failure-free 40-year-old individuals is 21% for men and 20.3% for women although women are at more than twice the risk (46% vs. 22% for men) of developing heart failure after a myocardial infarction [63]. A very recent Canadian study reported a higher mortality rate in women who have heart failure [64]. Whether differences in NHE-1 expression or activity profiles are involved in such differences is not known. Using cultured rat ventricular myocytes we have recently found that low levels of estrogen (1 pM) produce cardiomyocyte hypertrophy through ERK/NHE-1 activation and intracellular alkalini-

zation whereas an antihypertrophic effect is seen at high (1 nM) concentrations [65]. These results suggest that very low levels of estrogen may produce a prohypertrophic effect through an NHE-1 dependent pathway which may account for increased heart failure risk seen in postmenopausal females.

Potential Mechanisms Underlying the Role of NHE-1 in the Remodelling/Hypertrophic Process

Role of Intracellular Na^+

Despite the emerging strong evidence for NHE-1 involvement in the heart failure process and the prospect for novel therapeutic interventions, the mechanisms underlying the role of NHE-1 are presently unknown but likely involve multiple processes which will be discussed below. Although NHE-1 dependent pHi changes may be proposed in view of the role of pH in protein synthesis, this is unlikely since it would be expected that under long term NHE-1 blockade other pHi regulatory processes would likely compensate to ensure maintenance of physiological pHi levels. For example, in papillary muscles obtained from SHR it was shown that pHi is unchanged in bicarbonate-containing buffer despite increased NHE-1 activity reflecting enhanced compensatory activity by other pHi regulatory processes, particularly the Na^+-independent $Cl^-HCO_3^-$ anion exchanger [55]. Thus, simultaneous activation of both NHE-1 and the anion exchanger, as shown for angiotensin II, likely reflects the major mechanism by which pHi changes are prevented under physiological conditions when bicarbonate is present [55]. Moreover, it has recently been shown that improved function of failing cardiomyocytes by NHE-1 inhibition occurred through a mechanism independently of pHi [66]. It has been suggested that NHE-1 activation results in the influx of sodium ions which then in turn activate various PKC isozymes which then alter gene expression and protein synthesis [67]. The NHE-1 dependent elevation in intracellular Na$^+$ concentrations has been shown to contribute to defective ventricular cellular calcium handling in rabbits following pressure and volume overload induced heart failure [38]. However, it should be added that others have shown, using a rabbit pressure-overload heart failure model, that the elevation in intracellular Na$^+$ concentrations occurred primarily via a tetrodotoxin-dependent pathway with little contribution from NHE-1 [68].

The importance of Na$^+$ to NHE-1 mediated cardiotoxicity is further supported by our recent report showing that NHE-1 inhibition attenuates the hypertrophic effect of cardiac glycosides (ouabain or digoxin) while preserving the inotropic responses, effects which were associated with a diminution of glycoside-induced elevations in intracellular Na$^+$ concentrations [69].

Role of Mitochondria

Due to the multifunctional and putative roles of mitochondria in both cell life and death, an impairment of mitochondrial structure or function is fundamental for cardiac diseases. Progression of heart remodelling after myocardial infarction is accompanied by "mitochondrial remodelling" including both morphological and biochemical abnormalities in mitochondria due to their swelling, large ROS production and dysfunction of ATP synthesis and transport. Most likely, the development of the final phenotype during postinfarction remodelling depends on a balance of mitochondria-mediated pro- and antiremodelling signalling pathways. Thus, "mitochondrial remodelling" likely represents a key component of the extent of remodelling that may be detrimental for the reversibility of remodelling and functional recovery following infarction [70]. Therefore, cardioprotective effects of any pharmacological or conditional intervention during postinfarction remodelling and heart failure converge on mitochondria improving their functional and structural integrity.

We have shown that inhibition of NHE-1 by EMD improves mitochondrial respiratory function and reduces myocardial hypertrophy at 12 and 18 weeks after coronary artery ligation in rats [71]. Ca^{2+} overload in cardiac cells, especially when accompanied by oxidative stress and ATP depletion induces formation of nonspecific pores in the inner mitochondrial membrane called mitochondrial permeability transition (MPT) pores [70, 72–74]. MPT pore opening is detrimental to mitochondria by inducing matrix swelling and depolarization of the mitochondrial inner membrane leading to impairment of ATP synthesis. The functional recovery of the heart (e.g., during ischemia/reperfusion) correlates with the extent of the inhibition of MPT pore opening, that may be mediated either by a direct interaction with the MPT pores (e.g., by the immunosuppressant cyclosporine A), or indirectly by decreasing intracellular calcium overload and ROS production, or by lowering pHi, since MPT pore opening is blocked at low pH (<7). The latter concept is difficult to reconcile in view of the preceding discussion indicating a dissociation between NHE-1 activity and pHi; however, the possibility of heterogeneity in pHi changes following NHE-1 inhibition producing mitochondrial effects cannot be excluded at the present time. Irrespective of the precise mechanisms, we have suggested that, in addition to preventing Ca^{2+} overload, a beneficial effect of NHE-1-specific inhibitors may be due to inhibition of MPT pore opening, resulting in improvement of mitochondrial function during postinfarction remodelling [70, 71]. EMD-treated hearts demonstrated less opening of MPT pores. Furthermore, mitochondria isolated from EMD-treated coronary artery-ligated hearts were less sensitive to extramitochondrial Ca^{2+} than control hearts subjected to the same procedure indicating desensitization of the MPT pores to added Ca^{2+} and thus, reflecting less Ca^{2+} overload [71]. The protective effect of NHE-1 inhibition on mitochondria is unlikely to be direct because NHE-1 specific inhibitors do not exhibit any beneficial effect when isolated mitochondria were subjected to simulated ischemia [75] and Ca^{2+}-induced matrix swelling [76]. NHE-1 inhibition attenuated the downregulation of transcription factors responsible for mitochondrial biogenesis including peroxisome proliferators activated receptor gamma co-activator 1α (PGC-1α) and its downstream transcription factors such as mitochondrial transcription factor A (MTF A), nuclear respiratory factor 1 (NRF-1) and nuclear respiratory factor 2 (NRF-2) during postinfarction remodelling in rats [75]. In addition to its effects on postinfarction remodelling and heart failure, EMD attenuated MPT pore opening and mitochondrial membrane depolarization in cultured neonatal cardiomyocytes during phenylephrine-induced hypertrophy that was associated with reduced accumulation of mitochondria-generated ROS [77]. Recently, we have identified mitochondrial fission/fusion proteins, important for cellular metabolism as a potential target for the antihypertrophic effects of NHE-1 inhibitors [78]. Thus, the existing data demonstrate that NHE-1 inhibition improves mitochondrial function during postinfarction remodelling. The effect of NHE-1 inhibition on the mitochondria is most likely indirect and secondary to the attenuation of intracellular calcium overload, acidosis and ROS accumulation which are major inducers for MPT pore opening.

Critical Role of NHE-1 Dependent Calcineurin Activation and Nuclear Factor of Activated T Cells Translocation

The potential role of calcium in mediating the hypertrophic effect NHE-1 activation has received scant attention. Frey and Olson [79] first proposed that NHE-1 dependent hypertrophy reflects a Na^+-dependent reverse mode Na–Ca exchange (NCX) activity which results in elevations in intracellular Ca^{2+} concentrations and subsequent calcineurin activation. The role of calcineurin activation in cardiac hypertrophy has received extensive interest in the past number of years [80–83]. Briefly, calcineurin is a calmodulin-activated serine/threonine protein phosphatase which is activated by elevations in intracellular calcium concentrations and the resulting increase in the Ca^{2+}/calmodulin complex, thus allowing calmodulin binding to and activation of calcineurin. Once activated, calcineurin mediates

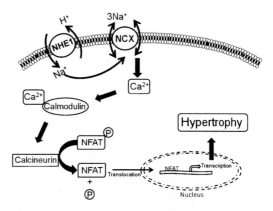

Fig. 1 Key role of NHE-1 in the stimulation of calcineurin activity by virtue of its ability to elevate intracellular calcium concentrations via NCX. Calcineurin activation results in NFAT dephosphorylation and its translocation into nuclei resulting in the hypertrophic phenotype. Please see text for discussion

hypertrophy by dephosphorylating its downstream transcriptional effector nuclear factor of activated T cells (NFAT) resulting in its nuclear translocation and subsequent initiation of transcription (Fig. 1). There is now strong evidence that calcineurin mediates cardiac hypertrophy and studies have shown that inhibition of calcineurin (either pharmacologically or genetically) reduces hypertrophy or heart failure. For example, the antihypertrophic effect of NHE-1 inhibition has been shown to be associated with regression of calcineurin activation. Furthermore, it has recently been reported that cardiac NHE-1 overexpression in mice results in the activation of the calcineurin/NFAT pathway which mediates the hypertrophic phenotype in these animals [84]. Thus, this study showed that cardiac NHE-1 overexpression per se produces the hypertrophic phenotype in the absence of insult which was associated with calcineurin activation and NFAT translocation which were inhibited by the NHE-1 inhibitor cariporide [84]. It is possible that this NHE-1/calcineurin pathway represents an attractive target for mitigating hypertrophic responses. Indeed, we have recently found that the antihypertrophic effects of a novel chimeric natriuretic peptide as well as ginseng are mediated by inhibition of the NHE-1/calcineurin pathways [85, 86].

Conclusions

Experimental studies using varied approaches have strongly implicated a role for NHE-1 in the myocardial remodelling and heart failure process. It appears that the major role for the antiporter lies in its ability to regulate cell growth thus contributing to chronic maladaptive hypertrophy. Although the precise mechanism of action of NHE-1 as a mediator of cardiac hypertrophy needs to be further examined, the role of the antiporter in regulation of transcription via calcineurin activation and resultant NFAT translocation appears to be a critical pathway. NHE-1 may indeed be a common downstream mediator for the hypertrophic effect of a significant number of hormonal, paracrine and autocrine factors. Indeed, the ability of NHE-1 inhibitors to attenuate remodelling and heart failure in a variety of experimental models strongly implicate the antiporter as a common pathway in the remodelling process irrespective of initiating factor(s). NHE-1 therefore appears to be a highly attractive therapeutic target for cardiac hypertrophy and heart failure.

Acknowledgements The work originating from the author's laboratory has been supported by the Canadian Institutes of Health Research.

References

1. Orlowski J, Grinstein S. Molecular and functional diversity of mammalian Na$^+$/H$^+$ exchangers In: Karmazyn M, Avkiran M, Fliegel L, editors. The sodium–hydrogen exchanger. From molecule to its role in disease. Chap. 2. Dordrecht: Kluwer; 2003. p. 17–34.
2. Orlowski J, Grinstein S. Diversity of the mammalian sodium/proton exchanger SLC9 gene family. Pflugers Arch. 2004;447:549–65.
3. Lee SH, Kim T, Park ES, et al. NHE10, an osteoclast-specific member of the Na$^+$/H$^+$ exchanger family, regulates osteoclast differentiation and survival. Biochem Biophys Res Commun. 2008;369:320–6.
4. Nakamura N, Tanaka S, Teko Y, et al. Four Na$^+$/H$^+$ exchanger isoforms are distributed to Golgi and post-Golgi compartments and are involved in organelle pH regulation. J Biol Chem. 2004;280:1561–72.
5. Karmazyn M, Gan XT, Humphreys RA, et al. The myocardial Na$^+$–H$^+$ exchange: structure, regulation and its role in heart disease. Circ Res. 1999;85:777–86.
6. Karmazyn M, Sostaric JV, Gan XT. The myocardial Na$^+$/H$^+$ exchanger: a potential therapeutic target for the prevention of myocardial ischaemic and reperfusion injury and attenuation of postinfarction heart failure. Drugs. 2001;61:375–89.
7. Putney LK, Denker SP, Barber DL. The changing face of the Na$^+$/H$^+$ exchanger, NHE1: structure, regulation, and cellular actions. Annu Rev Pharmacol Toxicol. 2002;42:527–52.
8. Bianchini L, Pouyssegur J. Regulation of the Na$^+$/H$^+$ exchanger isoform NHE1: role of phosphorylation. Kidney Int. 1996;49:1038–41.
9. Leem CH, Lagadic-Gossmann D, Vaughan-Jones RD. Characterization of intracellular pH regulation in the guinea-pig ventricular myocyte. J Physiol. 1999;517 (Pt 1):159–80.
10. Spitzer KW, Vaughan-Jones RD. Regulation of intracellular pH in mammalian cells. In: Karmazyn M, Avkiran M, Fliegel L, editors. The sodium–hydrogen exchanger. From molecule to its role in disease. Chap. 1. Dordrecht: Kluwer; 2003.
11. Wakabayashi S, Fafournoux P, Sardet S, et al. The Na$^+$/H$^+$ antiporter cytoplasmic domain mediates growth factor signals and controls "H" sensing. Proc Natl Acad Sci USA. 1992;89:2424–8.
12. Wakabayashi S, Hisamitsu T, Pang T, et al. Mutations of Arg440 and Gly455/Gly456 oppositely change pH sensing of Na$^+$/H$^+$ exchanger 1. J Biol Chem. 2003;278:11828–35.
13. Kinsella JL, Heller P, Frohlich JP. Na$^+$/H$^+$ exchanger: proton modifier site regulation of activity. Biochem Cell Biol. 1998;76:743–9.
14. Khandoudi N, Karmazyn M. Role of sodium/hydrogen exchange in mediating the effects of endothelin-1 on the normal and ischemic and reperfused heart. Circ Res. 1994;75:369–78.
15. Woo SH, Lee CO. Effects of endothelin-1 on Ca^{2+} signaling in guinea pig ventricular myocytes: role of protein kinase C. J Mol Cell Cardiol. 1999;31:631–43.
16. Matsui H, Barry WH, Livsey C, et al. Angiotensin II stimulates sodium–hydrogen exchange in adult rabbit ventricular myocytes. Cardiovasc Res. 1995;29:215–21.
17. Gunasegaram M, Haworth RS, Hearse DJ, et al. Regulation of sarcolemmal Na$^+$/H$^+$ exchanger activity by angiotensin II in adult rat ventricular myocytes: opposing actions via AT1 versus AT2 receptors. Circ Res. 1999;85:919–30.
18. Wallert MA, Frohlich O. α1-adrenergic stimulation of Na–H exchange in cardiac myocytes. Am J Physiol. 1992;263:C1096–102.
19. Yokoyame H, Yasutake M, Avkiran M. α1-adrenergic stimulation of sarcolemmal Na$^+$–H$^+$ exchanger activity in rat ventricular myocytes: evidence for selective mediation by the α1Aadrenoceptor subtype. Circ Res. 1998;82:1078–85.
20. Sabri A, Byron KL, Samarel AM, et al. Hydrogen peroxide activates mitogen-activated protein kinases and

Na$^+$–H$^+$ exchange in neonatal rat cardiac myocytes. Circ Res. 1998;82:1053–62.

21. Wang H, Silva NL, Lucchesi PA, et al. Phosphorylation and regulation of the Na$^+$/H$^+$ exchanger through mitogen-activated protein kinase. Biochemistry. 1997;29: 9151–8.

22. Moor AN, Fliegel L. Protein kinase-mediated regulation of the Na$^+$/H$^+$ exchanger in the rat myocardium by mitogen-activated protein kinase-dependent pathways. J Biol Chem. 1999;274:22985–92.

23. Sisczkowski M, Ng LL. Phorbol ester activation of the rat vascular myocyte Na$^+$/H$^+$ exchanger isoform I. Hypertension. 1996;27:859–66.

24. Moor AN, Gan XT, Karmazyn M, et al. Activation of Na$^+$/H$^+$ exchanger-directed protein kinases in the ischemic and ischemic-reperfused rat myocardium. J Biol Chem. 2001;276:16113–22.

25. Cuello F, Snabaitis AK, Cohen MS, et al. Evidence for direct regulation of myocardial Na$^+$/H$^+$ exchanger isoform 1 phosphorylation and activity by 90-kDa ribosomal S6 kinase (RSK): effects of the novel and specific RSK inhibitor fmk on responses to α1-adrenergic stimulation. Mol Pharmacol. 2007;71(3): 799–806.

26. Snabaitis AK, D'Mello R, Dashnyam S, et al. A novel role for protein phosphatase 2A in receptor-mediated regulation of the cardiac sarcolemmal Na$^+$/H$^+$ exchanger NHE1. J Biol Chem. 2006;281:20252–62.

27. Wu ML, Tseng YZ. The modulatory effects of endothelin-1, carbachol and isoprenaline upon Na$^+$–H$^+$ exchange in dog cardiac Purkinje fibers. J Physiol. 1993;471:583–97.

28. Ito N, Kagaya Y, Weinberg EO, et al. Endothelin and angiotensin II stimulation of Na$^+$–H$^+$ exchange is impaired in cardiac hypertrophy. J Clin Invest. 1997;99:125–35.

29. Boston DR, Koyama T, Rodriguez-Larrain J, et al. Effects of angiotensin II on intracellular calcium and contracture in metabolically inhibited cardiomyocytes. J Pharmacol Exp Ther. 1998;285:716–23.

30. Mattiazi A, Perez NG, Vila-Petrof MG, et al. Dissociation between positive inotropic and alkalinizing effects of angiotensin II in feline myocardium. Am J Physiol. 1997;272:H1131–6.

31. Puceat M, Vassort G. Neurohumoral modulation of intracellular pH in the heart. Cardiovasc Res. 1995;29:178–83.

32. Katz AM. Heart failure. Pathophysiology, molecular biology, and clinical management. Philadelphia, PA: Lippincott Williams & Wilkins; 2000.

33. Yamazaki T, Komuro I, Kudoh S, et al. Role of ion channels and exchanger in mechanical stretch-induced cardiomyocyte hypertrophy. Circ Res. 1998;82: 430–7.

34. Cingolani HE, Alvarez BV, Ennis IL, et al. Stretch-induced alkalinization of feline papillary muscle. An autocrine–paracrine system. Circ Res. 1998;83: 775–80.

35. Hori M, Nakatsubo B, Kagiya T, et al. The role of Na$^+$/H$^+$ exchange in norepinephrine-induced protein synthesis in neonatal cultured cardiomyocytes. Jpn Circ J. 1990;54:535–9.

36. Dostal DE, Baker KM. Angiotensin and endothelin: messengers that couple ventricular stretch to the Na$^+$/H$^+$ exchanger and cardiac hypertrophy. Circ Res. 1998;83:870–3.

37. Cingolani HE. Na$^+$/H$^+$ exchange hyperactivity and myocardial hypertrophy: are they linked phenomena? Cardiovasc Res. 1999;44:462–7.

38. Baartscheer A, Schumacher CA, van Borren MM, et al. Increased Na$^+$/H$^+$-exchange activity is the cause of increased (Na$^+$)i and underlies disturbed calcium handling in the rabbit pressure and volume overload heart failure model. Cardiovasc Res. 2003;57:1015–24.

39. Yokoyama H, Gunasegaram S, Harding SE, et al. Sarcolemmal Na$^+$/H$^+$ exchanger activity and expression in human ventricular myocardium. J Am Coll Cardiol. 2000;36:534–40.

40. Schluter KD, Schafer M, Balser C, et al. Influence of pHi and creatine phosphate on α-adrenoceptor-mediated cardiac hypertrophy. J Mol Cell Cardiol. 1998;30:763–71.

41. Ennis IL, Escudero EM, Console GM, et al. Regression of isoproterenol-induced cardiac hypertrophy by Na$^+$/H$^+$ exchanger inhibition. Hypertension. 2003;41: 1324–9.

42. Chen S, Khan ZA, Karmazyn M, et al. Role of endothelin-1, sodium hydrogen exchanger-1 and mitogen activated protein kinase (MAPK) activation in glucose-induced cardiomyocyte hypertrophy. Diabetes Metab Res Rev. 2007;23:356–67.

43. Karmazyn M, Liu Q, Gan XT, et al. Aldosterone increases NHE-1 expression and induces NHE-1-dependent hypertrophy in neonatal rat ventricular myocytes. Hypertension. 2003;42:1171–6.

44. Young M, Funder J. Mineralocorticoid action and sodium–hydrogen exchange: studies in experimental cardiac fibrosis. Endocrinology. 2003;144:3848–51.

45. Hasegawa S, Nakano M, Taniguchi Y, et al. Effects of Na$^+$–H$^+$ exchange blocker amiloride on left ventricular remodeling after anterior myocardial infarction in rats. Cardiovasc Drugs Ther. 1995;9:823–6.

46. Taniguchi Y, Nakano M, Hasegawa S, et al. Beneficial effect of amiloride, a Na$^+$–H$^+$ exchange blocker, in a murine model of dilated cardiomyopathy. Res Commun Chem Pathol Pharmacol. 1996;92:201–10.

47. Yoshida H, Karmazyn M. Na$^+$/H$^+$ exchange inhibition attenuates hypertrophy and heart failure in 1-wk postinfarction rat myocardium. Am J Physiol. 2000;278:H300–4.

48. Kusumoto K, Haist JV, Karmazyn M. Na$^+$/H$^+$ exchange inhibition reduces hypertrophy and heart failure after myocardial infarction in rats. Am J Physiol. 2001;280: H738–45.

49. Chen L, Chen CX, Gan XT, et al. Inhibition and reversal of myocardial infarction-induced hypertrophy and heart failure by NHE-1 inhibition. Am J Physiol. 2004;286:H381–7.

50. Aker S, Snabaitis AK, Konietzka I. Inhibition of the Na$^+$/H$^+$ exchanger attenuates the deterioration of

ventricular function during pacing-induced heart failure in rabbits. Cardiovasc Res. 2004;63:273–81.

51. Cingolani HE, Rebolledo OR, Portiansky EL, et al. Regression of hypertensive myocardial fibrosis by Na$^+$/H$^+$ exchange inhibition. Hypertension. 2003;41: 373–7.

52. Chen L, Gan XT, Haist JV, et al. Attenuation of compensatory right ventricular hypertrophy and heart failure following monocrotaline-induced pulmonary vascular injury by the Na$^+$–H$^+$ exchange inhibitor cariporide. J Pharmacol Exp Ther. 2001;298: 469–76.

53. Pérez NG, Piaggio MR, Ennis IL, et al. Phosphodiesterase 5A inhibition induces Na$^+$/H$^+$ exchanger blockade and protection against myocardial infarction. Hypertension. 2007;49:1095–103.

54. Schussheim AE, Radda GK. Altered Na$^+$–H$^+$-exchange activity in the spontaneously hypertensive rat. J Mol Cell Cardiol. 1995;27:1475–81.

55. Perez NG, Alvarez BV, Camilión de Hurtado MC, et al. pHi regulation in the myocardium of the spontaneously hypertensive rat. Compensated enhanced activity of the Na$^+$–H$^+$ exchanger. Circ Res. 1995; 77:1192–200.

56. Ennis IL, Alvarez BV, Camilión de Hurtado MC. Enalapril induces regression of cardiac hypertrophy and normalization of pHi regulatory mechanisms. Hypertension. 1998;31:961–7.

57. Engelhardt L, Hein U, Keller K, et al. Inhibition of Na$^+$–H$^+$ exchange prevents hypertrophy, fibrosis, and heart failure in β1-adrenergic receptor transgenic mice. Circ Res. 2002;90:814–9.

58. Chahine M, Bkaily G, Nader M, et al. NHE-1-dependent intracellular sodium overload in hypertrophic hereditary cardiomyopathy: prevention by NHE-1 inhibitor. J Mol Cell Cardiol. 2005;38:571–82.

59. Kilić A, Velic A, De Windt LJ, et al. Enhanced activity of the myocardial Na$^+$/H$^+$ exchanger NHE-1 contributes to cardiac remodeling in atrial natriuretic peptide receptor-deficient mice. Circulation. 2005;112: 2307–17.

60. Kilić A, Bubikat A, Gassner B, et al. Local actions of atrial natriuretic peptide counteract angiotensin II stimulated cardiac remodelling. Endocrinology. 2007; 148:4162–9.

61. Tajima M, Bartunek J, Weinberg EO, et al. Atrial natriuretic peptide has different effects on contractility and intracellular pH in normal and hypertrophied myocytes from pressure-overloaded hearts. Circulation. 1998;98:2760–4.

62. Darmellah A, Baetz D, Prunier F, et al. Enhanced activity of the myocardial Na$^+$/H$^+$ exchanger contributes to left ventricular hypertrophy in the Goto–Kakizaki rat model of type 2 diabetes: critical role of Akt. Diabetologia. 2007;50:1335–44.

63. American Heart Association. Women and cardiovascular disease statistics. http://www.americanheart.org/downloadable/heart/1199816973854FS10WM08.pdf.

64. Tu JV, Nardi L, Fang J, et al. Canadian Cardiovascular Outcomes Research Team. National trends in rates of death and hospital admissions related to acute myocardial infarction, heart failure and stroke, 1994–2004. CMAJ. 2009;180:E118–25

65. Kilić A, Javadov S, Karmazyn M. Estrogen exerts concentration-dependent pro-and anti-hypertrophic effects on adult cultured ventricular myocytes. Role of NHE-1 in estrogen-induced hypertrophy. J Mol Cell Cardiol. 2009;46:360–9.

66. Van Borren MM, Zegers JG, Baartscheer A, et al. Contribution of NHE-1 to cell shortening of normal and failing rabbit heart. J Mol Cell Cardiol. 2006;41:706–15.

67. Hayasaki-Kajiwara Y, Kitano Y, Iwasaki T, et al. Na$^+$ influx via Na$^+$/H$^+$ exchange activates protein kinase C isozymes δ and ε in cultured neonatal rat cardiac myocytes. J Mol Cell Cardiol. 1999;31:1559–72.

68. Despa S, Islam MA, Weber CR, et al. Intracellular Na$^+$ concentration is elevated in heart failure but Na/K pump function is unchanged. Circulation. 2002;105: 2543–8.

69. Gan XT, Gong XQ, Xue J, et al. Sodium–hydrogen exchange inhibition attenuates glycoside-induced hypertrophy in rat ventricular myocytes. Cardiovasc Res. 2010;85:79–89.

70. Javadov S, Karmazyn M. Mitochondrial permeability transition pore opening as an endpoint to initiate cell death and as a putative target for cardioprotection. Cell Physiol Biochem. 2007;20:1–22.

71. Javadov S, Huang C, Kirshenbaum LA, et al. NHE-1 inhibition improves impaired mitochondrial permeability transition and respiratory function during postinfarction remodelling in the rat. J Mol Cell Cardiol. 2005;38:135–43.

72. Crompton M. The mitochondrial permeability transition pore and its role in cell death. Biochem J. 1999;341:233–49.

73. Weiss JN, Korge P, Honda HM, et al. Role of the mitochondrial permeability transition in myocardial disease. Circ Res. 2003;93:292–301.

74. Halestrap AP, Clarke SJ, Javadov S. Mitochondrial permeability transition pore opening during myocardial reperfusion: a target for cardioprotection. Cardiovasc Res. 2004;61:372–85.

75. Javadov S, Purdham DM, Zeidan A, et al. NHE-1 inhibition improves cardiac mitochondrial function through regulation of mitochondrial biogenesis during postinfarction remodeling. Am J Physiol. 2006; 291:H1722–30.

76. Javadov S, Choi A, Rajapurohitam V, et al. NHE-1 inhibition-induced cardioprotection against ischemia/reperfusion is associated with attenuation of the mitochondrial permeability transition. Cardiovasc Res. 2008;77:416–24.

77. Javadov S, Baetz D, Rajapurohitam V, et al. Antihypertrophic effect of Na$^+$/H$^+$ exchanger isoform 1 inhibition is mediated by reduced mitogen-activated protein kinase activation secondary to improved mitochondrial integrity and decreased generation of mitochondrial-derived reactive oxygen species. J Pharmacol Exp Ther. 2006;317:1036–43.

78. Javadov S, Rajapurohitam V, Kilić A, et al. Expression of mitochondrial fusion-fission proteins during post-infarction remodeling: the effect of NHE-1 inhibition. Basic Res Cardiol. 2011;106(1):99–109.
79. Frey N, Olson EN. Cardiac hypertrophy: the good, the bad, and the ugly. Annu Rev Physiol. 2003;63:45–79.
80. Molkentin JD. Calcineurin-NFAT signaling regulates the cardiac hypertrophic response in coordination with the MAPKs. Cardiovasc Res. 2004;63:467–75.
81. Bueno OF, van Rooij E, Molkentin JD, et al. Calcineurin and hypertrophic heart disease: novel insights and remaining questions. Cardiovasc Res. 2002;53:806–21.
82. Wilkins BJ, Molkentin JD. Calcium-calcineurin signaling in the regulation of cardiac hypertrophy. Biochem Biophys Res Commun. 2004;322:1178–91.

83. Heineke J, Molkentin JD. Regulation of cardiac hypertrophy by intracellular signalling pathways. Nat Rev Mol Cell Biol. 2006;7:589–600.
84. Nakamura TY, Iwata Y, Arai Y, et al. Activation of Na^+/H^+ exchanger 1 is sufficient to generate Ca^{2+} signals that induce cardiac hypertrophy and heart failure. Circ Res. 2008;103:891–9.
85. Kilic A, Rajapurohitam V, Sandberg SM, et al. A novel chimeric natriuretic peptide reduces cardiomyocyte hypertrophy through the NHE-1-calcineurin pathway. Cardiovasc Res. 2010;88:434–42.
86. Guo J, Gan XT, Haist JV, et al. Ginseng Inhibits cardiomyocyte hypertrophy and heart failure via NHE-1 Inhibition and attenuation of calcineurin activation. Circ Heart Fail. 2011;4(1):79–88.

The Structural Basis of Cardiac Dysfunction in Human Heart Failure

Stefan Hein, Sawa Kostin, and Jutta Schaper

Abstract

In this chapter we describe the structural alterations observed in failing human myocardium. We review the current literature and compare these reports with our own findings. One of the earliest significant structural changes is the occurrence of myocyte hypertrophy and a significant degree of reactive fibrosis, which are the major factors causing diastolic dysfunction. Furthermore, we describe equivalents of systolic dysfunction: the ultrastructural changes indicating myocyte degeneration characterized by the reduction of myofilaments, an increase in cytoplasm, and the occurrence of small mitochondria with less cristae. The cytoskeleton: the microtubuli showed densification and desmin was augmented and irregularly arranged, most probably a mechanism compensatory for reduced cellular stability because of loss of sarcomeres. The remaining sarcomeres showed less elements of the sarcomeric skeleton, i.e., of titin, α-actinin, and myomesin, which contributes to sarcomeric instability. Membrane damage leads to ionic imbalance and is caused by either loss or increase of the membrane proteins dystrophin, the vinculin–talin– integrin complex, and of spectrin. The gap junctional protein connexin 43 of the intercalated disc is likewise reduced and represents the basis of defects of the excitation–contraction coupling. In the extracellular space, an accumulation of blood borne cells indicates a process of chronic low-grade inflammation, which is injurious to the sarcolemma of the myocyte. These different processes involving the interstitium as well as almost all cellular components of the cardiomyocytes will finally lead to myocyte death, either autophagic or oncotic but less apoptotic. It is postulated that fibrosis and myocyte hypertrophy combined with loss of sarcomeres are

J. Schaper (✉)
Max-Planck-Institute for Heart and Lung Research,
Bad Nauheim, Germany
e-mail: jutta.schaper@mpi-bn.mpg.de

N.S. Dhalla, M. Nagano, B. Ostadal (eds.), *Molecular Defects in Cardiovascular Disease*,
DOI 10.1007/978-1-4419-7130-2_15, © Springer Science+Business Media, LLC 2011

the structural equivalent of diastolic dysfunction. Systolic dysfunction occurs at a later stage of progression to heart failure and is caused by damage of the various components of the myocytes in addition to cellular hypertrophy and fibrosis. In conclusion, the development of heart failure is a multifactorial event involving the extracellular matrix and almost all cellular components of the myocytes. Therefore; fibrosis as well as myocyte degeneration and cell death are the structural factors determining cardiac dysfunction.

Keywords

Heart failure • Cardiac structure • Fibrosis • Myocyte degeneration • Cell death • Fibronectin • Collagen • Contractile filaments • Sarcomeric skeleton • Cytoskeleton • Dystrophin • T-tubules • Gap junctions • Ubiquitin • C9 • Extracellular matrix • Apoptosis • Diastolic dysfunction • Systolic dysfunction

Introduction

For more than 20 years, our group has studied failing myocardium of the human heart with the purpose of defining the characteristic changes in the left ventricular myocardium from patients with heart failure (HF) caused by a variety of cardiovascular diseases. We published our results in peer-reviewed journals and presented the data at international meetings. The present chapter represents a summary of our findings involving most of the structural components of the myocytes as well as of the extracellular matrix including the microvasculature and a discussion of the possible functional consequences of these structural alterations. This chapter starts with a description of the different structural components and their alterations in the diseased heart and ends with a discussion of the role of cell death followed by conclusion that surfaces from the data presented here.

The Extracellular Matrix-Fibrosis

Cardiac remodeling leading to HF is characterized by alterations in cardiomyocyte structure and function. The same is true for the accumulation of the different collagens, fibronectin, glycoproteins, and cellular elements including fibroblasts, fibromyoblasts, and microvessels in the extracellular space, which is commonly denominated as fibrosis. Reactive fibrosis occurs in the interstitium and in perivascular areas and is due to stimulated activity of fibroblasts, without the occurrence of cell death. Reparative or replacement fibrosis depicts the deposition of extracellular matrix proteins during the process of scar formation after cell injury and death. Fibrosis is multifactorial and can be caused by several processes including ischemia, senescence, inflammation, and various hormones, especially transforming growth factor ß (TGF-ß) and angiotensin II (see reviews by Swynghedauw [1], Spinale [2] and Creemers [3]).

Regardless of etiology, fibrosis results with time in decreased ventricular compliance and finally in diastolic and systolic dysfunction [4–6]. Clinically, this may present with symptoms of cardiac failure though often this is a subclinical disease, and cardiac dysfunction is noticeable only at later stages of remodeling [7].

Fibronectin is present as major matrix protein and may be used as indicator of the size of the interstitial space. We measured 10–12% of the normal human myocardial tissue to contain fibronectin. This can increase up to 40% of the myocardial tissue in HF [8]. In patients with

DCM, we found a significant upregulation of fibronectin protein and its mRNA which confirmed our histological findings [9].

The various collagens determine the degree of compliance of the cardiac ventricle and are therefore important to measure in diseased myocardium. The same is true for measurements of collagen synthesis and degradation, which can be studied using antibodies against their N-terminal propeptides (PINP for newly synthetized collagen I, PIIINP for collagen III), the aminoterminal telopeptide (IIINTP) for mature crosslinked collagen fibers, and the carboxyterminal telopeptides (ICTP) for the degradation product of collagen I [10]. Cardiac fibroblasts are involved in the production and degradation of the cardiac extracellular matrix through the production of collagens, proteoglycans, matrix metalloproteinases (MMPs), and their tissue inhibitors (TIMPs). Fibroblasts secrete various bioactive mediators e.g., VEGFα, FGFs, TGF-ß, and PDGF.

Their role has been discussed extensively by Krenning et al. who pointed out that fibroblasts might have different sources, that they represent a heterogeneous cell population, and that they not only determine extracellular protein production and degradation but also influence cardiac angiogenesis and myocyte proliferation [11].

A new aspect of fibroblast activity is the fact that there seems to exist a direct interplay between cellular changes such as sarcomeric protein mutations and the ECM as demonstrated recently in MHC[719/+] mice where activated proliferative and profibrotic signals in nonmyocyte cells mediated preferentially by TGF-ß were observed [12]. Furthermore, de Cavanagh et al. recently published a review discussing in depth the interaction between mitochondria, the cytoskeleton, and the ECM, and its regulation and various conditions in varying tissues and isolated cells [13].

Another new area in fibrosis research is centered on the role of mast cells that play a role in activating MMPs and stimulating myocardial fibrillar collagen degradation thereby causing fibrosis in the diseased heart and adverse ventricular remodeling [14].

The ECM in the remodeling process undergoes continuous synthesis and degradation by the action of MMPs and their TIMPs; however, under normal conditions the collagens are extremely stable and resistant to degradation. Therefore, the interplay and balance of MMPs and their TIMPs determine the maintenance of interstitial tissue homeostasis. The role of MMPs and TIMPs has been discussed recently in an excellent review by Spinale where he emphasized that the myocardial matrix is not a passive but a dynamic structure determining for a great part the remodeling process in various disease states, thereby offering a new goal for diagnostic and therapeutic strategies [2]. Our own studies confirm this view. We showed that in patients with aortic valve stenosis the amount and activity of several MMPs and TIMPs increased during the development of HF [15]. In another study, we showed that in human hearts with DCM or in the borderzone of infarcts or in myocarditis, the MMPs are activated, the TIMPs are upregulated and the number of fibroblasts is significantly increased. PINP was higher than ICTP in all groups, but PIIINP was only elevated in DCM and the infarct border zone but not in the other groups whereas IIINTP was augmented in all failing hearts [16]. This indicates that collagen metabolism was specifically altered to different degrees of severity in all groups, but generally collagen was accumulated and the degree of fibrosis was elevated to up to almost 30% in all groups. Furthermore, the expression of the cytokines fibrosin and activin was increased to different degrees but the fibroblast growth factors −1 and 2 expression was unchanged. However, we found a significant upregulation of angiotensin II and of TGF-ß in human myocardium during the progression to failure [8]. Our group believes, therefore, that collagen deposition in different cardiac diseases may be due to multiple mechanisms acting alone or in concert in fibrosis development in HF [16].

In general, we would like to conclude that fibrosis is an important factor with significant functional implications, i.e., loss of ventricular compliance and therefore diastolic dysfunction, in the development of HF.

Degeneration of the Myocytes

Contractile Filaments, Mitochondria, and Nuclei

Myocardial degeneration was defined as involvement of all cellular organelles in a chronic and in most cases slow process of degradation that finally results in cellular atrophy, cell death, and reparative as well as replacement fibrosis. In failing myocardium, hypertrophy of the cells, i.e., an increase in length and width, and degenerative changes of the myocytes are most obvious by light and electron microscopy. Degenerative changes include loss of myofibrils, nuclear aberrations with enlargement and bizarre shape, occurrence of large areas containing nonspecified sarcoplasm and inclusions such as autophagic vacuoles, numerous perinuclear lipofuscin granules as well as lysosomes, enlargement of the T-tubules, and very small mitochondria accumulated at the nuclear pole and between the sarcomeres [17]. One of the causes of myocardial degeneration appears to be defective lysosomal function and the hindrance of turnover of damaged cellular structures by an increased lipofuscin loading [18]. Furthermore, in a recent publication Maloyan and Robbins showed ultrastructural evidence of myocyte degeneration with mitochondrial abnormalities and scarcity of sarcomeres in mice with overexpression of mutated aB-crystallin (CryAB[R120G]), which acts as a chaperone to desmin [19]. These authors speculated that amplification of the autophagic response leads to promotion of autophagic cell death, which may be the case in human myocardium as well.

In our own study, the nuclear density in cardiomyocytes from failing human hearts was reduced by 18% but the nuclear profile area was significantly increased, i.e., the number of nuclei was reduced but they were larger than normal, which indicates an altered nucleus/cytoplasm relationship (1.0 in control and 0.85 in DCM) in cardiomyocytes from failing hearts [20]. In a later study in patients with aortic valvular stenosis, we determined the concentration of DNA and of the splicing factor Sc–35, and found a significant upregulation of both, even in nuclei from failing cardiomyocytes. In the presence of a disturbed nucleus/cytoplasm relationship this was interpreted as compensatory mechanism preserving the ability of the cardiomyocyte, even when injured, for ongoing transcription and translation [8, 20]. The increased synthesis of DNA might be necessary to avoid "dilution" of the genetic material in the enlarged cells and it permits DNA repair [8]. Data published by other groups support the notion that DNA synthesis occurs in the mammalian heart (overview by Soonpa and Field [21]).

Sarcomeres were significantly reduced to 42% (control 53%) in patients with a 40% mean left ventricular ejection fraction due to aortic valvular stenosis and to only 25% in patients with DCM [20, 22, 23]. The mitochondrial volume density was slightly reduced from 25% in control to 22% in decompensated pressure overload hypertrophy. The myocytes were significantly hypertrophic, normal in size, or atrophic without any direct contact with neighboring cardiomyocytes. These changes were described in detail in 1991 in failing myocardium from patients with dilated cardiomyopathy but they are characteristic as a consequence of chronic pressure overload as well [8, 17]. The functional consequences of myocyte degeneration, especially of the reduction of contractile material, are obvious. Already in 1975 Maron et al. claimed, that "degenerated cardiac muscle cells have poor contractile function and may be responsible for impaired cardiac performance" [24]. Furthermore, the ultrastructural data implicate that nuclear function is disturbed and that the cellular membrane including the T-tubular system is deranged. On the other hand, our group recently showed that the nuclei of degenerating cardiomyocytes are still viable and able to transcribe [8]. As mentioned above, this was measured by determination of the splicing factor Sc-35 and the DNA content in nuclei from failing hearts. The extremely small mitochondria exhibiting less cristae than those from normal tissue might be the cause for a disturbed energetic equilibrium (for a discussion of this problem see Braunwald and Bristow [25]). It was concluded that ongoing pressure induced hypertrophy finally resulting in HF is accompanied by compensatory mechanisms in the nuclei of cardiomyocytes, which therefore appear be a limiting factor for basic cellular function and survival only at late stages of progression to heart failure. On the other hand, a decrease in contractile filaments and mitochondrial changes are structural abnormalities that appear much earlier and most probably are responsible for diastolic dysfunction.

The Sarcomeric Skeleton

Titin

The sarcomeric skeleton comprises proteins that maintain the sarcomeric structure and function including the giant molecule titin, α-actinin, myomesin, the M- and C-proteins as well as others. Titin occurs in cardiac and skeletal muscle as well in a truncated form in smooth muscle cells [26]. The titin molecule spans the half-sarcomere from the Z-disk to the M-line as a spring-like filament with a length of 1.3 μm and its C-terminal regions overlap with the countertitin filament in the M-band [27, 28]; its extensible PEVK and N2B regions are situated in the I-band and are responsible for the passive and restoring force in stretched sarcomeres (reviewed in Granzier et al. [29] and in Tskhovrebova and Trinick [30]). By this action, the A-bands are maintained in a fixed position in the sarcomere and sarcomere length is homogeneous. Therefore, titin together with the connective tissue content determines the degree of diastolic filling [26]. Numerous publications have described the structure and function of titin but to cite them all would be beyond the limitations of this chapter. An excellent recent review by LeWinter and Granzier summarizes the history and major findings of this protein, important not only for the maintenance of the structural integrity of the sarcomere but also its role in determining diastolic function and its disturbances in HF [31]. Mutations of titin, changes in titin phosphorylation and in splicing were enumerated as being important for diastolic dysfunction and loss of compliance of failing cardiac ventricles [31]. In particular, truncation of the elastic PEVK region leads to cardiomyopathy and diastolic dysfunction as has been shown in mice, but not yet in human beings [26].

In an early publication our group described disorganization and lack of titin in myocytes in failing myocardium from patients with DCM, which occurred simultaneously with "myocyte degeneration", i.e., loss of contractile proteins indicating that the "third filament system" is involved in heart failure [32]. It was also shown that titin, acting in concert with α-actinin and myomesin, is necessary as template for the organization of newly synthesized myosin and actin filaments, i.e., in sarcomerogenesis [33].

α-Actinin

α-Actinin occurs in the I-band of the sarcomere and therefore appears in a regular cross-striation pattern by immunohistochemical methods using specific antibodies. Of the four isoforms of α-actinin (abbreviation ACTN 1–4), only α-actinin-2 (ACTN-2) occurs in cardiac muscle (for review, see Sjoblom et al. [34]). The Z-repeat of the N-terminal end of the titin filament binds to the N-termini of α-actinin in the I-band thereby ensuring the stability of the sarcomeric structure, especially by binding the actin filaments of neighboring sarcomeres. Because of the regular striated labeling pattern of α-actinin, we use this protein for the diagnosis of sarcomeric disorganization, i.e., myocyte degeneration [8, 35]. During the progression to HF, we find gross disorganization and accumulation of α-actinin, which might significantly contribute to loss of contractility because of the instability of contractile filaments and disturbance of sarcomerogenesis.

ACTN-1 is the isoform characteristic of smooth muscle cells and can be labeled with a specific antibody [34]. In failing myocardium we found perinuclear clusters of this protein in many myocytes, and this phenomenon was absent in normal myocardium. The accumulation of smooth muscle α-actinin is certainly an indicator of cellular degeneration but the numbers vary from 0 to 360 clusters per section. Colocalization with ubiquitin was not found (Hein, unpublished data). We believe that the occurrence of ACTN-1 is useful as an indicator of myocyte degeneration but its absence does not exclude degenerative processes in the myocardium [36].

Myomesin

Myomesin binds myosin and titin in the M-band region, and this process is regulated by myomesin phosphorylation. This interaction significantly contributes to the maintenance of the regular arrangement of thick filaments. Thus, α-actinin increases sarcomeric stability by the binding of adjacent actin filaments in the Z-band and the M-band-complex which further increases the stability by fixing myosin filaments [37, 38]. Interestingly, Gautel and his group identified obscurin which binds to M-band titin as well as to the M-band protein myomesin. In addition, obscurin interacts with Z-disk titin. Titin mutations lead to obscurin mislocalization, suggesting that the interaction of these proteins might be of relevance to human disease resulting in HF [39]. This very important and interesting observation, however, has yet to be proven in human myocardium.

In normal human myocardium, myomesin is localized in a clear cross-striation pattern in the center of the sarcomere, i.e., the M-band [38]. In failing human myocardium we observed irregular arrangement of myomesin indicating loss of stability of the sarcomere [35].

M-Protein in the M-Band

This is another protein increasing the stability of the M-band and binding to myosin filaments (review by Furst et al. [38]).

Myosin Binding Protein C

cMyBP-C is a sarcomeric thick filament protein that interacts with titin, myosin, and actin to regulate sarcomeric assembly, structure, and function. cMyBP-C phosphorylation regulates cross-bridge

formation by the action of several kinases. Moreover, dephosphorylation of cMyBP-C, which accelerates its degradation, has been shown to associate with the development of heart failure in mouse models and in humans (overview in Barefield and Sadayappan [40]).

In conclusion, the sarcomeric skeleton consists of several proteins that play an important role in maintaining sarcomeric stability. Disorganization of these proteins, at either the Z-disk or the M-line, as observed in myocardium in progression to HF will lead to decreased sarcomere stability and loss of contractile function of the cardiomyocyte.

The Cytoskeleton

The cytoskeleton comprises the microtubuli, the intermediate filament desmin, and F-actin.

The Microtubuli

The microtubuli are the largest parts of the cytoskeleton with a diameter of 25 nm. They consist of αß dimers that form a network with abundant longitudinal elements and some crossing structures. Next to their role in forming the spindle preceding cell division, their major role in association with dynein and kinesin is transportation of proteins, RNAs and of vesicles. Microtubuli are also partly responsible for maintaining cellular stability. Microtubuli undergo constant turnover by depolymerization and are therefore regarded as very dynamic structures. Since the early 1970s, Cooper in elegant experiments studied the role of microtubules in feline and canine overloaded myocardium [41]. This author in a recent review summarized his pioneering work on the relationship between changes of the microtubuli and cardiac function by stating that "The hypothesis that evolved was that microtubule network densification might be a culprit structural defect" and might significantly contribute to the progression to HF [42].

Our group was able to confirm this hypothesis in human myocardium [9]. We used quantitative protein and mRNA determinations as well as confocal microscopy and reported an increase in the expression of cytoskeletal proteins as well as disorganization in failing human myocardium. We put forward the hypothesis that this phenomenon represents a compensation of the loss of myofilaments with the purpose of maintaining the stability of the myocytes. This might even result in an overshoot reaction causing an elevation of cellular stiffness thereby contributing to diastolic and systolic dysfunction as postulated by Cooper's group [43–45].

Scholz working in G. Cooper's group approached the problem of microtubular changes in hypertrophy and failure from a different point of view. In an elegant study they showed in different experimental models that excessive decoration of microtubuli with microtubule associated protein 4 (MAP4) produces disruption of messenger ribonucleoprotein particle transport and protein synthesis. The dense MAP4 overdecorated microtubular system may cause contractile dysfunction and may prevent a fully compensatory growth response to hemodynamic overloading [46].

From Cooper's group and our own work, it appears, therefore, that densification of the microtubular network represents an important factor in producing disturbances of cardiac function.

The Intermediate Filament Desmin

Desmin belongs to the cytoskeletal system. In the myocardium, the main intermediate filaments are desmin and vimentin. Both are localized in fibroblasts, endothelial, and smooth muscle cells. Desmin occurs in cardiomyocytes where it surrounds the Z-disc and mutually connects the sarcomeres thus providing maintenance of cellular integrity, force transmission, and mechanochemical signaling. In the myocardium, 2% of the protein content consists of desmin indicating its abundance and importance for cellular stability [47] (see review by Goldfarb and Dalakes [48]). AB-crystallin, a member of the heat shock protein family, chaperones desmin and actin thereby participating in the maintenance of cellular stability. Its mutant $CryAB^{R120G}$ results in desminopathy and initiates protein microaggregates that

can be transported to the perinuclear area by the microtubular system to form depositions of misfolded proteins termed aggresomes. These might be harmful to cellular function, especially to the process of autophagy and cell death [19, 48]. Whether the accumulations of ACTN-1 observed by Hein in human myocardium are identical to these aggresomes observed in mouse myocardium has still to be determined [36].

Numerous mutations of desmin have been described that result in heart failure (see review by Goldfarb and Dalakas [48]) but large accumulations of desmin and a 2.1 fold elevated protein concentration were also observed by our group in failing hearts without any obvious desmin mutations [9]. In this study, a good correlation was found between the amount of cytoskeletal proteins and end-diastolic pressure in controls and DCM patients, indicating the importance of desmin and tubulin alterations for cardiac function.

F-actin is almost impossible to identify because of the lack of a specific antibody that allows a differentiation from contractile actin filaments.

The Membrane Associated Proteins

Dystrophin and Spectrin

The dystrophin–glycoprotein complex (DGC) and the vinculin–talin–integrin system are located at the cellular membrane of cardiac and skeletal muscle cells [49, 50]. The dystrophin gene is the largest gene known and mutations are common causing Duchenne muscular dystrophy and other muscular dystrophies (for review, see le Rumeur et al. [51]). The large DGC binds the cytoskeleton (F-actin binding at the N-terminal) to laminin in the extracellular basement membrane and therefore it plays an important role in maintaining membrane stability and lateral force-transduction as a structural and functional link between cytoskeleton and membrane [51].

The dystrophin network in human cardiomyocytes is present at the sarcolemma and locally enriched at costameres [52, 53]. The DGC consists of three different subcomplexes: the sarcoplasmic, the αß-dystroglycan complex, and the sarcoglycan $\alpha\delta$ transmembrane complex. The $\alpha\beta$-dystroglycan complex binds to laminin-2 in the basement membrane, i.e., the extracellular component, but it also binds to the sarcoglycans which in turn bind to the C-terminal of the intra-cytoplasmic dystrophin molecule. Prochniewicz et al. recently demonstrated that when dystrophin (and utrophin) binds to actin, these filaments become stronger and more resilient and that it furthermore acts as a stabilizing component at the sarcolemma [54].

It has been postulated that conditions in which the myocyte contractile apparatus and the internal cytoskeleton are disrupted, such as in remodeling in the development of heart failure, emphasize the vital role of the membrane cytoskeleton in cell survival [52]. In support of this notion, Toy-Oka and colleagues in hamsters which missed the delta-sarcoglycan gene found increased sarcolemmal fragility due to dystrophin cleavage by increased levels of calpain during the development of HF [55, 56]. The same group found dystrophin disruption in hearts from patients with intractable DCM confirming the importance of the intactness of dystrophin for sarcolemmal stability [56]. Our own studies showed reduction and disruption of dystrophin at the sarcolemma in human myocardium from hearts failing because of different etiologies [47].

Towbin postulated that hypertrophic cardio-myopathy might be a sarcomeric disease but that DCM might result from mutations or other dis-turbances of the cytoskeletal proteins [57, 58]. This is an interesting hypothesis; however, it might be too exclusive. As stated at the end of this chapter, HF might have a multifactorial origin involving almost all structural elements of the cardiomyocyte and the extracellular matrix.

The Vinculin–Talin–Integrin Complex (Focal Adhesion Molecules, FAMs)

The vinculin–talin–integrin complex connects the extracellular matrix with the cytoskeleton. Whereas MAPs are present at the free sarco-lemma, FAMs occur at the costameres and at the T-tubular membrane only [53]. Geiger et al. in

1980 using immunoferritin labeling and electron microscopy found that vinculin was also local-ized close to the transverse portions of the inter-calated disk membranes. Talin and the integrins are absent from the intercalated disc [59]. These investigators emphasized the absence of vinculin from any parts of the sarcomeres, especially from the Z-disk, which was confirmed by studies from our group [53]. Nowadays, several subgroups of integrins are known, but a detailed description exceeds the limitations of this chapter [60]. It was postulated that integrins function not only as structural receptors that connect the extracellular matrix, especially laminin, with the cytoskeleton but also acts as signaling receptor regulating intracellular pH and free Ca^{2+} concentration as well as phosphorylation of proteins [60, 61]. Recently, Anastasi et al. stated that all proteins of the DGC colocalized with the vinculin–talin–integrin system [49]. This review provides an excellent discussion of the localization and func-tion of the vinculin–talin–integrin complex. Furthermore, Wolfenson et al. in a review on the function of integrins emphasized the dependence of focal adhesion proteins on mechanical tension development and the central role of local mechan-ical forces in regulating the interplay between FAMs and the actin system, i.e., the cytoskeleton [62]. This might be important in the develop-ment of heart failure when the cardiomyocytes contract less and less and therefore mechanical tension is reduced.

It is interesting to note that vinculin and myo-mesin bind to the actin-based protein LIM-only protein MLP, which is present in the myofibril fraction of the cardiomyocyte and is essential for myocyte architecture in cardiomyocyte develop-ment and differentiation [63]. MLP-deficient mice reproduce the morphological and clinical picture of dilated cardiomyopathy and heart fail-ure in humans [63] which was confirmed in human patients suffering from either dilated or ischemic cardiomyopathy [64]. Whereas a metav-inculin missense mutation is associated with dilated and hypertrophic cardiomyopathy and a reduction of vinculin [65], an increased amount of vinculin but a decrease in myomesin in human hearts failing because of DCM was reported by our group [9, 47, 66]. We concluded from this work that abnormalities of the membrane bound proteins may play a causative role in cardiac remodeling and the origin of cardiac dysfunction.

The T-Tubular System

The cardiac T-tubules are specialized parts of the sarcolemma. They contain the MAPs dystrophin and spectrin, as well as the FAMs vinculin, talin, and the $\alpha_5\beta_1$ integrin. Costameres contain the same proteins but the free sarcolemma is devoid of vinculin, talin, and $\alpha_5\beta_1$ integrin. FAMs and MAPs were localized in the T-tubular membrane in a similar pattern: in longitudinally oriented myocytes as transverse punctuate lines at the Z-level and in transversally cut myocytes as a radial tubular network extending throughout the interior of the cell [53]. Furthermore, the T-tubules contain the basement membrane proteins fibronectin, laminin, and collagen IV. The elements of the sarcoplasmic reticulum (SR) are in close contact with the T-tubules and both are therefore responsible for the rapid propagation of the excitation impulse throughout the myocytes in skeletal and cardiac muscle. The T-tubules are the organelles responsible for excitation–contraction coupling. In the cardiac dyad, the tubules functionally couple the sarcolemmal L-type calcium channels (LCCs) to the sarcoplasmic reticulum ryanodine receptors (RyR) and this configuration controls calcium induced calcium release from the SR into the cytosol inducing myofilament contraction (reviewed in Bito et al. [67]). These authors present an extensive discussion of the different feedback mechanisms in the regulation of Ca^{2+} influx in normal and failing myocytes and they come to the conclusion that the coupling between LCC and RyR, essential for regular Ca^{2+} release and therefore for myofilament contractility, may be disturbed by functional as well as structural changes [67]. These might be the loss of T-Tubules as described by He et al. in failing canine myocardium, in pigs, and in mice or loss of channels or receptors as described by Song [68–71]. Song et al. examined the ratio between LLC and Ryr in failing rat myocardium and finding a reduction of

LCC they coined the expression "orphaned RyR". Their final conclusion was that the HF-associated Ca^{2+} instability arises from structural changes in the relationship between the T-tubules and the SR that disrupt the local control of RyRs by LCCs [71]. We would like to support this view.

In 1998, Kostin et al. reported that in diseased human myocardium the number of T-tubules was reduced but they were more dilated than in normal myocytes [53]. This structural abnormality is thought to be indicative of a disturbance of impulse conduction in cardiomyocytes. Lyon et al. in 2009 confirmed this finding by describing loss of T-tubules in ventricular myocytes from human myocardium failing because of either ischemic heart disease or dilated or hypertrophic obstructive cardiomyopathy [72]. In this study, the alterations in human myocardium were confirmed in rat myocytes from a postinfarction HF model, thus emphasizing the usefulness of a rat model in HF studies. Furthermore it was reported that in both models changes of the sarcolemma with flattening of the Z-grooves and partial loss of these structures occurred, again independent of the underlying etiology of cardiac disease resulting in HF. Because of the occurrence of the T-tubular changes in a diversity of cardiac pathologies, these authors conclude that the structural alterations are not the direct outcome of the initial specific insult but that they are rather the end-result of ongoing cellular adaptation during the process of HF development [72].

A more recent study aimed to determine the time-point of onset of T-tubular changes in relation to left ventricular function in a rat aortic banding model [73]. Using state-of-the-art confocal microscopy, these authors developed a quantitative T-tubule power index (TTpower) to represent the integrity of the T-tubule structure. The interesting results show that already in early compensated hypertrophy of the left ventricle a partial loss and global reorganization of the T-tubules occurs as indicated by a leftward shift of TTpower and that this T-tubular remodeling correlates with LV function, i.e., it is more pronounced in later stages of LV dysfunction. Spreading to the RV occurred later, i.e., at the early HF stage. Furthermore, this study was concerned with the function of the protein junctophilin (JP-2), a protein important for the formation of the T-tubule-SR junctions [74]. Data obtained on protein levels with Western blot and knock-out of JP-2 and using a knock-out procedure in isolated myocytes with lentivirus carrying JP-2 short hairpin (sh)RNA (gene silencing) showed that JP-2 is essential for T-tubule formation and that downregulation occurs at early stages of hypertrophy. The final conclusion of this innovative work was the assumption that T-tubule remodeling may constitute a key mechanism underlying the progression to HF.

Since the T-tubules are a specialized part of the sarcolemma it is obvious that alterations of the membrane associated proteins influence the function of the T-system. Kawada et al. studied the expression of dystrophin in the sarcolemma and found a patchy expression of dystrophin in cardiomyocytes from cardiomyopathic hamsters and in human failing hearts that possess a gene deletion or mutation of delta-sarcoglycan, a dystrophin related protein which might result in membrane instability [75]. In 2004, Toyo-Oka et al. found that cardio-selective cleavage of dystrophin may lead to progression of HF to an advanced stage [56] and later they reported increased expression of calpain most probably responsible for dystrophin cleavage in failing myocardium [55].

In our own studies in ischemic canine myocardium we observed depletion of dystrophin from the cellular membrane, which might be an active mechanism causing membrane instability in failing myocardium as well [76].

Changes of the Intercalated Disc Composition

Three types of membrane junctions exist within an intercalated disc: fascia adherens, macula adherens (desmosomes), and gap junctions. The fascia adherens connects to the sarcomere by binding to actin filaments. The macula adherens binds to the intermediate filaments desmin, and the gap junctions allow for the propagation of the excitation impulse by permitting the passage

of ions. The desmosomes contain the proteins desmoplakin, desmocollin, desmoglein, plakoglobin, and plectin. The fascia adherens contains cadherins, and its cytoplasmic part interacts with either desmoplakin or ß-catenin. These interact with α-catenin which binds to the actin cytoskeleton. Connexin 43 (Cx43) is the most abundant gap junction protein (for a recent review, see Li et al. [77]).

In 1990, Severs in his pioneering work on gap junctions emphasized that in human myocardium disease-related alterations occur due to the distribution of gap junctions as well as changes in the amount and type of connexins expressed. Alterations in Cx45 and Cx40 expression were also discussed [78].

In our own study in patients with aortic valve disease, we observed an increase in Cx43 protein in the early phase of compensated hypertrophy, which was reflected in an augmented number of gap junctions per intercalated disc area and an increased gap junction surface density. Decompensated LV hypertrophy was characterized by a reduction of the Cx43 signal per myocyte area or per intercalated disc. In addition, decompensated LV myocardium showed a markedly heterogeneous spatial distribution of Cx43. We speculated that upregulation of Cx43 in compensated hypertrophy may represent an immediate adaptive response to increased load, whereas diminished and heterogeneous Cx43 distribution in decompensated hypertrophy may play maladaptive roles culminating in heart failure and ventricular arrhythmias [79, 80].

Low-Grade Inflammation

Low-grade chronic inflammation is present in hearts failing because of either DCM, pressure overload, or ischemic heart disease; on the other hand, in myocarditis an acute or chronic inflammatory reaction is characteristic of the disease [81]. We showed that the ratio PECAM-1/ICAM-1 was elevated in all of these cardiac pathologies studied and the number of cells expressing CD11/CD18, the ICAM receptor, and that of lymphocytes (CD3), monocytes (CD14), and macrophages (CD68) was significantly upregulated. A slightly increased number of granulocytes (CD45) was also observed. Furthermore, the number of mast cells was elevated, which might cause fibrosis in the diseased heart [14]. It was hypothesized that degeneration of myocytes with the production and deposition of cellular debris in the extracellular space might be the common denominator for the inflammatory response and the development of fibrosis [81]. This was also emphasized by Kania et al. in a recent review [82].

Innate immunity plays an important role in the remodeling process towards heart failure but whether or not this reaction has beneficial (repair) or deleterious effects is still under debate [83]. It is evident, however, that numerous groups of bioactive molecules including various cytokines such as TNF-α and TGF-ß or angiotensin II, toll-like receptors, and the nuclear transcription kappa B and others are effective in causing an inflammatory reaction (Maisch et al. [84]; for a recent review, see Valen [83]). Our own data in patients with pressure overload hypertrophy showed an increased occurrence of leukocytes, lymphocytes, and macrophages as well as of angiotensin II and TGF-ß in early as well as late stages of heart failure development, which indicates that inflammation is continuously present and an important factor in the process of adverse remodeling [8].

The situation is particularly evident in myocarditis where large infiltrates containing granulocytes and CD3, CD11/CD18, CD14, and CD68 positive cells as well as remnants of myocytes are observed. Acute myocarditis and its sequela, dilated cardiomyopathy, are most often caused by cardiotropic viral infections resulting in later stages in transgression of myocarditis to dilated cardiomyopathy and heart failure (for overview, see Valen [83]). According to Maisch, inflammatory cardiomyopathy (DCMi) is a specific cardiomyopathy entity of DCM, being defined by the proof of intramyocardial inflammation and/or viral infection in endomyocardial biopsies [84]. This is in contrast to our own data showing that a low-grade inflammatory reaction is generally present in cardiac tissue during the development of HF.

Cell Death

At the end of adverse remodeling in the progression to HF, the degenerated cardiomyocytes die by different death mechanisms.

Three different types of cell death are known: Oncotic (necrotic, ischemic), autophagic, and apoptotic [85] (for review, see Whelan et al. [86]).

Oncosis (former term necrosis or ischemic cell death) results from increased leakage of the sarcolemma; therefore, the cellular uptake of complement 9 (C9) is a reliable marker of this type of cell death. The term oncosis seems to be more appropriate because necrosis is the state of the cell after cell death has occurred [85, 87]. It is interesting that the rate of oncosis was similar to that of autophagic cell death in our observations indicating the importance of both types of cell death [8].

Autophagy is an important process as evidenced by the occurrence of an increased number of ubiquitin–protein clusters in failing myocardium. Ubiquitin accumulation in the absence of a nucleus serves as a marker of autophagic cell death until a more specific marker has been found. Tests using monodansylcadaverine as marker of autophagic vacuoles demonstrated that ubiquitin is exclusively accumulated in myocytes positive for monodansylcadaverine, thus providing evidence for a link between ubiquitin accumulations and autophagy. Therefore, we hypothesized that myocytes often may die as a consequence of slow degenerative processes involving the ubiquitin/proteasomal pathway [85]. De Meyer et al. confirmed these findings and stated that accumulations of "garbage" including "intracellular protein aggegates" result in cell death (review by De Meyer et al. [88]).

Apoptosis is suicidal, programmed cell death and is characterized by DNA fragmentation. These fragments are evidenced by specific staining methods available nowadays as commercial kits (e.g., the in situ cell death detection kit TMR red by Roche) or by Southern blots [87]. Western blots of caspase 3, caspase 9, or bcl$_2$ provide further information on the apoptotic process. The calculation of exact numbers of apoptotic cells is hindered by the fact that the time course of the entire process is still partially unknown. How long

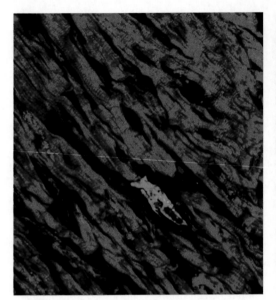

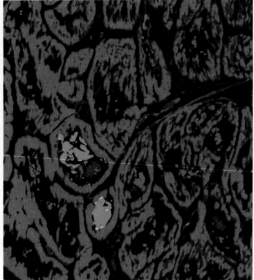

Fig. 1 Oncotic cell death identified by C9 (*green*). Counterstain for actin is by Phalloidin (*red*). Nuclei are *blue* with DAPI, lipofuscin is visible (*magenta*). The oncotic cell is smaller than normal and only a fragment of the nucleus is visible. Note the *large black central areas* in the myocytes where myofilaments are missing

Fig. 2 Autophagic cell death identified by ubiquitin staining (*green*).The upper myocyte shows ubiquitin clusters but the nucleus is still present. This cell was not counted (see text). The lower smaller myocyte showing *green* ubiquitin accumulations lacks a nucleus and was counted. Actin is *red* by Phalloidin, nuclei are *blue*, lipofuscin is present (*magenta*). Note the *large black areas* at the center of the myocytes where myofilaments are missing

does it take until the DNA is totally fragmented? How long is the interval from DNA fragmentation and removal of the cell? Maybe we count dead cells twice or even more often? Because of these uncertainties, there still exists a controversy regarding the rate and importance of apoptotic cell death in human myocardium [85]. This issue will only be solved when answers to the above questions have been provided.

In earlier studies using the electron microscope, we observed cardiomyocytes from failing hearts that did not contain a nucleus, which was interpreted as evidence for an ongoing process of cell death because in the absence of a nucleus the cell is unable to resynthesize the used materials such as contractile or signaling proteins and fragments are expelled into the extracellular space, the cell will shrink, and it will finally disappear [17]. In a more recent study, we quantitatively determined the rate of cell death in myocardium from patients with aortic valve defects undergoing valve replacement [8]. With increasing severity of the reduction of cardiac function, the rate of oncotic (Fig. 1) and autophagic (Fig. 2) cell death

increased significantly (up to 6‰ for ubiquitin positive cells without nuclei indicating autophagic cell death, and up to 4‰ for C9 positive cells indicating oncotic cell death). Apoptosis was observed at a negligible rate, with 0.02% as the highest value. Cardiomyocyte mitosis was never observed and therefore, as a consequence of cell death, the number of myocytes/mm^2 decreased significantly when compared to control.

Guerra et al. suggested that necrosis was more frequent than apoptosis in heart failure and they concluded that both myocyte necrosis and apoptosis affect the decompensated human heart and that each contributes to the evolution of cardiac failure, more so in men than in women [89]. These findings are somewhat in contrast with our own data showing the rates that in end-stage heart failure patients with DCM cell death by either oncosis or autophagy were ten times higher than in control hearts but apoptosis was very low [85]. Regarding autophagic cell death, the most important finding was the downregulation of the deubiquitination enzyme isopeptidase-T, which might lead to accumulation of ubiquitin–protein conjugates which in turn inhibit proteasomal activity [85].

In 1992, Meredith et al. reported that in endothelial cells the extracellular matrix serves as a cell survival factor inhibiting apoptosis and they suggested that integrin-mediated signals are required for maintaining cell viability [90]. Cellular attachment by integrin ß₁, which has a widespread distribution along the sarcolemma, seems to be especially important [91]. In later years, this important finding gained momentum and it was shown to occur in many different cell types including cancer metastasis, regression of the mammary gland after pregnancy, and many other situations (see the retrospective article by Schwartz [92]). In cardiac muscle, cell adhesion to the extracellular matrix was shown to be important in an experimental model of aortic stenosis in mice and the authors concluded that the disruption of normal myocyte anchorage to the neighboring extracellular matrix and cells, a process called anoikis, may signal apoptosis and may promote the transition from hypertrophy to early heart failure [93].

From these studies it is concluded that autophagy and cell death represent maladaptations to increased cardiac load and might contribute to a reduction in contractile function of the ventricles [8, 85, 88]. On the other hand, Piot states that necrosis "mediates" HF and Whelan et al. and others believe that cell death might be causal for heart failure [86, 94]. For a comprehensive discussion of the possible causes of heart failure see the following conclusions.

Conclusions

We would like to present an integrated view on the structural aspects as part of the cause of HF. In Fig. 3 all components of the cardiomyocyte investigated in our own studies are depicted and in Table 1 all structural alterations observed in our work are listed together with their functional consequences.

As can be seen from this table, the manifold structural defects which are the equivalent of the reduction of contractile force and of ventricular

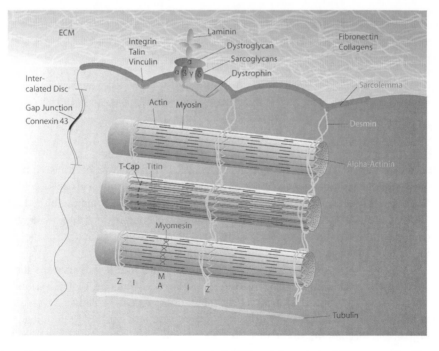

Fig. 3 Schematic drawing showing all structural components of the cardiomyocyte that were examined in our studies and discussed here (drawing by schaper-kommunikation.de)

Table 1 Structural alterations and functional consequences in failing myocardium

Component	Immunofluorescence/EM	Protein content/incidence	Functional consequence
ECM proteins	Perivascular and interstitial accumulations	⇑⇑	Reactive and replacement fibrosis, microscarring Diastolic dysfunction
Myofilaments	Disarranged, reduction	⇓⇓	Reduced systolic function
Nuclei	Enlarged and bizarre shape	⇓ DNA and Sc-35 because of reduced nucleus/cytoplasm ratio	Loss of transcription
Mitochondria	Small, less cristae	⇔	Energy imbalance
Sarcomeric skeleton			
Titin	All: disorganized, locally	⇓	Reduced stability of the
α-actinin	accumulated, mostly	⇓	sarcomeres, disturbed
Myomesin	reduced	⇓	sarcomerogenesis reduced systolic function
Cytoskeleton			
Desmin	Disarrangement and accumulation	⇑⇑	Cellular stability increased (stiffness), contributes mostly to diastolic dysfunction (compliance ⇓)
Tubulin		⇑⇑	
Membrane proteins			
DGC complex	Disorganized	Either ⇑ or ⇓	Membrane stability disturbed, specific properties lost
FAMs (vinculin)	⇑ later ⇓	⇑⇑	Impulse propagation disturbed
ID (Cx43)	Disorganized	Early HF ⇑ later ⇓	Arrhythmia
T-tubules	Dilated	⇓⇓	Disturbance of impulse conduction
Blood borne cells in interstitium	CD3–CD68 positive CD45 positive	⇑⇑ ⇑	Low-grade inflammation
Cell death			
Autophagy	Ubiquitin positive	⇑⇑	Loss of myocytes
Oncosis	Complement 9 positive	⇑⇑	Loss of systolic function, further increase of diastolic dysfunction
Apoptosis	TUNEL positive	(⇑)	

compliance will finally lead to cell death and fibrosis. These cellular injuries together with an augmentation of the extracellular matrix will slowly increase during the progression to heart failure and at a certain point in time they will result in diastolic and later also in systolic dysfunction [25].

The changes listed in Table 1 are considered to be the structural basis of multiple dysfunctions as observed in failing myocardium: disturbances of Ca²⁺-metabolism and receptor density in the case of membrane alterations including the T-tubular system, reduced contractile protein expression because of reduction of transcription (nuclei), disturbed energy balance because of mitochondrial abnormalities, and disturbed excitation–contraction coupling because of alterations of the sarcolemma in general and of the gap junctions in particular.

We would like to put forward the following scenario of interaction of the various structural alterations: As can be deduced from our work on progression to heart failure in human patients, it is obvious that hypertrophy of the overloaded heart and therefore of its myocytes is the first compensatory mechanism, especially visible in hearts with chronic pressure overload. Chronic cellular hypertrophy will produce injury including loss of contractile elements, nuclear changes with reduction of transcription, and a reduction of compliance because of a densification of the cytoskeleton as a compensatory mechanism counteracting the increased strain on the myocardium. The proteins of the sarcomeric skeleton (titin, α-actinin, myomesin), in contrast, are reduced and will contribute to sarcomeric instability, in addition to the loss of myofilaments. Simultaneously, this process is accompanied by the occurrence of reactive and later on also by replacement fibrosis.

The cytoskeleton is not only involved in the maintenance of cellular stability and integrity but it also plays a significant role in transmitting signals from the cellular membrane to the nucleus. Integrins can act as mechanoreceptors, and transfer of force from integrins to the cytoskeleton is thought to represent a proximal step in an intracellular mechanical signaling pathway. Binding of fibronectin to integrins furthermore enforces the interaction of the ECM with the cellular milieu. This, however, is defective because of the reduction of integrins in failing hearts. Increased sarcolemmal fragility due to loss of dystrophin as well as the loss of connexin 43 from gap junctions will produce a pronounced ionic imbalance and disturbances of excitation–contraction coupling. Chronic inflammation will further damage the already injured cardiomyocytes. Taken together, these different structural–functional factors will result in cell death, i.e., in disappearance of myocytes and an increase in fibrotic tissue.

To establish a definitive sequence of events is almost impossible at the present time. However, from our studies it became obvious that diastolic dysfunction appears first, at a stage when the entire process is still reversible [95]. The structural correlate of this clinical symptom is increased stiffness of individual myocytes and the occurrence of reactive fibrosis. Systolic dysfunction is evident at a later stage. The structural equivalent is prominent loss of myofilaments, failure of transcription, and loss of cells by cell death in addition to the above described structural changes

accompanied by reparative as well as replacement fibrosis [95].

Therefore, we conclude that the origin of heart failure is a multifactorial event involving almost all cellular components of the myocytes and the extracellular matrix.

References

1. Swynghedauw B. Molecular mechanisms of myocardial remodeling. Physiol Rev. 1999;79:215–62.
2. Spinale FG. Myocardial matrix remodeling and the matrix metalloproteinases: influence on cardiac form and function. Physiol Rev. 2007;87:1285–342.
3. Creemers EE, Pinto YM. Molecular mechanisms that control interstitial fibrosis in the pressure-overloaded heart. Cardiovasc Res. 2011;89:265–72.
4. Villari B, Hess OM, Piscione F, Vassalli G, Weber KT, Chiariello M. Heart function in chronic pressure overload caused by aortic stenosis: the role of collagen tissue. Cardiologia. 1994;39:411–20.
5. Weber KT, Sun Y, Tyagi SC, et al. Collagen network of the myocardium: function, structural remodeling and regulatory mechanisms. J Mol Cell Cardiol. 1994;26:279–92.
6. Brower GL, Gardner JD, Forman MF, et al. The relationship between myocardial extracellular matrix remodeling and ventricular function. Eur J Cardiothorac Surg. 2006;30:604–10.
7. Konstam MA, Udelson JE, Anand IS, et al. Ventricular remodeling in heart failure: a credible surrogate endpoint. J Card Fail. 2003;9:350–3.
8. Hein S, Arnon E, Kostin S, et al. Progression from compensated hypertrophy to failure in the pressure-overloaded human heart: structural deterioration and compensatory mechanisms. Circulation. 2003;107:984–91.
9. Heling A, Zimmermann R, Kostin S, et al. Increased expression of cytoskeletal, linkage, and extracellular proteins in failing human myocardium. Circ Res. 2000;86:846–53.
10. Risteli J, Risteli L. Analysing connective tissue metabolites in human serum. Biochemical, physiological and methodological aspects. J Hepatol. 1995;22 (2 Suppl):77–81.
11. Krenning G, Zeisberg EM, Kalluri R. The origin of fibroblasts and mechanism of cardiac fibrosis. J Cell Physiol. 2010;225:631–7.
12. Teekakirikul P, Eminaga S, Toka O, et al. Cardiac fibrosis in mice with hypertrophic cardiomyopathy is mediated by non-myocyte proliferation and requires Tgf-beta. J Clin Invest. 2010;120:3520–9.
13. de Cavanagh EM, Ferder M, Inserra F, et al. Angiotensin II, mitochondria, cytoskeletal, and extracellular matrix connections: an integrating viewpoint. Am J Physiol Heart Circ Physiol. 2009;296:H550–8.

14. Levick SP, Melendez GC, Plante E, et al. Cardiac mast cells: the centrepiece in adverse myocardial remodelling. Cardiovasc Res. 2011;89:12–9.

15. Polyakova V, Hein S, Kostin S. Matrix metalloproteinases and their tissue inhibitors in pressure-overloaded human myocardium during heart failure progression. J Am Coll Cardiol. 2004;44:1609–18.

16. Polyakova V, Loeffler I, Hein S, et al. Fibrosis in endstage human heart failure: Severe changes in collagen metabolism and MMP/TIMP profiles. Int J Cardiol. (2010), doi:10.1016/j.ijcard.2010.04.053 in press.

17. Schaper J, Froede R, Hein S, et al. Impairment of the myocardial ultrastructure and changes of the cytoskeleton in dilated cardiomyopathy. Circulation. 1991;83: 504–14.

18. Terman A, Kurz T, Gustafsson B, et al. The involvement of lysosomes in myocardial aging and disease. Curr Cardiol Rev. 2008;4:107–15.

19. Maloyan A, Sayegh J, Osinska H, et al. Manipulation of death pathways in desmin-related cardiomyopathy. Circ Res. 2010;106:1524–32.

20. Scholz D, Diener W, Schaper J. Altered nucleus/cytoplasm relationship and degenerative structural changes in human dilated cardiomyopathy. Cardioscience. 1994;5:127–38.

21. Soonpa MH, Field LJ. Survey of studies examining mammalian cardiomyocyte DNA synthesis. Circ Res. 1998;83:15–26.

22. Schwarz F, Schaper J, Kittstein D, et al. Reduced volume fraction of myofibrils in myocardium of patients with decompensated pressure overload. Circulation. 1981;63:1299–304.

23. Schwarz F, Schaper J, Kittstein D, et al. Quantitative ultrastructural findings of the myocardium in the failing heart. I. Aortic valve insufficiency. Z Kardiol. 1981;70:729–32.

24. Maron BJ, Ferrans VJ, Roberts WC. Myocardial ultrastructure in patients with chronic aortic valve disease. Am J Cardiol. 1975;35:725–39.

25. Braunwald E, Bristow MR. Congestive heart failure: fifty years of progress. Circulation. 2000;102(20 Suppl 4): IV14–23.

26. Granzier H, Labeit S. Structure-function relations of the giant elastic protein titin in striated and smooth muscle cells. Muscle Nerve. 2007;36:740–55.

27. Obermann WM, Gautel M, Steiner F, et al. The structure of the sarcomeric M band: localization of defined domains of myomesin, M-protein, and the 250-kD carboxy-terminal region of titin by immunoelectron microscopy. J Cell Biol. 1996;134:1441–53.

28. Van Der Ven PF, Obermann WM, Weber K, et al. Myomesin, M-protein and the structure of the sarcomeric M-band. Adv Biophys. 1996;33:91–9.

29. Granzier HL, Radke MH, Peng J, et al. Truncation of titin's elastic PEVK region leads to cardiomyopathy with diastolic dysfunction. Circ Res. 2009;105: 557–64.

30. Tskhovrebova L, Trinick J. Roles of titin in the structure and elasticity of the sarcomere. J Biomed Biotechnol. 2010;2010:612482.

31. LeWinter MM, Granzier H. Cardiac titin: a multifunctional giant. Circulation. 2010;121:2137–45.

32. Hein S, Scholz D, Fujitani N, et al. Altered expression of titin and contractile proteins in failing human myocardium. J Mol Cell Cardiol. 1994;26:1291–306.

33. Person V, Kostin S, Suzuki K, et al. Antisense oligonucleotide experiments elucidate the essential role of titin in sarcomerogenesis in adult rat cardiomyocytes in long-term culture. J Cell Sci. 2000;113(Pt 21): 3851–9.

34. Sjoblom B, Salmazo A, Djinovic-Carugo K. Alphaactinin structure and regulation. Cell Mol Life Sci. 2008;65:2688–701.

35. Kostin S, Hein S, Arnon E, et al. The cytoskeleton and related proteins in the human failing heart. Heart Fail Rev. 2000;5:271–80.

36. Hein S, Block T, Zimmermann R, et al. Deposition of nonsarcomeric alpha-actinin in cardiomyocytes from patients with dilated cardiomyopathy or chronic pressure overload. Exp Clin Cardiol. 2009;14:e68–75.

37. Obermann WM, Gautel M, Weber K, et al. Molecular structure of the sarcomeric M band: mapping of titin and myosin binding domains in myomesin and the identification of a potential regulatory phosphorylation site in myomesin. EMBO J. 1997;16:211–20.

38. Furst DO, Obermann WM, van der Ven PF. Structure and assembly of the sarcomeric M band. Rev Physiol Biochem Pharmacol. 1999;138:163–202.

39. Fukuzawa A, Lange S, Holt M, et al. Interactions with titin and myomesin target obscurin and obscurin-like 1 to the M-band: implications for hereditary myopathies. J Cell Sci. 2008;121(Pt 11):1841–51.

40. Barefield D, Sadayappan S. Phosphorylation and function of cardiac myosin binding protein-C in health and disease. J Mol Cell Cardiol. 2010;48:866–75.

41. Gt C. by Cooper, G. Cardiocyte adaptation to chronically altered load. Annu Rev Physiol. 1987;49:501–18.

42. Gt C. Cytoskeletal networks and the regulation of cardiac contractility: microtubules, hypertrophy, and cardiac dysfunction. Am J Physiol Heart Circ Physiol. 2006;291:H1003–14.

43. Tsutsui H, Ishihara K, Cooper GT. Cytoskeletal role in the contractile dysfunction of hypertrophied myocardium. Science. 1993;260:682–7.

44. Tsutsui H, Tagawa H, Kent RL, et al. Role of microtubules in contractile dysfunction of hypertrophied cardiocytes. Circulation. 1994;90:533–55.

45. Tagawa H, Wang N, Narishige T. Cytoskeletal mechanics in pressure-overload cardiac hypertrophy. Circ Res. 1997;80:281–9.

46. Scholz D, Baicu CF, Tuxworth WJ, et al. Microtubule-dependent distribution of mRNA in adult cardiocytes. Am J Physiol Heart Circ Physiol. 2008;294: H1135–44.

47. Hein S, Kostin S, Heling A, et al. The role of the cytoskeleton in heart failure. Cardiovasc Res. 2000; 45:273–8.

48. Goldfarb LG, Dalakas MC. Tragedy in a heartbeat: malfunctioning desmin causes skeletal and cardiac muscle disease. J Clin Invest. 2009;119:1806–13.

49. Anastasi G, Cutroneo G, Gaeta R, et al. Dystrophin-glycoprotein complex and vinculin-talin-integrin system in human adult cardiac muscle. Int J Mol Med. 2009;23:149–59.
50. Ervasti JM, Campbell KP. Membrane organization of the dystrophin-glycoprotein complex. Cell. 1991;66: 1121–31.
51. Le Rumeur E, Winder SJ, Hubert JF. Dystrophin: more than just the sum of its parts. Biochim Biophys Acta. 2010;1804:1713–22.
52. Kaprielian RR, Severs NJ. Dystrophin and the cardiomyocyte membrane cytoskeleton in the healthy and failing heart. Heart Fail Rev. 2000;5:221–38.
53. Kostin S, Scholz D, Shimada T, et al. The internal and external protein scaffold of the T-tubular system in cardiomyocytes. Cell Tissue Res. 1998;294:449–60.
54. Prochniewicz E, Henderson D, Ervasti JM, et al. Dystrophin and utrophin have distinct effects on the structural dynamics of actin. Proc Natl Acad Sci USA. 2009;106:7822–7.
55. Kawada T, Masui F, Tezuka A, et al. A novel scheme of dystrophin disruption for the progression of advanced heart failure. Biochim Biophys Acta. 2005;1751:73–81.
56. Toyo-Oka T, Kawada T, Nakata J, et al. Translocation and cleavage of myocardial dystrophin as a common pathway to advanced heart failure: a scheme for the progression of cardiac dysfunction. Proc Natl Acad Sci USA. 2004;101:7381–5.
57. Towbin JA. The role of cytoskeletal proteins in cardiomyopathies. Curr Opin Cell Biol. 1998;10:131–9.
58. Towbin JA, Bowles KR, Bowles NE. Etiologies of cardiomyopathy and heart failure. Nat Med. 1999; 5:266–7.
59. Geiger B, Tokuyasu KT, Dutton AH, et al. Vinculin, an intracellular protein localized at specialized sites where microfilament bundles terminate at cell membranes. Proc Natl Acad Sci USA. 1980;77:4127–31.
60. Hynes RO. Integrins: versatility, modulation, and signaling in cell adhesion. Cell. 1992;69:11–25.
61. Schwartz MA. Transmembrane signalling by integrins. Trends Cell Biol. 1992;2:304–8.
62. Wolfenson H, Henis YI, Geiger B, et al. The heel and toe of the cell's foot: a multifaceted approach for understanding the structure and dynamics of focal adhesions. Cell Motil Cytoskeleton. 2009;66:1017–29.
63. Arber S, Hunter JJ, Ross Jr J, et al. MLP-deficient mice exhibit a disruption of cardiac cytoarchitectural organization, dilated cardiomyopathy, and heart failure. Cell. 1997;88:393–403.
64. Zolk O, Caroni P, Bohm M. Decreased expression of the cardiac LIM domain protein MLP in chronic human heart failure. Circulation. 2000;101:2674–7.
65. Vasile VC, Will ML, Ommen SR, et al. Identification of a metavinculin missense mutation, R975W, associated with both hypertrophic and dilated cardiomyopathy. Mol Genet Metab. 2006;87:169–74.
66. Vasile VC, Edwards WD, Ommen SR, et al. Obstructive hypertrophic cardiomyopathy is associated with reduced expression of vinculin in the intercalated disc. Biochem Biophys Res Commun. 2006;349:709–15.
67. Bito V, Heinzel FR, Biesmans L, et al. Crosstalk between L-type Ca^{2+} channels and the sarcoplasmic reticulum: alterations during cardiac remodelling. Cardiovasc Res. 2008;77:315–24.
68. He J, Conklin MW, Foell JD, et al. Reduction in density of transverse tubules and L-type Ca^{2+} channels in canine tachycardia-induced heart failure. Cardiovasc Res. 2001;49:298–307.
69. Heinzel FR, Bito V, Biesmans L, et al. Remodeling of T-tubules and reduced synchrony of Ca^{2+} release in myocytes from chronically ischemic myocardium. Circ Res. 2008;102:338–46.
70. Louch WE, Mork HK, Sexton J, et al. T-tubule disorganization and reduced synchrony of Ca^{2+} release in murine cardiomyocytes following myocardial infarction. J Physiol. 2006;574:519–33.
71. Song LS, Sobie EA, McCulle S, et al. Orphaned ryanodine receptors in the failing heart. Proc Natl Acad Sci USA. 2006;103:4305–10.
72. Lyon AR, MacLeod KT, Zhang Y, et al. Loss of T-tubules and other changes to surface topography in ventricular myocytes from failing human and rat heart. Proc Natl Acad Sci USA. 2009;106: 6854–9.
73. Wei S, Guo A, Chen B, et al. T-tubule remodeling during transition from hypertrophy to heart failure. Circ Res. 2010;107:520–31.
74. Takeshima H, Komazaki S, Nishi M, et al. Junctophilins: a novel family of junctional membrane complex proteins. Mol Cell. 2000;6:11–22.
75. Kawada T, Hemmi C, Fukuda S, et al. Sarcolemmal fragility secondary to the degradation of dystrophin in dilated cardiomyopathy, as estimated by electron microscopy. Exp Clin Cardiol. 2003;8:67–70.
76. Rodriguez M, Cai WJ, Kostin S, et al. Ischemia depletes dystrophin and inhibits protein synthesis in the canine heart: mechanisms of myocardial ischemic injury. J Mol Cell Cardiol. 2005;38:723–33.
77. Li J, Radice GL. A new perspective on intercalated disc organization: implications for heart disease. Dermatol Res Pract. 2010;2010:207835.
78. Severs NJ. The cardiac gap junction and intercalated disc. Int J Cardiol. 1990;26:137–73.
79. Kostin S, Dammer S, Hein S, et al. Connexin 43 expression and distribution in compensated and decompensated cardiac hypertrophy in patients with aortic stenosis. Cardiovasc Res. 2004;62:426–36.
80. Kostin S. Zonula occludens-1 and connexin 43 expression in the failing human heart. J Cell Mol Med. 2007;11:892–5.
81. Devaux B, Scholz D, Hirche A, et al. Upregulation of cell adhesion molecules and the presence of low grade inflammation in human chronic heart failure. Eur Heart J. 1997;18:470–9.
82. Kania G, Blyszczuk P, Eriksson U. Mechanisms of cardiac fibrosis in inflammatory heart disease. Trends Cardiovasc Med. 2009;19:247–52.

83. Valen G. Innate immunity and remodelling. Heart Fail Rev. 2011;16:71–8.
84. Maisch B, Richter A, Sandmoller A, et al. Inflammatory dilated cardiomyopathy (DCMI). Herz. 2005; 30:535–44.
85. Kostin S, Pool L, Elsasser A, et al. Myocytes die by multiple mechanisms in failing human hearts. Circ Res. 2003;92:715–24.
86. Whelan RS, Kaplinskiy V, Kitsis RN. Cell death in the pathogenesis of heart disease: mechanisms and significance. Annu Rev Physiol. 2010;72: 19–44.
87. Majno G, Joris I. Apoptosis, oncosis, and necrosis. An overview of cell death. Am J Pathol. 1995;146: 3–15.
88. De Meyer GR, De Keulenaer GW, Martinet W. Role of autophagy in heart failure associated with aging. Heart Fail Rev. 2010;15:423–30.
89. Guerra S, Leri A, Wang X, et al. Myocyte death in the failing human heart is gender dependent. Circ Res. 1999;85:856–66.

90. Meredith Jr JE, Fazeli B, Schwartz MA. The extracellular matrix as a cell survival factor. Mol Biol Cell. 1993;4:953–61.
91. Saetersdal T, Larsen TH, Dalen H. The beta1 integrin subunit is not a specific component of the costamere domain in human myocardial cells. Histochem J. 2002;34:323–9.
92. Schwartz MA. Remembrance of dead cells past: discovering that the extracellular matrix is a cell survival factor. Mol Biol Cell. 2010;21:499–500.
93. Ding B, Price RL, Goldsmith EC, et al. Left ventricular hypertrophy in ascending aortic stenosis mice: anoikis and the progression to early failure. Circulation. 2000;101:2854–62.
94. Piot C, Croisille P, Staat P, et al. Effect of cyclosporine on reperfusion injury in acute myocardial infarction. N Engl J Med. 2008;359:473–81.
95. Hein S, Schaper J. Remodeling from compensated hypertrophy to heart failure. In: Greenberg B, editor. Cardiac remodeling mechanisms and treatment. New York/London: Taylor&Francis; 2006. p. 103–20.

Hormonal Mechanisms of Cardiac Remodeling in Heart Failure

Andrea P. Babick, Vijayan Elimban, and Naranjan S. Dhalla

Abstract

It is now generally accepted that cardiac dysfunction in congestive heart failure (CHF) is due to cardiac remodeling as a consequence of changes in the size and shape of the heart. Furthermore, both the sympathetic nervous system (SNS) and the renin–angiotensin system (RAS) are activated, and the circulating levels of catecholamines and angiotensin II are elevated in CHF. Experimental and clinical studies have revealed that the blockade of SNS by different adrenoceptor (AR) antagonists improve cardiac function and attenuate cardiac remodeling. In addition to modifying β-AR-mediated signal transduction, β-AR antagonists have been shown to depress the elevated levels of catecholamines in CHF. On the contrary, the improvement of cardiac function and cardiac remodeling in CHF due to the blockade of RAS by angiotensin-converting enzyme inhibitors and angiotensin receptor blockers were associated with a reduction in the formation of angiotensin and antagonism of the angiotensin-receptor-mediated signal transduction, respectively. Blockade of either SNS or RAS prevented subcellular remodeling upon modifying changes in cardiac gene expression, reduced the development of intracellular Ca^{2+}-overload, and attenuated the occurrence of oxidative stress in the failing heart. These observations are consistent with the view that the activation of both SNS and RAS plays a crucial role in the genesis of cardiac remodeling and cardiac dysfunction in CHF.

Keywords

Congestive heart failure • Sympathetic nervous system • Renin–angiotensin system • Catecholamines • Angiotensin II • Cardiac gene expression • Cardiac remodeling • β-Adrenoceptor antagonists • Angiotensin-receptor antagonists • Angiotensin-converting enzyme

N.S. Dhalla (✉)
Institute of Cardiovascular Sciences, St. Boniface
General Hospital Research Centre, Winnipeg, Canada

Department of Physiology, Faculty of Medicine,
University of Manitoba, Winnipeg, Canada
e-mail: nsdhalla@sbrc.ca

N.S. Dhalla, M. Nagano, B. Ostadal (eds.), *Molecular Defects in Cardiovascular Disease*,
DOI 10.1007/978-1-4419-7130-2_16, © Springer Science+Business Media, LLC 2011

Introduction

The inability of the myocardium to balance oxygen supply and oxygen demand, as well as to maintain efficient cardiac contractility during both rest and exercise, is the hallmark of congestive heart failure (CHF). In fact, it is the only cardiovascular problem that continues to increase in both incidence and prevalence [1]. Various organs such as the heart, brain, liver, kidneys, lungs, skeletal muscle, and blood vessels behave abnormally in CHF. Furthermore, the overload of fluid drowns the peripheral organs in the body. Accordingly, examination of the etiologies of CHF has become an area of intensive research [2]. It should be noted that CHF is commonly associated with peripheral edema, lung congestion, and/or liver enlargement. Particularly, CHF is the common concluding pathway for the majority of primary cardiovascular diseases such as hypertension, coronary atherosclerosis, cardiomyopathy, diabetes, myocarditis, and congenital heart malformations [3]. The progression of CHF emerges as a widespread and coordinated reaction to cardiac injury, giving a complex cascade of events that underlie changes in the failing myocardium [4]. As heart disease advances, the size of the heart increases, cardiac function begins to deteriorate, and the symptoms of CHF become increasingly apparent [1]. This cardiac remodeling is acknowledged as the prominent course of clinical CHF and is associated with molecular, cellular, and interstitial alterations that are evident as the myocardium changes in size, shape, and function upon experiencing pathophysiologic insult [3, 4].

Although several mechanisms have been proposed to explain the development of cardiac remodeling and heart dysfunction in CHF [1–13], elevation in the level of various hormones in the circulation appears to be of critical importance. Depression in cardiac function due to different pathological conditions is commonly associated with a decrease in blood pressure, and this has been considered to provide signal for the activation of sympathetic nervous system (SNS), release of norepinephrine from the adrenergic nerve endings, release of epinephrine from the adrenal medulla, and increase in the circulating levels of catecholamines in CHF. Depression in cardiac output has also been indicated to decrease blood flow in the kidney, and this ischemic insult is considered to activate the renin–angiotensin system (RAS) and thus increase the circulating levels of angiotensin II (ANG II) in CHF. The levels of several other hormones such as vasopressin, aldosterone, endothelin, and serotonin [5, 6, 12, 13] are also known to be elevated in the circulation in CHF; however, the exact mechanism of their release or their role in the genesis of heart dysfunction has not been clearly defined. Accordingly, the discussion in this article is focused on the roles of both SNS and RAS in the development of CHF as well as the mechanisms for the induction of cardiac remodeling and heart dysfunction.

SNS and the Cardiovascular System

The ability of the heart to markedly increase contractility and heart rate during periods of stress is facilitated by the SNS that innervates the myocardium [14]. To date, two different types of major adrenergic receptors (ARs) have been identified, namely, the α- and the β-ARs [15]; the α_1, β_1 and β_2 subtypes are expressed in the human heart [6–21]. Described as a transmembrane signaling system situated in the sarcolemma (SL) membrane, the G-protein family members are neighbors to the α- and β-ARs that couple different receptors via effector enzymes [22–24]. Upon stimulation of the SNS and release of norepinephrine, the stimulatory G-protein couples the β-AR with the activation of adenylyl cyclase to generate the second messenger cAMP, which activates the cAMP-dependent protein kinase to phosphorylate the sarcoplasmic reticulum (SR) protein phospholamban (PLB), the L-type Ca^{2+}-channel in the SL membrane, troponin 1 in the myofibrils, and some regulatory proteins of the nucleus [14]. The effect on slow inward Ca^{2+}-channel promotes the entry of Ca^{2+} in cardiomyocytes, whereas the phosphorylation of PLB enhances the uptake of Ca^{2+} in the SR and thus results in

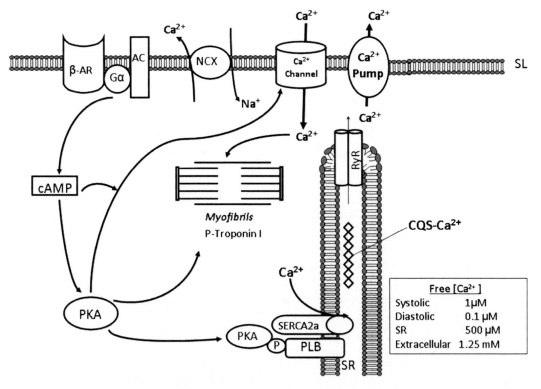

Fig. 1 Sympathetic system activation in cardiovascular system. *SL* sarcolemma, *SR* sarcoplasmic reticulum, *RYR* ryanodine receptor, *SERCA* sarcoplasmic reticulum Ca²⁺-ATPase pump, *PLB* phospholamban, *CQS* calsequestrin, *b-AR* β-adrenergic receptor, *Ga* G-coupled protein, *AC* adenylyl cyclase, *NCX* Na⁺/Ca²⁺ exchanger, *PKA* protein kinase A, *P* Phosphorylated, *CAMP* cyclic AMP

increasing the rates of cardiac contraction and relaxation; cardiac relaxation is also increased due to the phosphorylation of troponin I. These events form the molecular basis for the action of catecholamines on the heart (Fig. 1).

The cellular changes of the cardiomyocytes that are observed in the failing heart include cellular hypertrophy, irregularities in Ca²⁺-homeostasis, cross-bridge cycling, and electrical excitation–contraction coupling, as well as several alterations in the cytoskeletal framework. Recent reports have indicated that some of these changes are observed during the early stages of heart failure (HF), while remainder of the changes are developed in the overt decompensated stages of the failing heart and can be linked with abnormalities in both systolic and diastolic contractile function [25]. The SNS plays a vital role in regulating the cardiovascular system in both the healthy and diseased states [26–30], as it not only provides

appropriate vascular resistance through arteriolar constriction but also employs a sympathetic discharge on the heart to give enhanced chronotropic and intropic effects. Long-term blood pressure in the closed vasculature is also maintained for blood vessel growth and permeability by regulation of the RAS in the kidney [31]. During physiological conditions, these mechanisms act in harmony to regulate the cardiac, vascular, and renal entities for maintaining blood volume/pressure, perfusion pressure, cardiac output, and blood distribution [32]. However, in the event of the disruption of a healthy functioning myocardium that illustrates a decrease in cardiac output and subsequent blood supply to end organs, it is the action of neurohormones that are greatly amplified to provide a compensatory response to promptly support the essential circulatory function to maintain survival of the existing tissue and organs [32].

In response to myocardial ischemic insult, activation of the β-ARs by epinephrine and norepinephrine augments cardiac output and helps to maintain the blood pressure at an appropriate level. Simultaneous activation of α-ARs by the same hormones increase total peripheral resistance while shunting blood flow to organs of priority that include the heart and the brain [33]. The increase in cardiac output initially is compensatory; however, over a period of time it places an increased workload and oxygen demand on the heart. In the same way, an increased peripheral resistance initially is beneficial for maintaining blood pressure but its enhanced afterload effect induces an increased resistance against which the heart must pump [34–36]. These effects are a result of the stimulation of the sympathohumoral system that is originally focused to attenuate the ongoing systemic hypoperfusion, but eventually exacerbates the development of cardiac contractile dysfunction. This in turn enhances extracardiac irregularities to form a positive feedback of sequence of events that act continuously in a vicious cycle [37].

Notwithstanding the fact that the SNS offers a means of supporting cardiac contractile function, it has been documented that the failing human heart subjected to idiopathic dilated cardiomyopathy becomes less sensitive to stimulation of the SNS [38]. This observation can be partly explained by a selective loss of β_1-ARs that contribute to an overall reduction in the ratio of β_1/β_2, which ultimately gives rise to a decrease from 80:20 in the normal healthy heart to the approximate 60:40 in the failing myocardium [39]. In addition, the relative loss in β_1-ARs is proportional to the degree of CHF [40]; it has been suggested that chronic stimulation of the SNS accounts for the decrease in the level of β_1-AR mRNA [41]. Overstimulation of the SNS is also accompanied by other biochemical alterations including an increase in the expression of the α-subunit of inhibitory G-proteins, as well as attenuation of the positive inotropic effect of the β-AR activation [42, 43]. With respect to cardiac performance in conjunction with SR function, Stein et al. [44] have reported that chronic stimulation of the β-ARs enhanced the relaxation of

papillary muscle, and reduced the expression of protein levels of PLB and Ca^{2+}-pump ATPase (SERCA); the regulatory phosphorylation of PLB was also reduced. This was additionally supported by Linck et al. [45] who showed that the administration of the β-AR agonist, isoproterenol, gave rise to transiently increased relaxation due to an increase in the Ca^{2+}-uptake activity with consequent decreases in mRNA and protein levels of both PLB and SERCA. Isoproterenol has also been reported to increase heart weight [46, 47]. It has been shown that a strong negative correlation exists between catecholamine levels and life expectancy [45]. Lai et al. [48] have documented that norepinephrine infusion in dog hearts produced a decrease in the mRNA and protein levels of SERCA, which paralleled those hearts of pacing-induced heart failure, with no change in the mRNA levels of ryanodine receptor (RyR), calsequestrin (CQS), and PLB.

Blockade of the SNS in Myocardial Infarction

In the past, β-AR antagonists have been utilized for the remedy of several cardiovascular disorders including hypertension, angina pectoris, and myocardial infarction (MI) [49]. More specifically, the advantageous aspects of β-blockade in reducing mortality due to MI have been greatly acknowledged for a period of more than 10 years [50], whereby these benefits are observed in conditions of left ventricular dysfunction. Conventionally, the use of β-ARs have been considered a contraindication in CHF, primarily because of their characteristic negative inotropic effects, yet recent data clearly indicate that β-blockade significantly decreased mortality and improved the left ventricular function [50, 51]. As chronic heart failure progresses, myocardial contractile dysfunction occurs in response to the activation of the RAS and SNS, which inevitably releases various neurohormones to accelerate the downward slope of ventricular failure [52]. Although the initial stages of the SNS activation are considered as compensatory, it is the deleterious effects of the excess catecholamines that are

Table 1 Clinical trials of β-blockade in patients with MI

Clinical trial	Drug name	Human dose	Study highlights
BHAT [56]	Propanolol	180 mg/day	Significant ↓ in overall mortality. 240 mg/day
ISIS-1 [57]	Atenolol	100 mg/day	↓ overall vascular mortality at 1 year with ↓ risk of recurrent reinfarction, arrest and death from day 1–7.
MERIT-HF [58]	Metoprolol	200 mg/day	Metoprolol CR/XL with standard optimum therapy enhanced survival and was well tolerated.
CIBIS-II [59]	Bisoprolol	10 mg/day	Survival benefits in patients with stable HF only.
CAPRICORN [60]	Carvedilol	25 mg/twice daily	↓ both all cause and CV mortality + recurrent nonfatal MI in postacute MI with LV systolic dysfunction.
COPERNICUS [61]	Carvedilol	25 mg/twice daily	Alleviates severity of HF and ↓ risk of deterioration, hospitalization in euvolemic symptomatic patients at rest.

References to these clinical trials are given in brackets

BHAT β blocker heart attack trial, *CAPRICORN* carvedilol postinfarction survival control in left ventricular dysfunction, *CIBIS-II* Cardiac Insufficiency Bisoprolol Study II, *COPERNICUS* Carvedilol, prospective randomized cumulative survival, *CV* cardiovascular, *ISIS-1* First International Study of Infarct Survival; *LV* left ventricular, *MERIT-HF* Metoprolol CR/XL randomized intervention trial in congestive heart failure; *MI* myocardial infarction, ↓ decrease

produced during the advanced stages which are detrimental and in fact, directly relate to the severity of the disease process [53]. Moreover, it has been shown that increased levels of serum epinephrine are paralleled with the worst prognosis [54]. In view of these intriguing reports, it has been previously proposed that the blockade of the SNS in terms of the β-ARs may provide useful results in dampening the detrimental mechanisms triggered in myocardial injury [51]. This can be achieved with a long-term therapy that consists of an initial low dosage of β-blockers that is titrated slowly and gradually over the course of treatment [33].

Since the initial wave of Swedish studies [55], there have been a substantial number of placebo-controlled clinical trials that have verified the advantageous outcomes of β-blockers (Table 1, [56–61]). Particularly, single-center studies have continuously validated the usefulness of these compounds in chronic heart failure by showing improvements in ejection fraction as well as in overall clinical status in subjects, who were symptomatic with this disease [62–67]. Beneficial outcomes of reduced morbidity and mortality were also apparent from some clinical trials, namely, CIBIS-II with the drug bisoprolol [59], MERIT-HF with the drug metoprolol [58], and COPERNICUS with the drug carvedilol [68]. Now that β-blockers have proven to be of ultimate prognostic value in the long-term therapy of CHF, it is vastly accepted by the current medical community as a customary pharmacological remedy in subjects who continue to be symptomatic regardless of therapy with other medications such as ACE inhibitors and diuretics [55]. Several studies in experimental animals have also indicated the usefulness of β-AR blocking agents in attenuating the adverse effects of MI (Table 2, [69–75]).

RAS and the Cardiovascular System

RAS is a crucial element that plays a role in both the short- and long-term regulation of total body fluid, blood volume, overall electrolyte balance, arterial blood pressure, and mediation of disease pathophysiology [76, 77]. Particularly, the RAS is intimately involved in the regulation of cardiovascular function and structural remodeling, as its stimulation starts the pathway to deterioration

Table 2 Effects of β1-adrenergic antagonists in experimental MI animal models

Animal model	Drug	Dose	Therapeutic effects	References
Male SD Rats AB	Propranolol	40 mg/kg/day	↓ LV hypertrophy, dilation and lung congestion, but no significant improvement on survival.	Perlini et al. [69]
Male Wistar Rats CL	Metoprolol	250 mg/kg/day	↓ EF deterioration, post wall stress, LV dilation. ↓ NCX activity, ↑ Ca^{2+}-transient amplitude, Normalized Ca^{2+}-sensitivity of RyR.	Maczewski et al. [70]
Male SD Rats CL	Carvedilol	30 mg/kg/day	Improved LV+ RV wt and SERCA2a mRNA levels	Sun et al. [71]
	Metoprolol	60 mg/kg/day	Same effects as for carvedilol, but more significant improvement on SERCA2a mRNA expression.	
Male SD Rats CL	Metoprolol	1 mg/kg/h	Improved LV dimensions and volumes as well as ↓ plasma levels IL-6, but ↑ IL-1β. ↑↓ PCr/ATP.	Omerovic et al. [72]
Male SD Rats CL	Metoprolol	5 mg/kg/h	Normalization of phosphocreatine/ATP, ↑ SV & EF. ↓ plasma NE and brain natriuretic peptide.	Omerovic et al. [73]
Male SD Rats CL	Metoprolol	10 mg/kg/day	Attenuated LVEDP, ↓ collagen deposition, but did not affect plasma NE or urinary NE excretion.	Latini et al. [74]
Male SD Rats (CL)	Carvedilol	1 mg/kg	↓ infarct size by ~50%	Feuerstein et al. [75]

AB aortic banding, *CL* coronary ligation, *EF* ejection fraction, *LV* left ventricle, *LVEDP* left ventricular end diastolic pressure, *MI* myocardial infarction, *NCX* Na^+/Ca^{2+}-exchanger, *NE* norepinephrine, *PCr/ATP* phosphocreatine/ATP ratio, *RV* right ventricle, *SD* Sprague Dawley, *SV* stroke volume, ↓ decrease, ↑ increase, ↑↓ no change

of endothelial cell function, augmentation of growth, advancement of apoptosis, and the development of oxidative stress [78]. Irrespective of the etiology of CHF, major players stimulated in the development of CHF include the neurohormonal and cytokine systems [79–81]. Accordingly, the activation of the neurohormonal system occurs in a stepwise fashion, and is regarded as organ specific [82]. The detrimental cycle of CHF is initiated by a decrease in cardiac output that leads to the release of a variety of vasoconstrictor neurohormones, in addition to Na^+ and water retention [83, 84]. It has been well established that the most studied neurohormonal systems are the SNS and RAS [7]. Though these two complementary mechanistic pathways are required for optimal cardiac function, the result of cardiac injury causes these systems to pose a paradoxical degeneration in overall cardiac performance primarily through an increase in both preload and afterload [85]. The RAS is a critical entity in the regulation of cardiovascular function and structural remodeling in terms of everyday survival, as the transmitter

(Ang II) released from it acts primarily on the Ang II type 1 receptor (AT_1R) in the myocardium [86]. Accordingly, it has been shown by Ju et al. [87] that alterations in the mRNA levels of certain Ca^{2+}-transport proteins and the increased levels of mRNA for the $Na^+–Ca^{2+}$ exchanger, the RyR, and the SERCA proteins due to the presence of increased Ang II, were attenuated upon treatment with the Ang II receptor antagonist, losartan. The effects of Ang II are further reported in a study by Rouet-Benzineb et al. [88], who observed that the transcription factor, NF-κB, was translocated into the nucleus from the cytoplasm via the protein kinase C (PKC) pathway in neonatal rat cardiomyocytes subjected to Ang II stimulation and this process was blocked with the administration of calphostatin C, a specific PKC inhibitor.

Throughout these years of research, extensive efforts have been made to improve heart function in the infarcted animals upon treatments with various pharmacological interventions. Certain therapies include angiotensin-converting enzyme inhibitors (ACEIs) and angiotensin receptor blockers (ARBs). ARBs are a moderately new family of drugs that target diabetic nephropathy, CHF, and hypertension to produce physiological effects similar to those of ACEIs [89]. ACEI are directed against the active site of angiotensin-converting enzyme (ACE), whereby their beneficial effects are viewed through their ability to suppress Ang II formation, in addition to exerting arteriolar dilation, venodilation, and diuretic effects [90]. In a long-term study focusing on the effects of the ACEI captopril, on left ventricular remodeling of the myocardial infarcted canine model, Jugdutt et al. [91] revealed attenuation of early infarct expansion, the absence of late wall thinning, a reduction in the diastolic bulging, eradication of aneurysms, and a general restitution in overall cardiac systolic function, as well as a marked reduction in preload and afterload. In another study involving ACEI treatment, McDonald et al. [92] discovered that during progressive ventricular remodeling in the myocardial infarcted rat, late captopril therapy attenuated further increase in cell length, which is associated with myocyte hypertrophy and growth of the cardiac interstitium due to MI. In this regard, it is pointed out that a study by Dixon et al. [93] focused on the effects of the combination treatment of ramipril and losartan on collagen expression in the MI rat model and found that the administration of both the ACEI and AT_1R antagonist showed an overall reduction in cardiac fibrosis, which hypothesized that Ang II may be involved in the regulation of cardiac collagen synthesis after MI at the posttranscriptional site.

Blockade of RAS in Myocardial Infarction

Upregulation of the RAS is believed to be associated with the development of various cardiovascular pathologies that include atherosclerosis, hypertension, cardiac hypertrophy, heart failure, and neuropathies. Ang II, to some extent, is also produced by an ACE-independent pathway [94], and hence, ACEIs cannot completely block its production. Accordingly, ARBs, which are nonpeptide competitive AT_1R antagonists, were developed to prevent specifically the binding of Ang II to the AT_1R, thereby completely blocking the effect of the hormone. It has not yet been determined if the overwhelming receptor blockade of ARBs is due to a slow dissociation kinetics of Ang II from its receptor, from an internalization of the ARB-induced receptor, or to alternative binding sites on the AT_1R [89]. Supposedly, this prolonged receptor blockade can be beneficial in situations of increased levels of the endogenous ligand or in situations of missed doses in therapeutic drug treatment. Furthermore, ARBs have been anticipated to act superiorly to ACEIs. ARBs are a family of the drugs with evolving indications in hypertension, CHF and diabetic nephropathy, as their physiological effects are similar to those of ACEIs [95]. By blocking the actions of Ang II at the receptor level in blood vessels, adrenals, and tissues, these agents are able to induce dilation of arterioles and veins, to prevent pathological changes in cardiac structure, to reduce the release of aldosterone, to increase renal Na^+ and water excretion, to reduce plasma volume, and to decrease cellular hypertrophy. Several studies in experimental animals with MI have shown that ARBs produce beneficial effects in improving cardiac function (Table 3, [96–112]). Clinically ARBs are known to enhance left ventricular ejection fraction, improve CHF symptoms, increase exercise tolerance, and boost quality of life, in addition to reducing mortality and hospitalization (Table 4, [113–122]). However, the indication of ARBs in CHF was greatly ambiguous until the CHARM trials were published [95, 120, 121]. This study specifically established the value of these drugs in systolic CHF. In addition to CHARM, the initial trial of ELITE was also uniquely designed to compare the nephrotoxicity of the ARB losartan with the ACEI captopril in the elderly with CHF. The result showed a significant survival advantage in favor of the ARB [114, 116, 121]. However, the short-term study by Lang et al. [123] and the follow-up study of ELITE II [124], which was adequately powered to assess survival in a similar patient group, failed to confirm the superiority of losartan. In fact, it was observed that the ACEI

Table 3 Effects of $AT_1 R$ Antagonists in experimental animals with MI after coronary ligation

Animal model	Drug	Dose	Therapeutic effects	References
Male Wistar Rat	Losartan	1 mg/kg/day *icv*	Improved LV dimensions, EF, LVEDP, LVPSP and dP/dt$_{max/min}$ at 6 weeks.	Huang et al. [96]
		100 mg/kg/day *sc*	Only showed improvement of LVEDP at 6 weeks.	
		200 mg/kg/day *oral*	↓ $AT_1 R$ density in brain nuclei, improved LVEDP with an associated ↓ in LVPSP and dP/dt.	
Male SD Rats	Losartan	20 mg/kg/day	Improved LVSP, dP/dt$_{max/min}$, systolic/diastolic aortic pressure. Also ↓ TIMP-1 protein levels, mitigated expression of ACE, $AT_1 R$, attenuated myocardial fibrosis.	Xu et al. [97]
Male Wistar Rat	Irbesartan	50 mg/kg/day	Significantly ↓ LVEDP, LVESV, LVEDV, as well as ↓ interstitial fibrosis and expression of LV collagen I and III. Therapy combined with eplerenone ↑ α/β MHC, ANF, SERCA2a levels.	Fraccarollo et al. [98]
Male SD Rat	Losartan	20 mg/kg/day	Effectively ↓ HW, ascites, lung wet/dry wt ratio at 13 weeks. Attenuated LVSP, LVEDP, HR + Ca^{2+}-uptake as well as Ca^{2+}-stimulated ATP activity.	Shah et al. [99]
Male SD Rat	Losartan	20 mg/kg/day	Corrected HW, HW/BW, lung wet/dry wt ratio as well as heart function – LVEDP, dP/dt$_{max/min}$.↑ levels RyR, SERCA2a and PLB mRNA and protein.	Guo et al. [100]
Male SD Rat	Valsartan	15 mg/kg/day	Preserved LV FS%, systolic/diastolic diameters, and LVPW. Reversed changes in gene expression of muscle-specific, immune response, and fibrous tissue proliferation genes.	Gurevich et al. [101]
Female SD Rat	Losartan	3 mg/kg/twice daily	Marked ↑ binding affinities of Ang II for $AT_2 R$, with ↑↓ observed in $AT_1 R$ expression. Treatment also corrected HW/BW, LVW/BW, RVW/BW.	El-Sabban et al. [102]
Male Wistar Rat	Losartan	10 mg/kg/day	Significantly ↓ MAP, LVEDP. However, ↑↓ was observed in the mRNA levels of $AT_1 R$ and $AT_2 R$ levels at 30 min & 24 h post MI.	Zhu et al. [103]
Male Wistar Rat	Losartan	10 mg/kg/day	Attenuation of body characteristics of HW/BW in addition to improving LV dilatation & scar thinning.	Jain et al. [104]
Male SD Rat	Losartan	2 g/L water	↓ LV and RV weights and improves MAP, LVSP. Successfully decreases interstitial fibrosis.	Thai et al. [105]
Male SD Rat	Irbesartan	40 mg/kg/day	Reverses myocardial hypertrophy, attenuates ↑ *tau* time constant of isovolumic relaxation, ANP levels.	Ambrose et al. [106]
Female SD Rat	Losartan	2 g/L water	Effectively attenuates LV remodeling, inhibits elevation in TFG-β1 mRNA levels, ↓ interstitial fibrosis.	Youn et al [107]
Male Wistar Rat	Candesartan	1 mg/kg/day	Attenuates mRNA levels in LV and RV of ANP, α-skeletal actin, β-MHC, NCX, collagen I and III, and SERCA2a.	Hanatani et al. [108]
Male SD Rat	Losartan	40 mg/kg/day	Limits collagen deposition, improves HW/BW, but shows no benefits in nonmyocytes, collagen deposition.	Taylor et al. [109]
Male SD Rat	Losartan	2 g/L water	Similar effect as captopril in survival rate, yet linked with ↑ HR and ↓ peak developed pressure.	Milavetz et al. [110]
Male SD Rat	Losartan	3 mg/kg/day	Treatment ↓ myocardial hypertrophy, preserves minimal coronary vascular resistance, and reverses interstitial fibrosis in noninfarcted LV region.	Schieffer et al. [111]
Male Wistar Rat	Losartan	15 mg/kg/day	Significantly ↓ cardiac hypertrophy and fully inhibits deposition of collagen.	Smits et al. [112]
Male SD Rat	Losartan	40 mg/kg/day	Effectively ↑ venous compliance, ↓ LVEDP.	Raya et al. [113]

ANP atrial natriuretic peptide, AT_1R angiotensin II type 1 receptor, AT_2R angiotensin II type II receptor, *BW* body weight, *CL* coronary ligation, *EF* ejection fraction, *HR* heart rate, *HW* heart weight, *icv* intracerebroventricularly, *LV* left ventricle, *LVEDP* left ventricular end diastolic pressure, *LVEDV* left ventricular end diastolic volume, *LVESV* left ventricular end systolic volume, *LVPSP* left ventricular peak systolic pressure, *MHC* myosin heavy chain, *MI* myocardial infarction, *NCX* Na$^+$/Ca^{2+}-exchanger, *NE* norepinephrine, *PLB* phospholamban, *RV* right ventricle, *RyR* ryanodine receptor, *sc* subcutaneously, *SD* Sprague Dawley, *SERCA2a* sarco(endo)plasmic reticulum Ca^{2+}-ATPase, *wt* weight, ↓ decrease, ↑ increase, ↑↓ no change

Table 4 Clinical trials of AT$_1$R antagonists in patients with MI

Clinical trial	Drug name	Human dose	Study highlights
ELITE [114]	Losartan	50 mg/day	Losartan has unexpected ↓ mortality than ACEI, and was better tolerated with fewer discontinued therapies.
RESOLVD [115]	Candesartan	4, 8 or 16 mg/day	Alone was as efficient, tolerable and safe than ACEI, but in combination more beneficial to inhibit LV remodeling.
ELITE II [116]	Losartan	50 mg/day	Not chosen over BB for ↑ HF survival in elderly, but better tolerated.
LIFE [117]	Losartan	50 mg/day	Prevents more CV deaths than BB with a similar ↓ blood pressure and is better tolerated.
OPTIMAAL [118]	Losartan	50 mg/day	No significant difference in mortality than ACEI in patients with acute MI and proof of HF with LV dysfunction.
VALIANT [119]	Valsartan	20 mg/twice daily	Alone is as effective as ACEI for ↓ CV risks after MI. 160 mg/twice daily Combination with ACEI ↑ side effects without ↑ survival.
CHARM-Alternative [95]	Candesartan	32 mg/day	A well-tolerated drug that ↓ cardiovascular mortality and morbidity in patients with symptomatic chronic HF and intolerance ACE inhibitors.
CHARM-Preserved [120]	Candesartan	32 mg/day	The drug has moderate impact on inhibiting admissions for CHF with patients of HF and LVEF more than 40%.
CHARM-Added [121]	Candesartan	32 mg/day	Addition to ACEI gives clinically important ↓ in CV events in patients with CHF and ↓ LVEF.
ONTARGET [122]	Telmisartan	80 mg/day	Ongoing trial to see if ARB + Ramipril more effective than ramipril alone; if Telmisartan as effective as ACEI alone.
TRANSCEND [122]	Telmisartan	80 mg/day	Ongoing trial to see if ARB more effective than placebo in patients who cannot tolerate ACEI.

References to these clinical trials are given in brackets

ACEI Angiotensin-Converting Enzyme Inhibitor, *ARB* Angiotensin Receptor Blocker, *BB* β-blocker, *CHARM* Candesartan in Heart Failure, Assessment of Reduction in Mortality and Morbidity, *CHF* congestive heart failure, *CV* cardiovascular, *ELITE* Evaluation of Losartan in the Elderly, *HF* heart failure, *LIFE* Losartan Intervention for End point Reduction, *LV* left ventricular, *LVEF* left ventricular ejection fraction, *MI* myocardial infarction, *ONTARGET* Ongoing Telmisartan Alone and in Combination with Ramipril Global End point Trial, *OPTIMAAL* The Optimal Therapy in Myocardial Infarction with the Angiotensin II Antagonist Losartan, *RESOLVD* The Randomized Evaluation of Strategies for Left Ventricular Dysfunction, *TRANSCEND* The Telmisartan Randomized Assessment Study in ACE-1 Intolerant Subjects with Cardiovascular Disease, *VALIANT* Valsartan in Acute Myocardial Infarction, ↓ decrease, ↑ increase

reduced the onset of sudden death better than by the ARB but a meta-analysis of ARBs in CHF and high-risk MI revealed that ACEIs and ARBs do not differ in efficacy for reducing all-cause mortality and hospitalization for CHF [124–126], and therefore, ARBs are suitable alternatives to ACEIs in CHF or high-risk MI. Future works include an additional ongoing trial termed I-PRESERVE, which attempts to test the effects of ARBs in CHF with preserved systolic function [125]. The concern of using ARBs in combination with ACEIs still remains vague, and continues to pose a challenge to both clinicians and scientists. In some trials, the addition of ARBs to an ACEI did not provide any additional benefit in combating CHF [115, 119, 127]. Based on this finding, ARBs should not be routinely added to the otherwise stable CHF patient receiving a combination of an ACEI and a β-blocker. Nevertheless, the addition of ARBs can be beneficial in terms of reducing hospitalization for CHF and improving the quality of life [114, 128–130], with favorable effects on hemodynamics, ventricular remodeling, and neurohormonal profile [128]. The VALIANT trial [119] and a case-control study [122] attempted to clarify the relationship between ACEI and ARB in terms of use and risk of recurrence of MI, and found no significant differences regarding the risk for recurring MI among the two treatment regimens.

Conclusions

Both experimental and clinical studies have revealed that the SNS and RAS are activated and the circulating levels of both catecholamines and ANG II are elevated in CHF. Initially, the activation of these systems is associated with the maintenance of blood pressure and cardiac output; however, prolonged activation of both SNS and RAS results in cardiac remodeling and cardiac dysfunction in the failing heart [131–138]. It should be mentioned that cardiac dysfunction in CHF is associated with remodeling of one or more subcellular organelles depending upon the type and stage of the heart disease [139–147]. Furthermore, both catecholamines and ANG II have been shown to induce cardiac remodeling and subcellular alterations at the molecular and gene expression levels [148–152]. Although various β-AR antagonists and AT_1R antagonists are known to improve cardiac function as well as attenuate cardiac remodeling and subcellular alterations in CHF, the beneficial effects of these agents are also considered to be due to their actions on sites other than at the receptor and associated signal transduction levels [153–156]. It should be noted that different β-AR antagonists have been shown to lower the plasma level of catecholamine, whereas ACE inhibitors, which reduce the formation of ANG II, have been demonstrated to produce beneficial effects in CHF similar to those seen with AT_1R antagonists. In addition, the blockade of both SNS and RAS has been reported to be due to reduction in the intensity of oxidative stress [157–159]. Thus, it appears that different hormones such as catecholamines and ANG II, by virtue of the activation of SNS and RAS, induced cardiac remodeling,

subcellular alterations, and CHF by affecting various mechanisms in the myocardium.

Acknowledgments   The work in this article was supported by a grant from the Canadian Institutes of Health Research. The infrastructure support for this project was provided by the St. Boniface Hospital Research Foundation.

References

1. Dhalla NS, Afzal N, Beamish RE, et al. Pathophysiology of cardiac dysfunction in congestive heart failure. Can J Cardiol. 1993;9:873–87.
2. Cohn JN, Bristow MR, Chien KR, et al. Report of the national heart, lung, and blood institute special emphasis panel on heart failure research. Circulation. 1997;95:766–70.
3. Cohn JN, Ferrari R, Sharpe N. Cardiac remodeling – concepts and clinical implications: a consensus paper from an international forum on cardiac remodeling. J Am Coll Cardiol. 2000;35:569–82.
4. Fedak PWM, Verma S, Weisel RD, et al. Cardiac remodeling and failure from molecules to man (Part I). Cardiovasc Physiol. 2005;12:1–11.
5. Ortega Mateo A, de Artinano AA. Highlights on endothelins: a review. Pharm Res. 1997;36:339–51.
6. Declayre C, Swynghedauw B. Molecular mechanisms of myocardial remodeling. The role of aldosterone. J Mol Cell Cardiol. 2002;34:1577–84.
7. Rouleau JL. The neurohumoral hypothesis and the treatment of heart failure. Can J Cardiol. 1996;12(suppl F):3F–8.
8. Dhalla NS, Saini-Chohan HK, Rodriguez-Leyva D, et al. Subcellular remodelling may induce cardiac dysfunction in congestive heart failure. Cardiovasc Res. 2009;81:429–38.
9. Packer M. Neurohormonal interactions and adaptations in congestive heart failure. Circulation. 1998;77:721–30.
10. Swedberg K, Eneroth P, Kjekshus J, et al. Hormones regulating cardiovascular function in patients with severe congestive heart failure and their relation to mortality. CONSENSUS Trial Study Group. Circulation. 1990;82:1730–6.
11. Nicholls DP, Onuoha GN, McDowell G, et al. Neuroendocrine changes in chronic cardiac failure. Basic Res Cardiol. 1996;91 Suppl 1:13–20.
12. Birkeland JA, Sjaastad I, Brattelid T, et al. Effects of treatment with a 5-HT4 receptor antagonist in heart failure. Br J Pharmacol. 2007;150:143–52.
13. Rehsia NS, Dhalla NS. Potential of endothelin-1 and vasopressin antagonists for the treatment of congestive heart failure. Heart Fail Rev. 2010;15:85–101.
14. Feldman AM. Modulation of adrenergic receptors and G-transduction proteins in failing human ventricular myocardium. Circulation. 1993;87(suppl IV):IV27–34.

15. Ahlquist RP. A study of the adrenotropic receptors. Am J Physiol. 1948;I153:586–600.

16. Bohm M, Diett F, Feiler G, et al. α-Adrenoceptors and α-adrenoceptor-mediated positive inotropic effects in failing human myocardium. J Cardiovasc Pharmacol. 1988;12:357–64.

17. Braunwald E, Sonnenblick EH, Ross J. Mechanisms of cardiac contraction and relaxation. In: Braunwald E, editor. Heart disease, a textbook of cardiovascular medicine. Philadelphia: WB Saunders; 1988. p. 383–425.

18. Kurabayashi M, Shibasaki Y, Komuro I, et al. The myosin gene switching in human cardiac hypertrophy. Jpn Circ J. 1990;54:1192–205.

19. Ask JA, Stene-Larsen G, Helle KB, et al. Functional β_1 and β_2 adrenoceptors in the human myocardium. Acta Physiol Scand. 1985;123:81–8.

20. Mugge A, Posselt D, Reimer U, et al. Effects of the β_2-adrenoceptors agonists fenoterol and salbutamol on force of contraction in isolated human ventricular myocardium. Klin Wochenschr. 1985;63:26–31.

21. Bristow MR, Ginsburg R. β_2-receptors are present on myocardial cells in human ventricular myocardium. Am J Cardiol. 1986;57:3F–6.

22. Gilman AG. G proteins: transducers of receptor-generated signals. Annu Rev Biochem. 1987;56:615–49.

23. Johnson GL, Dhanasekaran N. The G-protein family and their interaction with receptors. Endocr Rev. 1989;10:317–31.

24. Birnbaumer L, Aramovitz J, Brown AM. Receptor-effector coupling by G proteins. Biochim Biophys. 1990;1031:163–224.

25. Piano MR, Kim SD, Jarvis C. Cellular events linked to cardiac remodeling in heart failure: targets for pharmacologic intervention. J Cardiovasc Nurs. 2000; 14:1–23.

26. Mark AL. The sympathetic nervous system in hypertension: a potential long-term regulator of arterial pressure. J Hypertens. 1996;14 suppl 5:159–65.

27. Mancia G. Bjorn Folkow Award Lecture: the sympathetic nervous system in hypertension. J Hypertens. 1997;15:1553–65.

28. Julius S, Nesbitt S. Sympathetic overactivity in hypertension. A moving target. Am J Hypertens. 1996;9: 113–20.

29. Esler M, Lambert G, Brunner-La Rocca HP, et al. Sympathetic nerve activity and neurotransmitter release in humans: translation from pathophysiology into clinical practice. Acta Physiol Scand. 2003;177: 275–84.

30. Narkiewicz K. Sympathetic nervous system and hypertension. Gdansk: Via Medica; 2001.

31. Sinski M, Lewandoski J, Abramczyk P, et al. Why study sympathetic nervous system? J Physiol Pharmacol. 2006;57 Suppl 11:79–92.

32. Summers RL, Amsterdam E. Pathophysiology of acute decompensated heart failure. Heart Fail Clin. 2009;5:9–17.

33. White CM. Catecholamines and their blockade in congestive heart failure. Am J Health Syst Pharm. 1998;55:676–82.

34. Lily LS, editor. Pathophysiology of heart disease. Malvern, PA: Lea & Febiger; 1993. p. 147–66.

35. Doval HC, Nul DR, Grancelli HO, et al. Randomised trial of low-dose amiodarone in severe congestive heart failure. Lancet. 1994;344:493–8.

36. Arrigoni LW, Depew CC. Intensive care therapeutics. In: Koda-Kimble M, Young L, editors. Applied therapeutics. 5th ed. Vancouver, WA: Applied therapeutics; 1992. p. 12.1–12.29.

37. Torres RA. Carotid body and sympathetic activation in heart failure: a story of sensors and sensitivity. Cardiovasc Res. 2009;81:633–4.

38. Bristow MR, Hershberger RE, Port JD, et al. β_1 and β_2-adrenergic receptor mediated adenylate cyclase stimulation in nonfailing and failing human ventricular myocardium. Mol Pharmacol. 1989;35:295–303.

39. Asano T, Kamiya N, Morishita R, et al. Immunoassay for the $\beta\gamma$-subunits of GTP-binding proteins and their regional distribution in bovine brain. J Biochem. 1988;103:950–3.

40. Fowler MB, Laser JA, Hopkins GL, et al. Assessment of the β-adrenergic receptor pathway in the intact failing human heart: progressive receptor downregulation and subsensitivity to agonist response. Circulation. 1986;74:1290–302.

41. Hadcock JR, Malbon CC. Down-regulation of β-adrenergic receptors: agonist-induced reduction in mRNA levels. Proc Natl Acad Sci USA. 1988;85:5021–5.

42. Chang HY, Klein RM, Kunos G. Selective desensitization of cardiac beta adrenoceptors by prolonged in vivo infusion of catecholamines in rats. J Pharmacol Exp Ther. 1982;221:784–9.

43. Eschenhagen T, Mende U, Diederich M, et al. Long term β-adrenoceptor-mediated up-regulation of $G_{i\alpha}$ and $G_{o\alpha}$ mRNA level and pertussis toxin-sensitive guanine nucleotide-binding proteins in rat heart. Mol Pharmacol. 1992;42:773–83.

44. Stein B, Bartel S, Kirchhefer U, et al. Relation between contractile function and regulatory cardiac proteins in hypertrophied hearts. Am J Physiol. 1996;270:H2021–8.

45. Linck B, Boknik P, Baba HA, et al. Long term beta adrenoceptor-mediated alteration in contractility and expression of phospholamban and sarcoplasmic reticulum Ca^{++}-ATPase in mammalian ventricle. J Pharmacol Exp Ther. 1998;286:531–8.

46. Leenen FHH, Harmsen E. Antihypertensive drugs and cardiac trophic mechanisms. J Cardiovasc Pharm. 1991;17:S50–7.

47. Zierhut W, Zimmer HG. Significance of myocardial α- and β-adrenoceptors in catecholamine-induced cardiac hypertrophy. Circ Res. 1989;65:1417–25.

48. Lai L, Raju VS, Delehanty JM, Yatani A, Liang C. Altered sarcoplasmic reticulum Ca^{2+} ATPase gene expression in congestive heart failure: effect of chronic norepinephrine infusion. J Mol Cell Cardiol. 1998;30:175–85.

49. Goldstein S. Clinical studies on beta blockers and heart failure preceding the MERIT-HF Trial. Am J Cardiol. 1997;80:501–3.

50. Goldstein S, Gottlieb SS. The impact of beta-blockade on mortality rates in patients with congestive heart failure. J Card Fail. 2000;6(2 suppl1):15–24.

51. Sallach JA, Goldstein S. Use of beta-blockers in congestive heart failure. Ann Med. 2003;35:259–66.

52. Eichorn EJ. Experience with beta-blockers in heart failure mortality trials. Clin Cardiol. 1999;22(Suppl V):V21–9.

53. Thomas J, Marks BH. Plasma norepinephrine in congestive heart failure. Am J Cardiol. 1978;41:233–43.

54. Cohn JN, Levine TB, Olivari MET, et al. Plasma norepinephrine as a guide to prognosis in patients with chronic congestive heart failure. N Engl J Med. 1984;311:819–23.

55. Krum H. Beta-blockers in heart failure. The 'new wave' of clinical trials. Drugs. 1999;58:203–10.

56. BHAT. A randomized trial of propranolol in patients with acute myocardial infarction. I. Mortality results. JAMA. 1982;247:1707–14.

57. ISIS-I. Randomised trial of intravenous atenolol among 16 027 cases of suspected acute myocardial infarction: ISIS-1. First International Study of Infarct Survival Collaborative Group. Lancet. 1986;2: 57–66.

58. MERIT-HF Study Group. Effect of metoprolol CRyXL in chronic heart failure: metoprolol CR/XL randomised intervention trial in congestive heart failure (MERIT-HF). Lancet. 1999;353:2001–7.

59. CIBIS-II Investigators. The Cardiac Insufficiency Bisoprolol Study II (CIBIS-II) : A randomised trial. Lancet. 1999;353:9–13.

60. Dargie HJ. Effect of carvedilol on outcome after myocardial infarction in patients with left-ventricular dysfunction: the CAPRICORN randomised trial. Lancet. 2001;357:1385–90.

61. Packer M, Fowler MB, Roecker EB, et al. Carvedilol Prospective Randomized Cumulative Survival (COPERNICUS) Study Group. Effect of carvedilol on the morbidity of patients with severe chronic heart failure: results of the carvedilol prospective randomized cumulative survival (COPERNICUS) study. Circulation. 2002;106:2194–9.

62. Anderson JL, Lutz JR, Gilbert EM, et al. A randomized trial of low-dose beta blockade therapy for idiopathic dilated cardiomyopathy. Am J Cardiol. 1985;55:471–5.

63. Engelmeier RS, O'Connell JB, Walsh R, et al. Improvement in symptoms and exercise tolerance by metoprolol in patients with dilated cardiomyopathy: a double-blind, randomised placebo-controlled trial. Circulation. 1985;72:536–46.

64. Gilbert EM, Anderson JL, Deitchman D, et al. Long-term β-blocker vasodilator therapy improves cardiac function in idiopathic dilated cardiomyopathy: a double-blind, randomised study of bucindolol versus placebo. Am J Med. 1990;88:223–9.

65. Krum H, Sackner-Bernstein JD, Goldsmith R, et al. Doubleblind, placebo-controlled study of the long-term efficacy of carvedilol in severe chronic heart failure. Circulation. 1995;92:1499–506.

66. Metra M, Nardi M, Giubbini R, et al. Effects of short-term and long-term carvedilol administration on rest and exercise hemodynamic variables, exercise capacity and clinical conditions in patients with idiopathic dilated cardiomyopathy. J Am Coll Cardiol. 1994;24:1678–87.

67. Olsen SL, Gilbert EM, Renlund DG, et al. Carvedilol improves left ventricular function and symptoms in chronic heart failure: a double-blind randomised study. J Am Coll Cardiol. 1995;25:1225–31.

68. Packer M, Coats AJ, Fowler MB, et al. Effect of carvedilol on survival in severe chronic heart failure. N Engl J Med. 2001;344:1651–8.

69. Perlini S, Ferrero I, Palladini G. Survival benefits of different antiadrenergic interventions in pressure overload left ventricular hypertrophy/failure. Hypertension. 2006;48:93–7.

70. Maczewski M, Mackiewicz U. Effect of metoprolol and ivabradine on left ventricular remodelling and Ca^{2+} handling in the post-infarction rat heart. Cardiovasc Res. 2008;79:42–51.

71. Sun YL, Hu SJ, Wang LH, et al. Effect of beta-blockers on cardiac function and calcium handling protein in postinfarction heart failure rats. Chest. 2005; 128:1812–21.

72. Omerovic E, Bollano E, Soussi B, et al. Selective beta1-blockade attenuates post-infarct remodelling without improvement in myocardial energy metabolism and function in rats with heart failure. Eur J Heart Fail. 2003;5:725–32.

73. Omerovic E, Bollano E, Mobini R, Madhu B, et al. Selective beta(1)-blockade improves cardiac bioenergetics and function and decreases neuroendocrine activation in rats during early postinfarct remodeling. Biochem Biophys Res Commun. 2001;281:491–8.

74. Latini R, Masson S, Jeremic G, et al. Comparative efficacy of a DA2/alpha2 agonist and a beta-blocker in reducing adrenergic drive and cardiac fibrosis in an experimental model of left ventricular dysfunction after coronary artery occlusion. J Cardiovasc Pharmacol. 1998;31:601–8.

75. Feuerstein GZ, Yue TL, Cheng HY, et al. Myocardial protection by the novel vasodilating beta-blocker, carvedilol: potential relevance of anti-oxidant activity. J Hyperten Suppl. 1993;11:S41–8.

76. Weir MR, Dzau VJ. The renin-angiotensin-aldosterone system: a specific target for hypertension management. Am J Hypertens. 1995;12:205S–13.

77. Sealey JH, Laragh JH. The renin-angiotensin-aldosterone system for normal regulation of blood pressure and sodium and potassium homeostasis. In: Laragh JH, Brenner BM, editors. Pathophysiology, diagnosis and management. New York: Raven; 1990. p. 1287–99.

78. Zhang W, Elimban V, Nijjar S. Role of renin-angiotensin system in the development of cardiav hypertrophy and heart failure. In: Hargens A, Takeda N, Singal PK, editors. Adaptation biology and medicine. Volume 4. Current concepts. New Dehli: Narosa; 2005. p. 239–57.

79. Francis GS, Cohn JN, Johnson G, et al. Plasma norepinephrine, plasma-renin activity, and congestive heart failure. Relations to survival and the effects of therapy in V-HeFT II. The V-HeFT VA Cooperative Studies Group. Circulation. 1993;87(suppl VI): 40–8.

80. Torre-Amione G, Kapadia S, Lee J, et al. Tumor necrosis factor-alpha and tumor necrosis factor receptors in the failing human heart. Circulation. 1996;93: 704–11.

81. Torre-Amione G, Kapadia S, Benedict C, et al. Proinflammatory cytokine levels in patients with depressed left ventricular ejection fraction: a report from the study of left ventricular dysfunction (SOLVD). J Am Coll Cardiol. 1996;27:1201–6.

82. Hasenfuss G. Animal models of human cardiovascular disease, heart failure and hypertrophy. Cardiovasc Res. 1998;39:60–76.

83. Francis GS, Goldsmith SR, Levine BT, et al. The neurohumoral axis in congestive heart failure. Ann Intern Med. 1984;101:370–7.

84. Mettauer B, Rouleau JL, Bichet D, et al. Sodium and water excretion abnormalities in congestive heart failure. Ann Intern Med. 1986;105:161–7.

85. Baig MK, Mahon N, McKenna WJ, et al. The pathophysiology of advanced heart failure. Am Heart J. 1998;135:S216–30.

86. Zhang J, Pfaffendorf M, van Zwietien PA. Positive inotropic action of angiotensin II in the pithed rat. Naunyn-Schmiedeberg's Arch Pharmacol. 1993;347:658–63.

87. Ju H, Scammell-La Fleur T, Dixon IMC. Altered mRNA abundance of calcium transport genes in cardiac myocytes induced by angiotensin II. J Mol Cell Cardiol. 1996;28:1119–28.

88. Rouet-Benzineb P, Gontero B, Dreyfus P, et al. Angiotensin II induces nuclear factor-κB activation in cultured neonatal rat cardiomyocytes through protein kinase C signaling pathway. J Mol Cell Cardiol. 2000;32:1767–78.

89. Mimran A, Ribstein J. Angiotensin receptor blockers: pharmacology and clinical significance. J Am Soc Nephrol. 1999;10:S273–7.

90. Leckie BJ. Targeting the renin-angiotensin system: what's new? Curr Med Chem Cardiovasc Hematol Agents. 2005;3:23–32.

91. Jugdutt BI, Schwarz-Michorowski BL, Khan MI. Effect of long-term captopril therapy on left ventricular remodeling and function during healing of canine myocardial infarction. J Am Coll Cardiol. 1992; 19:713–21.

92. McDonald KM, Chu C, Francis GS, et al. Effect of delayed intervention with ACE-inhibitor therapy on myocyte hypertrophy and growth of the cardiac interstitium in the rat model myocardial infarction. J Mol Cell Cardiol. 1997;29:3203–10.

93. Dixon IMC, Ju H, Jassal DS, et al. Effect of ramipril and losartan on collagen expression in right and left heart after myocardial infarction. Mol Cell Biochem. 1996;165:31–45.

94. McConnaughey MM, McConnaughey JS, Ingenito AJ. Practical considerations of the pharmacology of angiotensin receptor blockers. J Clin Pharmacol. 1999;39:547–59.

95. Granger CB, McMurray JJ, Yusuf S, et al. Effects of candesartan in patients with chronic heart failure and reduced left-ventricular systolic function intolerant to angiotensin-converting-enzyme inhibitors: the CHARM-Alternative trial. Lancet. 2003;362:772–6.

96. Huang BS, Ahmad M, Tan J, et al. Chronic central versus systemic blockade of AT1 receptors and cardiac dysfunction in rats post myocardial infarction. Am J Physiol Heart Circ Physiol. 2009;297: H968–75.

97. Xu X, Wan W, Ji L, et al. Exercise training combined with angiotensin II receptor blockade limits post-infarct ventricular remodelling in rats. Cardiovasc Res. 2008;78:523–32.

98. Fraccarollo D, Galuppo P, Schmidt I, et al. Additive amelioration of left ventricular remodeling and molecular alterations by combined aldosterone and angiotensin receptor blockade after myocardial infarction. Cardiovasc Res. 2005;67:97–105.

99. Shah KR, Ganguly PK, Netticadan T, et al. Changes in skeletal muscle SR Ca2+ pump in congestive heart failure due to myocardial infarction are prevented by angiotensin II blockade. Can J Physiol Pharmacol. 2004;82:438–47.

100. Guo X, Chapman D, Dhalla NS. Partial prevention of changes in SR gene expression in congestive heart failure due to myocardial infarction by enalapril or losartan. Mol Cell Biochem. 2003;254:163–72.

101. Gurevich AK, Falk SA, Nemenoff RA, et al. Effects of angiotensin receptor blockade on haemodynamics and gene expression after myocardial infarction. Drugs R D. 2002;3:239–49.

102. El-Sabban ME, Hassan KA, Birbari AE, et al. Angiotensin II binding and extracellular matrix remodelling in a rat model of myocardial infarction. J Renin Angiotensin Aldosterone Sys. 2000;1: 369–78.

103. Zhu YZ, Zhu YC, Li J, et al. Effects of losartan on haemodynamic parameters and angiotensin receptor mRNA levels in rat heart after myocardial infarction. J Renin Angiotensin Aldosterone Syst. 2000;1: 257–62.

104. Jain M, Liao R, Ngoy S, et al. Angiotensin II receptor blockade attenuates the deleterious effects of exercise training on post-MI ventricular remodelling in rats. Cardiovasc Res. 2000;46:66–72.

105. Thai HM, Van HT, Gaballa MA, et al. Effects of AT1 receptor blockade after myocardial infarct on myocardial fibrosis, stiffness, and contractility. Am J Physiol. 1999;276:H873–80.

106. Ambrose J, Pribnow DG, Giraud GD, et al. Angiotensin type 1 receptor antagonism with irbesartan inhibits ventricular hypertrophy and improves diastolic function in the remodeling post-myocardial infarction ventricle. J Cardiovasc Pharmacol. 1999; 33:433–9.

107. Youn TJ, Kim HS, Oh BH. Ventricular remodeling and transforming growth factor-beta 1 mRNA expression after nontransmural myocardial infarction in rats: effects of angiotensin converting enzyme inhibition and angiotensin II type 1 receptor blockade. Basic Res Cardiol. 1999;94:246–53.

108. Hanatani A, Yoshiyama M, Takeuchi K, et al. Angiotensin II type 1-receptor antagonist candesartan cilexitil prevents left ventricular dysfunction in myocardial infarcted rats. Jpn J Pharmacol. 1998;78:45–54.

109. Taylor K, Patten RD, Smith JJ, et al. Divergent effects of angiotensin-converting enzyme inhibition and angiotensin II-receptor antagonism on myocardial cellular proliferation and collagen deposition after myocardial infarction in rats. J Cardiovasc Pharmacol. 1998;31:654–60.

110. Milavetz JJ, Raya TE, Johnson CS, et al. Survival after myocardial infarction in rats: captopril versus losartan. J Am Coll Cardiol. 1996;27:714–9.

111. Schieffer B, Wirger A, Meybrunn M, et al. Comparative effects of chronic angiotensin-converting enzyme inhibition and angiotensin II type 1 receptor blockade on cardiac remodeling after myocardial infarction in the rat. Circulation. 1994;89:2273–82.

112. Smits JF, van Krimpen C, Schoemaker RG, et al. Angiotensin II receptor blockade after myocardial infarction in rats: effects on hemodynamics, myocardial DNA synthesis, and interstitial collagen content. J Cardiovasc Pharmacol. 1992;20:772–8.

113. Raya TE, Fonken SJ, Lee RW, et al. Hemodynamic effects of direct angiotensin II blockade compared to converting enzyme inhibition in rat model of heart failure. Am J Hyperten. 1991;4:334S–40.

114. Pitt B, Segal R, Martinez FA, et al. Randomised trial of losartan versus captopril in patients over 65 with heart failure (Evaluation of Losartan in the Elderly Study, ELITE). Lancet. 1997;349:747–52.

115. McKelvie RS, Yusuf S, Pericak D, et al. Comparison of candesartan, enalapril, and their combination in congestive heart failure: randomized evaluation of strategies for left ventricular dysfunction (RESOLVD) pilot study. The RESOLVD Pilot Study Investigators. Circulation. 1999;100:1056–64.

116. Pitt B, Poole-Wilson PA, Segal R, et al. Effect of losartan compared with captopril on mortality in patients with symptomatic heart failure: randomised trial – the Losartan Heart Failure Survival Study ELITE II. Lancet. 2000;355:1582–7.

117. Dahlöf B, Devereux RB, Kjeldsen SE, et al. LIFE Study Group. Cardiovascular morbidity and mortality in the Losartan Intervention For Endpoint reduction in hypertension study (LIFE): a randomised trial against atenolol. Lancet. 2002;359:995–1003.

118. Dickstein K, Kjekshus J. Effects of losartan and captopril on mortality and morbidity in high-risk patients after acute myocardial infarction: the OPTIMAAL randomised trial. Optimal Trial in Myocardial Infarction with Angiotensin II Antagonist Losartan. Lancet. 2002;360:752–60.

119. Solomon SD, Velazquez EJ, White H, et al. Hypertension and the risk of adverse cardiovascular outcomes following MI: the VALIANT experience. Program and abstracts of the European Society of Cardiology Congress 2004; 2004 Aug 28–Sep 1; Munich, Germany.

120. Yusuf S, Pfeffer MA, Swedberg K, et al. Effects of candesartan in patients with chronic heart failure and preserved left-ventricular ejection fraction: the CHARM-Preserved Trial. Lancet. 2003;362:777–81.

121. McMurray JJ, Ostergren J, Swedberg K, et al. Effects of candesartan in patients with chronic heart failure and reduced left-ventricular systolic function taking angiotensin-converting-enzyme inhibitors: the CHARM-Added trial. Lancet. 2003;362:767–71.

122. Yusuf S. From the HOPE to the ONTARGET and the TRANSCEND studies: challenges in improving prognosis. Am J Cardiol. 2002;89:18A–25. discussion 25A-26A.

123. Lang RM, Elkayam U, Yellen LG, et al. Comparative effects of losartan and enalapril on exercise capacity and clinical status in patients with heart failure. The Losartan Pilot Exercise Study Investigators. J Am Coll Cardiol. 1997;30:983–91.

124. Lee VC, Rhew DC, Dylan M, et al. Meta-analysis: angiotensin-receptor blockers in chronic heart failure and high-risk acute myocardial infarction. Ann Intern Med. 2004;141:693–704. Erratum in Ann Intern Med. 2005;42:391.

125. Carson P, Massie BM, McKelvie R, et al. The irbesartan in heart failure with preserved systolic function (I-Preserve). J Card Fail. 2005;11:576–85.

126. Murdoch DR, McDonagh TA, Farmer R, et al. ADEPT: Addition of the AT1 receptor antagonist eprosartan to ACE inhibitor therapy in chronic heart failure trial: hemodynamic and neurohormonal effects. Am Heart J. 2001;141:800–7.

127. Pfeffer MA, McMurray JJV, Velazquez EJ, et al. Valsartan, Captopril, or both in myocardial infarction complicated by heart failure, left ventricular dysfunction, or both. N Engl J Med. 2003;349:1893–906.

128. Hamroff G, Katz SD, Mancini D, et al. Addition of angiotensin II receptor blockade to maximal angiotensin-converting enzyme inhibition improves exercise capacity in patients with severe congestive heart failure. Circulation. 1999;99:990–2.

129. Blanchet M, Sheppard R, Currier D, et al. Dual angiotensin-II suppression with an angiotensin-converting enzyme inhibitor and irbesartan improves submaximal exercise time without changes in exercise-induced neurohormonal response in patients with CHF. Program and abstracts from the American College of Cardiology 53rd Annual Scientific Session; 2004; Abstract 1012–129.

130. Tatti P, Pahor M, Byington RP, et al. Outcome results of the Fosinopril Versus Amlodipine Cardiovascular Events Randomized Trial (FACET) in patients with hypertension and NIDDM. Diabetes Care. 1998;21:597–603.

131. Ren B, Shao Q, Ganguly PK, et al. Influence of long-term treatment of imidapril on mortality, cardiac function, and gene expression in congestive heart failure due to myocardial infarction. Can J Physiol Pharmacol. 2004;82:1118–27.

132. Yoshiyama M, Takeuchi K, Hanatani A, et al. Effect of cilazapril on ventricular remodeling assessed by Doppler-echocardiographic assessment and cardiac gene expression. Cardiovasc Drugs Ther. 1998;12:57–70.

133. Zhang G, Shen X, Pu S, et al. Comparative effects of losartan and captopril on ventricular remodeling and function after myocardial infarction in the rat. Chin Med Sci J. 1998;13:32–6.

134. Sethi R, Shao Q, Ren B, et al. Changes in beta-adrenoceptors in heart failure due to myocardial infarction are attenuated by blockade of renin-angiotensin system. Mol Cell Biochem. 2004;263:11–20.

135. Daniëls MC, Keller RS, de Tombe PP. Losartan prevents contractile dysfunction in rat myocardium after left ventricular myocardial infarction. Am J Physiol Heart Circ Physiol. 2001;281:H2150–8.

136. Esler M, Kaye D. Measurement of sympathetic nervous system activity in heart failure. Heart Fail Rev. 2005;5:17–525.

137. Takano H, Hasegawa H, Nagai T, et al. Implication of cardiac remodling in heart failure. Mechanisms and therapeutic strategies. Inter Med. 2003;42:465–9.

138. Dhalla NS, Heyliger CE, Beamish RE, et al. Pathophysiological aspects of myocardial hypertrophy. Can J Cardiol. 1987;4:183–96.

139. Pelouch V, Dixon IMC, Golfman L, et al. Role of extracellular matrix proteins in heart function. Mol Cell Biochem. 1994;129:101–20.

140. Dhalla NS, Wang X, Sethi R, et al. Beta-adrenergic linked signal transduction mechanisms in failing hearts. Heart Fail Rev. 1997;2:55–65.

141. Dhalla NS, Dent MR, Tappia PS, et al. Subcellular remodeling as a viable target for the treatment of congestive heart failure. J Cardiovasc Pharmacol Therapeut. 2006;11:31–45.

142. Spinale FG. Myocardial matrix remodeling and the matrix metalloproteinases: influence on cardiac form and function. Physiol Rev. 2007;87:1285–342.

143. Rysa J, Leskinen H, Ilves M, et al. Distinct upregulation of extra-cellulular matrix genes in transition from hypertrophy to hypertensive heart failure. Hypertension. 2005;45:927–33.

144. Weisser-Thomas J, Kubo H, Hefner CA, et al. The Na$^+$/Ca^{2+} exchanger/SR Ca^{2+} ATPase transport capacity regulates the contractility of normal and hypertrophied feline ventricular myocytes. J Card Fail. 2005;11:380–7.

145. Yano M, Yamamoto T, Ikemoto N, et al. Abnormal ryanodine receptor function in heart failure. Pharmacol Ther. 2005;107:377–91.

146. Machackova J, Barta J, Dhalla NS. Myofibrillar remodeling in cardiac hypertrophy, heart failure and cardiomyopathies. Can J Cardiol. 2006;22:953–68.

147. Babick AP, Dhalla NS. Role of subcellular remodeling in cardiac dysfunction due to congestive heart failure. Med Princ Prac. 2007;16:81–9.

148. Schillinger W, Schneider H, Minami K, et al. Importance of sympathetic activation for the expression of Na$^+$-Ca^{2+} exchanger in end-stage failing human myocardium. Eur Heart J. 2002;23:1118–24.

149. Sabbah HN. The cellular and physiologic effects of beta-blockers in heart failure. Clinical Cardiol. 1999;22 Suppl 5:V16–20.

150. Machackova J, Sanganalmath SK, Elimban V, et al. β-adrenergic blockade attenuates cardiac dysfunction and myofibrillar remodeling in congestive heart failure. J Cell Mol Med. 2011;15:545–54.

151. Satoh S, Ueda Y, Suematsu N, et al. Beneficial effects of angiotensin-coverting enzyme inhibition on sarcoplasmic reticulum function in the failing heart of the Dahl rat. Circ J. 2003;67:705–11.

152. Panagia V, Pierce GN, Dhalla KS, et al. Adaptive changes in subcellular calcium transport during catecholamine-induced cardiomyopathy. J Mol Cell Cardiol. 1985;17:411–20.

153. Machackova J, Sanganalmath SK, Barta J, et al. Amelioration of cardiac remodelling in congestive heart failure by beta-adrenoceptor blockade is associated with depression in sympathetic activity. Cardiovasc Toxicol. 2009;10:9–16.

154. Brophy JM, Joseph L, Rouleau JL. Beta-blockers in congestive heart failure. A Bayesian meta-analysis. Ann Intern Med. 2001;134:550–60.

155. Cleland JG, Bristow MR, Erdmann E, et al. Beta-blocking agents in heart failure. Should they be used and how? Eur Heart J. 1996;17:1629–39.

156. Hu K, Gaudron P, Ertl G. Long-term effects of beta-adrenergic blocking agent treatment on hemodynamic function and left ventricular remodeling in rats with experimental myocardial infarction. Importance of timing of treatment and infarct size. J Am Coll Cardiol. 1998;31:692–700.

157. Adameova A, Abdellatif Y, Dhalla NS. Role of the excessive amounts of circulation catrecholamines and glucocorticoids in stress-induced heart disease. Can J Phys Pharm. 2009;87:493–514.

158. Tsutsui H, Ide T, Kinugawa S. Mitochondrial oxidative stress, DNA damage and heart failure. Antioxid Redox Signal. 2006;8:1737–44.

159. Khaper N, Singal PK. Modulation of oxidative stress by a selective inhibition of angiotensin II type 1 receptors in MI rats. J Am Coll Cardiol. 2001;37:1461–6.

Modulators of Remodeling After Myocardial Infarction

Bodh I. Jugdutt

Abstract

Remodeling of the heart wounded by myocardial infarction (MI) refers to the sum total of adaptive and maladaptive changes in myocardial structure, geometric shape, and function that occur over time after the initial event. Its consequences are most sinister in the patient with a large anterior transmural MI, also clinically known as the ST-segment MI (STEMI) in the early hours or Q-wave MI in later stages. It is recognized that these infarcts undergo adverse remodeling that leads to progressive left ventricular (LV) remodeling, which is the central mechanism in the march to ventricular dilatation, ventricular dysfunction, congestive heart failure, disability, and death. Over time, remodeling in survivors extends to other cardiac chambers, tissues, cells, and molecules, resulting in a vicious cycle leading to end-stage heart disease with significant morbidity and mortality. Knowledge of the modulators of the remodeling process is critical in efforts to prevent, interrupt, or limit the progression toward end-stage heart failure or reverse it. The focus of this chapter is on some key modulators of the post-MI remodeling process.

Keywords

Aging • Cytokines • Fibrosis • Growth factors • Healing • Macrophages • Matrix proteases • Myocardial infarction • Remodeling • Reperfusion

Introduction

Remodeling of the heart wounded by myocardial infarction (MI) refers to the sum total of adaptive and maladaptive changes in myocardial structure, geometric shape, and function that occur over time after the initial event [1–5]. Its consequences are most sinister in the patient with a large anterior transmural MI, clinically known as the ST-segment

B.I. Jugdutt (✉)
Division of Cardiology, Department of Medicine,
University of Alberta and Hospitals,
Edmonton, Alberta, Canada
e-mail: bjugdutt@ualberta.ca

N.S. Dhalla, M. Nagano, B. Ostadal (eds.), *Molecular Defects in Cardiovascular Disease*,
DOI 10.1007/978-1-4419-7130-2_17, © Springer Science+Business Media, LLC 2011

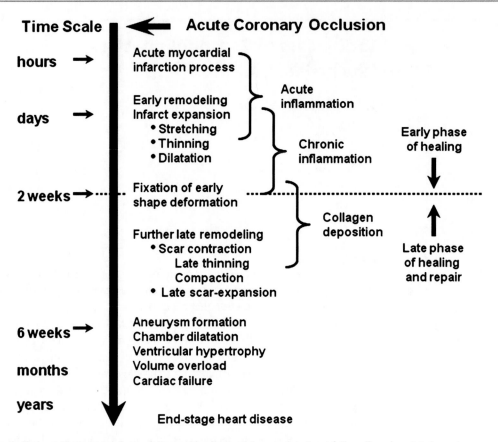

Fig. 1 Early and late stages of remodeling and healing and the march to heart failure. Based on data in canine myocardial infarction and supported by human data

MI (STEMI) in the early hours and Q-wave MI in later stages. Such infarcts result in adverse left ventricular (LV) remodeling and poor outcome [6–10]. Three decades of bench to bedside research have established that these infarcts undergo early infarct remodeling that leads to progressive remodeling of the entire left ventricle, which is the central mechanism in the relentless march to ventricular dilatation, dysfunction, heart failure, disability, and death (Fig. 1) [2–5]. Ventricular remodeling begins early during the infarction phase [6–12], and continues during the subsequent healing phase after MI and extends well beyond [2–5, 11–14]. Multiple factors modulate the postinfarction remodeling process and include changes in myocardium, vascular tissue, and the extracellular matrix (ECM) [1–5, 15–17]. Over time, the remodeling process in survivors of acute MI extends to other cardiac chambers, tissues, cells, and molecules, resulting in a vicious cycle leading to end-stage heart disease with significant morbidity and mortality (Fig. 2) [2–5]. Knowledge of the modulators of the post-MI remodeling process is therefore critical in efforts to prevent, interrupt or limit the progression toward end-stage heart failure or reverse it. Several key modulators of the post-MI remodeling process were identified previously [2–5, 11, 12], and several of them have received attention and have been applied in patients [1, 18, 19], but several others such as the healing process [2–5, 20–23] and impact of the aging process [24, 25] need intensive study.

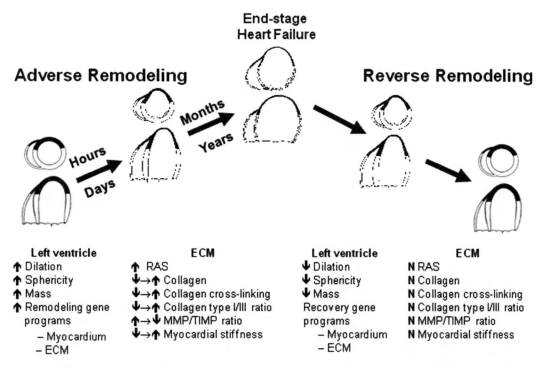

Fig. 2 Adverse ventricular and extracellular matrix remodeling and reversal. Schematic depicts the features of left ventricular and extracellular matrix (ECM) remodeling and geometric changes in long- and short-axis sections. *Dark areas* represent the area of myocardial infarction. *MMP* matrix metalloproteinase, *RAS* renin–angiotensin system, *TIMP* tissue inhibitor of matrix metalloproteinase, *N* normal

Modulators of Postinfarction Ventricular Remodeling

Our research over the last 3 decades has focused on ventricular and ECM remodeling during postinfarct healing, its mechanisms and reversal [2–5, 26–29]. We studied patients and experimental animals including dogs as a pertinent preclinical model [30, 31], as well as rats and mice to gain insight into basic mechanisms. Early studies identified five key modulators of structural postinfarction ventricular remodeling that proved useful for developing therapeutic strategies. These are the processes of infarction, regional shape deformation, ECM remodeling, healing, and progressive ventricular dilatation. Various aspects of these key structural modulators can be targeted for limiting LV remodeling and preserving shape, size, and systolic function after MI (Fig. 3) [2–5].

The Infarction Process and Early Remodeling

Pioneer work by Professor Eugene Braunwald and associates in the early- and mid-1970s identified major determinants of infarct size. They emphasized the concept of myocardial oxygen supply and demand that led to interventions for myocardial protection during early hours after coronary artery occlusion. Studies by Reimer and Jennings in the mid- and late-1970s showed that the acute infarction process involves a march to necrosis, with transmural progression from endocardium to epicardium over several hours [32]. We demonstrated that the march to and distribution of infarction depend on the transmural distribution of myocardial blood flow within the anatomical region at risk [33, 34]. The latter works led to the preclinical testing of several early interventions for modifying infarct size relative

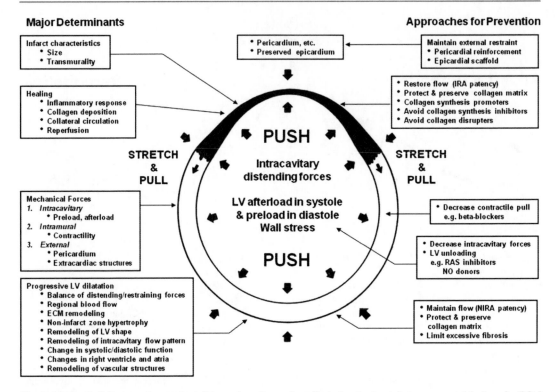

Fig. 3 Mechanical forces acting on the infarct and noninfarct segments and determinants of postinfarction ventricular remodeling. These forces acting on a beat-to-beat basis lead to remodeling of both infarct and noninfarct segments. Short-axis section of the left ventricle showing the diastolic bulge in the infarct segment (*darkened*). *ECM* extracellular matrix, *IRA* infarct-related artery, *LV* left ventricular, *NIRA* noninfarct-related artery, *NO* nitric oxide, *RAS* renin–angiotensin system

to the region at risk [35, 36]. Two-dimensional (2D) echocardiography was validated for the noninvasive assessment of infarct size [37], and for demonstrating the limitation of infarct size [38].

Also in the late 1970s, a pathological study by Bulkley and Hutchins first demonstrated that 50% of patients who died within 30 days of acute MI had infarct expansion, which was most severe in those with large, transmural, and anterior MI [39]. A subsequent clinical study first showed that 50% of patients with early infarct expansion on 2D echocardiography died by 8 weeks [40]. Our studies in the 1980s showed that infarct expansion with regional bulging of the infarct zone on 2D echocardiography was a marker for rupture of the ventricular septum [6] and aneurysm formation [7] and poor outcome in patients with MI [10]. Several studies in the 1980s helped to identify the determinants of early infarct expansion and its role in progressive LV remodeling

as well as potential approaches to limit it (Fig. 4) [2–5, 26–29].

Although infarct size and collateral blood flow are major determinants of LV remodeling and outcome, detailed studies showed that infarct limitation by vasodilator therapy may be jeopardized by excessive reduction of blood pressure resulting in impaired perfusion [13, 41, 42], suggesting the need for caution. Although reperfusion of the infarct-related artery, aimed at improving flow to myocardium at risk [32] became the undisputed early therapy of choice for acute MI in the mid-1980s and has proven benefits [43] in moderate to large MI, it is associated with significant reperfusion damage to myocardium through necrosis and apoptosis [44–46], ECM damage through increased matrix metalloproteinases (MMPs) [16, 47, 48], and microvasculature damage [44] leading to persistent LV dysfunction [44] and remodeling [49]. In addition,

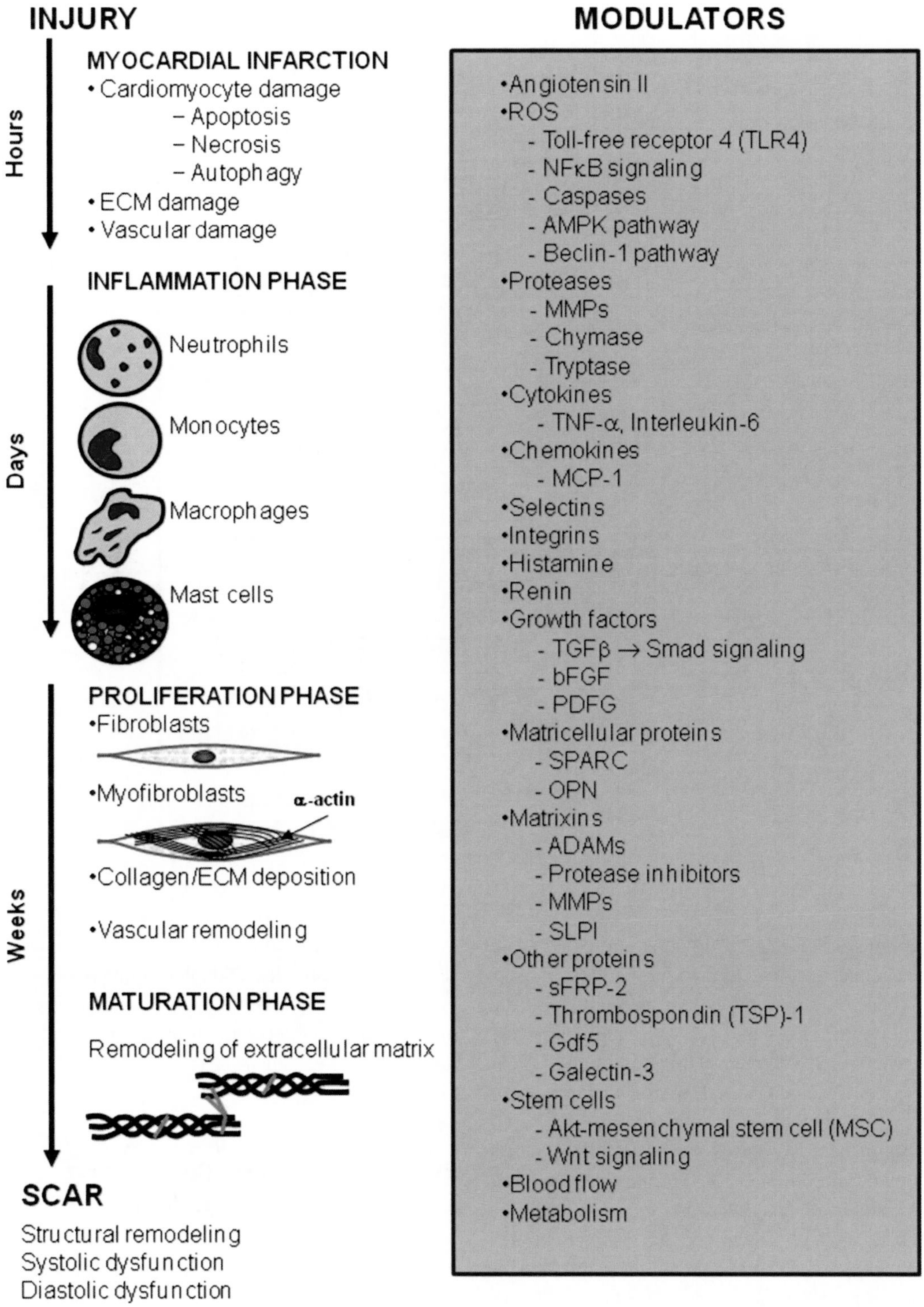

Fig. 4 Cellular and molecular changes during postinfarct healing and known modulators. *ADAM* a-disintegrin metalloproteinase, *AMPK* AMP-activated protein kinase, *bFGF* basic fibroblast growth factor, *ECM* extracellular matrix, *Gdf5* growth differentiation factor-5, *MCP-1* monocyte chemoattractant protein-1, *MMPs* matrix metalloproteinases, *OPN* osteopontin, *PDFG* platelet-derived growth factor, *ROS* reactive oxygen species, *sFRP-2* secreted frizzled-related protein-2, *SLPI* secretory leucocyte protease inhibitor, *SPARC* secreted protein acidic and rich in cysteine, *TGF-b* transforming growth factor-β, *TNF-a* tumor necrosis factor-α

Fig. 5 Potentially
targetable modulators
of postinfarct remodeling.
Abbreviations as in
Fig. 4 and in text

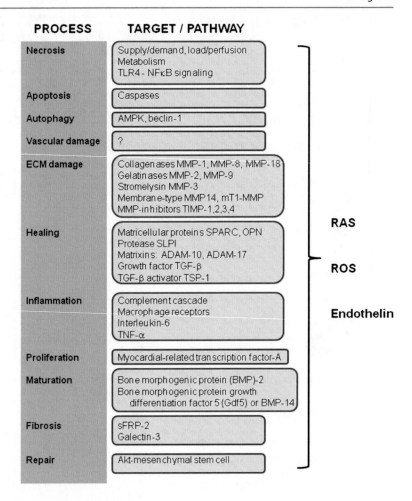

reperfusion enhances inflammation [25] and accelerates healing albeit in rats [50].

Four other points deserve mention. First, the infarction process and early remodeling process are both highly dynamic. It is important in translational research to allow for differences in temporal evolution of infarction and different rates of necrosis across species, namely, within about 30 min in mice, 30–90 min in rats, 30 min to hours in rabbits, 2–6 h in dogs, 4–8 h in pigs, and 6–14 h in humans [2, 5]. Second, besides physiological factors that influence infarct size, the renin–angiotensin system (RAS), with angiotensin II as the primary effector peptide, exerts an important regulatory role. Third, reactive oxygen species (ROS) and oxidative stress play an important role in modulation of necrosis. Fourth,

genetic and molecular studies have implicated several genes, proteins, and intersecting pathways that modulate the infarction process (Fig. 5) and may become targets for limiting remodeling through this mechanism.

Extracellular Matrix Remodeling and Progressive Remodeling

Four points deserve mention here. First, evidence [2–5, 20] indicates that ECM degradation after MI is a key factor in infarct remodeling and progressive LV enlargement, and angiotensin II, a cytokine and primary mediator of the RAS, plays a regulatory role in ECM and LV remodeling.

Although increased MMPs relative to tissue inhibitors of MMPs (TIMPs) is the widely accepted pathway to ECM degradation and LV remodeling [16, 17], failure of MMP inhibition initiated after acute STEMI to limit LV remodeling [51] suggests that ECM damage occurred earlier and/or other matrix proteins besides MMPs may contribute to damage [25].

Second, although over 20 MMPs and 4 TIMPs have been identified, some MMPs, such as MMP-2 and MMP-9, were shown to play a major role in LV remodeling [16, 17], and all four TIMPS have been implicated (Fig. 5). Evidence suggests that a balance between MMPs and TIMPs is critical for normal ECM remodeling. A sharp rise in MMPs post-MI and a high MMP/TIMP ratio result in rapid ECM degradation, decreased collagen, adverse ECM and LV remodeling, and LV dysfunction [16, 17, 52]. Although MMP and TIMP levels subside over days, a chronically high MMP–TIMP ratio may promote continued ECM degradation and contribute to progressive LV dilatation during healing, whereas a low MMP–TIMP ratio may contribute to increased ECM and fibrosis and diastolic dysfunction.

Third, emerging evidence suggests that interactions between matrix proteases and inflammatory cytokines may modulate ECM damage [25]. Fourth, studies in humans and genetic animal models have identified several proteins and pathways that may be potential targets for limiting ECM remodeling (Fig. 5).

The Healing Process and Progressive Remodeling

It is now accepted that infarct healing and LV remodeling are concurrent dynamic processes and LV remodeling progresses during healing [2–5]. Ten points deserve special emphasis. First, extensive studies in animals and humans have shown that healing after MI involves an orchestrated sequence of 3 sets of events over time: (1) inflammation - acute and chronic, (2) tissue repair – with fibroblast proliferation, deposition

of ECM (that consist mostly of collagen) by fibroblasts and myofibroblasts (that contain α-actin), and formation of a firm living scar, and (3) structural and functional remodeling of both infarcted and noninfarcted myocardium through dilatation followed by remote hypertrophy and angiogenesis (Figs. 1 and 4) [2–5, 16, 17].

Second, while considerable remodeling of damaged and preserved myocardium occurs in timed sequence, it is again important in translational research to recognize the different rates of healing across species [2–5, 29]. Thus, healing to the collagen plateau [15] takes about 1 week in mice, 3 weeks in rats, 6 weeks in dogs, and 6 weeks to 6 months in humans depending on infarct size [20, 21]. Evidence suggests that infarct size is a critical factor affecting the intensity and rate of healing, reparative and remodeling responses, and functional outcome [2, 16]. In dogs, small MIs usually heal within 6 weeks, with a firm scar and preservation of LV shape, size, and systolic function [16]; large MIs heal slowly, with impaired and delayed healing over months, resulting in adverse LV remodeling that negatively impacts function and clinical outcome [2, 16]. Importantly, reperfusion alters the healing substrate and accelerates infarct healing [50].

Third, regional differences have profound implications for pathophysiology and therapy and are often overlooked. For example, the regional distribution of fibrosis and the quality and quantity of collagen in infarct and noninfarct zones impact regional and global LV remodeling. Normally, the quantity of collagen and amount of fibrosis by the end of the healing phase are several times greater in infarct than noninfarct zones [16, 17]. The type of collagen that is deposited early during healing (i.e., type III collagen) is immature, weak, and distensible so that the healing infarct area is more susceptible to dilatation and thinning (Fig. 3). As this collagen matures to the stronger and less distensible type I collagen over weeks toward the end of the healing phase, the scar becomes less prone to dilatation from increased cardiac load [16, 53].

Fourth, a window of increased vulnerability for adverse remodeling develops during the healing phase. The window is the result of rapid ECM degradation early post-MI followed by slow synthesis, deposition of collagen type III and slow maturation to type I. This window provides opportunity for therapeutic interventions to limit remodeling.

Fifth, the decrease in ECM and mature collagen during early healing favors adverse LV remodeling, dysfunction and cardiac rupture, a most catastrophic complication of MI [16, 17]. Studies in young mice, in which post-MI rupture is very common, suggest that ECM damage through MMPs mediates both adverse LV remodeling and rupture [48]. In humans, thrombolytic therapy has been implicated in spontaneous rupture after reperfused-MI and involves MMP activation [17, 24, 48]. We have previously documented cardiac rupture and significant LV remodeling in patients with transmural MI, suggesting that infarct size and transmurality are contributing factors [6–9]. In the dog model, rupture induced by high afterload in healed infarcted hearts was also linked to decreased and defective collagen [53, 54].

Sixth, inflammatory mediators play a regulatory role in healing and remodeling. Evidence suggests that inflammatory, fibroblast and vascular cells, growth factors and cytokines influence remodeling during post-MI healing [16, 17, 55]. Fibrogenic growth factors such as transforming growth factor (TGF)-β1 and proinflammatory cytokines including angiotensin II, tumor necrosis factor (TNF)-α, and interleukin (IL)-6 are released into the interstitial space where they modulate MMPs and TIMPs, ECM degradation, interstitial fibrosis, and remodeling [16,17]. Anti-inflammatory cytokines, such as IL-10 and TGF-β1, released after MI may have favorable effects on LV remodeling and function. Importantly, angiotensin II modulates the inflammatory markers [25].

Seventh, evidence suggests that TGF-β signaling plays a very critical role in post-MI healing and remodeling but there are temporal differences [16, 21]. During early healing, TGF-β exerts anti-inflammatory effects with repression of inflammation, macrophage deactivation and resolution of inflammatory infiltrate; during late healing, TGF-β activates profibrotic pathways with fibroblast

activation and ECM deposition, and myocyte hypertrophy [21]. TGF-β null mice show excessive inflammation and early death [21]. Additionally, early TGF-β activation protects against early myocardial damage, whereas sustained activation leads to adverse LV remodeling and failure in later stages [21].

Eighth, the data underscore the importance of timing and differential temporal responses. Thus, increased TGF-β can promote ECM preservation through increased protease inhibitors (e.g., TIMPs) and suppression of inflammatory cytokines (e.g., TNF-α and IL-6) and ECM degradation during early healing. By contrast, TGF-β can promote ECM deposition by suppressing proteases (e.g., TIMPs) in later healing [21], which can lead to maladaptive remodeling. Other cytokines also show similar differential effects in early versus late stages of healing, with implications for therapy targeting TGF-β and cytokines.

Ninth, recent evidence suggests that several healing-specific matrix proteins can modulate ECM and LV remodeling during healing [13, 24]. For example, secretory leucocyte protease inhibitor (SLPI), a potent inhibitor of serine protease that upregulates production of anti-inflammatory cytokines can terminate MMP and inflammatory mediated proteolytic responses. Osteopontin (OPN), a matricellular protein, can interact with integrins and collagen, and promote collagen synthesis. Secreted protein acidic and rich in cysteine (SPARC), another matricellular protein, can modulate cell-matrix interactions and regulate fibroblast migration. A disintegrin and metalloproteinase (ADAM)-10 and ADAM-17, both matrixins, interact with inflammatory cytokines and alter MMPs. These matrix proteins are all upregulated post-MI [25] and can improve healing through the aforementioned interactions.

Tenth, emerging evidence suggests that aging can profoundly alter these healing and remodeling responses [22, 24, 25]. Aging affects most factors that modulate post-MI healing, including infarct size, angiogenesis and collateral flow, neurohormones such as angiotensin II, oxidative stress (via OFRs, NADPH oxidase and nuclear factor kappa B [NFκB] signaling), inflammation,

ECM, and other matrix proteins [24]. Aging may delay infarct healing after reperfusion, especially of large STEMI [23–25]. Our recent data suggest that aging increases myocardial and ECM damage, amplifies collagen alterations during healing, and may widen this window of vulnerability [25]. Clinical studies showed that age is a strong predictor of adverse events after MI and the elderly represent a high-risk group for heart failure and adverse remodeling, and recommended therapies do not target these issues in the elderly [24].

Progressive Ventricular Dilatation and its Limitation

Limitation and prevention of progressive LV dilatation post-MI is crucial for saving lives and reducing suffering. Six points deserve mention here. First, data from studies in humans have established that, untreated, adverse LV remodeling and dilatation may progress over years [1, 10, 13, 14], and lead to end-stage heart failure and death (Figs. 1 and 2). Data at both bench and bedside have underscored the regulatory role of the RAS and angiotensin II throughout and established the value of therapy with RAS-inhibitors [1, 26–28]. The value of early reperfusion has also been established. However, despite optimal medical therapy with angiotensin-converting enzyme (ACE) inhibitors, angiotensin II type 1 (AT_1) receptor blockers, statins, beta-blockers, and reperfusion, prognosis of post-STEMI patients is far from optimal and remodeling persists [16, 24, 49]. This suggests the need for developing improved therapies and/or strategies.

Second, while ACE-inhibitors, AT_1 blockers, statins and beta-blockers are recommended post-MI therapies [2–5, 26], they all decrease collagen synthesis, cytokines, MMP activation and inflammation in infarct regions [23, 24, 57]. Third, therapeutic drugs may have delayed and often undesirable effects during healing [56–58], suggesting the need for caution during this phase. Fourth, it should be noted that the effects of these drugs on inhibition of collagen synthesis would

be beneficial for hypertensive and other cardiac diseases with excessive fibrosis and in remote MI or healed post-MI hearts.

Fifth, data from our laboratory and others have shown that RAS-inhibitors have many benefits, including limitation of infarct size, LV dysfunction and remodeling, and improving metabolic proteins and MMP-9–TIMP-3 balance [1, 16, 28, 52, 54, 55]. Importantly, both ACE-inhibition and AT_1 receptor blockade attenuate TGF-β [21], and limit adverse ECM remodeling [59]. AT_1 receptor blockade also attenuates infarct size, inflammatory cytokines, TGF-β, MMPs, SLPI, OPN, SPARC, ADAM-10, and ADAM-17, and remodeling [25].

Sixth, the effect of aging on post-MI healing, remodeling, and outcome needs more study [24]. Most post-MI research studies have used young animals. Although clinical studies found that age is a strong predictor of adverse outcome after MI and the elderly represent a high risk group for adverse remodeling and heart failure [60], recommended therapies do not adequately target these issues [24]. We provided mechanistic evidence that elderly myocardium is a more vulnerable substrate to infarction and adverse remodeling, and this is likely due to amplified induction of intersecting pathways and signaling cascades and proteolytic events that contribute to an augmented and accelerated LV remodeling process [25]. Importantly, AT_1 receptor blockade attenuates these deleterious effects [25].

Conclusion

The collective evidence suggests that post-MI LV remodeling is a multifactorial, highly dynamic and time-dependent process. It begins after MI and may continue for years in survivors. It is most active during the infarction and healing phases. Besides remodeling of structure, shape, and systolic function, remodeling occurs at cellular, molecular, and biochemical levels. It involves the myocardium, ECM, and vascular tissues. It extends to other cardiac chambers and tissues, resulting on the long-term, in end-stage heart disease with inappropriate fibrosis and hypertrophy.

It is associated with remodeling of contractile proteins, RAS, and beta-adrenergic systems and changes in the kidneys. During the active infarction and healing phases, several genes and pathways are activated in timed sequence and thereby orchestrate the remodeling process. The RAS plays an important regulatory role. The RAS and other modulators can be favorably manipulated to limit infarction damage and optimize healing, and thereby limit adverse remodeling. Therapeutic manipulation of the genes and modulators may need to be appropriately timed for optimal benefit. Regional therapeutic approaches may need to be considered. Different approaches may be needed in elderly patients.

Acknowledgments This work was supported in part by grant # IAP99003 from the Canadian Institutes of Health Research, Ottawa, Ontario. I thank Catherine Jugdutt for assistance.

References

1. Pfeffer MA, Braunwald E. Ventricular remodelling after myocardial infarction. Circulation. 1990;81:1161–72.
2. Jugdutt BI. Prevention of ventricular remodelling post myocardial infarction: timing and duration of therapy. Can J Cardiol. 1993;9:103–14.
3. Jugdutt BI. Modification of left ventricular remodeling after myocardial infarction. In: Dhalla NS, Beamish RE, Takeda N, Nagano M, editors. The failing heart. Philadelphia, PA: Lippincot-Raven; 1995. p. 231–45.
4. Jugdutt BI. Prevention of ventricular remodeling after myocardial infarction and in congestive heart failure. Heart Fail Rev. 1996;1:115–29.
5. Jugdutt BI. Modification of left ventricular geometry and function during healing after acute myocardial infarction, vol. 1. DM thesis. Glasgow: University of Glasgow; 2006. p. 1–223.
6. Jugdutt BI, Michorowski B. Role of infarction expansion in rupture of the ventricular septum after acute myocardial infarction: a two-dimensional echocardiography study. Clin Cardiol. 1987;10:641–52.
7. Jugdutt BI, Basualdo CA. Myocardial infarct expansion during indomethacin and ibuprofen therapy for symptomatic post-infarction pericarditis: effect of other pharmacologic agents during early remodelling. Can J Cardiol. 1989;5:211–21.
8. Jugdutt BI, Khan MI. Impact of increased infarct transmurality on remodeling and function during healing after anterior myocardial infarction in the dog. Can J Physiol Pharmacol. 1992;70:949–58.
9. Jugdutt BI, Tang SB, Khan MI, et al. Functional impact on remodeling during healing after non-Q-wave versus Q-wave anterior myocardial infarction in the dog. J Am Coll Cardiol. 1992;20:722–31.
10. Jugdutt BI. Identification of patients prone to infarct expansion by the degree of regional shape distortion on an early two-dimensional echocardiogram after myocardial infarction. Clin Cardiol. 1990;13:28–40.
11. Michorowski B, Senaratne PJM, Jugdutt BI. Myocardial infarct expansion. Cardiovasc Rev Rep. 1987;8:42–7.
12. Michorowski B, Senaratne PJM, Jugdutt BI. Deterring myocardial infarct expansion. Cardiovasc Rev Rep. 1987;8:55–62.
13. Jugdutt BI, Warnica JW. Intravenous nitroglycerin therapy to limit myocardial infarct size, expansion and complications: effect of timing, dosage and infarct location. Circulation. 1988;78:906–19.
14. Gaudron P, Eilles C, Kugler I, et al. Progressive left ventricular dysfunction and remodeling after myocardial infarction. Potential mechanisms and early predictors. Circulation. 1993;87:755–63.
15. Jugdutt BI, Amy RW. Healing after myocardial infarction in the dog: changes in infarct hydroxyproline and topography. J Am Coll Cardiol. 1986;7:91–102.
16. Jugdutt BI. Ventricular remodeling post-infarction and the extracellular collagen matrix. When is enough enough? Circulation. 2003;108:1395–403.
17. Jugdutt BI. Remodeling of the myocardium and potential targets in the collagen degradation and synthesis pathways. Curr Drug Targets Cardiovasc Haematol Disord. 2003;3:1–30.
18. Sabbah HN. Global left ventricular remodeling with the acorn cardiac support device: hemodynamic and angiographic findings in dogs with heart failure. Heart Fail Rev. 2005;10:109–15.
19. Landa N, Miller L, Feinberg MS, et al. Effect of injectable alginate implant on cardiac remodeling and function after recent and old infarcts in rat. Circulation. 2008;117:1388–96.
20. Frangogiannis NG, Smith CW, Entman ML. The inflammatory response in myocardial infarction. Cardiovasc Res. 2002;53:31–47.
21. Bujak M, Frangogiannis NG. The role of TGF-β signaling in myocardial infarction and cardiac remodeling. Cardiovasc Res. 2007;74:184–95.
22. Bujak M, Kweon HJ, Chatila K, et al. Aging-related defects are associated with adverse cardiac remodeling in a mouse model of reperfused myocardial infarction. J Am Coll Cardiol. 2008;51:1384–92.
23. Ertl G, Franz S. Healing after myocardial infarction. Cardiovasc Res. 2005;66:22–32.
24. Jugdutt BI. Aging and remodeling during healing of the wounded heart: current therapies and novel drug targets. Curr Drug Targets. 2008;9:325–44.
25. Jugdutt BI, Jelani A, Palaniyappan A, et al. Aging-related changes in markers of ventricular and matrix remodelling after reperfused ST-segment elevation myocardial infarction in the canine model. Effect of

early therapy with an angiotensin II type 1 receptor blocker. Circulation. 2010;122:341–51.

26. Jugdutt BI. Pharmacological intervention in post-infarction wound healing. In: Karmazyn M, editor. Myocardial ischemia: mechanisms, reperfusion, protection. Basel: Birkhausser Verlag; 1996. p. 501–12.

27. Jugdutt BI. Role of AT_1 receptor blockade in reperfused myocardial infarction. In: Dhalla NS, Hryshko LV, Kardami E, Singal PK, editors. Signal transduction and cardiac hypertrophy. Boston, MA: Kluwer; 2003. p. 221–36.

28. Jugdutt BI. Valsartan in the treatment of heart attack survivors. Vasc Health Risk Manag. 2006;2:125–38.

29. Jugdutt BI. Extracellular matrix and cardiac remodeling. In: Villarreal FJ, editor. Interstitial fibrosis in heart failure. New York: Springer; 2004. p. 23–55.

30. Reimer KA, Jennings RB, Cobb FR, et al. Animal models for protecting ischemic myocardium: results of the NHLBI cooperative study. Comparison of unconscious and conscious dog models. Circ Res. 1985;56:651–65.

31. Bolli R, Becker L, Gross G, et al, NHLBI Working Group on the Translation of Therapies for Protecting the Heart from Ischemia. Myocardial protection at a crossroads: the need for translation into clinical therapy. Circ Res. 2004;95:125–34.

32. Reimer KA, Jennings RB. The "wavefront phenomenon" of myocardial ischemic cell death. II. Transmural progression of necrosis within the framework of ischemic bed size (myocardium at risk) and collateral flow. Lab Invest. 1979;40:633–44.

33. Jugdutt BI, Becker LC, Hutchins GM. Early changes in collateral blood flow during myocardial infarction in conscious dogs. Am J Physiol. 1979;237:H371–80.

34. Jugdutt BI, Hutchins GM, Bulkley BH, et al. Myocardial infarction in the conscious dog: three-dimensional mapping of infarct, collateral flow and region at risk. Circulation. 1979;60:1141–50.

35. Jugdutt BI, Hutchins GM, Bulkley BH, et al. Effect of indomethacin on collateral blood flow and infarct size in the conscious dog. Circulation. 1979;59:734–43.

36. Jugdutt BI, Becker LC, Hutchins GM, et al. Effect of intravenous nitroglycerin on collateral blood flow and infarct size in the conscious dog. Circulation. 1981;63:17–28.

37. Lieberman AN, Weiss JL, Jugdutt BI, et al. Two-dimensional echocardiography and infarct size: relationship of regional wall motion and thickening to the extent of myocardial infarction in the dog. Circulation. 1981;63:739–46.

38. Jugdutt BI, Sussex BA, Warnica JW, et al. Persistent reduction in left ventricular asynergy in patients with acute myocardial infarction with infusion of nitroglycerin. Circulation. 1983;68:1264–73.

39. Hutchins GM, Bulkley BH. Expansion versus extension. Two different complications of acute myocardial infarction. Am J Cardiol. 1978;41:1127–32.

40. Eaton LW, Weiss JL, Bulkley BH, et al. Regional cardiac dilation after acute myocardial infarction: recognition by two-dimensional echocardiography. N Engl J Med. 1979;300:57–62.

41. Jugdutt BI. Myocardial salvage by intravenous nitroglycerin in conscious dogs: loss of beneficial effect with marked nitroglycerin-induced hypotension. Circulation. 1983;68:673–84.

42. Jugdutt BI. Intravenous nitroglycerin unloading in acute myocardial infarction. Am J Cardiol. 1991;68:52D–63.

43. Jugdutt BI. Effect of reperfusion on ventricular mass, topography and function during healing of anterior infarction. Am J Physiol. 1997;272:H1205–11.

44. Kloner RA, Ellis SG, Lange R, et al. Studies of experimental coronary artery reperfusion: effects on infarct size, myocardial function, biochemistry, ultrastructure and microvascular damage. Circulation. 1983;68(Suppl I):I-8–15.

45. Ohno M, Takemura G, Ohno A. 'Apoptotic' myocytes in infarct area in rabbit hearts may be oncotic myocytes with DNA fragmentation: analysis by immunogold electron microscopy combined with In situ nick end-labeling. Circulation. 1998;98:1422–30.

46. Matsumura K, Jeremy RW, Schaper J, et al. Progression of myocardial necrosis during reperfusion of ischemic myocardium. Circulation. 1998;97:795–804.

47. Cleutjens JP, Kandala JC, Guarda E, et al. Regulation of collagen degradation in the rat myocardium after infarction. J Mol Cell Cardiol. 1995;27:1281–92.

48. Heymans S, Luttun A, Nuyens D, et al. Inhibition of plasminogen activators or matrix metalloproteinases prevents cardiac rupture but impairs therapeutic angiogenesis and causes cardiac failure. Nat Med. 1999;5:1135–42.

49. Bolognese L, Neskovic AN, Parodi G, et al. Left ventricular remodeling after primary coronary angioplasty: patterns of left ventricular dilation and long-term prognostic implications. Circulation. 2002;106:2351–7.

50. Boyle MP, Weisman HF. Limitation of infarct expansion and ventricular remodeling by late reperfusion. Study of time course and mechanism in a rat model. Circulation. 1993;88:2872–83.

51. Hudson MP, Armstrong PW, Ruzyllo W, et al. Effects of selective matrix metalloproteinase inhibitor (PG-116800) to prevent ventricular remodeling after myocardial infarction: results of the PREMIER (Prevention of Myocardial Infarction Early Remodeling) trial. J Am Coll Cardiol. 2006;48:15–20.

52. Sawicki G, Menon V, Jugdutt BI. Improved balance between TIMP-3 and MMP-9 after regional myocardial ischemia-reperfusion during AT_1 receptor blockade. J Card Fail. 2004;10:442–9.

53. Jugdutt BI. Left ventricular rupture threshold during the healing phase after myocardial infarction in the dog. Can J Physiol Pharmacol. 1987;65:307–16.

54. Jugdutt BI, Idikio H, Uwiera R. Therapeutic drugs during healing after myocardial infarction modify infarct collagens and ventricular distensibility at elevated pressures. Mol Cell Biochem. 2007;304: 79–91.

55. Jugdutt BI, Menon V, Kumar D, et al. Vascular remodeling during healing after myocardial infarction in the dog model. Effects of reperfusion, amlodipine and enalapril. J Am Coll Cardiol. 2002;39:1538–45.

56. Jugdutt BI. Pleiotropic effects of cardiac drugs on healing post MI. The good, bad and ugly. Heart Fail Rev. 2008;13:439–52.

57. Jugdutt BI. Delayed effects of early infarct-limiting therapies on healing after myocardial infarction. Circulation. 1985;72:907–14.

58. Jugdutt BI. Cyclooxygenase inhibition and ventricular remodeling after acute myocardial infarction. Circulation. 2007;115:288–91.

59. Jugdutt BI, Idikio H, Uwiera R. Angiotensin receptor blockade and ACE inhibition limit adverse collagen remodeling in the infarct zone and global diastolic dysfunction during healing after reperfused ST-elevation myocardial infarction. Mol Cell Biochem. 2007;303:27–38.

60. St John Sutton M, Pfeffer MA, Moye L, et al. Cardiovascular death and left ventricular remodeling two years after myocardial infarction: baseline predictors and impact of long-term use of captopril: information from the Survival and Ventricular Enlargement (SAVE) trial. Circulation. 1997;96: 3294–9.

Phosphodiesterase-5 Inhibitors in Protection Against Doxorubicin-Induced Cardiomyopathy

Saisudha Koka and Rakesh C. Kukreja

Abstract

Doxorubicin (DOX) is one of the most effective anticancer drugs. Despite its clinical efficacy, the therapeutic usage of DOX is restricted due its potential for causing dose-dependent cardiotoxicity. The mechanisms of DOX-induced cardiomyopathy remain unclear, but most of the evidence indicates enhanced oxidative stress, cardiomyocyte apoptosis, and subcellular changes in the myocardium eventually leading to the heart failure. Although numerous efforts have been made to develop effective therapeutic strategies to combat DOX-induced cardiomyopathy, cardiac transplantation still remains the only definitive option to treat DOX-induced heart failure in later stages. Hence, there is an ongoing need to further investigate and develop efficient therapeutic agents to combat DOX-induced cardiac damage. In this chapter, we focus on a novel application of phosphodiesterase-5 (PDE-5) inhibitors as potential agents in the treatment of DOX-induced cardiotoxicity and present an overview of our recent findings, as well as consider the potential mechanisms by which PDE-5 inhibitors mediate beneficial cardioprotective effects during DOX-induced cardiomyopathy. Several landmark studies from our laboratory showed that PDE-5 inhibitors induce powerful cardioprotective effects against ischemia–reperfusion injury and DOX-induced cardiomyopathy. PDE-5 inhibitors (sildenafil and tadalafil) attenuated DOX-induced apoptosis, depletion of prosurvival proteins including Bcl-2, and dissipation of mitochondrial membrane potential ($\Delta\psi$m) and improved cardiac contractile function, which was impaired by DOX. Cardiac oxidative stress was attenuated by tadalafil via upregulation of MnSOD and direct scavenging of reactive oxygen species (ROS). Moreover, tadalafil treatment increased cardiac cGMP level and protein kinase G (PKG) activity and

R.C. Kukreja (✉)
Division of Cardiology, Department of Internal Medicine,
Pauley Heart Center, Virginia Commonwealth University
Medical Center, Richmond, VA, USA
e-mail: rakesh@vcu.edu

N.S. Dhalla, M. Nagano, B. Ostadal (eds.), *Molecular Defects in Cardiovascular Disease*,
DOI 10.1007/978-1-4419-7130-2_18, © Springer Science+Business Media, LLC 2011

restored the depletion of GATA-4 in the DOX treated myocardium. Based on these compelling studies, we speculate that the class of PDE-5 inhibitors can represent an attractive therapeutic approach for managing DOX-induced cardiotoxicity in patients.

Keywords

Phosphodiesterase inhibitors • Doxorubicin • Cardiomyopathy • ROS • PKG

Introduction

Anthracycline antibiotics such as doxorubicin (DOX), epirubicin, daunorubicin, pirarubicin, and idarubicin are highly effective chemotherapeutic agents. However, despite their excellent antitumor efficacy, these drugs are potentially cardiotoxic to varying degrees, depending on the dosage, method of administration, the patient's age and cardiovascular history, and previous cytotoxic and concomitant treatments. DOX is a prototype among this class of drugs and is a potent, broad-spectrum antibiotic that has been widely used as a chemotherapeutic agent since late 1960s in the treatment of many hematologic and solid malignancies, including acute leukemias, lymphomas, stomach, breast and ovarian cancers, Kaposi's sarcoma, and bone tumors [1, 2]. Unfortunately, the clinical use of DOX is limited by its dose-dependent cardiotoxicity [3]. The overall prevalence of DOX-induced cardiomyopathy is 1.7–6.8% and is highly dependent on the total cumulative dose [4]. DOX is known to cause irreversible cardiomyopathy and heart failure predominately at cumulative doses of 500 mg/m^2 or higher [3, 5]. Although recent evidence shows that less toxic doses of DOX can be used effectively, heart failure in DOX-treated patients can go undetected for up to 20 years even after cessation of treatment, causing some cancer patients to be unwilling to use DOX [6]. The cardiotoxic effects of DOX in adults are progressively manifested as congestive heart failure within weeks or months after the end of treatment, while the delayed effects of DOX are more prominent in children [7]. At any given cumulative dose,

children were shown to have an increased risk of cardiomyopathy when compared to adults [8].

Clinical Manifestations of DOX-Induced Cardiotoxicity

Acute cardiotoxic effects of DOX are usually infrequent and normally occur within a week after the initiation of an anthracycline regimen. They are reversible and are clinically manifested as tachycardia, arterial hypotension, arrhythmias, shortness of breath, and depression of contractile function and occur in less than 1% of the patients undergoing the treatment. An even rarer acute complication is the development of myocarditis and pericardial effusion, usually occurring a few weeks after DOX administration [9]. Chronic symptoms are marked by ventricular dilatation and cardiac dysfunction eventually leading to heart failure. Reduction in fractional shortening and abnormalities in nonspecific T wave and ST-T segment of ECG are typically observed in DOX-induced ventricular dysfunction [10] .

As shown in Fig. 1, the ultrastructural features of DOX-induced cardiomyopathy include the extensive fibrosis accompanied with cytoplasmic vacuolization [11], disintegration of the myofibrillar array, loss of myofibrils, dilation of the sarcoplasmic reticulum, swelling of mitochondria followed by mitochondrial injury, increased number of lysosomes, and cardiomyocyte apoptosis leading to the loss of the myofibrils. These deleterious morphologic changes are species-independent as indicated by studies in various animal models [12].

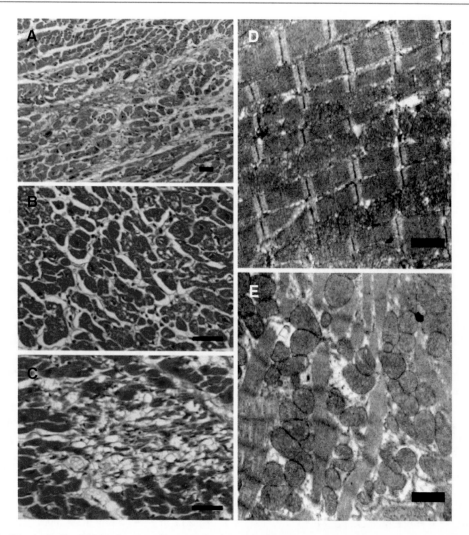

Fig. 1 Histologically, DOX-induced cardiomyopathy is characterized by extensive fibrosis (**a**) and scattered cardiomyocytes with vacuolar degeneration (Adria cells) (**b**); foci of necrotic cardiomyocytes may be encountered, though rarely (**c**). Bars (**a–c**) 20 μm. (**a**) Masson's trichrome stain; (**b**, **c**) Hematoxylin–eosin stain. Electron micrographs of cardiac specimens. (**d**) Specimen from a healthy mouse heart. (**e**) Specimen from a heart affected by DOX-induced cardiomyopathy. Note the vacuolization and marked myofibrillar loss in the cardiomyopathic cell. Bars (**d**, **e**), 1 μm (reprinted from Takemura and Fujiwara [11] with permission)

Mechanisms of DOX-Induced Cardiomyopathy

A variety of mechanisms have been suggested to contribute to DOX-induced cardiomyopathy and heart failure. These include free radical formation, lipid peroxidation, inhibition of nucleic acid and protein synthesis, mitochondrial dysfunction, calcium overloading, cardiomyocyte apoptosis, and release of vasoactive amines. Among the diverse set of mechanisms described [13], three major mechanisms that play a key role in the pathogenesis of DOX-induced cardiomyopathy are discussed below.

(a) Oxidative stress: DOX-induced cardiomyopathy occurs primarily via the generation of reactive oxygen species (ROS) in the cardiomyocyte – a mechanism that is separate from its antineoplastic activity, which occurs primarily through inhibition of topoisomerase II [14]. Previous studies detected DOX-generated ROS using electron spin resonance spectroscopy, which provide direct evidence for the role of oxidative stress in DOX-induced cardiotoxicity [15]. Furthermore, many studies have reported increased levels of intracellular peroxynitrite, hydrogen peroxide formation [16] and tissue malondialdehyde, a product of lipid peroxidation [17], all of which conceptually support the role of oxidative stress in DOX-induced cardiotoxicity. In addition, the myocardium exhibits antioxidant deficit because of the low levels of catalase and glutathione peroxidase, and this GSH-peroxidase-1 enzyme is also inactivated by DOX which further reduces the levels of superoxide dismutases, thus creating an antioxidant enzyme deficit environment that promotes hydroxyl radical formation. Moreover, the unique chemical structure of DOX makes it more susceptible to redox cycling under aerobic conditions and leads to the formation of a semiquinone free radical, which donates its unpaired electron to oxygen (O_2), forming a superoxide radical. This enhanced oxidative stress correlates with cellular injury and leads to a variety of subcellular changes in the myocardium, including the slow loss of myofibrils and vacuolization of myocardial cells, changes typical of DOX-induced cardiomyopathy. Thus, an increase in ROS and a decrease in antioxidants levels result in increased oxidative stress in myocardium, leading to the development of cardiomyopathy and heart failure [18].

(b) Cardiomyocyte apoptosis and mitochondrial damage: Although, several studies provide ample evidence on various molecular mechanisms underlying the DOX-induced apoptosis of cardiomyocytes [19, 20], hydrogen peroxide production remains to be the primary cause of DOX-induced cardiomyocyte apoptosis. DOX is known to induce apoptosis both by extrinsic and intrinsic pathways. The target organ of DOX-induced toxicity is

the myocardium enriched with mitochondria. Cardiomyocytes are particularly more susceptible to apoptosis than other tissues, as they rely on oxidative phosphorylation and require continuous supply of high energy phosphates. Earlier reports have shown that the intramitochondrial concentration of DOX is almost double its extracellular concentration in culture [21]. Various studies have shown that in the intrinsic pathway, cytochrome c is released from mitochondria, leading to activation of caspase-9 through formation of apoptosome complexes composed of apoptosis-activating factor-1, cytochrome c, and procaspase-9 through upregulation of Bax [22] or by depletion of Bcl-xl [23]. In line with the above observations, the activation of p53 further induces activation of Bax gene. Together, all these apoptotic responses such as redox cycling of DOX, induction of p53 by superoxide and hydrogen peroxide and transcriptional activation of Bax gene seem to be interlinked and contribute to the opening of mitochondrial permeability transition pore (MPTP) by DOX [24]. Additionally, numerous studies involving both in vitro and in vivo models of heart failure linked ROS to cardiomyocyte apoptosis [25, 26]. It is well recognized that apoptosis plays a role in the development of heart failure via mechanisms that contribute to cardiomyocyte loss, eventually leading to structural changes maladaptive to normal cardiac physiological demands [13].

(c) Reduction in the expression of cardiospecific proteins: A variety of cardiac specific proteins including contractile proteins (α-actinin, myosin light and heavy chains, troponin I, desmin), sarcoplasmic reticulum proteins (Ca^{2+}ATPase, ryanodine receptor 2), mitochondrial proteins (iron–sulfur protein, ADP/ATP translocase, phosphofructokinase, Mt-CK), and others [creatine kinase, phospholamban, calsequestrin, phospholipase A2, brain natriuretic peptide (BNP)] have been reported to be downregulated by DOX. DOX-mediated suppression of mitochondrial proteins impairs myocardial energy production, and its inhibition of sarcoplasmic reticulum Ca^{2+}-ATPase interferes with the sequestration of cytosolic free Ca^{2+} after systole, thereby causing diastolic dysfunction. Reductions in the cardiac muscle proteins are coupled with reduced contractility of cardiomyocytes and would explain the pathologic features of myofibrillar loss in DOX-induced cardiomyopathy. Recent reports have shown that DOX treatment depletes GATA-4 [27], a key transcriptional factor known to regulate myocardial expression of sarcomeric proteins such as myosin heavy chain and troponin I. However, it remains unknown whether the altered expression of specific proteins or transcription factors is directly mediated by ROS.

Management of DOX-Induced Cardiomyopathy

Over the past few decades numerous attempts have been made to develop effective protective strategies against DOX-induced cardiotoxicity. Administration of free radical scavengers and antioxidants such as probucol, amifostine, and dexrazoxane has demonstrated protection from DOX-induced cardiotoxicity, further substantiating the role of ROS in DOX-induced cardiotoxicity [28, 29]. However, all of these agents have pronounced clinical disadvantages including a significant decline in high-density lipoprotein levels, inability to prevent DOX-induced mortality, weight loss, and potentiation of DOX-induced myelosuppression [30]. Additional therapeutic strategies such as administration of β-blockers, inhibitors of renin–angiotensin system have been employed to reduce DOX-induced cardiotoxicity at early stages; however, all of these approaches have been limited by their marked side effects and demerits. The development of anthracycline analogues and alternative methods of drug delivery such as liposomal and nanosomal encapsulated DOX might be some of the promising approaches aimed at improving the antitumor efficacy and attenuating the toxic effects of DOX. However, at present, cardiac transplantation remains as the only definitive option to treat DOX-induced heart failure in later stages. Hence,

there is an ongoing need to further investigate and develop efficient therapeutic agents to combat DOX-induced cardiac damage.

Phosphodiesterase-5 Inhibitors in the Attenuation of DOX Cardiotoxicity

Phosophodiesterase-5 (PDE-5) inhibitors are a class of vasoactive drugs that were developed for treatment of erectile dysfunction (ED) in men. The mechanism of action involves active inhibition of the PDE-5A enzyme and resulting increase in cGMP and smooth muscle relaxation in the penis. Sildenafil and tadalafil had also been approved for pulmonary hypertension, but cardiac indications were still considered unlikely given its modest impact on arterial tone and low expression and activity in resting myocytes. This view began to change with the publication of several preclinical landmark studies from our laboratory showing a powerful protective effect of PDE-5 inhibitors including sildenafil (Viagra), vardenafil (Levitra) and tadalafil (Cialis) against ischemia–reperfusion injury in the rabbit and mouse hearts [31–33]. We demonstrated that sildenafil and other PDE-5 inhibitors increase eNOS/iNOS in the heart, which leads to downstream protective mechanisms involving cGMP-dependent activation of protein kinase G (PKG) and opening of mitochondrial K_{ATP} channels [34, 35]. Opening the mitoK$_{ATP}$ channel partially compensates the membrane potential, which enables additional protons to be pumped out to form an H^+ electrochemical gradient for both ATP synthesis and Ca^{2+} transport. The mitochondrial stabilizing effect of sildenafil was further confirmed in our isolated cardiomyocyte study [36], which showed an increase of Bcl-2–Bax ratio and preservation of mitochondrial membrane potential ($\Delta\psi$m), in the sildenafil-pretreated myocytes. Because DOX-induced cardiotoxicity involves the generation of ROS in the mitochondria, we hypothesized that cardiomyocyte protection by PDE-5 inhibition via opening of mitoK$_{ATP}$ channels, may be extended in demonstrating the prevention of cardiomyocyte apoptosis and subsequent development of cardiomyopathy. Previous studies have

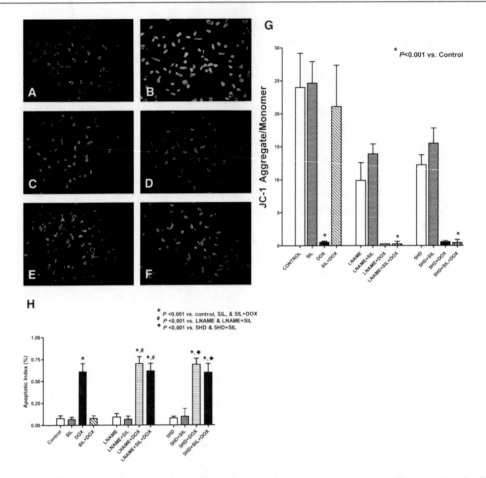

Fig. 2 Effect of sildenafil on $\Delta\psi$m and apoptosis in adult mouse ventricular myocyte cultures. (**a–f**) JC-1 staining of cardiomyocytes. Red fluorescence represents the mitochondrial aggregate form of JC-1, indicating intact mitochondrial membrane potential. Green fluorescence represents the monomeric form of JC-1, indicating dissipation of $\Delta\psi$m. (**a**) Control; (**b**) sildenafil (1 μmol/L); (**c**) DOX (1 μmol/L); (**d**) sildenafil (1 μmol/L) plus DOX (1 μmol/L); (**e**) L-NAME (100 μmol/L) plus sildenafil plus DOX; (**f**) 5-HD (100 μmol/L) plus sildenafil plus DOX; (**g**) ratio of mitochondrial aggregates to monomeric form of JC-1; (**h**) apoptotic index for TUNEL-positive cardiomyocytes. Data are mean±SEM ($n=3$; magnification ×200) (reprinted from Fisher et al. [38] with permission)

shown that the accumulation of ROS results in dissipation of the $\Delta\psi$m, direct activation of the MPTP, and cytochrome c release followed by caspase-3 activation and DNA fragmentation consistent with apoptosis [37].

In another landmark investigation form our laboratory [38], we demonstrated that in vivo treatment of mice with sildenafil before DOX administration conferred protective effects in the heart (Fig. 2a, b). We observed significant attenuation of cardiomyocyte apoptosis, preservation of myofibrillar integrity, prevention of left ventricular dysfunction, and ST prolongation consistent with chronic DOX-induced toxicity 8 weeks after

the final of three treatments. Sildenafil inhibited DOX-induced $\Delta\psi$m dissipation, caspase-3 activation, and cardiomyocyte apoptosis [38]. Moreover, exposure of adult mouse ventricular myocytes to DOX resulted in dissipation of $\Delta\psi$m, as illustrated via JC-1 immunofluorescent staining (Fig. 2c). By contrast, myocytes pretreated with sildenafil before the treatment with DOX demonstrated preservation of the $\Delta\psi$m (Fig. 2d, g). This protection of sildenafil in DOX-damaged cardiomyocytes was completely abolished by a nitric oxide synthase (NOS) inhibitor (L-NAME) and 5-hydroxydecanoate 5-HD (Fig. 2e–g). These findings implied that sildenafil-mediated protection from DOX-induced cardiomyocyte apoptosis was NOS-dependent and opening of $mitoK_{ATP}$ channel played critical role in attenuation of damage caused by DOX. Additionally, we observed a significant decline in Bcl-2 expression at both 2 and 8 weeks after treatment in the DOX group compared with the sildenafil + DOX and control groups, suggesting a pivotal role of Bcl-2 in altering the pathological process leading to end-stage heart failure.

There is increasing evidence that intermediate filaments such as desmin are involved in cardiomyopathy. Heling et al. [39] illustrated the disorganization and accumulation of desmin in explanted human heart specimens from patients with dilated cardiomyopathy (Fig. 3). Moreover, desmin-related cardiomyopathy in the knockout (desmin$^{-/-}$) mice was prevented by Bcl-2 overexpression, as evidenced by prevention of cardiomyocyte apoptosis and preservation of cardiac contractility [40]. Consistent with findings by Heling et al. [39] and Wang et al. [41], we observed disruption of desmin distribution in the DOX group compared with the sildenafil + DOX and control groups. Additionally, because desmin is known to adhere to the mitochondria in the same location where the MPTP is formed, it is conceivable that disruption of desmin either through repeated strain on the contractile apparatus resulting from impaired contractility or through direct cleavage from activated caspases may contribute to MPTP formation, cytochrome c release, and apoptosis.

In a more recent study, we demonstrated that the long acting PDE-5 inhibitor tadalafil also attenuated cardiac dysfunction in DOX-induced cardiomyopathy [42]. Although both PDE-5 inhibitors sildenafil and tadalafil, demonstrated protective effects against DOX-induced cardiomyopathy in mice, tadalafil appears to be the preferred choice for long-term management of patients receiving DOX for malignant tumors owing to its favorable pharmacokinetic properties, relatively slow metabolism, and greater selectivity for PDE-5 enzyme. Moreover, the rate and extent of tadalafil absorption is unaffected by food and hence it could be used at a relatively lower dosage regimen during chronic treatment. In a recent study [42], we demonstrated that tada-

lafil significantly improved the cardiac contractile function impaired by DOX treatment. Similar to sildenafil, tadalafil cotreatment with DOX improved survival of mice, restored the depletion of antiapoptotic protein Bcl-2, and decreased TUNEL-positive apoptotic cells (Figs. 4 and 5). GATA-4 is a key transcriptional factor that plays a pivotal role in controlling embryonic development, cardiomyocyte differentiation, and stress responsiveness of the heart. It has recently been shown that cardiac-specific deletion of GATA-4 resulted in a progressive and dose-dependent deterioration in cardiac function and dilation in adulthood [43]. In response to pressure overload, the GATA-4-deficient mice developed rapid decompensation and heart failure. These detrimental phenotypes were associated with increased cardiomyocyte apoptosis [43]. We also observed significant downregulation of GATA-4 expression after DOX treatment, which confirmed the previous reports [44], and GATA-4 expression was significantly preserved by cotreatment with tadalafil (Fig. 4b).

Our study also demonstrated that tadalafil treatment inhibited DOX-induced increase in lipid peroxidation (Fig. 5d). Antioxidant enzymes including Cu/ZnSOD (cytosolic) and MnSOD (mitochondrial) play a critical role in detoxification of ROS. Tadalafil did not affect the regulation of cytoplasmic Cu/ZnSOD, but MnSOD was significantly increased (Fig. 4c, d). These data imply that mitochondrial elimination of ROS contribute to the cardioprotective effects of tadalafil during DOX-induced toxicity. Previous studies have also shown that MnSOD overexpression can exert cardioprotection against DOX-induced injury and ischemia–reperfusion injury [45]. The antioxidant properties of PDE-5 inhibitors have not yet been well understood. Fernandes et al. [46] reported that the physiological concentrations of sildenafil (<50 μmol/L) decreased both H_2O_2 generation by mitochondria respiring glutamate/malate. Moreover, it was shown that sildenafil decreased superoxide radical generated by hypoxanthine–xanthine oxidase system, without affecting either mitochondrial bioenergetics or Ca^{2+}-induced mitochondrial permeability transition [46]. Most recently, in a rat model of traumatic spinal cord injury, Serarslan et al. demonstrated that tadalafil

Fig. 3 Desmin is
significantly increased on
the mRNA and protein
levels as shown by
Northern (**a**) and Western
(**b**) blot analysis (con
indicates control).
(**c, d**) Confocal microscopy
for desmin. (**c**) Normal
human myocardium shows
a regular cross-striation at
the Z-level and distinct
intercalated disk labeling.
(**d**) In failing myocardium,
the cross-striation pattern
is disturbed and desmin is
accumulated in many
irregularly shaped cells.
Nuclei are *red* (reprinted
from Heling et al. [39]
with permission)

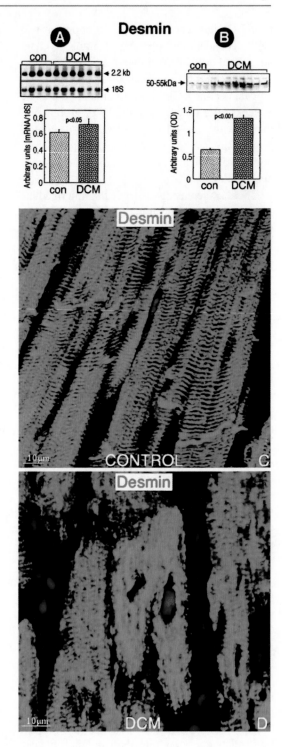

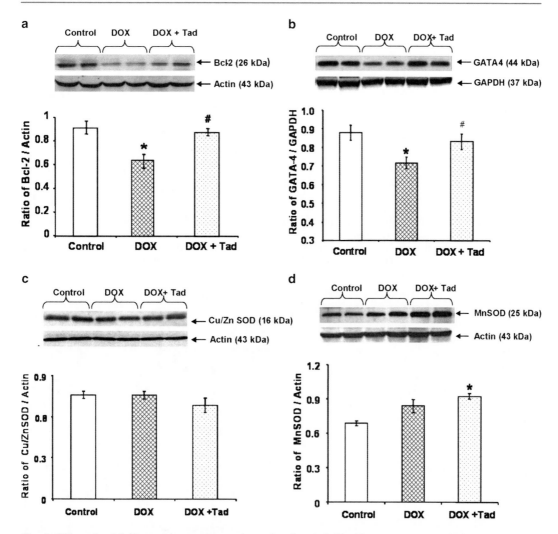

Fig. 4 Effect of tadalafil on antiapoptotic proteins and superoxide dismutases (SOD) after DOX treatment. Representative Western blots with specific bands of (**a**) Bcl-2, (**b**) GATA-4, (**c**) Cu/ZnSOD, and (**d**) MnSOD are shown. *Bar graphs* show densiometric quantification from four individual hearts per group, which was normalized against actin or glyceraldehyde 3-phosphate dehydrogenase (GAPDH) level for each sample. Data were expressed as mean ± SE. *$p < 0.05$ vs. Control, #$p < 0.05$ vs. DOX (reprinted from Koka et al. [42] with permission)

reduced the spinal cord injury via increasing tissue/serum levels of nitric oxide and serum activity of SOD [47]. Interestingly, our results demonstrated that co-treatment with tadalafil attenuated DOX-induced apoptosis as well lipid peroxidation (Fig. 5a, b), suggesting that tadalafil might have potent antioxidant-like effect, either through upregulation of MnSOD or by direct scavenging of ROS. Based on current state of knowledge, we propose that PDE-5 inhibitors could generate therapeutic levels of NO that result in enhanced formation of cGMP. cGMP may activate PKG that can subsequently open mitoK$_{ATP}$ channels resulting in protective effect against apoptosis by preservation of GATA-4 and Bcl-2, upregulation of MnSOD, attenuation of ROS generation, and inhibition of MPTP opening in the mitochondria as outlined in Fig. 6.

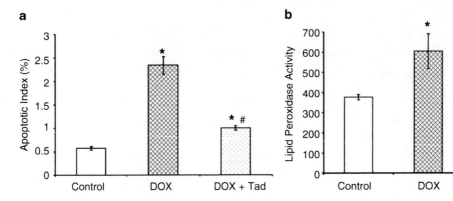

a

b

Fig. 5 Effect of tadalafil on ROS production, apoptosis, and lipid peroxidation after DOX treatment. (**a**) Cardiac tissue apoptosis quantified using TUNEL staining and expressed as apoptotic index for TUNEL-positive cells. (**b**) Lipid peroxidation activity was quantified using a commercial kit. Data are represented as mean ± SE ($n = 8$/ group). *$p < 0.05$ vs. Control, #$p < 0.05$ vs. DOX (reprinted from Koka et al. [42] with permission)

Fig. 6 Proposed pathway of inhibition of apoptosis by PDE-5 inhibitors. See text for details. *ROS* reactive oxygen species, *NO* nitric oxide, *PKG* protein kinase G, *mitoK_{ATP}* mitochondrial ATP-sensitive potassium channels, *MPTP* mitochondrial permeability transition pore

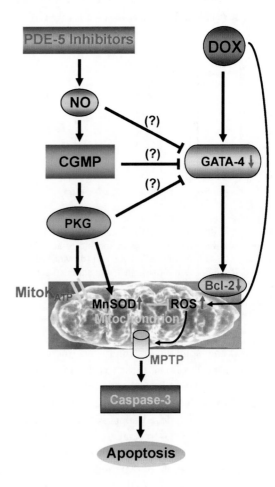

Conclusions

DOX remains a powerful anthracycline antibiotic used to treat many human neoplasms. However, its dose-dependent cardiotoxicity often leads to irreversible cardiomyopathy and ultimately congestive heart failure. Over the past 15 years, enormous progress has been made in our understanding of the basic biochemical and molecular mechanisms that underlie the cardiotoxicity associated with DOX. Currently, there is no optimal therapeutic intervention for protecting the heart against the DOX-cytotoxicity. Over the past decade, experimental and clinical studies have reported on the efficacy of PDE-5 inhibition to treat various forms of heart disease including myocardial infarction [34, 35], heart failure [48] and hypertrophy [49]. These studies have helped in the creation of ongoing NIH multicenter trial (RELAX: Evaluating the Effectiveness of Sildenafil at Improving Health Outcomes and Exercise Ability in People With Diastolic Heart Failure; NCT00763867) in patients with heart failure and a preserved ejection fraction (i.e., EF > 50%). We believe that these drugs have great potential to offer a novel and effective therapeutic approach for managing clinical concern of the DOX-induced cardiotoxicity. The time is ripe for a series of carefully designed clinical trials on the FDA-approved PDE-5 inhibitors, which hopefully could expedite their expanding nonurological therapeutic use in patients.

Acknowledgments This work was supported by grants from the National Institutes of Health (HL51045, HL79424, and HL93685) to Dr. Rakesh C. Kukreja.

Conflicts of Interest No potential conflicts of interest to disclose.

References

1. Bristow MR, Billingham ME, Mason JW, et al. Clinical spectrum of anthracycline antibiotic cardiotoxicity. Cancer Treat Rep. 1978;62:873–9.
2. Hortobagyi GN. Anthracyclines in the treatment of cancer: an overview. Drugs. 1997;54 Suppl 4:1–7.
3. Lefrak EA, Pitha J, Rosenheim S, et al. A clinicopathologic analysis of adriamycin cardotoxicity. Cancer. 1973;32:302–14.
4. Praga C, Beretta G, Vigo PL, et al. Adriamycin cardiotoxicity: a survey of 1273 patients. Cancer Treat Rep. 1979;63:827–34.
5. Minotti G, Menna P, Salvatorelli E, et al. Anthracyclines: molecular advances and pharmacologic developments in antitumor activity and cardiotoxicity. Pharmacol Rev. 2004;56:185–229.
6. Steinherz LJ, Steinherz PG, Tan C. Cardiac failure and dysrhythmias 6–19 years after anthracycline therapy: a series of 15 patients. Med Pediatr Oncol. 1995;24:352–61.
7. Fu LX, Waagstein F, Hjalmarson A. A new insight into adriamycin-induced cardiotoxicity. Int J Cardiol. 1990;29:15–20.
8. Von Hoff DD, Layard MW, Basa P, et al. Risk factors for doxorubicin-induced congestive heart failure. Ann Intern Med. 1979;91:710–7.
9. Zucchi R, Danesi R. Cardiac toxicity of antineoplastic anthracyclines. Curr Med Chem Anticancer Agents. 2003;3:151–71.
10. Friess GG, Boyd JF, Geer MR, et al. Effects of first-dose doxorubicin on cardiac rhythm as evaluated by continuous 24-hour monitoring. Cancer. 1985;56:2762–4.
11. Takemura G, Fujiwara H. Doxorubicin-induced cardiomyopathy from the cardiotoxic mechanisms to management. Prog Cardiovasc Dis. 2007;49:330–52.
12. Singal PK, Li T, Kumar D, et al. Adriamycin-induced heart failure: mechanism and modulation. Mol Cell Biochem. 2000;207:77–86.
13. Singal PK, Iliskovic N. Doxorubicin-induced cardiomyopathy. N Engl J Med. 1998;339:900–5.
14. Myers C. The role of iron in doxorubicin-induced cardiomyopathy. Semin Oncol. 1998;25(4 Suppl 10):10–4.
15. Alegria AE, Samuni A, Mitchell JB, et al. Free radicals induced by adriamycin-sensitive and adriamycin-resistant cells: a spin-trapping study. Biochemistry. 1989;28:8653–8.
16. Vasquez-Vivar J, Martasek P, Hogg N, et al. Endothelial nitric oxide synthase-dependent superoxide generation from adriamycin. Biochemistry. 1997;36:11293–7.
17. Singal PK, Pierce GN. Adriamycin stimulates low-affinity Ca2+ binding and lipid peroxidation but depresses myocardial function. Am J Physiol Heart Circ Physiol. 1986;250:H419–25.
18. Singal PK, Iliskovic N, Li T, et al. Adriamycin cardiomyopathy: pathophysiology and prevention. FASEB J. 1997;11:931–6.
19. Kang PM, Izumo S. Apoptosis and heart failure: a critical review of the literature. Circ Res. 2000;86:1107–13.
20. Sawyer DB, Fukazawa R, Arstall MA, et al. Daunorubicin-induced apoptosis in rat cardiac

myocytes is inhibited by dexrazoxane. Circ Res. 1999;84:257–65.

21. Konorev EA, Kennedy MC, Kalyanaraman B. Cell-permeable superoxide dismutase and glutathione peroxidase mimetics afford superior protection against doxorubicin-induced cardiotoxicity: the role of reactive oxygen and nitrogen intermediates. Arch Biochem Biophys. 1999;368:421–8.

22. Wang L, Ma W, Markovich R, et al. Insulin-like growth factor I modulates induction of apoptotic signaling in H9C2 cardiac muscle cells. Endocrinology. 1998;139:1354–60.

23. Kim Y, Ma AG, Kitta K, et al. Anthracycline-induced suppression of GATA-4 transcription factor: implication in the regulation of cardiac myocyte apoptosis. Mol Pharmacol. 2003;63:368–77.

24. Green PS, Leeuwenburgh C. Mitochondrial dysfunction is an early indicator of doxorubicin-induced apoptosis. Biochim Biophys Acta. 2002;1588: 94–101.

25. Kim SY, Kim SJ, Kim BJ, et al. Doxorubicin-induced reactive oxygen species generation and intracellular Ca^{2+} increase are reciprocally modulated in rat cardiomyocytes. Exp Mol Med. 2006;38:535–45.

26. Olson RD, Mushlin PS. Doxorubicin cardiotoxicity: analysis of prevailing hypotheses. FASEB J. 1990;4:3076–86.

27. Murphy AM, Thompson WR, Peng LF, et al. Regulation of the rat cardiac troponin I gene by the transcription factor GATA-4. Biochem J. 1997;322:393–401.

28. Kumar D, Kirshenbaum LA, Li T, et al. Apoptosis in adriamycin cardiomyopathy and its modulation by probucol. Antioxid Redox Signal. 2001;3:135–45.

29. Nazeyrollas P, Prevost A, Baccard N, et al. Effects of amifostine on perfused isolated rat heart and on acute doxorubicin-induced cardiotoxicity. Cancer Chemother Pharmacol. 1999;43:227–32.

30. Liu X, Chen Z, Chua CC, et al. Melatonin as an effective protector against doxorubicin-induced cardiotoxicity. Am J Physiol Heart Circ Physiol. 2002;283:H254–63.

31. Kukreja RC, Ockaili R, Salloum F, et al. Sildenafil-induced cardioprotection in rabbits. Cardiovasc Res. 2003;60:700–1.

32. Ockaili R, Salloum F, Hawkins J, et al. Sildenafil (Viagra) induces powerful cardioprotective effect via opening of mitochondrial K(ATP) channels in rabbits. Am J Physiol Heart Circ Physiol. 2002;283:H1263–9.

33. Salloum F, Yin C, Xi L, et al. Sildenafil induces delayed preconditioning through inducible nitric oxide synthase-dependent pathway in mouse heart. Circ Res. 2003;92:595–7.

34. Kukreja RC, Ockaili R, Salloum F, et al. Cardioprotection with phosphodiesterase-5 inhibi-tion: a novel preconditioning strategy. J Mol Cell Cardiol. 2004;36:165–73.

35. Kukreja RC, Salloum F, Das A, et al. Pharmacological preconditioning with sildenafil: basic mechanisms and clinical implications. Vascul Pharmacol. 2005;42:219–32.

36. Das A, Xi L, Kukreja RC. Phosphodiesterase-5 inhibitor sildenafil preconditions adult cardiac myocytes against necrosis and apoptosis. Essential role of nitric oxide signaling. J Biol Chem. 2005;280:12944–55.

37. Childs AC, Phaneuf SL, Dirks AJ, et al. Doxorubicin treatment in vivo causes cytochrome C release and cardiomyocyte apoptosis, as well as increased mitochondrial efficiency, superoxide dismutase activity, and Bcl-2:Bax ratio. Cancer Res. 2002;62:4592–8.

38. Fisher PW, Salloum F, Das A, et al. Phosphodiesterase-5 inhibition with sildenafil attenuates cardiomyocyte apoptosis and left ventricular dysfunction in a chronic model of doxorubicin cardiotoxicity. Circulation. 2005;111:1601–10.

39. Heling A, Zimmermann R, Kostin S, et al. Increased expression of cytoskeletal, linkage, and extracellular proteins in failing human myocardium. Circ Res. 2000;86:846–53.

40. Weisleder N, Taffet GE, Capetanaki Y. Bcl-2 overexpression corrects mitochondrial defects and ameliorates inherited desmin null cardiomyopathy. Proc Natl Acad Sci USA. 2004;101:769–74.

41. Wang X, Osinska H, Dorn GW, et al. Mouse model of desmin-related cardiomyopathy. Circulation. 2001;103:2402–7.

42. Koka S, Das A, Zhu SG, et al. Long-acting phosphodiesterase-5 inhibitor tadalafil attenuates doxorubicin-induced cardiomyopathy without interfering with chemotherapeutic effect. J Pharmacol Exp Ther. 2010;334:1023–30.

43. Oka T, Maillet M, Watt AJ, et al. Cardiac-specific deletion of Gata4 reveals its requirement for hypertrophy, compensation, and myocyte viability. Circ Res. 2006;98:837–45.

44. Aries A, Paradis P, Lefebvre C, et al. Essential role of GATA-4 in cell survival and drug-induced cardiotoxicity. Proc Natl Acad Sci USA. 2004;101: 6975–80.

45. Yen HC, Oberley TD, Vichitbandha S, et al. The protective role of manganese superoxide dismutase against adriamycin-induced acute cardiac toxicity in transgenic mice. J Clin Invest. 1996;98:1253–60.

46. Fernandes MA, Marques RJ, Vicente JA, et al. Sildenafil citrate concentrations not affecting oxidative phosphorylation depress H_2O_2 generation by rat heart mitochondria. Mol Cell Biochem. 2008;309:77–85.

47. Serarslan Y, Yonden Z, Ozgiray E, et al. Protective effects of tadalafil on experimental spinal cord injury in rats. J Clin Neurosci. 2010;17:349–52.

48. Salloum FN, Abbate A, Das A, et al. Sildenafil (Viagra) attenuates ischemic cardiomyopathy and improves left ventricular function in mice. Am J Physiol Heart Circ Physiol. 2008;294:H1398–406.

49. Takimoto E, Champion HC, Li M, et al. Chronic inhibition of cyclic GMP phosphodiesterase 5A prevents and reverses cardiac hypertrophy. Nat Med. 2005;11:214–22.

Part III

Hypertension and Diabetes

Molecular Basis of Pulmonary Hypertension in Left Heart Failure

Binil Raj, Harikrishnan Sivadasanpillai, and Chandrasekharan Cheranellore Kartha

Abstract

Pulmonary hypertension (PH) predicts poor outcome in patients with left heart failure. PH is associated with systolic and diastolic left heart failure. PH in association with left heart failure occurs initially as pulmonary venous hypertension as a result of backward transmission of elevated left ventricular filling pressure. Over a period of time, partly as an adaptive mechanism against pulmonary edema, remodeling of pulmonary vasculature occurs. The adaptive change includes pulmonary vasoconstriction and vascular remodeling, which result in sustained elevation of pulmonary vascular resistance and reduced response to vasodilatory drugs. Endothelial dysfunction is considered as a major cause for this response of pulmonary vasculature, which is characterized by altered production of vasoactive medators such as nitric oxide, endothelin-1, prostacyclin, and thromboxane. The imbalance in these molecules mediate vasoconstriction and leads to structural changes in the vessel wall. Currently, no specific therapy is available for PH associated with left heart failure. Pulmonary vasodilator drugs found effective for idiopathic pulmonary arterial hypertension are being tried recently in PH associated with left heart failure, but the results are not very promising. The clinical features, current therapeutic strategies, and molecular basis of pulmonary hypertension associated with left heart failure are reviewed in this article.

Keywords

Left heart failure • Pulmonary venous hypertension • Pulmonary vascular remodeling • Pulmonary vascular resistance • Endothelial dysfunction • Nitric oxide • Endothelin-1

C.C. Kartha (✉)
Division of Cardiovascular Disease Biology,
Rajiv Gandhi Center for Biotechnology,
Trivandrum, India
e-mail: cckartha@rgcb.res.in

N.S. Dhalla, M. Nagano, B. Ostadal (eds.), *Molecular Defects in Cardiovascular Disease*,
DOI 10.1007/978-1-4419-7130-2_19, © Springer Science+Business Media, LLC 2011

Introduction

Pulmonary vasculature is a low-resistance, low-pressure, high-capacity system that can accommodate large increases in blood flow [1]. Excess flow in the pulmonary circulation exceeding the compensatory capacity will result in PH [pulmonary artery pressure above 25 mmHg] [2]. Left heart failure (LHF) is associated with both functional and structural changes in the lung, which happen as an integrated response to chronic pressure induced insult to pulmonary circulation. Elevation in pulmonary artery pressure (PAP) may be either hyperkinetic or passive. Hyperkinetic PH results from excess blood flow through the pulmonary arteries (e.g., congenital systemic to pulmonary shunts), and passive PH occurs as a result of impedance to the pulmonary venous drainage (e.g., chronic LHF or mitral valve disease). Left-sided ventricular or valvular disease may produce an increase in left heart filling pressure, with backward transmission of the pressure leading to increased pulmonary venous hypertension and ultimately a passive pulmonary arterial hypertension. Long-standing high pressure in pulmonary vasculature leads to progressive morphological and functional changes in the pulmonary vasculature with resultant elevation in pulmonary vascular resistance (PVR>3 Wood units). The increased vascular resistance and ensuing elevation in pulmonary arterial pressure induce structural and functional changes in the lung.

Pathophysiology of PH in LHF

PH linked with LHF is a predictor of poor outcome in patients with heart failure [3–5]. A wide variety of abnormalities can cause LHF and coupled PH. The population of such patients includes heart failure patients with left ventricular systolic dysfunction, heart failure with preserved ejection (diastolic heart failure), valvular heart disease, and restrictive or infiltrative cardiomyopathies. Pulmonary capillary wedge pressure (PCWP), an indirect measure of left atrial pressure, is a prognostic marker in PH associated with LHF. It is a

hemodynamic indicator that can also be used to differentiate PH linked to LHF from pulmonary arterial hypertension [6]. In patients with LHF and PH, PCWP will be more than 15 mmHg [7].

In patients with LHF, elevated PCWP results in a passive increase in pulmonary venous pressure. This "passive" component represents the backward transmission of the elevated left atrial pressure. In the initial phase, elevation in PAP is caused solely by higher PCWP, without any intrinsic involvement of pulmonary vasculature. Parallel elevation of PCWP and mean PAP keeps the transpulmonary gradient (mean PAP-PCWP) normal. In this passive stage, interventions that lower PCWP can normalize PAP without any structural and functional abnormality in the pulmonary vasculature.

Chronic exposure to elevated left atrial pressures will, however, result in development of a "reactive" stage with structural and or functional defects in pulmonary circulation. This "reactive" phase have vasoconstrictive and fixed component because of the structural remodeling of the vascular wall [8]. Structural changes occur at the level of small peripheral pulmonary arteries; these include abnormalities of elastic fibers, intimal fibrosis, medial hypertrophy and muscularization of peripheral small vessels, and proliferation of vascular smooth muscle cells (SMCs). Lung changes also include remodeling of alveolar-capillary structure and function, which comprises thickening of capillary endothelial and alveolar epithelial cell basement membranes, endothelial and alveolar cell breaks, and impairment of cellular pathways involved in fluid filtration and reabsorption. This alveolar-capillary abnormality increases resistance to gas transfer, reducing membrane conductance and capillary blood volume, resulting in reduction of lung diffusion capacity [9]. The feature of severe end-stage disease is the development of plexiform lesions [10], characterized by over proliferation of endothelial like cells invading upon the vessel lumen. Compared to idiopathic pulmonary arterial hypertension, plexiform lesions are rare in secondary PH associated with LHF.

During the "reactive" stage, because of the intrinsic structural and functional impairment of

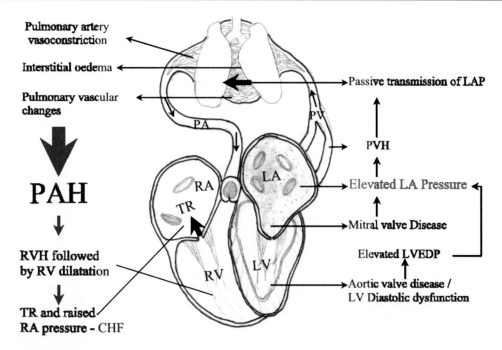

Fig. 1 Pathophysiology of pulmonary hypertension in left heart failure. *LV* left ventricle, *LVEDP* left ventricular end-diastolic pressure, *LA* left atrial, *PVH* pulmonary venous hypertension, *LAP* left atrial pressure, *PV* pulmonary veins, *PA* pulmonary artery, *PAH* pulmonary arterial hypertension, *RVH* right ventricular hypertrophy, *RV* right ventricular, *TR* tricuspid regurgitation, *RA* right atrium, *CHF* congestive heart failure. Reproduced with permission from ref. [11]

pulmonary vasculature, PAP does not merely reflect PCWP. Transpulmonary gradient will be higher since the mean PAP poorly correlates with PCWP. Interventions that lower the PCWP may not lower PAP readily as PAP is out of proportion. Only component that can come down is the vasoreactive or vasoconstrictive element, which takes even up to few weeks. Pulmonary vasculature partly loses its vasodilatory capacity and become much less sensitive to pharmacological agents. Pathophysiological mechanisms of PH in LHF are depicted in Fig. 1.

Development of reactive PH as a result of structural remodeling increases PVR and reduces vascular permeability. This is a compensatory mechanism to protect from fluid over load and pulmonary edema in presence of chronically elevated left ventricular filling pressure [11]. Pulmonary circulation is a primary factor that controls right ventricular afterload and regulates right ventricular output. As a consequence of elevated PVR, right ventricular afterload increases

with a reduction in right ventricular output. Persistent PH leads to right ventricular hypertrophy initially followed by right ventricular dilation and dysfunction and right heart failure. The combination of PH and right ventricular failure is a strong predictor of adverse outcome in patients with heart failure [12].

According to World Health Organization 2008 Dana Point World Symposium on PH, PH is classified into five different categories (Table 1) [13]. This classification is based on different manifestations of the disease, sharing similarities in pathological mechanisms, clinical presentation, and therapeutic approaches. PH associated with LHF is grouped under category II in the current classification. PH caused by left heart disease can be subdivided based on the nature of left heart disease, viz, systolic dysfunction, diastolic dysfunction, and valvular disease. Despite different origins, in the chronic stages they all share a common structural abnormality in pulmonary vessels [1].

Table 1 Clinical classification of pulmonary hypertension (Dana Point, 2008)

1. Pulmonary arterial hypertension
2. Pulmonary hypertension owing to left heart disease
(a) Systolic dysfunction
(b) Diastolic dysfunction
(c) Valvular disease
3. Pulmonary hypertension owing to lung diseases and/or hypoxia
4. Chronic thromboembolic pulmonary hypertension
5. Pulmonary hypertension with unclear multifactorial mechanisms

Reproduced with permission from ref. [13]

Clinical Implications of PH in LHF

PCWP is the characteristic diagnostic marker of PH associated with LHF. The clinical signs and symptoms of PH in LHF include dyspnea with effort, orthopnea, and paroxysmal nocturnal dyspnea [14]. In the later stages, they develop features of congestive heart failure when the right ventricle dilates and fails. Doppler echocardiography studies are used to obtain a reasonable approximation of the left ventricular filling pressure and left ventricular diastolic dysfunction [15]. Demonstration of an elevated PCWP at cardiac catheterization would confirm PH secondary to LHF and differentiate it from pulmonary arterial hypertension [16]. Measurement of B-type natriuretic peptide levels in the blood will also help to differentiate PH associated with LHF from idiopathic pulmonary arterial hypertension [17].

The degree of secondary pulmonary hypertension is a determinant of morbidity and mortality in patients with LHF. Impact of secondary PH was first recognized in heart transplant recipients. In patients with chronic heart failure, who were referred to as potential heart transplant candidates, but were selected for medical management, mean PAP and pulmonary systolic and diastolic pressures correlated significantly with selection for heart transplantation [18]. PH, secondary to LHF, represents a major risk factor for morbidity and mortality following heart transplantation [19]. Data from the International Society of Heart and Lung Transplantation indicate that approximately 50% of all cardiac complications and 20% of early deaths after cardiac complications all attributable to right ventricular failure [20]. In heart transplantation patients, transpulmonary gradient >12 mmHg and/or precapillary PVR>2.5 Wood Units are the limit for risk, above which the risk of death after transplantation increases [21]. According to the International Society of Heart and Lung Transplantation, PVR>5 Wood Units or PVR index>6 or transpulmonary gradient >16–20 mmHg is considered to be a relative contraindication to cardiac transplantation [22]. Hence, pulmonary hemodynamic assessment is considered essential in patients undergoing heart transplantation.

In patients with reduced left ventricular ejection fraction (systolic heart failure), PH is particularly common with a frequency of 68–76% [3, 4]. In patients with dilated cardiomyopathy, mortality and rate of hospitalization for heart failure are significantly more in patients with echocardiographic evidence of pulmonary hypertension [23]. Ghio et al. found that right ventricular dysfunction secondary to PH is also a strong predictor of morbidity and mortality in patients with chronic LHF [4]. In a community-based study, Lam et al. reported that 83% of patients with left ventricular failure and preserved ejection fraction (diastolic heart failure) have PH and that PH strongly predicted mortality in this group [24]. The potent association between PH and mortality suggests that PH may also contribute to the progression of heart failure.

A reduction in exercise capacity may occur in patients with heart disease of many causes and is expressed as a reduced peak oxygen uptake. Remodeling of alveolar-capillary membrane is one of the major causes of exercise intolerance in patients with heart failure [25]. In patients with chronic left ventricular failure, Franciosa et al. observed that during exercise, maximal oxygen consumption is correlated with pulmonary wedge pressure, pulmonary arterial mean pressure, and total pulmonary resistance, suggesting an important role of the pulmonary circulation in exercise capacity [26]. In patients with heart failure, there exists an inverse relation between peak oxygen consumption and resting pulmonary arterial pressure or PVR [3]. Right ventricular ejection fraction at rest is more predictive of exercise capacity than left ventricular ejection fraction [27]. These data suggest that elevation in right ventricular afterload causes a reduction in exercise capacity in patients with left ventricular failure.

Factors Determining PH in LHF

The progress and magnitude of PH in left ventricular dysfunction is more strongly associated with diastolic dysfunction than systolic dysfunction. Enriquez-Sarano et al. assessed systolic PAP in patients with primary left ventricular dysfunction by Doppler echocardiography [28]. They found out that PH is frequent, but highly variable in patients with left ventricular dysfunction. PH is not independently related to the degree of left ventricular systolic dysfunction but is strongly associated with diastolic dysfunction and the degree of functional mitral regurgitation. Neuman et al. evaluated the correlation between diastolic dysfunction and pulmonary arterial hypertension in patients with normal left ventricular wall motion [29]. Left ventricular diastolic dysfunction is associated with an increase in PAP in subjects with normal systolic function. In addition, PAP is significantly increased for each step-up in diastolic dysfunction grade. Interestingly, in patients with chronic heart failure, venous pulmonary congestion is an important determinant of systolic pulmonary artery hypertension [30].

Many patients with PH due to LHF have obesity, hypertension, diabetes mellitus, and hypercholesterolemia, which are clinical features of the metabolic syndrome, a cause for systemic vascular disease. Compared to patients with pulmonary arterial hypertension, patients with pulmonary venous hypertension have associated metabolic syndrome, suggesting that the metabolic syndrome may predispose patients to pulmonary vascular disease [31].

Carolyn et al. provided the first population-based evidence for age-associated increases in PAP [32]. Increase in PAP with age, is related at least in part to age-associated vascular stiffening

and pulmonary venous hypertension from left ventricular diastolic dysfunction. PH is also highly prevalent among patients with chronic renal failure [33].

Molecular Mechanisms of PH in LHF

Pathophysiology of PH associated with LHF is a complex and multifactorial process (Fig. 2). Left ventricular or valvular disease results in passive backward transmission of elevated left atrial pressure and partial obstruction to pulmonary venous drainage. This hemodynamic disturbance in circulation causes increased shear stress and turbulent flow in pulmonary circulation. Vascular endothelium senses this hemodynamic stress acting on luminal surface, initiating signals that adapt vasculature to its new environment by functional and

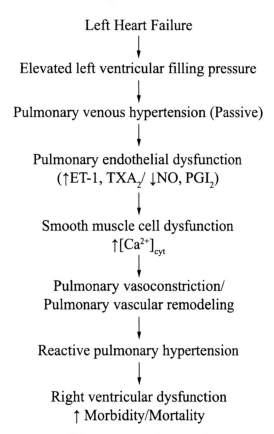

Fig. 2 Mechanism of pulmonary hypertension in left heart failure. *ET* endothelin, *TXA* thromboxane, *NO* nitric oxide, *PGI* prostacycline, *Ca* Calcium, *cyt* cytosole

structural changes [34]. Normally in the vasculature, endothelium plays a significant role in local control of vascular tone and cell proliferation through regulated release of various vasoactive mediators and growth factors [35]. Various reports suggest that chronic heart failure results in endothelial dysfunction, which in turn leads to dysregulation of counterbalancing mediators in pulmonary vascular endothelium. Defective endothelial response is the major factor that causes progression from passive PH to the deleterious pulmonary vascular disease. Ineffective production or response to endothelium-dependent vasodilators or excessive production or responsiveness to endothelium-dependent vasoconstrictors and/or mitogenic substances may all contribute to the development of pulmonary vascular disease. Various endothelium-dependent mediators such as nitric oxide (NO), endothelin-1 (ET-1), prostacyclin, thromboxane, and vascular endothelial growth factor (VEGF) have a pathological role in the development of PH associated with LHF. Most of these mediators affect growth of SMCs and facilitate development of pulmonary vascular hypertrophy and structural remodeling characteristic of PH in LHF.

Nitric Oxide

NO is one of the major determinants of basal pulmonary vascular tone [36] and alterations in their endogenous production are associated with development of PH. In the endothelium, NO is synthesized by a constitutive isoform of nitric oxide synthase [known as endothelial nitric oxide synthase (eNOS/NOS3)] by catalyzing the conversion of L-arginine to L-citrulline [37]. It is a potent pulmonary vasodilator and inhibits platelet activation and vascular SMC proliferation [38]. eNOS activity is regulated by different vasoactive factors and physiological stimuli such as shear stress, increased pulmonary blood flow, hypoxia, inflammation, and oxidative stress [39].

Once produced, NO diffuses to neighboring SMCs and readily activates soluble guanylate cyclase, and increases intracellular cGMP concentration. Intracellular cGMP induces vasodilation via many mechanisms; it activates cGMP-dependent protein kinase, which reduces the intracellular Ca^{2+} levels. In addition, intracellular cGMP activates myosin light chain phosphatase, reduces phosphorylation in the myosin, thereby sustaining the vascular smooth muscle tone and producing vasodilation [37].

Results from various clinical and preclinical studies suggest that NO-dependent pulmonary vasodilation is impaired in heart failure. In pulmonary artery segments from rats with chronic LHF, Ontkean et al. found that vasodilator response to acetylcholine was impaired, whereas that for nitroglycerin was normal [40]. In another study, Cooper et al. observed in control subjects or patients with heart failure and a normal PAP, infusion of L-NMMA (an analogue of L-arginine that inhibits eNOS) caused vasoconstriction. In patients with heart failure and pulmonary hypertension, the vasoconstrictor response to L-NMMA was attenuated, suggesting impaired endothelium-dependent relaxation. NO inhalation has been used as a therapeutic strategy to selectively decrease PVR in patients with heart failure. Short-term inhalation of NO lowers PVR in patients with left ventricular dysfunction and the magnitude of response to inhaled NO is strongly dependent on baseline PVR [41]. In patients with secondary PH, sildenafil (a phosphodiesterase V inhibitor), which indirectly augments the action of NO, reduced PVR and improved exercise capacity and quality of life [42]. These data suggest that relative deficiency of endothelium dependent NO production and related impaired pulmonary vascular relaxation contribute to the development and progression of pulmonary hypertension secondary to heart failure.

In a rat model of chronic heart failure, Alexander et al. demonstrated a novel mechanism of pulmonary endothelial dysfunction and lack of endothelial NO production [43]. These effects resulted from impaired regulation of endothelial NO synthase by cytosolic Ca^{2+}; pulmonary endothelial cells showed a deficient Ca^{2+} response to appropriate stimulation. Impaired Ca^{2+} signaling is attributed as a cause for massive upregulation and remodeling of endothelial actin cytoskeleton.

Endothelin-1

ET-1 is a 21 residue vasoactive peptide, and the most potent vasoconstrictor ever identified [44]. Various physiological stimuli such as low shear stress, turbulent flow, hypoxia, cytokines, reactive oxygen species, and catecholamines can stimulate ET-1 production. By contrast, high shear stress, NO, prostacyclin, and natriuretic peptides suppress ET-1 production [45]. The effect of ET-1 is mediated by two different G protein coupled receptors, namely, ET_A and ET_B. ET_A receptors are situated mainly on vascular SMCs and ET_B receptors on both endothelial and vascular SMCs. ET-1 mediates vasoconstriction and SMC proliferation through ET_A receptors. By contrast, binding of ET-1 to ET_B receptors on endothelium produce vasodilation by the release of NO and prostacyclin [46]. ET_B receptors are also found to play a significant role in ET-1 clearance. ET_B receptor located on vascular SMCs differ from those on endothelial cells as they mediate smooth muscle contraction [47]. The ratio of ET_A to ET_B in human pulmonary arteries is approximately 9:1, and hence, the net effect of ET-1 in pulmonary arteries is vasoconstriction [15]. ET-1 is also a known mitogen and mediates its effects through ET_A or ET_B receptors. The contribution of ET receptors to mitogenesis is dependent upon their relative distribution in the pulmonary vasculature. For example, ET_A predominantly mediates mitogenesis in main pulmonary artery, whereas both ET_A and ET_B mediate resistance in arteries [39]. The actions of ET-1 is mediated by increase in intracellular calcium, along with activation of protein kinase C, mitogen-activated protein kinase (MAP kinase), and the early growth response genes *c-fos* and *c-jun* [48].

ET-1 can produce dose-dependent contraction in pulmonary arteries and veins resulting in elevated PVR [49, 50]. An increase in preproendothelin-1 mRNA and ET-1 levels has been found in rats with chronic heart failure and pulmonary hypertension [51]. ET-1 immunoreactivity is also much higher in pulmonary vascular endothelial cells from patients with primary and secondary pulmonary hypertension [52]. In patients with congestive heart failure and elevated capillary wedge pressure, endothelin levels are found to have a strong correlation with PAP and PVR [53]. These data suggest that ET-1 has a important role in the development and progression of PH associated with LHF. The overactivity of ET-1 in PH associated LHF may be because of increased ET-1 production and or decreased pulmonary clearance.

Prostacyclin and Thromboxane

Prostacyclin (PGI_2) and thromboxane A_2 are two major vasoactive arachidonic acid metabolites synthesized in vascular endothelium. Prostacyclin is a potent vasodilator that inhibits platelet activation and has antiproliferative properties. It is synthesized by cyclooxygenase enzyme in the arachidonic acid pathway and the action is mediated mainly by stimulating cAMP production in vascular SMCs and platelets. In contrast to prostacyclin, thromboxane A_2 is a potent vasoconstrictor and platelet-aggregating agent [54]. An analysis of urine of patients with secondary pulmonary hypertension revealed that the level of prostacyclin metabolite 6-keto-prostaglandin F1 alpha is decreased where as the level of thromboxane A_2 metabolite dehydrothromboxane B_2 is increased, suggesting elevated production of thromboxane A_2 [55]. Thus, in PH associated with LHF there is an imbalance between these two mediators, which may remodel pulmonary vasculature to a vasoconstrictive and prothrombotic state.

Vascular Endothelial Growth Factor

Studies in experimental models and humans demonstrate the role of various endothelium-mediated growth factors in pulmonary arterial hypertension but comprehensive data are lacking with respect to PH secondary to LHF. In a canine model of PH secondary to overpacing-induced heart failure, Ray et al. discovered an increased expression of genes encoding VEGF and its receptors VEGFR1 and VEGFR2 [56]. In normal endothelial cells, VEGF is a survival and differentiating factor for lung endothelial cells and VEGF elevation in PH may represent a protective response [57, 58]. In diseased settings, VEGF may, however, be a primary growth promoting factor, thereby contributing to endothelial cell clustures or plexiform lesion formation [39]. VEGF also restores endothelial vasoreactivity in injured tissue [59] and induces production of NO and prostacyclin [60]. VEGF, hence, may be protective against some of the early pathological changes in the development of secondary PH.

Increased Thrombogenicity of Endothelium

Endothelial dysfunction causes hypercoagulability and thrombus formation in pulmonary vasculature. Normally, endothelium maintains a nonthrombogenic milieu by the regulated expression of various endothelium-derived agents such as heparan sulfate, thrombomodulin, plasminogen activator, von Willebrand factor, etc. [61]. Elevated levels of P-selectin and von Willebrand factor and decreased levels of thrombomodulin are found in patients with primary as well as secondary PH causing the vessels to be thrombogenic [62]. Deficiency of antithrombotic molecules such as NO and prostacyclin and slowing of blood flow in pulmonary circulation because of luminal narrowing further enhances thrombogenicity [63].

Smooth Muscle Dysfunction

Cross talk between pulmonary endothelial cells and SMCs is critical in pulmonary vasoconstriction and remodeling. Normal adult pulmonary artery SMCs usually do not proliferate, migrate, or produce extracellular matrix. Endothelial cells maintain SMC quiescence by regulated release of various mediators [64]. Phenotypical alteration of endothelium during chronic heart failure affects quiescent stage of SMCs. The SMCs become dysfunctional and starts proliferating, migrating, and synthesizing extracellular matrix, resulting in pulmonary vascular remodeling.

Constant shear stress affects barrier function of endothelium resulting in exposure of underlying SMCs to higher concentrations of plasma factors that can also stimulate SMCs [65].

Vasoconstrictive mediators from endothelium usually increase the cytosolic Ca^{2+} concentration in SMCs. This increase in cytosolic calcium would contribute not only to smooth muscle contraction but also to their growth and proliferation. As the intracellular Ca^{2+} increases, calmodulin binds to Ca^{2+} activating myosin light chain kinases. The phosphorylated myosin light chain kinases stimulate activity of myosin ATPase, hydrolyzing ATP to release energy for the subsequent cycling of myosin cross bridges with actin filaments [66]. Formation of these cross bridges underlies SMC contraction leading to vasoconstriction. The extent of pulmonary vasoconstriction is dependent on the level of cytosolic Ca^{2+}. Abnormal signals from endothelium elevate cytosolic Ca^{2+} concentration resulting in enhanced basal tone and contractility of pulmonary vasculature. Calcium–calmodulin complex also stimulates some of the cytoplasmic signal transduction proteins, propels quiescent cells into cell cycle, promoting cellular proliferation [67].

The increased contractility of the pulmonary arteries in pulmonary arterial hypertension has been attributed to reduced expression and activity of voltage gated potassium channels (K_V). Reduced K_V channel activity leads to depolarization of cell membranes, increased calcium influx through voltage gated channels, and further vasoconstriction [68]. The K_V channels may also have a role in PH associated with LHF, but there is no experimental evidence to confirm the phenomenon.

Treatment of Pulmonary Hypertension in Patients with LHF

Presence of PH is independently linked with morbidity and mortality in patients with LHF. Hence, a strong rationale exists for the treatment of PH in LHF patients. Presently, there is no approved specific therapy for the treatment of PH associated with heart failure [69]. When PH is passive, treatment is generally limited to improvement of left ventricular function by various medical, interventional, or electrophysiological approaches. Improvement of left ventricular function can significantly reverse passive PH in patients with LHF. For example, in a patient with severe aortic stenosis, relief of the obstruction by balloon valvotomy or surgical valve replacement leads to reduction in pulmonary pressure. In patients with significant pulmonary vascular disease, improvement of left ventricular function alone will not be sufficient to reverse pulmonary vascular changes. This condition demands selective pulmonary vasodilators that can reduce the elevated PVR. Drugs with a "selective" vasodilatory effect in the pulmonary vasculature and those that are useful in idiopathic pulmonary arterial hypertension have been tested in PH secondary to LHF.

The problem of using pulmonary vasodilator therapy such as inhaled NO and prostacyclin in PH related to LHF is that these drugs reduces the PVR and transpulmonary pressure gradient with an improvement in cardiac output. The increase in pulmonary venous return to left ventricle will result in increased left ventricular filling pressure and can precipitate acute left ventricular failure [70, 71].

The prostacyclin analogue epoprostenol is a potent vasodilator that has been used most successfully in the treatment of primary arterial hypertension. Prostacyclin, though very useful in the evaluation of vasoreactivity of the pulmonary vascular bed in heart failure, is associated with increased mortality in treated patients, when administered for a long time [72–75].

Different selective ET_A receptor antagonists (Darusentan and Tezosentan) and nonselective endothelin receptor antagonists (Bosentan) have been evaluated for their efficacy in PH associated with LHF. Bosentan did not provide any measurable hemodynamic benefit and was associated with more frequent adverse events requiring drug discontinuation [76, 77]. The results from these studies have cast doubt on the potential benefits of nonspecific endothelin receptor blockade in LHF. Darusentan and tezosentan also did not improve the symptoms or clinical outcomes in patients with heart failure [72–80].

Sildenafil is a promising candidate for therapy in PH associated with LHF and may be a potent novel agent in the management of the disease [42, 81, 82]. Sildenafil is a selective potent inhibitor of type 5 phosphodiesterse, the predominant phosphodiesterase isoform responsible for hydrolysis of intracellular cGMP in the pulmonary vasculature. Sildenafil lowers PVR in pulmonary hypertension by augmenting intracellular levels of the nitric oxide second messenger, cyclic GMP. The drug acts as a selective pulmonary vasodilator at rest and during exercise. Presently, the efficacy of sildenafil is being evaluated for the treatment of PH in diastolic heart failure patients in the RELAX (Phosphodiesterase-5 Inhibition to Improve Clinical Status and Exercise Capacity in Diastolic Heart Failure) study [7].

Various ionotropic agents are used for unloading the left ventricle, which can decrease PCWP, thus reducing PAP. Milrinone is one such drug, a phosphodiesterase type 3 inhibitor with vasodilating and inotropic properties. A bolus of milrinone consistently decreases PVR in patients with pulmonary hypertension secondary to severe heart failure. The reduction in PVR is associated with an increase in cardiac output and decrease of mean pulmonary artery and pulmonary artery wedge pressures, with no change in transpulmonary pressure gradient [83]. Milrinone acts both as an inotropic agent and a direct vasodilator, and thus may obviate the need for mechanical support for right ventricular failure due to residual pulmonary hypertension after left ventricular assist device implantation [84].

In a study by O'Dell et al., addition of Nesiritide (recombinant form of human B-type natriuretic peptide) to standard therapy and positive inotropic agents improved hemodynamic measures and clinical symptoms in patients with end-stage heart failure and secondary pulmonary hypertension [85]. However, long-term trials are required to confirm efficacy of these agents in secondary PH.

Left ventricular assist devices are used successfully in conditions where sufficient decrease in PVR is not achieved by pharmacological agents. Left ventricular assist devices will help in unloading the left ventricle, resulting in a reduction of PCWP, leading to a drop in PAP [86].

Among the new agents that are investigated for the treatment of PH in LHF are rho-kinase inhibitors and soluble guanylate cyclase stimulators. Rho-kinases are effectors of the small G-protein RhoA, which is involved in a variety of cellular functions including muscle contraction, proliferation and vascular inflammation through inhibition of myosin light chain phosphatase and activation of downstream mediators [87]. Soluble guanylate cyclase stimulators such as riociguat and cinaciguat can mimic NO-mediated signal transduction and NO-independent activation of soluble guanylate cyclase stimulators is a promising therapeutic strategy for PH [88, 89].

There is abundant presence of angiotensin-converting enzyme 2 in the lungs and its impressive effect in the prevention of experimental pulmonary arterial hypertension has led to the suggestion that pulmonary overexpression of this enzyme could be beneficial against secondary pulmonary hypertension [90].

In patients with rheumatic mitral valve disease and pulmonary hypertension, higher serum levels of normal T-cell-expressed and secreted chemokine (RANTES) and interleukin-6 (IL-6) have been observed. Based on these observations, Serag et al. recommend that RANTES and IL-6 should be investigated as potential targets in the control of rheumatic pulmonary arterial hypertension [91].

None of the abovementioned treatment modalities are truly effective in improving the outcome in patients with PH and LHF. Only definitive treatment that has been found to be effective is to improve the LV function, whether there is diastolic or systolic dysfunction. There appears to be a need for refinement of treatment strategies, where we can achieve a proportional decrease in PVR in addition to improvement of left ventricular function. Similar to the strategy in the treatment of pulmonary arterial hypertension, a combination of different agents can be employed in the management of PH associated with LHF where we can aim at a range of molecular targets.

The complete upstream pathogenic mechanisms that result in endothelial dysfunction and dysregulated signaling cascade in PH secondary to LHF are yet unknown. In contrast to the body of literature that has been published on pulmonary arterial hypertension, only a few studies have focused on PH in LHF. Given the minimal advances in treatment options for PH with left-sided heart disease, studies that can delineate molecular mechanisms of secondary PH and those that will help to identify novel drug targets for effective management of PH associated with LHF are mandated.

Conclusions

PH is an independent predictor of morbidity and mortality in patients with LHF. Despite being the primary therapeutic strategy to correct the underlying cardiac defect, modulation of pulmonary vascular function will be a supportive measure in disease management in patients with LHF. The pathophysiology of PH associated with LHF is a complex process, and no one factor identified so far is sufficient alone to explain the pathogenic process. Present knowledge strongly suggests a vital role for endothelial dysfunction in the development and progression of the disease. Maintenance of endothelial function and restoration of altered balance of endothelium-derived vasoactive mediators constitute the current treatment strategy for PH secondary to LHF. Drugs that modify pulmonary endothelial function found to be effective in idiopathic pulmonary arterial hypertension are, however, less effective in PH associated with LHF. This emphasizes the need for development of an alternative therapeutic approach in the treatment of PH secondary to LHF. Further studies are required to delineate the molecular basis of endothelial dysfunction and dysregulated signaling associated with PH in LHF, for developing more efficient therapeutic strategies for this condition.

References

1. Mandegar M, Fung YC, Huang W, et al. Cellular and molecular mechanisms of pulmonary vascular remodeling: role in the development of pulmonary hypertension. Microvasc Res. 2004;68:75–103.
2. Badesch DB, Champion HC, Sanchez MA, et al. Diagnosis and assessment of pulmonary arterial hypertension. J Am Coll Cardiol. 2009;54(1 Suppl): S55–66.

3. Butler J, Chomsky DB, Wilson JR. Pulmonary hypertension and exercise intolerance in patients with heart failure. J Am Coll Cardiol. 1999;34:1802–6.

4. Ghio S, Gavazzi A, Campana C, et al. Independent and additive prognostic value of right ventricular systolic function and pulmonary artery pressure in patients with chronic heart failure. J Am Coll Cardiol. 2001;37:183–8.

5. Kjaergaard J, Akkan D, Iversen KK, et al. Prognostic importance of pulmonary hypertension in patients with heart failure. Am J Cardiol. 2007;99:1146–50.

6. Flores ED, Lange RA, Hillis LD. Relation of mean pulmonary arterial wedge pressure and left ventricular end-diastolic pressure. Am J Cardiol. 1990;66:1532–3.

7. Bonderman D, Martischnig AM, Moertl D, et al. Pulmonary hypertension in chronic heart failure. Int J Clin Pract Suppl. 2009;161:4–10.

8. Moraes DL, Colucci WS, Givertz MM. Secondary pulmonary hypertension in chronic heart failure: the role of the endothelium in pathophysiology and management. Circulation. 2000;102:1718–23.

9. Gehlbach BK, Geppert E. The pulmonary manifestations of left heart failure. Chest. 2004;125:669–82.

10. Cool CD, Stewart JS, Werahera P, et al. Three-dimensional reconstruction of pulmonary arteries in plexiform pulmonary hypertension using cell-specific markers. Evidence for a dynamic and heterogeneous process of pulmonary endothelial cell growth. Am J Pathol. 1999;155:411–9.

11. Harikrishnan S, Kartha CC. Pulmonary hypertension in rheumatic heart disease. PVRI Rev. 2009;1:13–9.

12. Haddad F, Doyle R, Murphy DJ, et al. Right ventricular function in cardiovascular disease, part II: pathophysiology, clinical importance, and management of right ventricular failure. Circulation. 2008;117:1717–31.

13. Simonneau G, Robbins IM, Beghetti M, et al. Updated clinical classification of pulmonary hypertension. J Am Coll Cardiol. 2009;54(1 Suppl):S43–54.

14. Rich S, Dantzker DR, Ayres SM, et al. Primary pulmonary hypertension. A national prospective study. Ann Intern Med. 1987;107:216–23.

15. McLaughlin VV, Archer SL, Badesch DB, et al. ACCF/AHA 2009 expert consensus document on pulmonary hypertension: a report of the American College of Cardiology Foundation Task Force on Expert Consensus Documents and the American Heart Association: developed in collaboration with the American College of Chest Physicians, American Thoracic Society, Inc., and the Pulmonary Hypertension Association. Circulation. 2009;119:2250–94.

16. Rich S, Rabinovitch M. Diagnosis and treatment of secondary (non-category 1) pulmonary hypertension. Circulation. 2008;118:2190–9.

17. Tsutamoto T, Wada A, Maeda K, et al. Attenuation of compensation of endogenous cardiac natriuretic peptide system in chronic heart failure: prognostic role of plasma brain natriuretic peptide concentration in patients with chronic symptomatic left ventricular dysfunction. Circulation. 1997;96:509–16.

18. Rickenbacher PR, Trindade PT, Haywood GA, et al. Transplant candidates with severe left ventricular dysfunction managed with medical treatment: characteristics and survival. J Am Coll Cardiol. 1996;27:1192–7.

19. Delgado JF, Conde E, Sanchez V, et al. Pulmonary vascular remodeling in pulmonary hypertension due to chronic heart failure. Eur J Heart Fail. 2005;7:1011–6.

20. Stobierska-Dzierzek B, Awad H, Michler RE. The evolving management of acute right-sided heart failure in cardiac transplant recipients. J Am Coll Cardiol. 2001;38:923–31.

21. Delgado JF. The right heart and pulmonary circulation (III). The pulmonary circulation in heart failure. Rev Esp Cardiol. 2010;63:334–45.

22. Mehra MR, Kobashigawa J, Starling R, et al. Listing criteria for heart transplantation: International Society for Heart and Lung Transplantation guidelines for the care of cardiac transplant candidates–2006. J Heart Lung Transplant. 2006;25:1024–42.

23. Abramson SV, Burke JF, Kelly Jr JJ, et al. Pulmonary hypertension predicts mortality and morbidity in patients with dilated cardiomyopathy. Ann Intern Med. 1992;116:888–95.

24. Lam CS, Roger VL, Rodeheffer RJ, et al. Pulmonary hypertension in heart failure with preserved ejection fraction: a community-based study. J Am Coll Cardiol. 2009;53:1119–26.

25. Guazzi M. Alveolar gas diffusion abnormalities in heart failure. J Card Fail. 2008;14:695–702.

26. Franciosa JA, Baker BJ, Seth L. Pulmonary versus systemic hemodynamics in determining exercise capacity of patients with chronic left ventricular failure. Am Heart J. 1985;110:807–13.

27. Baker BJ, Wilen MM, Boyd CM, et al. Relation of right ventricular ejection fraction to exercise capacity in chronic left ventricular failure. Am J Cardiol. 1984;54:596–9.

28. Enriquez-Sarano M, Rossi A, Seward JB, et al. Determinants of pulmonary hypertension in left ventricular dysfunction. J Am Coll Cardiol. 1997;29:153–9.

29. Neuman Y, Kotliroff A, Bental T, et al. Pulmonary artery pressure and diastolic dysfunction in normal left ventricular systolic function. Int J Cardiol. 2008;127:174–8.

30. Capomolla S, Febo O, Guazzotti G, et al. Invasive and non-invasive determinants of pulmonary hypertension in patients with chronic heart failure. J Heart Lung Transplant. 2000;19:426–38.

31. Robbins IM, Newman JH, Johnson RF, et al. Association of the metabolic syndrome with pulmonary venous hypertension. Chest. 2009;136:31–6.

32. Lam CS, Borlaug BA, Kane GC, et al. Age-associated increases in pulmonary artery systolic pressure in the general population. Circulation. 2009;119:2663–70.

33. Havlucu Y, Kursat S, Ekmekci C, et al. Pulmonary hypertension in patients with chronic renal failure. Respiration. 2007;74:503–10.

34. Davies PF. Flow-mediated endothelial mechanotransduction. Physiol Rev. 1995;75:519–60.

35. Aird WC. Endothelial cell dynamics and complexity theory. Crit Care Med. 2002;30(5 Suppl):S180–5.

36. Cooper CJ, Landzberg MJ, Anderson TJ, et al. Role of nitric oxide in the local regulation of pulmonary vascular resistance in humans. Circulation. 1996;93:266–71.

37. Moncada S, Palmer RM, Higgs EA. Nitric oxide: physiology, pathophysiology, and pharmacology. Pharmacol Rev. 1991;43:109–42.

38. Radomski MW, Palmer RM, Moncada S. An L-arginine/nitric oxide pathway present in human platelets regulates aggregation. Proc Natl Acad Sci USA. 1990;87:5193–7.

39. Chan SY, Loscalzo J. Pathogenic mechanisms of pulmonary arterial hypertension. J Mol Cell Cardiol. 2008;44:14–30.

40. Ontkean M, Gay R, Greenberg B. Diminished endothelium-derived relaxing factor activity in an experimental model of chronic heart failure. Circ Res. 1991;69:1088–96.

41. Loh E, Stamler JS, Hare JM, et al. Cardiovascular effects of inhaled nitric oxide in patients with left ventricular dysfunction. Circulation. 1994;90:2780–5.

42. Guazzi M, Samaja M, Arena R, et al. Long-term use of sildenafil in the therapeutic management of heart failure. J Am Coll Cardiol. 2007;50:2136–44.

43. Kerem A, Yin J, Kaestle SM, et al. Lung endothelial dysfunction in congestive heart failure: role of impaired Ca^{2+} signaling and cytoskeletal reorganization. Circ Res. 2010;106:1103–16.

44. Abman SH. Role of endothelin receptor antagonists in the treatment of pulmonary arterial hypertension. Annu Rev Med. 2009;60:13–23.

45. Iglarz M, Clozel M. Mechanisms of ET-1-induced endothelial dysfunction. J Cardiovasc Pharmacol. 2007;50:621–8.

46. Fukuroda T, Kobayashi M, Ozaki S, et al. Endothelin receptor subtypes in human versus rabbit pulmonary arteries. J Appl Physiol. 1994;76:1976–82.

47. Dupuis J, Goresky CA, Fournier A. Pulmonary clearance of circulating endothelin-1 in dogs in vivo: exclusive role of ETB receptors. J Appl Physiol. 1996;81:1510–5.

48. Jeffery TK, Morrell NW. Molecular and cellular basis of pulmonary vascular remodeling in pulmonary hypertension. Prog Cardiovasc Dis. 2002;45:173–202.

49. Zellers TM, McCormick J, Wu Y. Interaction among ET-1, endothelium-derived nitric oxide, and prostacyclin in pulmonary arteries and veins. Am J Physiol Heart Circ Physiol. 1994;267:H139–47.

50. Lippton HL, Pellett A, Cairo J, et al. Endothelin produces systemic vasodilation independent of the state of consciousness. Peptides. 1989;10:939–43.

51. Sakai S, Miyauchi T, Sakurai T, et al. Pulmonary hypertension caused by congestive heart failure is ameliorated by long-term application of an endothelin receptor antagonist. Increased expression of endothelin-1 messenger ribonucleic acid and endothelin-1-like immunoreactivity in the lung in congestive heart failure in rats. J Am Coll Cardiol. 1996;28:1580–8.

52. Giaid A, Yanagisawa M, Langleben D, et al. Expression of endothelin-1 in the lungs of patients with pulmonary hypertension. N Engl J Med. 1993;328:1732–9.

53. Stewart DJ, Kubac G, Costello KB, et al. Increased plasma endothelin-1 in the early hours of acute myocardial infarction. J Am Coll Cardiol. 1991;18:38–43.

54. Gerber JG, Voelkel N, Nies AS, et al. Moderation of hypoxic vasoconstriction by infused arachidonic acid: role of PGI2. J Appl Physiol. 1980;49:107–12.

55. Christman BW, McPherson CD, Newman JH, et al. An imbalance between the excretion of thromboxane and prostacyclin metabolites in pulmonary hypertension. N Engl J Med. 1992;327:70–5.

56. Ray L, Mathieu M, Jespers P, et al. Early increase in pulmonary vascular reactivity with overexpression of endothelin-1 and vascular endothelial growth factor in canine experimental heart failure. Exp Physiol. 2008;93:434–42.

57. Le Cras TD, Markham NE, Tuder RM, et al. Treatment of newborn rats with a VEGF receptor inhibitor causes pulmonary hypertension and abnormal lung structure. Am J Physiol Lung Cell Mol Physiol. 2002;283:L555–62.

58. Partovian C, Adnot S, Raffestin B, et al. Adenovirus-mediated lung vascular endothelial growth factor overexpression protects against hypoxic pulmonary hypertension in rats. Am J Respir Cell Mol Biol. 2000;23:762–71.

59. Asahara T, Bauters C, Pastore C, et al. Local delivery of vascular endothelial growth factor accelerates reendothelialization and attenuates intimal hyperplasia in balloon-injured rat carotid artery. Circulation. 1995;91:2793–801.

60. He H, Venema VJ, Gu X, et al. Vascular endothelial growth factor signals endothelial cell production of nitric oxide and prostacyclin through flk-1/KDR activation of c-Src. J Biol Chem. 1999;274:25130–5.

61. Bombeli T, Mueller M, Haeberli A. Anticoagulant properties of the vascular endothelium. Thromb Haemost. 1997;77:408–23.

62. Sakamaki F. Coagulation and fibrinolytic abnormality related to endothelial injury in pulmonary arterial hypertension. Nippon Rinsho. 2001;59:1053–8.

63. Budhiraja R, Tuder RM, Hassoun PM. Endothelial dysfunction in pulmonary hypertension. Circulation. 2004;109:159–65.

64. Clowes AW, Reidy MA, Clowes MM. Kinetics of cellular proliferation after arterial injury. I. Smooth muscle growth in the absence of endothelium. Lab Invest. 1983;49:327–33.

65. Botney MD. Role of hemodynamics in pulmonary vascular remodeling: implications for primary pulmonary hypertension. Am J Respir Crit Care Med. 1999;159:361–4.

66. Somlyo AP, Somlyo AV. Signal transduction and regulation in smooth muscle. Nature. 1994;372:231–6.

67. Hardingham GE, Cruzalegui FH, Chawla S, et al. Mechanisms controlling gene expression by nuclear calcium signals. Cell Calcium. 1998;23:131–4.

68. Rhodes CJ, Davidson A, Gibbs JS, Wharton J, et al. Therapeutic targets in pulmonary arterial hypertension. Pharmacol Ther. 2009;121:69–88.

69. Galie N, Hoeper MM, Humbert M, et al. Guidelines for the diagnosis and treatment of pulmonary hypertension: The Task Force for the Diagnosis and Treatment of Pulmonary Hypertension of the European Society of Cardiology (ESC) and the European Respiratory Society (ERS), endorsed by the International Society of Heart and Lung Transplantation (ISHLT). Eur Heart J. 2009;30:2493–537.

70. Hare JM, Shernan SK, Body SC, et al. Influence of inhaled nitric oxide on systemic flow and ventricular filling pressure in patients receiving mechanical circulatory assistance. Circulation. 1997;95:2250–3.

71. Bocchi EA, Bacal F, Auler Junior JO, et al. Inhaled nitric oxide leading to pulmonary edema in stable severe heart failure. Am J Cardiol. 1994;74:70–2.

72. Yui Y, Nakajima H, Kawai C, et al. Prostacyclin therapy in patients with congestive heart failure. Am J Cardiol. 1982;50:320–4.

73. Haraldsson A, Kieler-Jensen N, Ricksten SE. Inhaled prostacyclin for treatment of pulmonary hypertension after cardiac surgery or heart transplantation: a pharmacodynamic study. J Cardiothorac Vasc Anesth. 1996;10:864–8.

74. Langer F, Wendler O, Wilhelm W, et al. Treatment of a case of acute right heart failure by inhalation of iloprost, a long-acting prostacyclin analogue. Eur J Anaesthesiol. 2001;18:770–3.

75. Califf RM, Adams KF, McKenna WJ, et al. A randomized controlled trial of epoprostenol therapy for severe congestive heart failure: The Flolan International Randomized Survival Trial (FIRST). Am Heart J. 1997;134:44–54.

76. Kalra PR, Moon JC, Coats AJ. Do results of the ENABLE (Endothelin Antagonist Bosentan for Lowering Cardiac Events in Heart Failure) study spell the end for non-selective endothelin antagonism in heart failure? Int J Cardiol. 2002;85:195–7.

77. Kaluski E, Cotter G, Leitman M, et al. Clinical and hemodynamic effects of bosentan dose optimization in symptomatic heart failure patients with severe systolic dysfunction, associated with secondary pulmonary hypertension – a multi-center randomized study. Cardiology. 2008;109:273–80.

78. Anand I, McMurray J, Cohn JN, et al. Long-term effects of darusentan on left-ventricular remodelling and clinical outcomes in the Endothelin A Receptor Antagonist Trial in Heart Failure (EARTH): randomised, double-blind, placebo-controlled trial. Lancet. 2004;364:347–54.

79. Luscher TF, Enseleit F, Pacher R, et al. Hemodynamic and neurohumoral effects of selective endothelin A (ET(A)) receptor blockade in chronic heart failure: the Heart Failure ET(A) Receptor Blockade Trial (HEAT). Circulation. 2002;106:2666–72.

80. McMurray JJ, Teerlink JR, Cotter G, et al. Effects of tezosentan on symptoms and clinical outcomes in patients with acute heart failure: the VERITAS randomized controlled trials. JAMA. 2007;298:2009–19.

81. Angel Gomez-Sanchez M, Saenz De La Calzada C, Escribano Subias P, et al. Pilot assessment of the response of several pulmonary hemodynamic variables to sublingual sildenafil in candidates for heart transplantation. Eur J Heart Fail. 2004;6:615–7.

82. Lewis GD, Shah R, Shahzad K, et al. Sildenafil improves exercise capacity and quality of life in patients with systolic heart failure and secondary pulmonary hypertension. Circulation. 2007;116:1555–62.

83. Givertz MM, Hare JM, Loh E, et al. Effect of bolus milrinone on hemodynamic variables and pulmonary vascular resistance in patients with severe left ventricular dysfunction: a rapid test for reversibility of pulmonary hypertension. J Am Coll Cardiol. 1996;28:1775–80.

84. Kihara S, Kawai A, Fukuda T, et al. Effects of milrinone for right ventricular failure after left ventricular assist device implantation. Heart Vessels. 2002;16:69–71.

85. O'Dell KM, Kalus JS, Kucukarslan S, et al. Nesiritide for secondary pulmonary hypertension in patients with end-stage heart failure. Am J Health Syst Pharm. 2005;62:606–9.

86. Martin J, Siegenthaler MP, Friesewinkel O, et al. Implantable left ventricular assist device for treatment of pulmonary hypertension in candidates for orthotopic heart transplantation – a preliminary study. Eur J Cardiothorac Surg. 2004;25:971–7.

87. Barman SA, Zhu S, White RE. RhoA/Rho-kinase signaling: a therapeutic target in pulmonary hypertension. Vasc Health Risk Manag. 2009;5:663–71.

88. Murthy SN, Nossaman BD, Kadowitz PJ. New approaches to the treatment of pulmonary hypertension: from bench to bedside. Cardiol Rev. 2010;18:76–84.

89. Ghofrani HA, Voswinckel R, Gall H, et al. Riociguat for pulmonary hypertension. Future Cardiol. 2010;6:155–66.

90. Yamazato Y, Ferreira AJ, Hong KH, et al. Prevention of pulmonary hypertension by Angiotensin-converting enzyme 2 gene transfer. Hypertension. 2009;54:365–71.

91. Serag AR, Hazaa SM, Afifi IK, et al. Regulated upon activation, normal T-cell expressed and secreted chemokine and interleukin-6 in rheumatic pulmonary hypertension, targets for therapeutic decisions. Eur J Cardiothorac Surg. 2010;37:853–8.

Modulation of Gi Protein Expression in Hypertension: Molecular Mechanisms

Madhu B. Anand-Srivastava

Abstract

Guanine nucleotide regulatory proteins (G proteins) play a key role in the regulation of various signal transduction systems including adenylyl cyclase–cAMP and phospholipase C (PLC)–phosphatidylinositol turnover (PI). These proteins are implicated in the modulation of a variety of physiological functions such as platelet functions, including platelet aggregation, secretion, and clot formation, and cardiovascular functions, including arterial tone and reactivity. Several abnormalities in adenylyl cyclase activity, cAMP levels, G proteins, and PLC/PKC have shown to be responsible for the altered cardiac performance and vascular functions observed in cardiovascular disease states. The enhanced or unaltered levels of inhibitory G proteins (Giα-2 and Giα-3) and mRNA have been reported in different models of hypertension, whereas Gsα levels were shown to be unaltered. These changes in G protein were associated with functions. The enhanced levels of Giα proteins precede the development of blood pressure and suggest that overexpression of Gi proteins may be one of the contributing factors for the pathogenesis of hypertension. The augmented levels of Giα proteins and associated adenylyl cyclase signaling in hypertension were shown to be attributed to the enhanced levels of vasoactive peptides. In addition, enhanced oxidative stress in hypertension may also be responsible for the enhanced expression of Giα proteins observed in hypertension. The augmented levels of Giα(alpha) proteins and associated adenylyl cyclase signaling in hypertension appear to be attributed to the enhanced levels of vasoactive peptides, which by increasing oxidative stress and transactivating growth factor receptors enhance MAP kinase activity that contributes to the enhanced expression of Giα proteins observed in hypertension.

M.B. Anand-Srivastava (✉)
Department of Physiology, Faculty of Medicine,
University of Montreal, Montreal, Quebec, Canada
e-mail: madhu.anand-srivastava@umontreal.ca

N.S. Dhalla, M. Nagano, B. Ostadal (eds.), *Molecular Defects in Cardiovascular Disease*,
DOI 10.1007/978-1-4419-7130-2_20, © Springer Science+Business Media, LLC 2011

Keywords

G proteins • Adenylyl cyclase • Vasoactive peptides • Growth factor receptors • Oxidative stress • MAP kinase • Hypertension

Introduction

Guanine nucleotide regulatory proteins (G proteins) are a family of guanosine triphosphate (GTP) binding proteins that play a key regulatory role as transducers in a variety of signal transduction system. These include adenylyl cyclase–cAMP system [1], the receptor-mediated activation of phospholipase C and A2 [2, 3], and a number of hormone and neurotransmitter-regulated ionic channels [4, 5] G proteins are heterotrimetric proteins composed of three distinct subunits: α (alpha), β (beta), and γ (gamma) subunits [6]. The α-subunits bind and hydrolyze GTP and confer specificity in receptor and effector interactions [6]. The GDP bound form of α binds tightly to $\beta\gamma$ (beta gamma) and is inactive, whereas the GTP bound form of α dissociates from $\beta\gamma$ and serves as a regulator of effector proteins. All α-subunits possess intrinsic GTPase activity and hydrolyze the terminal phosphate of bound GTP to yield bound GDP and free inorganic phosphate (Pi). Upon hormone binding and receptor activation, the receptor interacts with the heterotrimeric protein to promote a conformational change and dissociation of bound GDP from the guanine nucleotide binding site. GDP is released and replaced by GTP. Binding of GTP to α-subunit induces a conformational change and promotes the dissociation of hormone receptor complex and the holo G protein into α and $\beta\gamma$. Both α-GTP and $\beta\gamma$ subunits can interact with effectors. This activation cycle is terminated by intrinsic GTPase activity of α-subunit. The GDP-bound form of α-subunit has high affinity for $\beta\gamma$ and then reassociates with the $\beta\gamma$ dimer to form the heterotrimer in the basal resting state. The family of G protein α-subunits can be subclassified according to functional or structural relationship. More than 20 mammalian Gα gene

products and several alternatively spliced isoforms have been identified. These can be divided into four major subfamilies according to amino-acid homology and are represented by Gsα, Giα, Gqα/α11 and α12/α13. The G proteins Gsα and Giα are implicated in the regulation of adenylyl cyclase–cAMP signal transduction system.

The hormone-sensitive adenylyl cyclase system is composed of three components: the receptor, the catalytic subunit, and G proteins-stimulatory (Gs) and inhibitory (Gi). Molecular cloning has revealed four different forms of Gsα having molecular weights of 45, 45, and 52 kD resulting from the different splicing of one gene [7–9]. Gsα is positively coupled to adenylyl cyclase and mediates the stimulatory responses of hormones on adenylyl cyclase [10, 11]. The Gs-mediated activation of adenylyl cyclase results in the increase formation of cAMP. cAMP activates cAMP-dependent protein kinase A that induces the phosphorylation of contractile filaments, sarcolemmal and sarcoplasmic proteins, and regulates intracellular calcium homeostasis [12]. In addition, Gsα was also shown to open the Ca^{2+} channels directly by cAMP-independent mechanism [13]. By contrast, Giα protein is associated with adenylyl cyclase inhibition [10, 11]. Three distinct forms of Giα, namely, Giα-1, Giα-2, and Giα-3, have been cloned and encoded by three distinct genes [14–16]. All three forms of Giα (Giα 1–3) have been shown to be implicated in adenylyl cyclase inhibition [17] and activation of atrial Ach-K^+ channels [18]. Both the Gα and G$\beta\gamma$ dimers mediate G protein signaling. Five different β subunits of 35–36 kDa and 12 γ-subunits of 8–10 kDa have been identified by molecular cloning. The $\beta\gamma$ dimer is tightly associated with GDP bound chain and facilitates interaction of G protein with a receptor molecule. The effectors regulated by G$\beta\gamma$ include K^+ channels, phospholipase C-β, and adenylyl cyclase

[19–21]. Like α-subunit, the γ-subunit is subject to a cascade of posttranscriptional modification including isoprenylation and myristoylation that contributes to βγ membrane association and the interaction of the subunits [22].

G protein α-subunits also possess specific residues that can be covalently modified by bacterial toxins. Cholera toxin catalyzes the transfer of ADP-ribose moiety of NAD to a specific arginine residue in certain α-subunits, whereas pertussis toxin ADP-ribosylates those α-subunits that contain a specific cysteine residue near to carboxy terminus. Modification of α-subunit by cholera toxin persistently activates these protein by inhibiting their GTPase activity, whereas pertussis toxin inactives Giα protein and thereby results in the uncoupling of receptor from the effector. G protein α-subunits are regulated by covalent modifications by fatty acids myristate and palmate. These lipid modifications serve to anchor the subunits to the membrane and increase the interaction with other protein and also increase the affinity of α-subunit for βγ. In this regard, the myristoylation of Giα is required for adenylyl cyclase inhibition in cell-free assay [23].

G Proteins and Membrane Signaling in Cardiovascular Disease

A number of cardiovascular disease states that eventually result in chronic congestive heart failure are associated with alterations in cardiac performance. Several hormonal factors such as angiotensin II, endothelin and alterations in signal transduction mechanisms including adenylyl cyclase and phospholipase C (PLC) have been reported to play an important role in the alterations of cardiac performance.

Alterations in G-protein levels and functions such as altered adenylyl cyclase responsiveness to various agonists have also been demonstrated in cardiovascular and noncardiovascular tissues from genetic as well as experimental hypertensive rats [24–30].

G Proteins and Signal Transduction in Hypertension

An overexpression of Giα-2 and Giα-3 proteins as well as their genes was shown in hearts and aorta from spontaneously hypertensive rats (SHRs), deoxycorticosterone acetate (DOCA)-salt hypertensive rats (HR), N-[Omega]-nitro-L-arginine methylester (L-NAME) HR, and one kidney one clip (1K1C) HR [24, 26–29, 31–35], whereas Gsα protein and its gene was not altered in SHRs, 1K1C and L-NAME HR, and was decreased in DOCA-salt HRs [24–27, 32–35]. In addition, the levels of Goα in heart were also not altered [25]. Alterations in Gi protein levels have been shown to be reflected in altered responsiveness of adenylyl cyclase to stimulatory and inhibitory hormones in SHRs, and experimental models of HR [24, 25]. However, a decreased expression of Giα proteins was also shown in different tissues from different model of HR including Milan hypertensive rats (MHS) [30, 36–38]. The VSMC from MHS exhibit enhanced basal adenylyl cyclase activity as compared to control normotensive rats (MNS). The number of β-adrenoceptors and the stimulations exerted by isoproterenol and prostaglandin E1 (PGE₁) were significantly increased in MHS than in MNS. On the contrary, platelets from SHRs [27] as well as from hypertensive patients [39] exhibited a decreased expression of Giα-2 and Giα-3 proteins as compared to WKY and to normotensive control subjects, respectively, whereas the levels of Gsα protein were not altered. The decreased expression of Giα-2 and Giα-3 was correlated with adenylyl cyclase inhibition by inhibitory hormones. The ANP and Ang II-mediated inhibitions were completely attenuated in platelets from SHRs and hypertensive patients, whereas the stimulatory effects of PGE₁, NECA and forskolin were augmented [27, 39]. However, McLellan et al. [40] were unable to show any changes in the levels of Gsα, Giα-2, and Gβ in platelets from hypertensive patients as compared to normotensive subjects, whereas an enhanced stimulation of adenylyl cyclase by PGE₁ was observed in hypertensive patients as compared to normotensive subjects. On the contrary, lymphocytes from SHRs [41] and hypertensive patients [42] showed a decreased responsiveness of adenylyl cyclase to stimulatory hormones, which may be attributed to the alterations in Gs and Gi proteins. The potentiation of stimulatory responses of several hormones on adenylyl cyclase has also been demonstrated in platelets from SHRs [43]. In addition, antihypertensive drug therapy (a combination of β-blockers Ca^{2+} channel blocker and ACE inhibitor) partially restored Giα-2 levels toward normotensive subjects by about 60–70%. Furthermore, the enhanced stimulation of adenylyl cyclase by GTPγS, NECA and PGE$_1$ was partially corrected by about 50–80% in the patients under antihypertensive drug therapy [39]. These results suggest that the altered responsiveness of platelet adenylyl cyclase to hormones in hypertension and the normalization of the response with antihypertensive drug therapy could partially be due to the ability of the latter to modulate Giα protein expression. These effects on platelet function may underlie the beneficial effects of antihypertensive agents on some of the complications of hypertension.

The levels of Gsα, Giα-1, Giα-2, Giα-3, Goα, and Gβ were shown to be unaltered in myocardium from SHRs, and adenylyl cyclase activity stimulated by PGE1, glucagon, and isoproterenol was reduced in SHRs, whereas FSK-stimulated enzyme activity was greater in SHRs as compared to WKY [40]. On the contrary, a diminished stimulation of adenylyl cyclase by stimulatory hormones, guanine nucleotides, forskolin (FSK), and NaF in aorta and heart sarcolemma from SHRs [25], renal HR [44], 1K1C HR [34, 35], and DOCA-salt HR [28] has been demonstrated The reduction in the hormone receptor binding sites may be one of the possible mechanisms responsible for such an impaired response of hormones [45–47]. However, the decreased stimulation of adenylyl cyclase by dopamine D-1 receptors in the kidney tubules from SHRs was shown to be attributed to the defective coupling and not to the changes in the receptor number [48].

Furthermore, the increased levels of Giα were shown to be associated with hypertension and not with hypertrophy, due to the fact that heart and aorta from Nω(omega)-nitro-L-arginine methyl ester-(L-NAME)-induced HR, which do not have cardiac hypertrophy exhibited enhanced levels of Giα-2 and Giα-3 proteins as well as mRNA, whereas the levels of Gsα protein were unaltered [32, 33]. The increased levels of Giα-2 and Giα-3 proteins and their mRNA in heart and aorta precedes the development of blood pressure in SHRs [49], and DOCA-salt HR [50], suggesting that the enhanced levels of Giα proteins which result in the decreased levels of cAMP may be one of the contributing factors in the pathogenesis of hypertension. This was further supported by the recent studies showing that the inactivation of Giα protein in prehypertensive rats (2-week-old SHR) by single injection of pertussis toxin (PT) (1.5 μg/100 gm body weight) prevented the development of high blood pressure [51] which was associated with PT-induced decreased levels of Giα proteins.

Implication of Vasoactive Peptides and Growth Factor Receptors in Enhanced Expression of Giα Protein and Adenylyl Cyclase Signaling in Hypertension

The levels of vasoactive peptides such as angiotensin II (Ang II), endothelin (ET-1) and arginine vasopressin (AVP) as well as growth factors that have been reported to be augmented in various models of hypertension [52–60] may be responsible for the enhanced expression of Giα proteins in hypertension. In this regard, a role of Ang II in enhanced expression of Giα protein in SHR and 1K1C HR has been suggested by the studies showing that captopril, an angiotensin converting enzyme (ACE) inhibitor, treatment of the SHR and 1K1C HR decreased the blood pressure and also restored the enhanced levels of Giα protein to control levels [35, 61]. Similarly, the increased blood pressure and enhanced expression of Giα proteins in L-NAME hypertensive rats was also shown to be restored to control levels by losartan, an AT1 receptor antagonist [62], suggesting the

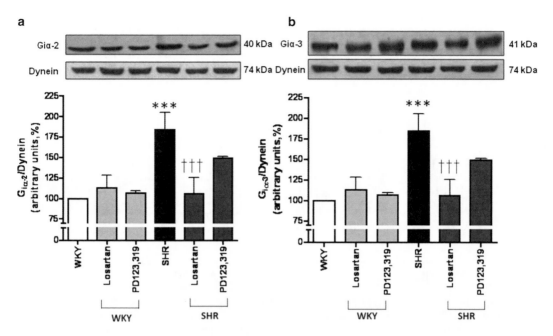

Fig. 1 Effect of losartan and PD123,319 on the expression of Giα-2 and Giα-3 proteins in VSMC from 12-week SHR and age-matched WKY. Confluent VSMC from 12-week-old SHR and age-matched WKY rats were incubated at 37°C in the absence or presence of losartan (100 μmol/l) and PD123,319 (100 μmol/l) for 16 h. Cell lysates were subjected to Western blot analysis using specific antibodies against Giα-2 (**a**, *top panel*) and Giα-3 (**b**, *top panel*) as described earlier [65]. The proteins were quantified by densitometric scanning (**a**, **b**, *bottom panels*). The results are expressed as percentage of WKY control. Values are means ± SE of five separate experiments. ***$P < 0.001$ vs. WKY and †††$P < 0.001$ vs. SHR

implication of Ang II in increased levels of Giα proteins and increased blood pressure in L-NAME-induced hypertension also. These treatments were also shown to restore the diminished stimulation of adenylyl cyclase by stimulatory hormones and enhanced inhibition by inhibitory hormones observed in SHRs, 1K1C, and L-NAME HR [34, 61, 62]. In addition, infusion of Ang II in rats that increased blood pressure has also been reported to enhance the levels of Giα proteins [63]. Similarly, nitrendipin and fosinopril treatments have also been reported to have similar effects on Gi proteins and functions in hearts from SHRs [64] and further support the implication of Ang II in enhanced levels of Giα protein in SHR. We also show that treatment of VSMC from SHR with AT1 receptor antagonist, losartan restored the enhanced expression of Giα proteins to WKY levels (Fig. 1) and

suggest the implication of endogenous Ang II in the enhanced expression of Giα proteins in VSMC from SHR. In addition, the inhibitors of endothelin ET_A and ET_B receptors, BQ123 and BQ788, respectively, were also shown to restore the enhanced expression of Giα proteins in VSMC from SHR to WKY levels [65], which suggest the role of endogenous endothelin that is increased in hypertension in enhanced expression of Giα proteins in VSMC from SHR [65]. In addition, growth factor receptors have also been shown to contribute to the enhanced expression of Giα proteins in VSMC from SHR, since the inhibitors of growth factor receptors attenuated the augmented expression of Giα proteins to control levels (Fig. 2). The activation of ET_A/ET_B by ET-1 has also been reported to enhance the activation of growth factor receptors, such as the platelet-derived growth factor receptor (PDGFR),

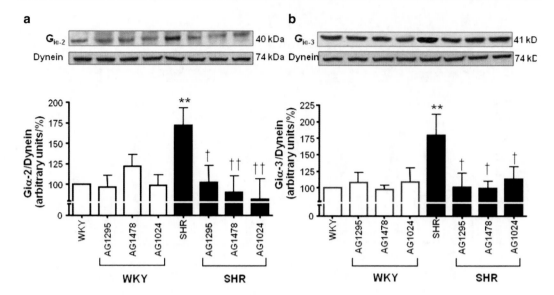

Fig. 2 Effect of PDGF-R, IGF-1R, and EGF-R antagonists on the expression of Giα-2 and Giα-3 proteins in VSMC from 12-week-old SHR and age-matched WKY. Confluent VSMC from 12-week-old SHR and age-matched WKY rats were incubated at 37°C in the absence or presence of AG1295 (5 μM), AG1478 (1 μM), and AG1024 (5 μM) for 16 h. Cell lysates were prepared and subjected to Western blot analysis using specific antibodies against Giα-2 (**a**, *top panel*) and Giα-3 (**b**, *top panel*) as described earlier [65]. The proteins were quantified by densitometric scanning (**a**, **b**, *bottom panels*). The results are expressed as percentage of WKY control. Values are means ± SE of five separate experiments. **$P < 0.01$ vs. WKY, †$P < 0.05$ vs. SHR and ††$P < 0.01$ vs. SHR

epidermal growth factor receptor (EGFR) and the insulin-like growth factor 1 receptor (IGF-1R), in a variety of cell types [66–68], a phenomenon termed transactivation [67]. We also showed that the enhanced phosphorylation of EGF-R in VSMC from SHR was attenuated by captopril, losartan, as well as BQ123 and BQ788 to control levels [69] and suggested the transactivation of EGF-R by endogenous Ang II and ET-1 in VSMC from SHR.

Implication of Oxidative Stress and MAP Kinase in Enhanced Expression of Giα Protein in Hypertension

A role of MAP kinase and PI3K signaling as well as oxidative stress in Ang II-induced enhanced levels of Giα proteins has also been reported [70, 71]. In addition, the studies showing that MEK inhibitor [72] as well as antioxidants such as diphenyleneiodonium (DPI) and N-acetyl cysteine

(NAC) [72] restored the enhanced levels of Giα proteins in SHR further suggest the implication of MAP kinase and oxidative stress in the enhanced expression of Giα protein in SHR. Furthermore, the enhanced phosphorylation of ERK1/2 in SHR was shown to be restored to WKY levels by antioxidants [72] as well as by the inhibitor of EGF-R [69] and suggested that the enhanced oxidative stress and EGF-R through MAP kinase signaling may contribute to the enhanced expression of Giα protein in SHR. The implication of Giα proteins in the regulation of blood pressure was further demonstrated by the studies showing that nitric oxide (NO) donors, SNAP and sodium nitroprusside (SNP), that have been reported to decrease blood pressure also attenuated the expression of Giα proteins and associated functions [73]. In addition, cGMP, which is the second messenger of NO action, also decreased the levels of Giα proteins and functions in VSMC [74]. These results indicate that the decreased levels of NO in L-NAME HR may be responsible for the enhanced expression

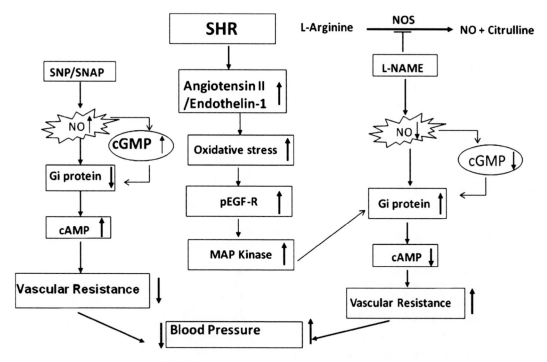

Fig. 3 Possible mechanisms involving angiotensin II or ET-1, oxidative stress, and nitric oxide in enhanced Gi protein expression in hypertension. Gi protein expression is enhanced in genetic (SHR) and experimental hypertension including L-NAME-induced hypertension. Inhibition of nitric oxide synthase (NOS) by L-NAME activates renin–angiotensin system, and also decreases the level of NO. Hypertensive rats including SHR also exhibit enhanced levels of Ang II and ET-1. Ang II and ET-1 increase oxidative stress that through EGF-R activation increases MAP kinase activity and results in enhanced expression of Giα proteins and thereby hypertension. On the contrary, increased level of NO and cGMP decreases the expression of Giα proteins in VSMC, which may be an additional mechanism through which NO decreases blood pressure in L-NAME-induced HR

of Giα proteins and also suggest that NO-induced decreased levels of Giα proteins may represent an additional mechanism through which NO decreases the blood pressure (Fig. 3).

Conclusions

We discuss the alterations in G proteins and associated functions in hypertension as well as their regulation by different modulators. We have mainly focused on Gi and Gs proteins, which are implicated in the regulation of the adenylyl cyclase–cAMP signal transduction system that plays an important role in the regulation of cardiovascular functions, including vascular tone and reactivity and cell proliferation. The levels of Giα-2 and Giα-3 proteins and mRNA are increased in hearts and aorta from genetic and

experimentally induced HR, whereas the levels of Gsα are unaltered in genetic and decreased in experimentally induced HR with established hypertrophy. The increased levels of Giα-2 and Giα-3 are associated with increased Gi functions, resulting in greater decreases in cAMP levels, which may partly explain the increased vascular resistance in hypertension. On the contrary, the decreased levels of Gsα and decreased formation of cAMP in hypertension associated with hypertrophy may also contribute to the increased vascular reactivity in hypertension. The increased levels of Giα-2 and Giα-3 may contribute to the pathogenesis of hypertension, whereas the decreased levels of Gsα may be associated with hypertrophy and not with hypertension. This notion is substantiated by our recent studies, showing that enhanced expression of Giα-2 and Giα-3 proteins and mRNA precede the development of blood pressure. The role of enhanced levels of Giα proteins in the pathogenesis of hypertension was further supported by our studies showing that inactivation of Giα proteins by pertussis toxin treatment in prehypertensive SHR prevented the development of blood pressure. However, the levels of Gs were decreased only in 15 weeks of SHRs with established hypertrophy. Similarly, L-NAME HR that do not have cardiac hypertrophy exhibited enhanced expression of Giα-2 and Giα-3 and no changes in Gsα, whereas hypertrophied rats with volume-overload hypertrophy, which do not have hypertension, exhibited decreased levels of Gsα and no augmentation in Giα-2 or Giα-3 proteins. The increased levels of endogenous Ang II and ET-1 through increased oxidative stress and transactivation of growth factor receptors and associated MAP kinase signaling may contribute to the enhanced expression of Giα proteins in VSMC from SHR (Fig. 3). Thus, it can be concluded that decreased formation of cAMP levels, either by increased levels and function of Gi or by decreased levels of Gsα and associated functions, may be responsible for the altered cardiac performance and vascular reactivity in cardiovascular disease.

References

1. Rodbell M, Krans HM, Pohl SL, et al. The glucagon-sensitive adenylyl cyclase system in plasma membranes of rat liver. IV. Effects of guanylnucleotides on binding of 125I-glucagon. J Biol Chem. 1971;246:1872–6.
2. Cockcroft S, Gomperts BD. Role of guanine nucleotide binding protein in the activation of polyphosphoinositide phosphodiesterase. Nature. 1985;314:534–6.
3. Litosch I, Wallis C, Fain JN. 5-Hydroxytryptamine stimulates inositol phosphate production in a cell-free system from blowfly salivary glands. Evidence for a role of GTP in coupling receptor activation to phosphoinositide breakdown. J Biol Chem. 1985;260:5464–71.
4. Breitwieser GE, Szabo G. Uncoupling of cardiac muscarinic and beta-adrenergic receptors from ion channels by a guanine nucleotide analogue. Nature. 1985;317:538–40.
5. Pfaffinger PJ, Martin JM, Hunter DD, et al. GTP-binding proteins couple cardiac muscarinic receptors to a K channel. Nature. 1985;317:536–8.
6. Gilman AG. G proteins and dual control of adenylate cyclase. Cell. 1984;36:577–9.
7. Bray P, Carter A, Simons C, et al. Human cDNA clones for four species of G alpha s signal transduction protein. Proc Natl Acad Sci USA. 1986;83:8893–7.
8. Robishaw JD, Smigel MD, Gilman AG. Molecular basis for two forms of the G protein that stimulates adenylate cyclase. J Biol Chem. 1986;261:9587–90.
9. Murakami T, Yasuda H. Rat heart cell membranes contain three substrates for cholera toxin-catalyzed ADP-ribosylation and a single substrate for pertussis toxin-catalyzed ADP-ribosylation. Biochem Biophys Res Commun. 1986;138:1355–61.
10. Stryer L, Bourne HR. G proteins: a family of signal transducers. Annu Rev Cell Biol. 1986;2:391–419.
11. Spiegel AM. Signal transduction by guanine nucleotide binding proteins. Mol Cell Endocrinol. 1987;49:1–16.
12. Wankerl M, Schwartz K. Calcium transport proteins in the nonfailing and failing heart: gene expression and function. J Mol Med. 1995;73:487–96.
13. Yatani A, Brown AM. Rapid beta-adrenergic modulation of cardiac calcium channel currents by a fast G protein pathway. Science. 1989;245:71–4.
14. Itoh H, Kozasa T, Nagata S, et al. Molecular cloning and sequence determination of cDNAs for alpha subunits of the guanine nucleotide-binding proteins Gs, Gi, and Go from rat brain. Proc Natl Acad Sci USA. 1986;83:3776–80.
15. Jones DT, Reed RR. Molecular cloning of five GTP-binding protein cDNA species from rat olfactory neuroepithelium. J Biol Chem. 1987;262:14241–9.
16. Itoh H, Toyama R, Kozasa T, et al. Presence of three distinct molecular species of Gi protein alpha subunit. Structure of rat cDNAs and human genomic DNAs. J Biol Chem. 1988;263:6656–64.
17. Wong YH, Conklin BR, Bourne HR. Gz-mediated hormonal inhibition of cyclic AMP accumulation. Science. 1992;255:339–42.
18. Kirsch GE, Yatani A, Codina J, et al. Alpha-subunit of Gk activates atrial K⁺ channels of chick, rat, and guinea pig. Am J Physiol Heart Circ Physiol. 1988;254:H1200–5.
19. Simon MI, Strathmann MP, Gautam N. Diversity of G proteins in signal transduction. Science. 1991;252:802–8.
20. Tang WJ, Gilman AG. Type-specific regulation of adenylyl cyclase by G protein beta gamma subunits. Science. 1991;254:1500–3.
21. Wickman KD, Iniguez-Lluhl JA, Davenport PA, et al. Recombinant G-protein beta gamma-subunits activate the muscarinic-gated atrial potassium channel. Nature. 1994;368:255–7.
22. Wedegaertner PB, Wilson PT, Bourne HR. Lipid modifications of trimeric G proteins. J Biol Chem. 1995;270:503–6.
23. Taussig R, Iniguez-Lluhi JA, Gilman AG. Inhibition of adenylyl cyclase by Gi alpha. Science. 1993;261:218–21.

24. Anand-Srivastava MB, Picard S, Thibault C. Altered expression of inhibitory guanine nucleotide regulatory proteins (Gi alpha) in spontaneously hypertensive rats. Am J Hypertens. 1991;4:840–3.

25. Anand-Srivastava MB. Enhanced expression of inhibitory guanine nucleotide regulatory protein in spontaneously hypertensive rats. Relationship to adenylate cyclase inhibition. Biochem J. 1992;288:79–85.

26. Thibault C, Anand-Srivastava MB. Altered expression of G-protein mRNA in spontaneously hypertensive rats. FEBS Lett. 1992;313:160–4.

27. Anand-Srivastava MB. Platelets from spontaneously hypertensive rats exhibit decreased expression of inhibitory guanine nucleotide regulatory protein. Relation with adenylyl cyclase activity. Circ Res. 1993;73:1032–9.

28. Anand-Srivastava MB, de Champlain J, Thibault C. DOCA-salt hypertensive rat hearts exhibit altered expression of G-proteins. Am J Hypertens. 1993;6: 72–5.

29. Bohm M, Gierschik P, Knorr A, et al. Cardiac adenylyl cyclase, beta-adrenergic receptors, and G proteins in salt-sensitive hypertension. Hypertension. 1993;22: 715–27.

30. Li P, Zou AP, al-Kayed NJ, et al. Guanine nucleotide-binding proteins in aortic smooth muscle from hypertensive rats. Hypertension. 1994;23:914–8.

31. Bohm M, Gierschik P, Knorr A, et al. Desensitization of adenylate cyclase and increase of Gi alpha in cardiac hypertrophy due to acquired hypertension. Hypertension. 1992;20:103–12.

32. Di Fusco F, Anand-Srivastava MB. Nitric oxide synthase inhibition by N(omega)-nitro-L-arginine methyl ester modulates G-protein expression and adenylyl cyclase activity in rat heart. Am J Hypertens. 1997;10: 471–5.

33. Di Fusco F, Anand-Srivastava MB. Enhanced expression of Gi proteins in non-hypertrophic hearts from rats with hypertension-induced by L-NAME treatment. J Hypertens. 2000;18:1081–90.

34. Ge C, Garcia R, Anand-Srivastava MB. Altered expression of Gi-protein and adenylyl cyclase activity in hearts from one kidney one clip hypertensive rats: effect of captopril. J Hypertens. 1999;17:1617–26.

35. Ge C, Garcia R, Anand-Srivastava MB. Enhanced expression of Gialpha protein and adenylyl cyclase signaling in aortas from 1 kidney 1 clip hypertensive rats. Can J Physiol Pharmacol. 2006;84:739–46.

36. Clark CJ, Milligan G, Connell JM. Guanine nucleotide regulatory protein alterations in the Milan hypertensive rat strain. J Hypertens. 1993;11:1161–9.

37. Michel MC, Farke W, Erdbrugger W, et al. Ontogenesis of sympathetic responsiveness in spontaneously hypertensive rats. II. Renal G proteins in male and female rats. Hypertension. 1994;23:653–8.

38. Kanagy NL, Webb RC. Increased responsiveness and decreased expression of G proteins in deoxycorticosterone hypertension. Hypertension. 1996;27:740–5.

39. Marcil J, Schiffrin EL, Anand-Srivastava MB. Aberrant adenylyl cyclase/cAMP signal transduction and G protein levels in platelets from hypertensive patients improve with antihypertensive drug therapy. Hypertension. 1996;28:83–90.

40. McLellan AR, Milligan G, Houslay MD, et al. G-proteins in essential hypertension: a study of human platelet plasma membranes. J Hypertens. 1993;11: 543–9.

41. Marcil J, Anand-Srivastava MB. Lymphocytes from spontaneously hypertensive rats exhibit enhanced adenylyl cyclase-Gi protein signaling. Cardiovasc Res. 2001;49:234–43.

42. Feldman RD, Tan CM, Chorazyczewski J. G protein alterations in hypertension and aging. Hypertension. 1995;26:725–32.

43. Hamet P, Franks DJ, Adnot S, et al. Cyclic nucleotides in hypertension. Adv Cyclic Nucleotide Res. 1980;12: 11–23.

44. Anand-Srivastava MB. Altered responsiveness of adenylate cyclase to adenosine and other agents in the myocardial sarcolemma and aorta of spontaneously-hypertensive rats. Biochem Pharmacol. 1988;37: 3017–22.

45. Limas C, Limas CJ. Reduced number of beta-adrenergic receptors in the myocardium of spontaneously hypertensive rats. Biochem Biophys Res Commun. 1978;83:710–4.

46. Woodcock EA, Funder JW, Johnston CI. Decreased cardiac beta-adrenergic receptors in deoxycorticosterone-salt and renal hypertensive rats. Circ Res. 1979;45:560–5.

47. Bhalla RC, Sharma RV, Ramanathan S. Ontogenetic development of isoproterenol subsensitivity of myocardial adenylate cyclase and beta-adrenergic receptors in spontaneously hypertensive rats. Biochim Biophys Acta. 1980;632:497–506.

48. Kinoshita S, Sidhu A, Felder RA. Defective dopamine-1 receptor adenylate cyclase coupling in the proximal convoluted tubule from the spontaneously hypertensive rat. J Clin Invest. 1989;84:1849–56.

49. Marcil J, Thibault C, Anand-Srivastava MB. Enhanced expression of Gi-protein precedes the development of blood pressure in spontaneously hypertensive rats. J Mol Cell Cardiol. 1997;29:1009–22.

50. Marcil J, de Champlain J, Anand-Srivastava MB. Overexpression of Gi-proteins precedes the development of DOCA-salt-induced hypertension: relationship with adenylyl cyclase. Cardiovasc Res. 1998;39: 492–505.

51. Li Y, Anand-Srivastava MB. Inactivation of enhanced expression of G(i) proteins by pertussis toxin attenuates the development of high blood pressure in spontaneously hypertensive rats. Circ Res. 2002;91:247–54.

52. Trinder D, Phillips PA, Risvanis J, et al. Regulation of vasopressin receptors in deoxycorticosterone acetate-salt hypertension. Hypertension. 1992;20:569–74.

53. Wahlander H, Wickman A, Isgaard J, et al. Interaction between the renin-angiotensin system and insulin-like growth factor I in aorto-caval fistula-induced cardiac hypertrophy in rats. Acta Physiol Scand. 1999;165: 143–54.

54. Kagiyama S, Eguchi S, Frank GD, et al. Angiotensin II-induced cardiac hypertrophy and hypertension are attenuated by epidermal growth factor receptor antisense. Circulation. 2002;106:909–12.

55. Kagiyama S, Qian K, Kagiyama T, et al. Antisense to epidermal growth factor receptor prevents the development of left ventricular hypertrophy. Hypertension. 2003;41:824–9.

56. Iglarz M, Schiffrin EL. Role of endothelin-1 in hypertension. Curr Hypertens Rep. 2003;5:144–8.

57. Kirchengast M, Witte K, Stolpe K, et al. Effects of chronic endothelin ET(A) receptor blockade on blood pressure and vascular formation of cyclic guanosine-3′,5′-monophosphate in spontaneously hypertensive rats. Arzneimittelforschung. 2005;55:498–504.

58. Schermuly RT, Dony E, Ghofrani HA, et al. Reversal of experimental pulmonary hypertension by PDGF inhibition. J Clin Invest. 2005;115:2811–21.

59. Morishita R, Higaki J, Miyazaki M, et al. Possible role of the vascular renin-angiotensin system in hypertension and vascular hypertrophy. Hypertension. 1992;19(2 Suppl):II62–7.

60. Jesmin S, Zaedi S, Maeda S, et al. Endothelin antagonism suppresses plasma and cardiac endothelin-1 levels in SHRSPs at the typical hypertensive stage. Exp Biol Med (Maywood). 2006;231:919–24.

61. Pandey SK, Anand-Srivastava MB. Modulation of G-protein expression by the angiotensin converting enzyme inhibitor captopril in hearts from spontaneously hypertensive rats. Relationship with adenylyl cyclase. Am J Hypertens. 1996;9:833–7.

62. Hashim S, Anand-Srivastava MB. Losartan-induced attenuation of blood pressure in L-NAME hypertensive rats is associated with reversal of the enhanced expression of Gi alpha proteins. J Hypertens. 2004;22:181–90.

63. Sims C, Ashby K, Douglas JG. Angiotensin II-induced changes in guanine nucleotide binding and regulatory proteins. Hypertension. 1992;19:146–52.

64. Bohm M, Kirchmayr R, Erdmann E. Myocardial Gi alpha-protein levels in patients with hypertensive cardiac hypertrophy, ischemic heart disease and cardiogenic shock. Cardiovasc Res. 1995;30:611–8.

65. Gomez Sandoval YH, Anand-Srivastava MB. Enhanced levels of endogenous endothelin-1 contribute to the over expression of Gialpha protein in vascular smooth muscle cells from SHR: role of growth factor receptor activation. Cell Signal. 2011;23:354–62.

66. Jankov RP, Kantores C, Belcastro R, et al. A role for platelet-derived growth factor beta-receptor in a newborn rat model of endothelin-mediated pulmonary vascular remodeling. Am J Physiol Lung Cell Mol Physiol. 2005;288:L1162–70.

67. Daub H, Weiss FU, Wallasch C, et al. Role of transactivation of the EGF receptor in signalling by G-protein-coupled receptors. Nature. 1996;379:557–60.

68. Sumitomo M, Milowsky MI, Shen R, et al. Neutral endopeptidase inhibits neuropeptide-mediated transactivation of the insulin-like growth factor receptor-Akt cell survival pathway. Cancer Res. 2001;61:3294–8.

69. Li Y, Levesque LO, Anand-Srivastava MB. Epidermal growth factor receptor transactivation by endogenous vasoactive peptides contributes to hyperproliferation of vascular smooth muscle cells of SHR. Am J Physiol Heart Circ Physiol. 2010;299:H1959–67.

70. Ge C, Anand-Srivastava MB. Involvement of phosphatidylinositol 3-kinase and mitogen-activated protein kinase pathways in AII-mediated enhanced expression of Gi proteins in vascular smooth muscle cells. Biochem Biophys Res Commun. 1998;251:570–5.

71. Li Y, Lappas G, Anand-Srivastava MB. Role of oxidative stress in angiotensin II-induced enhanced expression of Gi(alpha) proteins and adenylyl cyclase signaling in A10 vascular smooth muscle cells. Am J Physiol Heart Circ Physiol. 2007;292:H1922–30.

72. Lappas G, Daou GB, Anand-Srivastava MB. Oxidative stress contributes to the enhanced expression of Gialpha proteins and adenylyl cyclase signaling in vascular smooth muscle cells from spontaneously hypertensive rats. J Hypertens. 2005;23:2251–61.

73. Bassil M, Anand-Srivastava MB. Nitric oxide modulates Gi-protein expression and adenylyl cyclase signaling in vascular smooth muscle cells. Free Radic Biol Med. 2006;41:1162–73.

74. Bassil M, Anand-Srivastava MB. Cyclic GMP modulates the expression of Gi protein and adenylyl cyclase signaling in vascular smooth muscle cells. Cell Biochem Biophys. 2007;47:99–108.

Vascular Dysfunction in Heart Disease

Raissa Perrault and Peter Zahradka

Abstract

Vascular dysfunction is the underlying cause of almost 80% of heart disease cases. As the incidence of heart disease has now reached epidemic proportions, research into the mechanisms responsible for the initiation and progression of vascular disease is becoming critically important. The topic of prevention is addressed via a review of both modifiable and nonmodifiable risk factors, followed by a survey of recent advances in diagnostic approaches. Progression of the disease is thoroughly described at the molecular level, from the early dysfunctional endothelium, through a series of steps involving complex interactions between resident and circulating cell and LDL particles. Consequences of the altered microenvironment on subendothelial smooth muscle and inflammatory cells are subsequently described, with a focus on exacerbating events such as oxidation and inappropriate growth factor secretion. Finally, the controversial role of endothelial and smooth muscle progenitors in the development of atherosclerosis is presented and discussed.

Keywords

Atherosclerosis • Oxidized LDL, risk factors • Diagnosis • Smooth muscle cells • Endothelial dysfunction • Vascular inflammatory responses • Growth factors • Vascular progenitor cells

P. Zahradka (✉)

Department of Physiology, University of Manitoba and Canadian Centre for Agrifood Research in Health and Medicine, St. Boniface Hospital Research Centre, Winnipeg, Manitoba, Canada

e-mail: peterz@sbrc.ca

Introduction

Cardiovascular (CV) disease morbidity and mortality have now reached epidemic proportions. As a result, the importance of prevention of the disease, in addition to the treatment of the clinical outcome of the existing disease, has emerged as a priority in the field. These efforts

N.S. Dhalla, M. Nagano, B. Ostadal (eds.), *Molecular Defects in Cardiovascular Disease*,
DOI 10.1007/978-1-4419-7130-2_21, © Springer Science+Business Media, LLC 2011

have turned to what is in fact the underlying cause of myocardial infarctions and the resulting heart disease, namely, atherosclerotic vascular disease. This vascular condition affects the entire vascular tree and, thus, is also the cause of cerebrovascular and peripheral vascular disease (PAD), as well as the reason for major clinical complications such as restenosis and vein graft arterialisation [1]. The development of atherosclerotic vascular disease involves a complex interplay of genetic, metabolic, cellular, and immunological factors [2], and understanding these factors is the first step in targeting heart disease.

Vascular Dysfunction

Pathology of Atherosclerosis

Atherosclerosis is a form of arteriosclerosis, which signifies thickening (sclerosis) of the arteries (arterio). Atherosclerosis specifically refers to thickening and loss of elasticity in the walls of the large to medium-sized arteries [3, 4]. Atherosclerosis manifests as lesions, which are most intense in the coronary arteries and abdominal aorta. Though the onset of the clinical manifestations tends to occur in middle-aged individuals, the evolution of atherosclerosis is chronic and is believed to initiate as early as in childhood [5]. It is now thought to be the major cause of death, not only in the Western world but also worldwide [6]. Indeed, the costs of atherosclerosis and cardiovascular disease are staggering and ever increasing, now reaching 400 billion dollars annually in USA alone [7].

The starting point for gross evolution of atherosclerotic lesions is the "fatty streak," a region of intimal thickening due to an accumulation of inflammatory cells and lipid deposits on the arterial wall [8]. From the initial lesions, a "fibrous plaque" may develop. These consist of raised intimal lesions made up of a lipid core surrounded by vascular SMCs (VSMCs) that have migrated from the media to the subendothelial space and started secreting excess extracellular matrix proteins and collagen [9]. The lipid core of the lesion consists of foam cells formed from

accumulated macrophages and SMCs, which have taken up oxidized low-density lipoprotein (LDL) via the scavenger receptor [10, 11]. This oxidized LDL (oxLDL) originated as LDL, which remained trapped in the subendothelial space, where it was oxidized by reactive oxygen species, first to minimally modified (or oxidized) LDL (mmLDL) and further to oxLDL [12]. Evolution of a vascular lesion past a fibrous plaque leads to the formation of a "complicated lesion." Such a lesion is altered by hemorrhage, calcification, and neovascularization. The lesion core often becomes necrotic, leading to erosion and mural thrombosis [13]. In fact, although angina pectoris is usually a symptom of vessel narrowing, acute cardiovascular events are generally thought to result from plaque rupture and thrombosis [14, 15]. A general overview of atherogenesis and its progression is provided in Fig. 1.

The crucial importance of oxLDL in every step of atherogenesis is still being elucidated. Oxidative stress in the vessel wall is crucial to its function when present at physiological levels, but is detrimental at higher levels, having the ability to cause considerable biological damage. In accordance with this, studies have consistently reported increased oxidative stress and attenuated antioxidative stress mechanisms in patients with CV disease [16–18]. The lipid components of the LDL particle itself can vary, creating a range of size and density. It was found that small, dense LDL particles are more atherogenic, as they are more likely to be taken up by the artery wall [19] and have increased oxidative susceptibility [20]. In fact, an even greater correlation was found between oxLDL and CVD than was found with hypercholesterolemia [21].

As mentioned above, the modification of LDL is thought to occur as a two step process, first to mmLDL, then to oxLDL. In fact, there exist various degrees of oxidation separating these states. LDL first enters vessel walls by passive diffusion, a process dependent on ApoB and the LDL receptor. Local oxidative stress leads to the oxidation and the formation of mmLDL, which is chemically and biologically distinct from unmodified LDL, but retains the

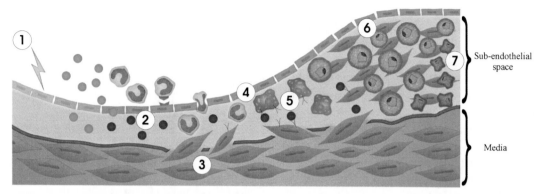

Fig. 1 Vascular events in atherogenesis. An injury affecting the intact, functional endothelium initiates the process (1). This insult can take many forms, including disturbed flow, increases in oxidative stress, and infectious agents. The resulting endothelial dysfunction (2) is demonstrated by major changes in EC phenotype. Increased expression of chemokines, growth factors, and adhesion molecules is observed and accompanied by LDL uptake and attenuation of antioxidant mechanisms. The result is the presence of inflammatory cells, such as monocytes, as well as large quantities of oxLDL in the subendothelial space. Chemokine expression leads to (a) a switch in SMC phenotype, which begin secreting proteases to digest the internal elastic lamina and migrate out of the media (3), and (b) monocyte differentiation into macrophages (4). Both synthetic SMCs and macrophages begin expressing the scavenger receptor and become capable of absorbing oxLDL, which leads to the formation of foam cells (5). Lipid-laden foam cells accumulate within ECM- and collagen-secreting SMCs to create a raised lesion covered by a fibrous cap (6). The process continues to feed-forward, thereby enlarging the lesion. Advanced lesions can often become necrotic at their core (7). Adapted from Faxon et al. [29]

ability to bind the LDL receptor [22]. It activates antiapoptotic signals and stimulates endothelial arterial wall cells to express inflammatory cytokines and adhesion molecules, thus promoting monocyte recruitment [22, 23]. Further oxidation leads to the formation of fully oxidized LDL, which is no longer recognized by the LDL receptor. Its subsequent uptake into macrophages and resultant conversion of macrophages to foam cells are mediated via scavenger receptors, in a manner that is modulated by a feed-forward mechanism, with oxLDL increasing scavenger receptor expression [24, 25], as opposed to the physiological negative feedback mechanism. In fact, studies with double knockout ApoE(−/−)/scavenger receptor-A (SRA) (−/−) mice show that disruption of the SRA gene is sufficient to significantly attenuate atherosclerotic lesion development [26]. Clearly then, the presence of LDL in the subendothelial space is crucial to the maintenance of the chronic degenerative environment created within the atherosclerotic plaque.

Risk Factors

A number of factors are associated with an elevated risk of developing atherosclerosis and are used to assess individual risk. These risk factors were established thanks to large-scale studies such as the Framingham Heart Study [27] and the Atherosclerosis Risk in Communities (ARIC) Study [28]. The risk factors that are most highly correlated with the development of atherosclerosis differ slightly with respect to the different vascular beds [29], a phenomenon that is not well understood. In accordance with this, diabetes mellitus and cigarette smoking are more strongly correlated with PAD, while hypertension is more strongly correlated with cerebrovascular disease leading to stroke [29].

Classical risk factors are divided into categories based on their potential for intervention. "Nonmodifiable risk factors" include age, gender, and heredity. The latter includes both race and genetics. These are predetermined and thus cannot be targeted to reduce the incidence of

CV events. Conversely, those risk factors that are potential targets for therapeutic interventions, either via pharmaceuticals or via lifestyle changes, are categorized as "modifiable risk factors." These are tobacco smoke, dyslipidemia, hypertension, diabetes mellitus, obesity, and inactivity [30]. Other notable factors that do not fall within these categories are stress and alcohol. However, the effects of the latter are thought to be secondary to the primary factors.

Nonconventional risk factors that are independent of the existing factors are also continuously studied to explain the proportion of CV events occurring in patients without the established risk factors (reviewed by Hackam and Anand [31]). One in particular, high sensitivity (hs)-C-reactive protein (CRP), has emerged in a variety of studies as a promising means of predicting vascular disease [32, 33]. It has also been shown that decreasing hs-CRP in patients with elevated circulating concentrations decreased the risk of future MI by nearly 60% [32]. Thus, the Centers for Disease Control and Prevention and the AHA have specified that, of the novel factors, CRP is the most conducive to use in clinical practice and was recognized as an independent marker to be used at physicians' discretion [33]. The acknowledgement of this factor accompanies the recognition of the role of inflammation in atherosclerotic disease. However, it presents limitations due to nonspecificity, since its levels may be elevated because of coexisting inflammatory states [34].

Diagnostic Approaches

Risk factor assessment has become an important tool in determining whether an individual requires a lifestyle or pharmacological intervention to prevent disease progression and onset of symptoms. At the same time, the presence of one or more risk factors does not indicate presence of disease. Indeed, approximately 10% of serious cardiovascular events (death, heart attack) occur in individuals who do not exhibit any risk factors [35], which indicates that the absence of risk factors does not mean absence of disease. Consequently, various technologies have been developed to monitor structural and functional changes in the blood vessels that are associated with the onset of atherosclerotic disease. It is anticipated that these new methods will eventually be used as screening tools in conjunction with risk factor assessment to aid in diagnosis and selection of appropriate treatments.

The inability to dilate is considered among the first signs of vascular dysfunction leading to atherosclerosis. Vasodilation can be measured with flow-mediated dilatation (FMD). This method uses Doppler ultrasound to monitor both the diameter and the mean flow velocity of the brachial artery before and after occlusion with a blood pressure cuff [36]. The greater the dilation, the better is the vessel function. Alternative detection methods that replaced the Doppler probe have been developed, with the most popular instruments (e.g., Itamar's EndoPAT, Endothelix's VENDY) employing fingertip probes to measure peripheral arterial tone. These instruments provide greater sensitivity and require less operator experience than standard FMD. Interestingly, it has recently been suggested that induction of hyperemia via occlusion may not be necessary. Instead, passive leg raising is sufficient to induce dilation of the brachial artery, and this approach has been shown to correlate with FMD [37].

A reduction in arterial compliance is a central feature of atherosclerosis. Increased stiffness of small arteries is considered a very early stage marker of disease, and this change can be monitored via funduscopic examination. Instrumentation to visualize the retinal vasculature enables direct measurement of arteriolar wall thickening. Similarly, alterations in large artery compliance are indicative of more extensive disease. Two methods of assessment have been developed to examine aortic stiffening. Pulse wave analysis (PWA) examines the pressure wave as it travels along the radial artery, although the use of other arteries is also possible [38]. The instrument, which uses a tonometer to capture the wave form, subsequently estimates stiffness from the degree of wave reflectance. A more direct measure of compliance is obtained with pulse wave velocity (PWV). The standard approach measures the speed at which the pressure wave travels along the aorta from the carotid to the femoral artery, with higher velocities indicating greater stiffness. Instruments that monitor brachial to ankle velocity have also been developed [39]. The prognostic value of both PWA and PWV with adverse cardiovascular outcomes has been established in a number of studies [40].

Decreased blood flow to the lower limbs can be detected with the ankle-brachial index (ABI), a ratio of the systolic blood pressure at the ankle and the upper arm. Although this method applies primarily to peripheral artery disease, an ABI less than 0.9 also suggests the presence of either asymptomatic coronary or cerebrovascular disease [41]. Consequently, these individuals have a five- to tenfold higher risk of heart attack or stroke.

Advances in arterial wall imaging have enabled monitoring of disease progression through greater resolution of atherosclerotic plaque burden [42–45]. In most cases, a correlation with disease pathology has also been obtained. The carotid thickness (IMT) can be obtained by high-resolution Doppler ultrasonography. This technique directly measures plaque thickness. However, since several positions along the artery can be employed, the utility of this method is limited as a result of differences in arterial uniformity, and it is highly reliant upon operator expertise. Similar measurements can be obtained in smaller vessels by intravascular ultrasound (IVUS), but this invasive method requires outpatient hospitalization and cannot be conducted in a clinic setting. By contrast, noninvasive CT (computer tomography angiography) or MRI (magnetic resonance imaging) scans provide enhanced sensitivity, but instrument availability is a limiting factor. Newer imaging methods are also being evaluated (e.g., near infrared spectroscopy, optical coherence tomography). However, as in the case of CT and MRI, these will not be suitable for the clinic setting.

The advantage of these techniques is associated with their ability to measure atherosclerotic disease directly, in contrast to risk factor assessment, thus enabling monitoring of disease burden at the level of the individual. Several unique circulating biomarkers of changes in arterial structure have also been identified [46–49], although their validity still requires confirmation. Thus the risk of a serious event can be determined for each person rather than being based on population-wide statistics. However, several of the techniques are limited due to the need for trained personnel (e.g., ultrasound-based methods) or due to the fact that the parameter under observation may not change rapidly (e.g., IMT). In the latter case, however, it is possible to monitor progression if a sufficiently long observation period is used, and this may be advisable for the purpose of including primary measures of disease, namely, death, myocardial infarction, and stroke. Regardless, identification of a panel of methods may still be more reliable than employing a single measure of disease, according to the principles originally outlined by Wilson [50], and several candidate combinations have already been proposed [51, 52].

Important Cell Types

A normal artery wall is made up of three tubular layers surrounding a central lumen. The tunica intima is the innermost layer, consisting of a thin sheet of endothelial cells (ECs) supported on a basement membrane. The middle layer, the tunica media, consists largely of many overlapping layers of smooth muscle cells. It is separated from the other layers by the internal and external elastic laminae, which are sheets primarily consisting of the extracellular matrix protein elastin. The final and outermost layer is called the tunica externa (or adventitia) and is composed primarily of collagen fibers for vessel support [53]. Both the ECs and SMCs within the artery wall are involved in vascular dysfunction leading to atherosclerosis, in conjunction with circulating inflammatory cells. Their contribution to normal arterial function and to progression of atherosclerotic disease is directly related to the modulation of their physical and functional characteristics (Fig. 2).

Endothelial Cells

The endothelial layer, which makes up the tunica intima, was long thought to simply act as an inert

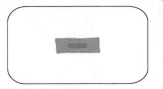
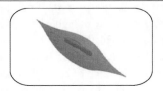

Healthy
- Anti-coagulant
- Anti-inflammatory
- Inhibition of leukocyte
  adhesion
- Vasodilatory

Diseased
- Platelet activation
- ↑ ROS → ↑ oxidation &
  inflammation
- ↑ leukocyte adhesion and
  activation
- ↑ NO & ↑ production of AngII
  & ET-1 → ↑ Vasoconstriction

Heathy
- Contractile
- Small, spindle shaped
- Low proliferative activity
- Low synthetic activity

Diseased
- ↑ Migration
- Hyperproliferative
- ↓contractile protein expression
- ↑ cell size
- ↑ response to GFs
- Disordered ECM synthesis

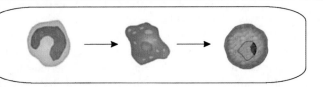

Healthy
- Originate from the bone marrow
- Non-proliferative
- Resident tissue penetration
- Differentiation to macrophages → phagocytosis of infections
  agents

Diseased
- $CD14^{hi}CD16^{lo}$
- Sub-endothelial penetration
- ↑ production of inflammatory cytokines, ROS & MMPs
- Differentiation to macrophages → ↑ expression of scavenger
  receptor
- Ox-LDL uptake → foam cell formation → ↑ ROS, MMP &
  GF production

Fig. 2 Characteristics of the major vascular cell types in healthy and diseased states. The ability to modulate cellular properties is important for maintaining vascular homeostasis in response to injury. However, progression of vascular disease occurs when the balance between these states is lost due to suppression of the negative feedback mechanisms that promote return of the cells to their healthy state

barrier that separated the vessel wall from the circulating blood components. It is now known to be an important and dynamic organ, playing a crucial role in the regulation of vascular tone and homeostasis [54]. Its homeostatic role encompasses regulation of VSMC proliferation and migration, as well as the delicate equilibriums maintaining the body's inflammatory, thrombogenic and coagulative responses [55, 56]. A damaged or dysfunctional endothelial layer can undergo functional and structural alterations, which can lead to disruption of this balance, predisposing the vasculature to an increasingly atheroprone phenotype that exhibits more vasoconstriction, leukocyte adhesion, platelet activation, mitogenesis, oxidation, thrombosis, and vascular inflammation [56, 57]. Indeed, endothelial dysfunction has been closely associated with cardiovascular events [58]. In addition, it has been associated with the presence of all established risk factors for coronary heart disease and precedes the development of atherosclerosis [55].

The defining feature of what is known as "endothelial dysfunction" is impaired nitric oxide (NO) bioavailability, leading to impaired endothelium-dependent vasodilation, and resulting most frequently from increased breakdown of endothelial NO synthase (eNOS) by reactive oxygen species [54]. However, the term also encompasses general defects in all of the homeostatic mechanisms. In particular, dysfunction is accompanied by higher turnover rates [59], secondary to increased apoptosis [60]. EC dysfunction is thought to be the initial step in the continuous cycle leading to the development of atherosclerotic lesions [61]. Increased synthesis of adhesion molecules such as vascular cell adhesion molecule (VCAM) and intercellular adhesion molecule (ICAM), as well as inflammatory cytokines such as monocyte chemoattractant protein (MCP-1), is part of the local inflammatory microenvironment created by the dysfunctional endothelium [62]. Together with increased formation of reactive oxygen species (ROS), penetration of monocytes into the subendothelial space sets the stage for differentiation into macrophages, foam cell formation, and VSMC phenotypic switching.

While the mechanisms behind endothelial dysfunction are not fully known, mechanical forces are thought to play an important role, since arterial branch points are highly susceptible to plaque development [63]. Here, shear flow, which triggers vascular endothelial cells to release NO [64], is disturbed [3]. This disturbed flow includes pulsatile [65] and turbulent flow, as well as low shear flow. These flow patterns can be further exacerbated by pathology such as hypertension, which affects encountered pressure. It has been suggested that these branch sites are susceptible to a chronic maladaptive response, being unable to adapt to disturbed flow and leading to failure of the ECs to maintain their normal quiescent phenotype and function. This disturbed flow also results in the higher cell turnover rates which accompany EC dysfunction [66]. Though it is not yet clear how forces are transduced to biochemical signals, potential mechanotransducers include the cytoskeleton [67], adhesion receptors [68], and other luminal membrane proteins such as G proteins [69] and ion channels [70].

Vascular Smooth Muscle Cells

The highly specialized environment that is the arterial vessel wall maintains its intrinsic ability to respond to injury, thus enabling repair and restoration of vessel integrity, primarily due to VSMCs. While their principal function lies in resistance vessel contraction for regulation of blood pressure and blood flow distribution [71], they also have a prominent role in this repair process, as they are recruited from the existing contractile coat and are also responsible for the production of new connective tissue [72]. An important repercussion of this, however, is that SMCs must retain the ability to reenter the cell cycle and proliferate [73, 74], a characteristic that has implicated them in the development of vascular diseases and postsurgery repair.

Even terminally differentiated smooth muscle cells retain remarkable phenotypic plasticity, a fact that has confounded the process of deciphering the molecular events in their differentiation.

Indeed, changes in local environmental cues can greatly influence cellular phenotype, inducing profound and reversible changes in gene expression and, therefore, in phenotype. This bidirectional switch in phenotype was suggested in 1967 by Wissler [75], and was based on the assumption that SMCs are integral to atherosclerosis. While two extreme phenotypes are commonly described, a range of more subtly altered, intermediate phenotypes is also seen. The first extreme phenotypic state is termed the "contractile" phenotype, most commonly seen in adult vessels, which defines a cell of small size, with a spindle-like, elongated morphology. The SMCs in this state have elevated levels of contractile proteins and maintain a very low proliferation rate as well as a low synthetic activity [76, 77]. The second state is referred to as the "synthetic" phenotype. A synthetic SMC is characterized by increased cell size and extracellular matrix production as well as decreased contractile protein expression. For this reason, a cell in this state is often termed as being "undifferentiated." A synthetic SMC is also hyperproliferative, has increased migration, and is exquisitely responsive to circulating vascular growth factors [78]. While this phenotypic plasticity is crucial for development of the vascular system and vessel remodeling after injury, it predisposes the cell to adverse phenotypic switching due to pathogenic environmental cues [79, 80].

An important study by Katsuda et al. [81] revealed that, with respect to numbers, smooth muscle cells were by far the predominant cell type found in atherosclerotic plaques. However, the implication that SMCs are important in lesion formation was first outlined in 1973 in a landmark paper by Ross and colleagues [13], who proposed a breakthrough hypothesis, namely, the "SMC response to injury." They argued that focal accumulation of SMCs is central to the process of lesion development, since it is involved in both the deposition of lipid and the accumulation of extracellular connective tissue. It is now thought that endothelial dysfunction, as previously described, precedes and possibly activates these SMC responses.

The origin of the SMCs that participate in intimal lesion formation has recently deviated from the long-standing belief that intimal SMCs are derived solely from preexisting medial SMCs. Evidence now suggests that ECs [82] and adventitial fibroblasts [83] may give rise to SMC-like cells within the intima that contribute to injury repair.

The role of the SMCs in atherosclerosis appears to vary with the stage of the disease. In early events, SMCs are involved in a maladaptive role in lesion development and progression via their proliferative and migratory responses. However, over 50% of acute cardiac events occur in arteries having a nonsignificant degree of stenosis ($\leq$50%), underlying the relatively minor role of plaque size in determining stability [84]. Thus, in late-stage disease, SMCs likely play a beneficial role within the fibrous plaque, forming a physiological, stabilizing cap. Indeed, it has been shown that rupture-prone vulnerable plaques are characterized by a necrotic core and a very thin fibrous cap containing reduced numbers of SMCs, and that plaques specifically tend to rupture at sites of reduced SMC content [85]. Vascular SMC apoptosis has been shown to occur in advanced atherosclerotic lesions [86] and is thought to be a prominent pathway leading to plaque destabilization [87]. Thus, agents that are present and involved in regulating apoptosis within the plaque remain attractive targets for acute MI research.

Inflammatory Cells

In the past, it was suggested that the two major characteristics of atherosclerotic lesions included the intimal proliferation of SMCs, as described above, and the inflammatory response [88]. These two characteristics are, in fact, not mutually exclusive, as both SMCs and ECs secrete and respond to cytokines involved in the inflammatory process, which further activates the proliferative response [88].

Indeed, it is now well established that circulating inflammatory cells play an important part in both the initiation and the progression of vascular disease. There is substantial evidence that inflammatory cascades are initiated by a wide range of cellular effectors that promote atherogenesis [89]. In addition, inflammation is now seen as a key regulatory process linking multiple risk factors for atherosclerosis [90]. Though macrophages are thought to be the predominant inflammatory species, T cells [81, 91], B cells [92, 93], neutrophils [94], mast cells [95], and dendritic cells [96] have also been detected in both human and mouse aortae. Some, such as the B cells and neutrophils, may be at least partially atheroprotective, while the T cells and mast cells, as well as the very important monocyte-derived macrophages, are negatively involved in every step of atherogenesis.

In the middle of the nineteenth century, the German scientist Rudolf Virchow studied and described inflammatory changes in atherosclerotic vessel walls, and postulated their role as being critical for atherogenesis [97]. Subsequently, however, the direction of atherosclerotic plaque research took a turn and became focused on cholesterol, metabolism and diet. Thus, it was not until much later that this aspect of vascular disease was further investigated [98].

The presence of leukocytes within atherosclerotic plaque was first characterized by Gerrity et al. [99] who studied the aortic intima of cholesterol-fed pigs. They found monocytes to be present in the very earliest stages of developing plaque. Monocytes under homeostasis represent 10% of circulating leukocytes [100], originate from the bone marrow [101] and do not proliferate [10]. However, during inflammation, they can migrate from the blood to the subendothelial space in response to tissue-derived signals [102], among which is the very potent monocyte chemoattractant protein-1 (MCP-1). MCP-1 can be produced by a variety of cells, including ECs [103] and SMCs [104], is present in plaque as early as the fatty streak [105], and is upregulated in these cells in response to oxidized lipids [106]. Once infiltrated, monocytes can phagocytose other cells and toxic molecules and produce inflammatory cytokines [107]. In addition, they can differentiate into inflammatory dendritic cells or macrophages, and further into foam cells, as determined by the inflammatory milieu [108].

Heterogeneity within the monocyte population has led to the study and identification of monocyte subtypes in both mice and humans, with each defined by variations in chemokine receptor and adhesion molecule expression. The most proinflammatory subtype, recognized by high levels of a marker known as Ly6C in mice [109], homes to the atherosclerotic plaque, where it expresses high levels of proinflammatory cytokines and other macrophage mediators, including matrix metalloproteinases (MMPs) [90]. Although a corresponding human subtype has not yet been identified, the CD14[hi]CD16[lo] monocytes, which express CCR2, CD62L, and CD64A, have been associated with the inflammatory subset [10, 110]. A study by Swirski et al. [111] found that monocytes were continually recruited to plaque, and that this accumulation increased proportionally with lesion size. This study directly correlated monocyte recruitment with progression of atherosclerosis. A second very interesting study found that inhibition of the potent MCP-1/CCR2 axis via a gene-eluting anti-MCP-1 stenting strategy in rabbits and monkeys [112] significantly decreased neointimal formation. Conversely, another study found that emigration of monocyte-derived DC-like cells was found in regressing lesions, and that increased differentiation into these cells decreased lesion size [113]. Together, these studies suggest that plaque progression may be the result of both increased monocyte recruitment and decreased monocyte emigration from lesions. Thus, the importance of monocytes in atherogenesis has been well documented. However, while the initial infiltration step is important, it is the subsequent differentiation to macrophages that is recognized as crucial for plaque progression.

Monocyte to macrophage differentiation is a process dependent on a combination of both the distinct subtype and the inflammatory milieu. Interactions with the extracellular matrix as well as with the cytokines Macrophage colony stimulating factor (MCSF) and members of the Tumor Necrosis Factor (TNF) family are known to drive the process [114]. This differentiation is characterized by significant changes in the gene expression program, including increases in scavenger receptors. They, along with smooth muscle cells, are able to take up oxidized LDL, which accumulates as cholesteryl esters in characteristic foamy deposits [115]. These foam cells then become a major contributor to pathology via ROS production and increased expression of cytokines, including TNFs, Interleukins (ILs) and Interferons (IFNs), of enzymes, including serine/cysteine proteinases and MMPs, and of growth factors, including platelet-derived growth factor (PDGF), vascular endothelial growth factor (VEGF), epidermal growth factor (EGF), and insulin-like growth factor (IGF) [23]. Through this degenerative cycle, the macrophage has been implicated in every stage of atherogenesis, from the early inflammatory events to the late-stage necrotic and ruptured plaque, which often contains high numbers of prothrombotic MMP- and tissue factor-secreting macrophages [85].

The Role of Vascular Growth Factors

Vascular growth factors (GFs) are important environmental factors that play a major role in atherogenesis, in particular via their actions on SMC phenotypic modulation. Some have been shown to promote the differentiated and anti-atherogenic contractile phenotype, while others tip the equilibrium toward an undifferentiated, proliferative, and migratory phenotype. Others still have indirect effects through surrounding cells, including ECs. While some are cytokines that act systemically on atheroprone sites as they circulate through the body, it is thought that many act in an autocrine and paracrine manner. These GFs become an integral part of the lesion microenvironment by exerting local effects on both the cells that synthesize them and those in the immediate surroundings. GFs are numerous and have proven to be effective cell communication tools, each one acting through specific and complex pathways. In addition, implication of one factor in a certain stage of the disease does not necessarily implicate it in all stages. Thus,

our current understanding of their actions within lesions is incomplete with respect to phenotypic modulation as well as with respect to interactions with inflammatory cell mediators, lipids, lipid peroxidation products, and ROS. However, certain GFs have been identified as potentially important and, through extensive studies, have provided some clues to their role in lesion development.

Platelet-Derived Growth Factor

PDGF is a potent chemoattractant and mitogen for cells of mesenchymal origin, such as fibroblasts and SMCs. It is produced by activated platelets and released during blood clotting or when platelets adhere at sites of vessel injury to initiate vessel repair [116]. Interestingly, it has also been shown to be secreted by lesion macrophages and by a number of both normal and transformed cell types [117, 118]. PDGF consists of either disulfide linked homo- or heterodimers of two chains, A and B, or of homodimers exclusively of two other chains, C and D [119]. It acts through two tyrosine kinase receptors, PDGFR-α and PDGFR-β, which initiate similar but nonidentical cellular responses [120]. These dimerize following activation, and hybrid receptor formation is also thought to occur. PDGF has been shown to induce rapid downregulation of SM-selective markers in cultured SMCs [121, 122], and importantly, several human postinjury models have detected PDGF chains as well as their receptors in coronary arteries [123, 124]. Sano et al. [125] suggested a critical role for PDGF in atherogenesis when they used antibodies against PDGFR-α and -β in ApoE(−/−) mice fed a Western diet. Their results showed a 67% reduction in lesion size and 80% reduction in SMC neointimal investment with PDGFR-β blockage, as compared to control ApoE(−/−) mice. Another study by Kozaki et al. [126] looked at these same ApoE(−/−) mice long-term, after a lethal irradiation and reconstitution of blood cells using PDGF-deficient embryonic liver cells.

They found an interesting temporal importance for the PDGF axis in lesion development, with lesion differences at 35 weeks, which were indistinguishable at 45 weeks.

Vascular Endothelial Growth Factor

The VEGF family of growth factors is a subfamily of the PDGF family. The major member, VEGF-A is a 165 amino acid (aa) peptide, which signals through the tyrosine kinase receptors VEGF receptor (VEGFR)-1/2. It is known as an important physiological mediator of angiogenesis, with a particularly potent effect on endothelial cells, as well as an important effect on inflammatory cells [127]. The role of VEGF also appears to be two-fold. It plays a role in plaque development, stimulating the formation of immature neovessels [128], which not only provide nutrients to the plaque but also contribute, either via hemorrhage or via invasion of inflammatory cells, to plaque instability [129]. However, it is also important for reendothelialization after injury, as well as maintenance of endothelial integrity, as VEGF gene-eluting stents have been shown to decrease NI formation [130–132], thus resulting in long-term decrease of SMC proliferation and inflammatory activity.

Transforming Growth Factor-β

Transforming Growth Factor beta (TGF-β (beta)) is a 390 aa peptide that signals through any one of the two receptor tyrosine kinase subtypes I and II. It has been shown to promote SMC differentiation via upregulation of SMC markers [133]. In addition, its levels are rapidly increased after balloon injury in animal models [134]. Though its role in lesion formation remains unclear, there is evidence suggesting a protective role for TGF-β. Patients with unstable angina will often present with severely low levels of plasma TGF-β [135], and studies in ApoE(−/−) mice have presented convincing evidence that TGF-β may be critical for SMC matrix production and the development of a stable plaque [136–138].

Epidermal Growth Factor

Epidermal Growth Factor (EGF) is a 53 aa polypeptide, one of six family members that originate as a transmembrane glycoprotein precursor with an extracellular growth factor sequence. Cleavage by MMPs releases the active growth factor, which acts on many cell types through the EGF receptor (EGFR), a member of the tyrosine kinase receptor family [139]. EGF, and other family members such as heparin binding-EGF (HB-EGF) and TGF-alpha (TGF-α), are expressed by cells involved in atherogenesis, including ECs [140], SMCs [141], and T lymphocytes [142]. In addition, they have been shown to contribute to phenotypic switching [143], and, while EGF is thought to be important for monocyte chemotaxis and macrophage proliferation [144], HP-EGF is thought to be an important chemoattractant and mitogen [145]. Furthermore, in differentiated macrophages and SMCs, it is upregulated in response to oxLDL [146] and upregulates other growth factors [147]. The EGFR and other family members also appear to be central in the growth responses of other important vascular factors including angiotensin II (AngII) [148] and endothelin-1 (ET-1) [149] via guanine nucleotide-binding protein (G protein) EGFR transactivation [150]. Thus, EGF appears to contribute to atherogenesis via many different mechanisms.

Basic Fibroblast Growth Factor/ Fibroblast Growth Factor-2

Basic Fibroblast Growth Factor (bFGF), also known as FGF-2, is a heparin-binding factor, part of the FGF family, which binds the tyrosine kinase FGF receptors. It is thought to act on SMCs and ECs to stimulate angiogenesis [151], through a synergistic effect with VEGF [130]. As with VEGF, the role of FGF-2 in atherogenesis remains elusive. While it may have a pro-atherogenic role as it has been shown to promote SMC proliferation [152], an experimental model has suggested a protective effect by reversing endothelial dysfunction [153]. A more recent study of diet-induced atherosclerosis further supported a protective role for FGF-2 in the early stages of plaque development, showing improved endothelium dependent relaxation and decreased plaque macrophage content with bFGF administration [154].

Insulin-Like Growth Factor-1

IGF-1 is a single chain, 70 aa peptide cytokine that is highly homologous to insulin in sequence, which translates to considerable similarity in three-dimensional structure [155]. Along with IGF-2, it is part of a growth factor family termed the IGFs that has effects on most cell types primarily via the tyrosine kinase IGF-1 receptor (IGF-1R) [156]. In the vascular system and with respect to atherosclerosis, IGF-1 has a strong influence on SMCs [157], inflammatory cells [158], and ECs [159]. IGF-1 is primarily known as a survival factor [160] but is also a chemoattractant and a mitogen [161, 162]. In addition, it is involved in the regulation of many crucial processes in VSMCs including contractility, protein synthesis, differentiation, and glucose uptake [163, 164]. Its role as a survival factor was first extensively studied in the cancer field for its oncogenic potential. However, this role takes on a different outlook in vascular disease where the balance between cell survival and cell death contributes to atherosclerotic plaque stability [165]. Indeed, it has been shown that in advanced atherosclerotic plaques, IGF-1 and IGF-1R expression is low or absent in intimal regions with macrophage infiltration, thereby contributing to increased apoptosis [166].

The Role of Vascular Progenitor Cells

Endothelial Progenitor Cells

Endothelial progenitor cells (EPCs) were first identified in 1997 by Asahara et al. [167], who isolated CD34+ hematopoietic progenitors from peripheral blood. However, an exact definition for EPCs has not yet been agreed upon, resulting in the term being used for a variety of cell types that are capable of differentiating into ECs, but with differing surface marker signatures. Generally accepted surface markers are CD34+ and VEGFR-2+ (CD309) [168], while a more immature subtype also expresses CD133 [169]. One group has reported a functionally different subgroup of CD34- EPCs [170], indicating that exceptions to the rule do occur. In addition, some subtypes can be further separated based on the presence or absence of other markers including CD45, CD14, and CD146. The different subpopulations are also likely to participate in different stages of vascular remodeling and repair, with early EPCs likely contributing indirectly via secretion of angiogenic factors [171], and late EPCs directly contributing to vessel growth [172].

As endothelial injury plays a primary role in the development of CVD, endothelial progenitor cells have become a major area of vascular research. It is thought that the repair of damaged endothelium, which often occurs at branch points, depends on both resident ECs and circulating EPCs [173], and that increased EPCs can directly restore the endothelial lining [174] (Fig. 3). In addition, it has been suggested that poor EPC numbers, or impaired function, are a better predictor of endothelial integrity than the presence of traditional risk factors [175]. In support of this view, EPCs from individuals with severe atherosclerosis show reduced colony forming and functional activity [176]. With respect to CV risk directly, a number of cardiovascular risk factors have been correlated with decreased number and impaired function, including smoking [177], age [178, 179], and type 2 diabetes [180]. However, a major population-study by Xiao et al. [181] overturned the developing views of EPCs by showing a positive correlation between EPC number and many risk factors. This study also suggested that the ability to mobilize EPCs may in fact be more important than any end-point measurement. With respect to the clinical potential of EPCs, it has repeatedly been shown that infusion of EPCs into ApoE knockout mice is detrimental, increasing plaque size and decreasing stability via thinner fibrous caps [182, 183]. Thus, the use of EPCs remains unclear, as controversy remains with respect to the effect of increasing EPC numbers on CV disease.

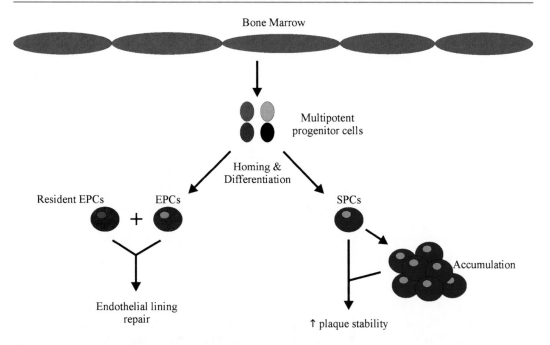

Fig. 3 Current most supported hypotheses of the roles of bone-marrow-derived EPCs and SPCs in atherosclerotic disease. Bone-marrow-derived progenitor cells are thought to home to sites of vascular injury and to acquire specific lineage markers for EPCs and SPCs. BM-EPCs cooperate with resident ECs to aid in the repair of the endothelial lining, as they fully differentiate into mature ECs. Alternatively, SPCs may or may not fully differentiate to mature SMCs and are thought to stabilize existing plaque via collagen synthesis. Adapted from Satoh and Berk [212]

Since EPCs originate from within the bone marrow (BM), homing to the site of injury must occur for vascular repair to be initiated, and differentiation into mature ECs is crucial for vessel integrity to be restored. The production of VEGF [184] and stromal-cell-derived factor-1 (SFD-1) [185] by damaged or ischemic areas is important as both factors result in an increase in circulating EPC numbers. The mechanisms underlying this are not fully elucidated, but it is thought to occur via MMP-9 activation at the level of the BM. MMP-9-driven conversion of the insoluble factor membrane-bound (mb)-KitL to soluble KitL may lead to progenitor cell transition from the quiescent to the proliferation niche, and subsequent mobilization from the BM [186]. Once released into the circulation, many adhesion and signaling events are involved in directing EPCs to an injury site. Of particular importance are platelet factors, which appear to be crucial, as they are involved in every step including homing, activation, and maturation of the EPCs [168].

Of note, while most research has focused on BM-derived cells, it has also been reported that EPCs can originate from other organs including the spleen [174], the intestine and liver [187], as well as adipose tissue [188].

SMC Progenitor Cells

Although a more recent concept, these is accumulating evidence that circulating BM-derived cells invest in the intima following injury and express at least some SMC markers [189–191], despite a few studies that deny their implication [192, 193]. Several studies have also raised doubts as to whether these undergo full differentiation into mature SMCs [189, 194]. In addition, their contribution to NI formation is controversial, as tracking the cells in vivo remains extremely difficult, and it has been shown that NI can form in cultured vessels, in the complete absence of any blood elements [195]. This was addressed in a study by Han et al. [196], who conducted a study of scratch induced vascular injuries of varying degrees. They found major investment of bone marrow-derived cells in severe injury, but none in minor injury cases where there was endothelial denudation but minimal damage to the medial SMCs, suggesting that bone marrow-derived cells may be recruited only to complement resident SMCs.

As with EPCs, the therapeutic potential of SPCs is under debate. A study in immune intolerant ApoE knockout mice found that chronic injections of SPCs promoted a change in plaque composition, stabilizing plaque via increased collagen content (Fig. 3), early on in disease development. This beneficial effect, however, was lost after 12 weeks, where there was no change in progression. They also extended their research to study SPC numbers in human patients and found that adults with acute cardiovascular symptoms have reduced peripheral blood-derived progenitor cells expressing SMC marker as compared to adults with angina [197]. However, there is not yet enough data regarding SPC function to draw significant conclusions.

The origin of SPCs is extremely variable. Some have been isolated directly from human peripheral blood [190], and these cells display a highly proliferative and proinflammatory phenotype, similar to that of dedifferentiated SMCs [198]. Mesenchymal stem cells isolated from the BM have been shown to differentiate into cells expressing SMC markers in varying conditions such as direct injection into mouse hearts [199], or when cultured on laminin, in which case they also retained these markers when implanted in vivo [200]. SMC progenitors have also been identified from many non-BM sites including the media [201, 202] and adventitia [203] of the vessel wall itself, adipose tissue [204], lymphoid follicular dendritic cells [205], and even myocardial tissue [206]. There is, however, very little evidence of their function past the expression of SMC markers and contraction, or of their contribution to the disease process.

It is unclear whether the cellular signals leading to differentiation of either BM or non-BM SPCs are the same as those involved during embryogenesis or whether they are specific to injury repair. The coagulation protein thrombin, which is generated as a response to vascular injury, can promote MSC differentiation into SMCs via myocardin [207], a signal that is not necessary for embryonic stem cell differentiation into SMCs [208]. Conversely, increased Hedgehog and Notch-1 signaling has been observed in the SMCs of carotid arteries after vascular injury [209], a signal that results in the expression of the SMC markers SM-α (alpha)-actin [210] and SM-myosin heavy chain [211].

Conclusions

Vascular disease is the root cause of the majority of the morbidity and mortality resulting from heart disease. Targeting the vasculature is, therefore, an important part of any treatment and prevention plan to help control the epidemic. Like heart disease itself, it is complex and multifactorial and will require many more years of research. Specifically, a better understanding of the consequences of the interactions between the major players in a nonisolated context will be crucial in creating a complete view of the disease. However, the progress in the last few years is indeed encouraging and has already led to the most promising treatments to date with respect to treating MIs and strokes.

Acknowledgements We would like to thank Robert Blaich for his assistance in the preparation of Figure 1 and Figure 2.

References

1. Fuster JJ, Fernandez P, Gonzalez-Navarro H, et al. Control of cell proliferation in atherosclerosis: insights from animal models and human studies. Cardiovasc Res. 2009;86:254–64.
2. Siu D. A new way of targeting to treat coronary artery disease. J Cardiovasc Med (Hagerstown). 2010;11:1–6.
3. Hahn C, Schwartz MA. Mechanotransduction in vascular physiology and atherogenesis. Nat Rev Mol Cell Biol. 2009;10:53–62.
4. Ross R. Atherosclerosis – an inflammatory disease. N Engl J Med. 1999;340:115–26.

5. Santos MG, Pegoraro M, Sandrini F, et al. Risk factors for the development of atherosclerosis in childhood and adolescence. Arq Bras Cardiol. 2008;90:276–83.

6. Hof D, von Eckardstein A. Risk factors in atherosclerotic coronary heart disease. Ther Umsch. 2009;66:253–9.

7. Lands B. Planning primary prevention of coronary disease. Curr Atheroscler Rep. 2009;11:272–80.

8. Katsiki N, Tziomalos K, Chatzizisis Y, et al. Effect of HMG-CoA reductase inhibitors on vascular cell apoptosis: beneficial or detrimental? Atherosclerosis. 2009;211:9–14.

9. Stoneman VE, Bennett MR. Role of apoptosis in atherosclerosis and its therapeutic implications. Clin Sci (Lond). 2004;107:343–54.

10. Woollard KJ, Geissmann F. Monocytes in atherosclerosis: subsets and functions. Nat Rev Cardiol. 2010;7:77–86.

11. Yu J, Li Y, Li M, et al. Oxidized low density lipoprotein-induced transdifferentiation of bone marrow-derived smooth muscle-like cells into foam-like cells in vitro. Int J Exp Pathol. 2010;91:24–33.

12. Gleissner CA, Leitinger N, Ley K. Effects of native and modified low-density lipoproteins on monocyte recruitment in atherosclerosis. Hypertension. 2007;50:276–83.

13. Ross R, Glomset JA. Atherosclerosis and the arterial smooth muscle cell: Proliferation of smooth muscle is a key event in the genesis of the lesions of atherosclerosis. Science. 1973;180:1332–9.

14. Shah PK. Mechanisms of plaque vulnerability and rupture. J Am Coll Cardiol. 2003;41:15S–22.

15. Davies MJ, Thomas A. Thrombosis and acute coronary-artery lesions in sudden cardiac ischemic death. N Engl J Med. 1984;310:1137–40.

16. Wang XL, Adachi T, Sim AS, et al. Plasma extracellular superoxide dismutase levels in an Australian population with coronary artery disease. Arterioscler Thromb Vasc Biol. 1998;18:1915–21.

17. McMurray J, McLay J, Chopra M, et al. Evidence for enhanced free radical activity in chronic congestive heart failure secondary to coronary artery disease. Am J Cardiol. 1990;65:1261–2.

18. Akkus I, Saglam NI, Caglayan O, et al. Investigation of erythrocyte membrane lipid peroxidation and antioxidant defense systems of patients with coronary artery disease (CAD) documented by angiography. Clin Chim Acta. 1996;244:173–80.

19. Bjornheden T, Babyi A, Bondjers G, et al. Accumulation of lipoprotein fractions and subfractions in the arterial wall, determined in an in vitro perfusion system. Atherosclerosis. 1996;123:43–56.

20. Tribble DL, Rizzo M, Chait A, et al. Enhanced oxidative susceptibility and reduced antioxidant content of metabolic precursors of small, dense low-density lipoproteins. Am J Med. 2001;110:103–10.

21. Gardner CD, Fortmann SP, Krauss RM. Association of small low-density lipoprotein particles with the incidence of coronary artery disease in men and women. JAMA. 1996;276:875–81.

22. Berliner JA, Territo MC, Sevanian A, et al. Minimally modified low density lipoprotein stimulates monocyte endothelial interactions. J Clin Invest. 1990;85:1260–6.

23. Saha P, Modarai B, Humphries J, et al. The monocyte/macrophage as a therapeutic target in atherosclerosis. Curr Opin Pharmacol. 2009;9:109–18.

24. Tsimikas S, Witztum JL. The oxidative modification hypothesis of atherosclerosis. In: Keaney JF, editor. Oxidative stress and vascular disease. Norwell, MA: Kluwer; 2000. p. 49–56.

25. Stocker R, Keaney Jr JF. Role of oxidative modifications in atherosclerosis. Physiol Rev. 2004;84:1381–478.

26. Suzuki H, Kurihara Y, Takeya M, et al. A role for macrophage scavenger receptors in atherosclerosis and susceptibility to infection. Nature. 1997;386:292–6.

27. Kannel WB, McGee D, Gordon T. A general cardiovascular risk profile: the Framingham Study. Am J Cardiol. 1976;38:46–51.

28. The Atherosclerosis Risk in Communities (ARIC) Study: design and objectives. Am J Epidemiol. 1989;129:687–702.

29. Faxon DP, Fuster V, Libby P, et al. Atherosclerotic Vascular Disease Conference: Writing Group III: pathophysiology. Circulation. 2004;109:2617–25.

30. American Heart Association. Risk Factors and Coronary Heart Disease. http://www.americanheart.org/presenter.jhtml?identifier=4726. Updated 2010. Accessed 13 Sep 2010.

31. Hackam DG, Anand SS. Emerging risk factors for atherosclerotic vascular disease: a critical review of the evidence. JAMA. 2003;290:932–40.

32. Ridker PM, Cushman M, Stampfer MJ, et al. Inflammation, aspirin, and the risk of cardiovascular disease in apparently healthy men. N Engl J Med. 1997;336:973–9.

33. Pearson TA, Mensah GA, Alexander RW, et al. Markers of inflammation and cardiovascular disease: application to clinical and public health practice: a statement for healthcare professionals from the Centers for Disease Control and Prevention and the American Heart Association. Circulation. 2003;107:499–511.

34. Ridker PM. High-sensitivity C-reactive protein: potential adjunct for global risk assessment in the primary prevention of cardiovascular disease. Circulation. 2001;103:1813–8.

35. Lown B. Sudden cardiac death: the major challenge confronting contemporary cardiology. Am J Cardiol. 1979;43:313–28.

36. Urbina EM, Williams RV, Alpert BS, et al. Noninvasive assessment of subclinical atherosclerosis in children and adolescents: recommendations for standard assessment for clinical research: a scientific statement from the American Heart Association. Hypertension. 2009;54:919–50.

37. Kamran H, Salciccioli L, Namana V, et al. Passive leg raising induced brachial artery dilation: is an old

technique a simpler method to measure endothelial function? Atherosclerosis. 2010;212:188–92.

38. Vyssoulis GP, Pietri PG, Karpanou EA, et al. Differential impact of metabolic syndrome on arterial stiffness and wave reflections: focus on distinct definitions. Int J Cardiol. 2010;138:119–25.

39. Tsuchikura S, Shoji T, Kimoto E, et al. Brachial-ankle pulse wave velocity as an index of central arterial stiffness. J Atheroscler Thromb. 2010;17:658–65.

40. Nelson MR, Stepanek J, Cevette M, et al. Noninvasive measurement of central vascular pressures with arterial tonometry: clinical revival of the pulse pressure waveform? Mayo Clin Proc. 2010;85:460–72.

41. Paraskevas KI, Kotsikoris I, Koupidis SA, et al. Ankle–brachial index: a marker of both peripheral arterial disease and systemic atherosclerosis as well as a predictor of vascular events. Angiology. 2010;61:521–3.

42. Lane HA, Smith JC, Davies JS. Noninvasive assessment of preclinical atherosclerosis. Vasc Health Risk Manag. 2006;2:19–30.

43. Uno K, Bayturan O, Lavoie A, et al. Rationale and approach to evaluation of the impact of medical therapies on progression of atherosclerosis with arterial wall imaging. Curr Med Res Opin. 2010;26:737–44.

44. Eijgelaar WJ, Heeneman S, Daemen MJ. The vulnerable patient: refocusing on the plaque? Thromb Haemost. 2009;102:231–9.

45. Bayturan O, Uno K, Lavoie A, et al. Future requirement for arterial wall imaging modalities in the evaluation of novel anti-atherosclerotic therapies. Curr Med Res Opin. 2010;26:753–7.

46. Mori K, Emoto M, Araki T, et al. Association of serum fetuin-A with carotid arterial stiffness. Clin Endocrinol (Oxf). 2007;66:246–50.

47. Roos M, Richart T, Kouznetsova T, et al. Fetuin-A and arterial stiffness in patients with normal kidney function. Regul Pept. 2009;154:39–43.

48. Borissoff JI, Heeneman S, Kilinc E, et al. Early atherosclerosis exhibits an enhanced procoagulant state. Circulation. 2010;122:821–30.

49. Zagura M, Serg M, Kampus P, et al. Association of osteoprotegerin with aortic stiffness in patients with symptomatic peripheral artery disease and in healthy subjects. Am J Hypertens. 2010;23:586–91.

50. Wilson JM. The evaluation of the worth of early disease detection. J R Coll Gen Pract. 1968;16:S48–57.

51. Hurks R, Peeters W, Derksen WJ, et al. Biobanks and the search for predictive biomarkers of local and systemic outcome in atherosclerotic disease. Thromb Haemost. 2009;101:48–54.

52. Cohn JN, Duprez DA, Grandits GA. Arterial elasticity as part of a comprehensive assessment of cardiovascular risk and drug treatment. Hypertension. 2005;46:217–20.

53. Moyes CD, Schulte PM. Chapter 9: Circulatory systems. In: Berriman L, Maloy S, Robbins B, Shaw R,

editors. Principles of animal physiology. San Francisco: Pearson-Benjamin Cummings; 2006. p. 340.

54. Versari D, Daghini E, Virdis A, et al. Endothelial dysfunction as a target for prevention of cardiovascular disease. Diabetes Care. 2009;32:S314–21.

55. Mensah GA. Healthy endothelium: the scientific basis for cardiovascular health promotion and chronic disease prevention. Vascul Pharmacol. 2007;46:310–4.

56. Verma S, Anderson TJ. Fundamentals of endothelial function for the clinical cardiologist. Circulation. 2002;105:546–9.

57. Bai X, Wang X, Xu Q. Endothelial damage and stem cell repair in atherosclerosis. Vascul Pharmacol. 2010;52:224–9.

58. Landmesser U, Drexler H. The clinical significance of endothelial dysfunction. Curr Opin Cardiol. 2005;20:547–51.

59. Foteinos G, Hu Y, Xiao Q, et al. Rapid endothelial turnover in atherosclerosis-prone areas coincides with stem cell repair in apolipoprotein E-deficient mice. Circulation. 2008;117:1856–63.

60. Dimmeler S, Hermann C, Zeiher AM. Apoptosis of endothelial cells. Contribution to the pathophysiology of atherosclerosis? Eur Cytokine Netw. 1998;9:697–8.

61. Chien S. Effects of disturbed flow on endothelial cells. Ann Biomed Eng. 2008;36:554–62.

62. Doran AC, Meller N, McNamara CA. Role of smooth muscle cells in the initiation and early progression of atherosclerosis. Arterioscler Thromb Vasc Biol. 2008;28:812–9.

63. Chien S. Role of shear stress direction in endothelial mechanotransduction. Mol Cell Biomech. 2008;5:1–8.

64. Jin ZG, Ueba H, Tanimoto T, et al. Ligand-independent activation of vascular endothelial growth factor receptor 2 by fluid shear stress regulates activation of endothelial nitric oxide synthase. Circ Res. 2003;93:354–63.

65. Ku DN, Giddens DP, Zarins CK, et al. Pulsatile flow and atherosclerosis in the human carotid bifurcation. Positive correlation between plaque location and low oscillating shear stress. Arteriosclerosis. 1985;5:293–302.

66. Davies PF, Remuzzi A, Gordon EJ, et al. Turbulent fluid shear stress induces vascular endothelial cell turnover in vitro. Proc Natl Acad Sci USA. 1986;83:2114–7.

67. Hartog H, Wesseling J, Boezen HM, et al. The insulin-like growth factor 1 receptor in cancer: old focus, new future. Eur J Cancer. 2007;43:1895–904.

68. Tzima E, Irani-Tehrani M, Kiosses WB, et al. A mechanosensory complex that mediates the endothelial cell response to fluid shear stress. Nature. 2005;437:426–31.

69. Gudi S, Nolan JP, Frangos JA. Modulation of GTPase activity of G proteins by fluid shear stress

and phospholipid composition. Proc Natl Acad Sci USA. 1998;95:2515–9.

70. Maroto R, Raso A, Wood TG, et al. TRPC1 forms the stretch-activated cation channel in vertebrate cells. Nat Cell Biol. 2005;7:179–85.

71. Hilgers RH, Webb RC. Molecular aspects of arterial smooth muscle contraction: focus on Rho. Exp Biol Med (Maywood). 2005;230:829–35.

72. Ross R, Fuster V. Chapter 25: The pathogenesis of atherosclerosis. In: Fuster V, Ross R, Topol EJ, editors. Atherosclerosis and coronary artery disease. Philadelphia: Lippincott-Raven; 1996. p. 441.

73. Mallika V, Goswami B, Rajappa M. Atherosclerosis pathophysiology and the role of novel risk factors: a clinicobiochemical perspective. Angiology. 2007;58:513–22.

74. Muto A, Fitzgerald TN, Pimiento JM, et al. Smooth muscle cell signal transduction: implications of vascular biology for vascular surgeons. J Vasc Surg. 2007;45:A15–24.

75. Wissler RW. The arterial medial cell, smooth muscle, or multifunctional mesenchyme? Circulation. 1967;36:1–4.

76. Rzucidlo EM, Martin KA, Powell RJ. Regulation of vascular smooth muscle cell differentiation. J Vasc Surg. 2007;45:A25–32.

77. Rudd JHF, Weissberg PL. Atherosclerosis. In: Hunt BJ, Poston L, Schachter M, Halliday A, editors. An introduction to vascular biology. 2nd ed. Cambridge: Cambridge University Press; 2002. p. 302.

78. Owens GK. Chapter 23: Role of alterations in the differentiated state of vascular smooth muscle cells in atherogenesis. In: Fuster V, Ross R, Topol EJ, editors. Atherosclerosis and coronary artery disease. Philadelphia: Lippincott-Raven; 1996. p. 401.

79. Ohlsson C, Mohan S, Sjogren K, et al. The role of liver-derived insulin-like growth factor-I. Endocr Rev. 2009;30:494–535.

80. Owens GK. Regulation of differentiation of vascular smooth muscle cells. Physiol Rev. 1995;75: 487–517.

81. Katsuda S, Boyd HC, Fligner C, et al. Human atherosclerosis. III. Immunocytochemical analysis of the cell composition of lesions of young adults. Am J Pathol. 1992;140:907–14.

82. DeRuiter MC, Poelmann RE, VanMunsteren JC, et al. Embryonic endothelial cells transdifferentiate into mesenchymal cells expressing smooth muscle actins in vivo and in vitro. Circ Res. 1997; 80:444–51.

83. Sartore S, Chiavegato A, Faggin E, et al. Contribution of adventitial fibroblasts to neointima formation and vascular remodeling: from innocent bystander to active participant. Circ Res. 2001;89:1111–21.

84. Versari D, Lerman LO, Lerman A. The importance of reendothelialization after arterial injury. Curr Pharm Des. 2007;13:1811–24.

85. Davies MJ, Richardson PD, Woolf N, et al. Risk of thrombosis in human atherosclerotic plaques: role of extracellular lipid, macrophage, and smooth muscle cell content. Br Heart J. 1993;69:377–81.

86. Han DK, Haudenschild CC, Hong MK, et al. Evidence for apoptosis in human atherogenesis and in a rat vascular injury model. Am J Pathol. 1995;147:267–77.

87. Bennett MR. Apoptosis of vascular smooth muscle cells in vascular remodelling and atherosclerotic plaque rupture. Cardiovasc Res. 1999;41:361–8.

88. Nilsson J. Cytokines and smooth muscle cells in atherosclerosis. Cardiovasc Res. 1993;27:1184–90.

89. Weber C, Zernecke A, Libby P. The multifaceted contributions of leukocyte subsets to atherosclerosis: lessons from mouse models. Nat Rev Immunol. 2008;8:802–15.

90. Libby P, Ridker PM, Hansson GK, et al. Inflammation in atherosclerosis: from pathophysiology to practice. J Am Coll Cardiol. 2009;54:2129–38.

91. Munro JM, van der Walt JD, Munro CS, et al. An immunohistochemical analysis of human aortic fatty streaks. Hum Pathol. 1987;18:375–80.

92. Caligiuri G, Nicoletti A, Poirier B, et al. Protective immunity against atherosclerosis carried by B cells of hypercholesterolemic mice. J Clin Invest. 2002;109:745–53.

93. Zhou X, Hansson GK. Detection of B cells and proinflammatory cytokines in atherosclerotic plaques of hypercholesterolaemic apolipoprotein E knockout mice. Scand J Immunol. 1999;50:25–30.

94. Zernecke A, Bot I, Djalali-Talab Y, et al. Protective role of CXC receptor 4/CXC ligand 12 unveils the importance of neutrophils in atherosclerosis. Circ Res. 2008;102:209–17.

95. Sun J, Sukhova GK, Wolters PJ, et al. Mast cells promote atherosclerosis by releasing proinflammatory cytokines. Nat Med. 2007;13:719–24.

96. Bobryshev YV, Lord RS. S-100 positive cells in human arterial intima and in atherosclerotic lesions. Cardiovasc Res. 1995;29:689–96.

97. Virchow R. Cellular pathology. As based upon physiological and pathological histology. Lecture XVI– Atheromatous affection of arteries. 1858. Nutr Rev. 1989;47:23–5.

98. Mayerl C, Lukasser M, Sedivy R, et al. Atherosclerosis research from past to present – on the track of two pathologists with opposing views, Carl von Rokitansky and Rudolf Virchow. Virchows Arch. 2006;449:96–103.

99. Gerrity RG, Naito HK, Richardson M, et al. Dietary induced atherogenesis in swine. Morphology of the intima in prelesion stages. Am J Pathol. 1979;95: 775–92.

100. Auffray C, Sieweke MH, Geissmann F. Blood monocytes: development, heterogeneity, and relationship with dendritic cells. Annu Rev Immunol. 2009;27:669–92.

101. Fogg DK, Sibon C, Miled C, et al. A clonogenic bone marrow progenitor specific for macrophages and dendritic cells. Science. 2006;311:83–7.

102. Ley K, Laudanna C, Cybulsky MI, et al. Getting to the site of inflammation: the leukocyte adhesion cascade updated. Nat Rev Immunol. 2007;7:678–89.

103. Rollins BJ, Yoshimura T, Leonard EJ, et al. Cytokine-activated human endothelial cells synthesize and secrete a monocyte chemoattractant, MCP-1/JE. Am J Pathol. 1990;136:1229–33.

104. Valente AJ, Graves DT, Vialle-Valentin CE, et al. Purification of a monocyte chemotactic factor secreted by nonhuman primate vascular cells in culture. Biochemistry. 1988;27:4162–8.

105. Gosling J, Slaymaker S, Gu L, et al. MCP-1 deficiency reduces susceptibility to atherosclerosis in mice that overexpress human apolipoprotein B. J Clin Invest. 1999;103:773–8.

106. Cushing SD, Berliner JA, Valente AJ, et al. Minimally modified low density lipoprotein induces monocyte chemotactic protein 1 in human endothelial cells and smooth muscle cells. Proc Natl Acad Sci USA. 1990;87:5134–8.

107. Geissmann F, Auffray C, Palframan R, et al. Blood monocytes: distinct subsets, how they relate to dendritic cells, and their possible roles in the regulation of T-cell responses. Immunol Cell Biol. 2008;86:398–408.

108. Tacke F, Randolph GJ. Migratory fate and differentiation of blood monocyte subsets. Immunobiology. 2006;211:609–18.

109. Swirski FK, Libby P, Aikawa E, et al. Ly-6Chi monocytes dominate hypercholesterolemia-associated monocytosis and give rise to macrophages in atheromata. J Clin Invest. 2007;117:195–205.

110. Weber C, Belge KU, von Hundelshausen P, et al. Differential chemokine receptor expression and function in human monocyte subpopulations. J Leukoc Biol. 2000;67:699–704.

111. Swirski FK, Pittet MJ, Kircher MF, et al. Monocyte accumulation in mouse atherogenesis is progressive and proportional to extent of disease. Proc Natl Acad Sci USA. 2006;103:10340–5.

112. Egashira K, Nakano K, Ohtani K, et al. Local delivery of anti-monocyte chemoattractant protein-1 by gene-eluting stents attenuates in-stent stenosis in rabbits and monkeys. Arterioscler Thromb Vasc Biol. 2007;27:2563–8.

113. Llodra J, Angeli V, Liu J, et al. Emigration of monocyte-derived cells from atherosclerotic lesions characterizes regressive, but not progressive, plaques. Proc Natl Acad Sci USA. 2004;101:11779–84.

114. Choudhury RP, Lee JM, Greaves DR. Mechanisms of disease: macrophage-derived foam cells emerging as therapeutic targets in atherosclerosis. Nat Clin Pract Cardiovasc Med. 2005;2:309–15.

115. Li AC, Glass CK. The macrophage foam cell as a target for therapeutic intervention. Nat Med. 2002;8:1235–42.

116. Deuel TF, Huang JS. Platelet-derived growth factor. Structure, function, and roles in normal and transformed cells. J Clin Invest. 1984;74:669–76.

117. Ross R, Raines EW, Bowen-Pope DF. The biology of platelet-derived growth factor. Cell. 1986;46:155–69.

118. Martinet Y, Bitterman PB, Mornex JF, et al. Activated human monocytes express the c-sis proto-oncogene and release a mediator showing PDGF-like activity. Nature. 1986;319:158–60.

119. Reigstad LJ, Varhaug JE, Lillehaug JR. Structural and functional specificities of PDGF-C and PDGF-D, the novel members of the platelet-derived growth factors family. FEBS J. 2005;272:5723–41.

120. Heldin CH, Ostman A, Ronnstrand L. Signal transduction via platelet-derived growth factor receptors. Biochim Biophys Acta. 1998;1378:F79–113.

121. Corjay MH, Thompson MM, Lynch KR, et al. Differential effect of platelet-derived growth factor- versus serum-induced growth on smooth muscle alpha-actin and nonmuscle beta-actin mRNA expression in cultured rat aortic smooth muscle cells. J Biol Chem. 1989;264:10501–6.

122. Blank RS, Owens GK. Platelet-derived growth factor regulates actin isoform expression and growth state in cultured rat aortic smooth muscle cells. J Cell Physiol. 1990;142:635–42.

123. Ueda M, Becker AE, Kasayuki N, et al. In situ detection of platelet-derived growth factor-A and -B chain mRNA in human coronary arteries after percutaneous transluminal coronary angioplasty. Am J Pathol. 1996;149:831–43.

124. Tanizawa S, Ueda M, van der Loos CM, et al. Expression of platelet derived growth factor B chain and beta receptor in human coronary arteries after percutaneous transluminal coronary angioplasty: an immunohistochemical study. Heart. 1996;75:549–56.

125. Sano H, Sudo T, Yokode M, et al. Functional blockade of platelet-derived growth factor receptor-beta but not of receptor-alpha prevents vascular smooth muscle cell accumulation in fibrous cap lesions in apolipoprotein E-deficient mice. Circulation. 2001;103:2955–60.

126. Kozaki K, Kaminski WE, Tang J, et al. Blockade of platelet-derived growth factor or its receptors transiently delays but does not prevent fibrous cap formation in ApoE null mice. Am J Pathol. 2002;161:1395–407.

127. Holm PW, Slart RH, Zeebregts CJ, et al. Atherosclerotic plaque development and instability: a dual role for VEGF. Ann Med. 2009;41:257–64.

128. Dunmore BJ, McCarthy MJ, Naylor AR, et al. Carotid plaque instability and ischemic symptoms are linked to immaturity of microvessels within plaques. J Vasc Surg. 2007;45:155–9.

129. Virmani R, Kolodgie FD, Burke AP, et al. Atherosclerotic plaque progression and vulnerability to rupture: angiogenesis as a source of intraplaque hemorrhage. Arterioscler Thromb Vasc Biol. 2005;25:2054–61.

130. Asahara T, Bauters C, Zheng LP, et al. Synergistic effect of vascular endothelial growth factor and basic fibroblast growth factor on angiogenesis in vivo. Circulation. 1995;92:II365–71.

131. Asahara T, Chen D, Tsurumi Y, et al. Accelerated restitution of endothelial integrity and endothelium-dependent function after phVEGF165 gene transfer. Circulation. 1996;94:3291–302.

132. Walter DH, Cejna M, Diaz-Sandoval L, et al. Local gene transfer of phVEGF-2 plasmid by gene-eluting stents: an alternative strategy for inhibition of restenosis. Circulation. 2004;110:36–45.

133. Hautmann MB, Madsen CS, Owens GK. A transforming growth factor beta (TGFbeta) control element drives TGFbeta-induced stimulation of smooth muscle alpha-actin gene expression in concert with two CArG elements. J Biol Chem. 1997;272: 10948–56.

134. Majesky MW, Lindner V, Twardzik DR, et al. Production of transforming growth factor beta 1 during repair of arterial injury. J Clin Invest. 1991;88:904–10.

135. Grainger DJ, Kemp PR, Metcalfe JC, et al. The serum concentration of active transforming growth factor-beta is severely depressed in advanced atherosclerosis. Nat Med. 1995;1:74–9.

136. Lutgens E, Gijbels M, Smook M, et al. Transforming growth factor-beta mediates balance between inflammation and fibrosis during plaque progression. Arterioscler Thromb Vasc Biol. 2002;22:975–82.

137. Owens GK, Kumar MS, Wamhoff BR. Molecular regulation of vascular smooth muscle cell differentiation in development and disease. Physiol Rev. 2004;84:767–801.

138. Mallat Z, Gojova A, Marchiol-Fournigault C, et al. Inhibition of transforming growth factor-beta signaling accelerates atherosclerosis and induces an unstable plaque phenotype in mice. Circ Res. 2001;89:930–4.

139. Dreux AC, Lamb DJ, Modjtahedi H, et al. The epidermal growth factor receptors and their family of ligands: their putative role in atherogenesis. Atherosclerosis. 2006;186:38–53.

140. Gospodarowicz D, Brown KD, Birdwell CR, et al. Control of proliferation of human vascular endothelial cells. Characterization of the response of human umbilical vein endothelial cells to fibroblast growth factor, epidermal growth factor, and thrombin. J Cell Biol. 1978;77:774–88.

141. Bhargava G, Rifas L, Makman MH. Presence of epidermal growth factor receptors and influence of epidermal growth factor on proliferation and aging in cultured smooth muscle cells. J Cell Physiol. 1979;100:365–74.

142. Blotnick S, Peoples GE, Freeman MR, et al. T lymphocytes synthesize and export heparin-binding epidermal growth factor-like growth factor and basic fibroblast growth factor, mitogens for vascular cells and fibroblasts: differential production and release

143. Yamanaka Y, Hayashi K, Komurasaki T, et al. EGF family ligand-dependent phenotypic modulation of smooth muscle cells through EGF receptor. Biochem Biophys Res Commun. 2001;281:373–7.

144. Lamb DJ, Modjtahedi H, Plant NJ, et al. EGF mediates monocyte chemotaxis and macrophage proliferation and EGF receptor is expressed in atherosclerotic plaques. Atherosclerosis. 2004;176: 21–6.

145. Higashiyama S, Abraham JA, Miller J, et al. A heparin-binding growth factor secreted by macrophage-like cells that is related to EGF. Science. 1991;251: 936–9.

146. Ouchi N, Kihara S, Yamashita S, et al. Role of membrane-anchored heparin-binding epidermal growth factor-like growth factor and CD9 on macrophages. Biochem J. 1997;328:923–8.

147. Peifley KA, Alberts GF, Hsu DK, et al. Heparin-binding epidermal growth factor-like growth factor regulates fibroblast growth factor-2 expression in aortic smooth muscle cells. Circ Res. 1996;79: 263–70.

148. Eguchi S, Numaguchi K, Iwasaki H, et al. Calcium-dependent epidermal growth factor receptor transactivation mediates the angiotensin II-induced mitogen-activated protein kinase activation in vascular smooth muscle cells. J Biol Chem. 1998;273: 8890–6.

149. Iwasaki H, Eguchi S, Marumo F, et al. Endothelin-1 stimulates DNA synthesis of vascular smooth-muscle cells through transactivation of epidermal growth factor receptor. J Cardiovasc Pharmacol. 1998;31: S182–4.

150. Kalmes A, Daum G, Clowes AW. EGFR transactivation in the regulation of SMC function. Ann N Y Acad Sci. 2001;947:42–54. discussion 54–5.

151. Przybylski M. A review of the current research on the role of bFGF and VEGF in angiogenesis. J Wound Care. 2009;18:516–9.

152. Lindner V, Lappi DA, Baird A, et al. Role of basic fibroblast growth factor in vascular lesion formation. Circ Res. 1991;68:106–13.

153. Meurice T, Bauters C, Auffray JL, et al. Basic fibroblast growth factor restores endothelium-dependent responses after balloon injury of rabbit arteries. Circulation. 1996;93:18–22.

154. Six I, Mouquet F, Corseaux D, et al. Protective effects of basic fibroblast growth factor in early atherosclerosis. Growth Factors. 2004;22:157–67.

155. Rinderknecht E, Humbel RE. The amino acid sequence of human insulin-like growth factor I and its structural homology with proinsulin. J Biol Chem. 1978;253:2769–76.

156. Laviola L, Natalicchio A, Giorgino F. The IGF-I signaling pathway. Curr Pharm Des. 2007;13:663–9.

157. Pfeifle B, Ditschuneit H. Receptors for insulin and insulin-like growth factor in cultured arterial smooth

muscle cells depend on their growth state. J Endocrinol. 1983;96:251–7.

158. Hochberg Z, Hertz P, Maor G, et al. Growth hormone and insulin-like growth factor-I increase macrophage uptake and degradation of low density lipoprotein. Endocrinology. 1992;131:430–5.

159. Bar RS, Boes M. Distinct receptors for IGF-I, IGF-II, and insulin are present on bovine capillary endothelial cells and large vessel endothelial cells. Biochem Biophys Res Commun. 1984;124:203–9.

160. Bai H, Pollman MJ, Inishi Y, et al. Regulation of vascular smooth muscle cell apoptosis. Modulation of bad by a phosphatidylinositol 3-kinase-dependent pathway. Circ Res. 1999;85:229–37.

161. Bornfeldt KE, Raines EW, Nakano T, et al. Insulin-like growth factor-I and platelet-derived growth factor-BB induce directed migration of human arterial smooth muscle cells via signaling pathways that are distinct from those of proliferation. J Clin Invest. 1994;93:1266–74.

162. Hsieh T, Gordon RE, Clemmons DR, et al. Regulation of vascular smooth muscle cell responses to insulin-like growth factor (IGF)-I by local IGF-binding proteins. J Biol Chem. 2003;278:42886–92.

163. Sowers JR. Insulin and insulin-like growth factor in normal and pathological cardiovascular physiology. Hypertension. 1997;29:691–9.

164. Boulware SD, Tamborlane WV, Matthews LS, et al. Diverse effects of insulin-like growth factor I on glucose, lipid, and amino acid metabolism. Am J Physiol. 1992;262:E130–3.

165. Jia G, Cheng G, Agrawal DK. Autophagy of vascular smooth muscle cells in atherosclerotic lesions. Autophagy. 2007;3:63–4.

166. Okura Y, Brink M, Zahid AA, et al. Decreased expression of insulin-like growth factor-1 and apoptosis of vascular smooth muscle cells in human atherosclerotic plaque. J Mol Cell Cardiol. 2001;33:1777–89.

167. Asahara T, Murohara T, Sullivan A, et al. Isolation of putative progenitor endothelial cells for angiogenesis. Science. 1997;275:964–7.

168. Zeoli A, Dentelli P, Brizzi MF. Endothelial progenitor cells and their potential clinical implication in cardiovascular disorders. J Endocrinol Invest. 2009;32:370–82.

169. Handgretinger R, Gordon PR, Leimig T, et al. Biology and plasticity of CD133+ hematopoietic stem cells. Ann N Y Acad Sci. 2003;996:141–51.

170. Friedrich EB, Walenta K, Scharlau J, et al. CD34-/CD133+/VEGFR-2+ endothelial progenitor cell subpopulation with potent vasoregenerative capacities. Circ Res. 2006;98:e20–5.

171. Rehman J, Li J, Orschell CM, et al. Peripheral blood "endothelial progenitor cells" are derived from monocyte/macrophages and secrete angiogenic growth factors. Circulation. 2003;107:1164–9.

172. Hur J, Yoon CH, Kim HS, et al. Characterization of two types of endothelial progenitor cells and their different contributions to neovasculogenesis. Arterioscler Thromb Vasc Biol. 2004;24:288–93.

173. Op den Buijs J, Musters M, Verrips T, et al. Mathematical modeling of vascular endothelial layer maintenance: the role of endothelial cell division, progenitor cell homing, and telomere shortening. Am J Physiol Heart Circ Physiol. 2004;287:H2651–8.

174. Wassmann S, Werner N, Czech T, et al. Improvement of endothelial function by systemic transfusion of vascular progenitor cells. Circ Res. 2006;99:e74–83.

175. Hill JM, Zalos G, Halcox JP, et al. Circulating endothelial progenitor cells, vascular function, and cardiovascular risk. N Engl J Med. 2003;348:593–600.

176. Heeschen C, Lehmann R, Honold J, et al. Profoundly reduced neovascularization capacity of bone marrow mononuclear cells derived from patients with chronic ischemic heart disease. Circulation. 2004;109:1615–22.

177. Kondo T, Hayashi M, Takeshita K, et al. Smoking cessation rapidly increases circulating progenitor cells in peripheral blood in chronic smokers. Arterioscler Thromb Vasc Biol. 2004;24:1442–7.

178. Heiss C, Keymel S, Niesler U, et al. Impaired progenitor cell activity in age-related endothelial dysfunction. J Am Coll Cardiol. 2005;45:1441–8.

179. Rauscher FM, Goldschmidt-Clermont PJ, Davis BH, et al. Aging, progenitor cell exhaustion, and atherosclerosis. Circulation. 2003;108:457–63.

180. Tepper OM, Galiano RD, Capla JM, et al. Human endothelial progenitor cells from type II diabetics exhibit impaired proliferation, adhesion, and incorporation into vascular structures. Circulation. 2002;106:2781–6.

181. Xiao Q, Kiechl S, Patel S, et al. Endothelial progenitor cells, cardiovascular risk factors, cytokine levels and atherosclerosis – results from a large population-based study. PLoS One. 2007;2:e975.

182. George J, Afek A, Abashidze A, et al. Transfer of endothelial progenitor and bone marrow cells influences atherosclerotic plaque size and composition in apolipoprotein E knockout mice. Arterioscler Thromb Vasc Biol. 2005;25:2636–41.

183. Silvestre JS, Gojova A, Brun V, et al. Transplantation of bone marrow-derived mononuclear cells in ischemic apolipoprotein E-knockout mice accelerates atherosclerosis without altering plaque composition. Circulation. 2003;108:2839–42.

184. Asahara T, Takahashi T, Masuda H, et al. VEGF contributes to postnatal neovascularization by mobilizing bone marrow-derived endothelial progenitor cells. EMBO J. 1999;18:3964–72.

185. Hattori K, Heissig B, Tashiro K, et al. Plasma elevation of stromal cell-derived factor-1 induces mobilization of mature and immature hematopoietic progenitor and stem cells. Blood. 2001;97:3354–60.

186. Heissig B, Hattori K, Dias S, et al. Recruitment of stem and progenitor cells from the bone marrow niche requires MMP-9 mediated release of kit-ligand. Cell. 2002;109:625–37.

187. Aicher A, Rentsch M, Sasaki K, et al. Nonbone marrow-derived circulating progenitor cells contribute

to postnatal neovascularization following tissue ischemia. Circ Res. 2007;100:581–9.

188. Miranville A, Heeschen C, Sengenes C, et al. Improvement of postnatal neovascularization by human adipose tissue-derived stem cells. Circulation. 2004;110:349–55.

189. Sata M, Saiura A, Kunisato A, et al. Hematopoietic stem cells differentiate into vascular cells that participate in the pathogenesis of atherosclerosis. Nat Med. 2002;8:403–9.

190. Simper D, Stalboerger PG, Panetta CJ, et al. Smooth muscle progenitor cells in human blood. Circulation. 2002;106:1199–204.

191. Caplice NM, Bunch TJ, Stalboerger PG, et al. Smooth muscle cells in human coronary atherosclerosis can originate from cells administered at marrow transplantation. Proc Natl Acad Sci USA. 2003;100:4754–9.

192. Bentzon JF, Weile C, Sondergaard CS, et al. Smooth muscle cells in atherosclerosis originate from the local vessel wall and not circulating progenitor cells in ApoE knockout mice. Arterioscler Thromb Vasc Biol. 2006;26:2696–702.

193. Bentzon JF, Sondergaard CS, Kassem M, et al. Smooth muscle cells healing atherosclerotic plaque disruptions are of local, not blood, origin in apolipoprotein E knockout mice. Circulation. 2007;116:2053–61.

194. Hu Y, Davison F, Ludewig B, et al. Smooth muscle cells in transplant atherosclerotic lesions are originated from recipients, but not bone marrow progenitor cells. Circulation. 2002;106:1834–9.

195. Wilson DP, Saward L, Zahradka P, et al. Angiotensin II receptor antagonists prevent neointimal proliferation in a porcine coronary artery organ culture model. Cardiovasc Res. 1999;42:761–72.

196. Han CI, Campbell GR, Campbell JH. Circulating bone marrow cells can contribute to neointimal formation. J Vasc Res. 2001;38:113–9.

197. Zoll J, Fontaine V, Gourdy P, et al. Role of human smooth muscle cell progenitors in atherosclerotic plaque development and composition. Cardiovasc Res. 2008;77:471–80.

198. Sugiyama S, Kugiyama K, Nakamura S, et al. Characterization of smooth muscle-like cells in circulating human peripheral blood. Atherosclerosis. 2006;187:351–62.

199. Gojo S, Gojo N, Takeda Y, et al. In vivo cardiovasculogenesis by direct injection of isolated adult mesenchymal stem cells. Exp Cell Res. 2003;288:51–9.

200. Suzuki S, Narita Y, Yamawaki A, et al. Effects of extracellular matrix on differentiation of human bone marrow-derived mesenchymal stem cells into smooth muscle cell lineage: utility for cardiovascular tissue engineering. Cells Tissues Organs. 2010;191:269–80.

201. Sainz J, Al Haj Zen A, Caligiuri G, et al. Isolation of "side population" progenitor cells from healthy arteries of adult mice. Arterioscler Thromb Vasc Biol. 2006;26:281–6.

202. Tintut Y, Alfonso Z, Saini T, et al. Multilineage potential of cells from the artery wall. Circulation. 2003;108:2505–10.

203. Hu Y, Zhang Z, Torsney E, et al. Abundant progenitor cells in the adventitia contribute to atherosclerosis of vein grafts in ApoE-deficient mice. J Clin Invest. 2004;113:1258–65.

204. Rodriguez LV, Alfonso Z, Zhang R, et al. Clonogenic multipotent stem cells in human adipose tissue differentiate into functional smooth muscle cells. Proc Natl Acad Sci USA. 2006;103:12167–72.

205. Munoz-Fernandez R, Blanco FJ, Frecha C, et al. Follicular dendritic cells are related to bone marrow stromal cell progenitors and to myofibroblasts. J Immunol. 2006;177:280–9.

206. Bearzi C, Leri A, Lo Monaco F, et al. Identification of a coronary vascular progenitor cell in the human heart. Proc Natl Acad Sci USA. 2009;106:15885–90.

207. Martin K, Weiss S, Metharom P, et al. Thrombin stimulates smooth muscle cell differentiation from peripheral blood mononuclear cells via protease-activated receptor-1, RhoA, and myocardin. Circ Res. 2009;105:214–8.

208. Pipes GC, Sinha S, Qi X, et al. Stem cells and their derivatives can bypass the requirement of myocardin for smooth muscle gene expression. Dev Biol. 2005;288:502–13.

209. Morrow D, Cullen JP, Liu W, et al. Sonic Hedgehog induces Notch target gene expression in vascular smooth muscle cells via VEGF-A. Arterioscler Thromb Vasc Biol. 2009;29:1112–8.

210. Noseda M, Fu Y, Niessen K, et al. Smooth Muscle alpha-actin is a direct target of Notch/CSL. Circ Res. 2006;98:1468–70.

211. Doi H, Iso T, Sato H, et al. Jagged1-selective notch signaling induces smooth muscle differentiation via a RBP-Jkappa-dependent pathway. J Biol Chem. 2006;281:28555–64.

212. Satoh K, Berk BC. Circulating smooth muscle progenitor cells: novel players in plaque stability. Cardiovasc Res. 2008;77:445–7.

Cellular and Molecular Mechanisms Associated with Salicylate Inhibition of Intimal Hyperplasia Following Balloon Catheter-Induced Vascular Injury

S.N. Murthy, P.J. Kadowitz, and D.B. McNamara

Abstract

Angioplasty followed by stent placement, bare or drug-eluting, proved to be a major step forward in the treatment of coronary and carotid artery disease. It was soon recognized that patients undergoing these procedures presented with restenosis within 6 months. The cause of these failures was the development of intimal hyperplasia. Aspirin, acetylsalicylic acid, soon became a focus of therapeutic intervention alone or in combination with other drugs due to its antiplatelet properties. When it was recognized that inflammation is a primary underlying factor in vascular disease, the use of aspirin was further encouraged. More recently, the anti-inflammatory proprieties of aspirin other than inhibition of cyclooxygenase activity have been described, namely, alterations in the expression and formation of proinflammatory molecules such as NF-κB. However, aspirin has gastrointestinal side effects and bleeding problems. Salicylates became the drug of interest, and more recently salsalate, the dimeric form of salicylic acid, is being recognized for similar anti-inflammatory actions as well as for lowering hyperglycemic glucose levels in type 2 diabetics without the deleterious side effects of aspirin. As revascularization procedures in type 2 diabetics have proven to produce a greater degree of intimal hyperplasia and, therefore, procedure failures, the effect of salsalate on the development of intimal hyperplasia in animals exhibiting symptoms of the metabolic syndrome was studied; the authors reported salsalate decreased intimal hyperplasia, increased eNOS expression, decreased NF-κB and VEGF expression. It is concluded in this chapter that clinical trials are indicated to define the effect of salsalate on the development of intimal hyperplasia and inflammation.

D.B. McNamara (✉)
Department of Pharmacology, Tulane University School
of Medicine, New Orleans, LA, USA
e-mail: dmcnama@tulane.edu

N.S. Dhalla, M. Nagano, B. Ostadal (eds.), *Molecular Defects in Cardiovascular Disease*,
DOI 10.1007/978-1-4419-7130-2_22, © Springer Science+Business Media, LLC 2011

Keywords

Angioplasty • Vascular injury • Intimal hyperplasia • Metabolic syndrome • Type 2 diabetes • Salsalate • NF-κB • VEGF • Inflammation • Aspirin • Salicylates • IL-6 • Nitric oxide • eNOS • p-eNOS • MnSOD

Introduction

The treatment and understanding of the etiology of coronary artery disease took a major step forward with the first successful balloon angioplasty by Andreas Gruentzig in 1977 [1, 2]. Angioplasty is a procedure in which blood vessels with a narrowed lumen due to atherosclerosis and/or calcium deposits are opened as evidenced by the restoration of adequate blood flow. This procedure employs a catheter that is fluoroscopically guided to the site of the occlusion, and the balloon on the end of the catheter is inflated producing a widening of the vessel. The elastic artery rebounds upon deflation of the balloon, thereby decreasing the gain in lumen size. In 1986, the first metallic stent was implanted in a human coronary artery to provide scaffold for the vessel and prevent elastic rebound at the site of the occlusion following inflation of the balloon [3]. In addition, drills or lasers can be used to remove the plaque.

Vascular injury occurs due to intramural pressure generated by balloon inflation with and without stent deployment. Injury also occurs during coronary bypass surgery and indwelling catheter placement. These procedures denude the endothelium and initiate thromboxane A2 generation, platelet aggregation, and thrombus formation, as well as a cascade of growth factors from aggregating platelets, e.g., platelet-derived growth factor, basic fibroblast growth factor. In response, the smooth muscle cells in the media change phenotype from contractile to secretory. This dedifferentiation process allows for the proliferation and subsequent migration of vascular smooth muscle cells through openings in the external lamina produced by activation of metalloproteinases. The proliferating cells synthesize cytokines, which act in an autocrine manner to promote further development of the lesion.

An inflammatory cascade develops when endothelial denudation exposes collagen on the subendothelial surface resulting in the recruitment of monocytes; with time, monocyte recruitment is maintained by the neointimal and neoendothelial cells. The net result is intimal thickening (intimal hyperplasia), which is a fibrocellular mass composed primarily of secreted glycoproteins and to a lesser extent of migrated cells (vascular smooth muscle and inflammatory) and local inflammation.

Intimal hyperplasia (constrictive remodeling) often develops in response to revascularization attempts such as angioplasty, stent deployment, endarterectomy, and bypass surgery employing arterial, venous, or synthetic grafts. Intimal hyperplasia is the main limiting factor in the long-term success of these revascularization procedures. The intima–media ratio is a surrogate marker of cardiovascular disease [4, 5]. We and others have proposed that the mechanisms promoting restenosis/vascular injury can be different in the presence or combination of other risk factors [6–8] (Fig. 1). Differences could be shear stress, differences in the repair processes as well as in the initiating processes, e.g., angioplasty or stent emplacement or venin graft injury.

The metabolic syndrome (Fig. 1) is a cluster of metabolic factors, and its definition may vary based on the organization defining the syndrome, e.g., American vs. European. A prothrombotic state and a proinflammatory state are observed. This syndrome is also known as the insulin-resistant syndrome. Individuals exhibiting several of these factors are at increased risk of coronary heart disease, atherogenesis, and type 2 diabetes. Patients with the metabolic syndrome are at greater risk for perioperative morbidity and stroke. Insulin resistance has a primary role in the pathogenesis of type 2 diabetes [6]. The mechanisms causing the hyperplastic response to injury

Metabolic Syndrome

❖ **Raised triglycerides > 150 mg/dL**

❖ **Reduced HDL**
   Women < 50 mg/dL
   Men   < 40 mg/dL

❖ **Raised blood pressure =/> 130/85 mm Hg**
   or use of medication for
hypertension

❖ **Elevated fasting glucose =/> 100 mg/dL**
   or use of medication for
hyperglycemia

❖ **Elevated waist circumfence**
   Women   =/> 35" (88 cm)
   Men   =/> 41" (102 cm)

Fig. 1

are not well understood, as the signal transduction pathways involved in the development of intimal hyperplasia following revascularization procedures appear to diverge based on the intervention employed, transmural pressure exerted, and individual comorbidities such as diabetes, hypertension, and hyperlipidemia. While the development of these fibroproliferative pathologies can be modulated by coexisting pathologies, following the injury it has been suggested there is a cascade of factors that is initially common [7]. These factors include endothelial injury, platelet aggregation, increased expression and activity of NF-κB-light chain-enhancer of activated B cells (NF-κB [9]), increased production of vascular endothelial growth factor (VEGF) and thrombin formation, expression and synthesis of growth factors and cytokines, and decreased formation of nitric oxide, all of which result in inflammatory cell recruitment and increased oxidative stress and inflammation ([10], Fig. 2). Targeting early changes that are common to many comorbidities exhibited by patients who undergo revascularization procedures seems logical.

Recently, Brito and Amiji [11] have suggested the key to a successful nanoparticle carrier therapy for restenosis is to promote reendothelialization while attenuating vascular smooth muscle growth/remodeling. Others have shown that delayed reendothelization after deployment of bare metal stents results in a marked increase in cell proliferation in the vessel wall [12]. We have shown that somatostatin inhibits catheter-induced intimal hyperplasia and promotes growth of a neoendothelial layer over the area denuded by balloon inflation; however, this neoendothelium exhibits dysfunction, as it cannot support nitric-oxide-dependent relaxation in response to acetylcholine as compared to control [13]. Thus, the attenuation of intimal hyperplasia associated with growth of a neoendothelium is not necessarily dependent on recovery of nitric oxide generating capability. Nevertheless, it is well described that nitric oxide inhibits vascular smooth muscle cell proliferation, platelet aggregation, adhesion molecule expression, and other mediators of the hyperplastic response to injury. An improvement in endothelial nitric oxide generating capacity is widely thought to have beneficial effects on hyperplastic responses as well as on the pathology associated with comorbidities.

The response of the vascular wall to injury is also characterized by the development and expansion of underlying inflammation associated with atherosclerosis. Metabolic factors that are part of the insulin resistance syndrome such as obesity, type 2 diabetes have been shown to induce underlying low-level vascular inflammation [9]. The potential for suppression of inflammation in the treatment of these conditions is under extensive investigation. Additionally, inflammatory responses have been linked to the production of reactive oxygen species and a deficiency in the antioxidant capacity of cells [14].

More than 17 million patients in USA suffer from type 1 or 2 diabetes and this number is rapidly expanding. In addition, the prediabetic population is thought to be a major undiagnosed group of thousands of individuals. Type 2 diabetes is an independent risk factor for heart disease [15], and it has been reported that cardiovascular disease accounts for as much as 80% additional mortality in patients with type 2 diabetes. Further, these patients have a twofold increased risk of death

Cascade of Events in Vascular Injury

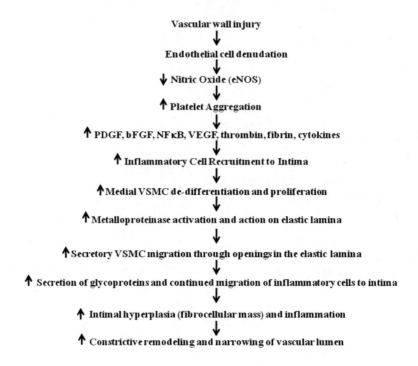

Fig. 2

independent of other known cardiovascular risk factors [16]. Moreover, not only cardiovascular disease but also other pathologies coexist with type 2 diabetes, e.g., Alzheimer's disease [17]. In patients with diabetes, interventional vascular procedures such as balloon angioplasty and stent placement, with or without drug-eluting coatings, have been shown to result in greater rates of restenosis. These procedures cause transmural mechanical injury and endothelial denudation of the arterial wall, leading to a cascade of cellular and inflammatory events with intimal hyperplasia being the primary underlying cause of the resulting restenosis and vessel narrowing. The role of the treatment of diabetes on the progression of cardiovascular disease is a major focus in cardiovascular medicine. As mentioned above cardiovascular disease is comorbidity with type 2 diabetes, insulin resistance and obesity [18, 19]. Clinical trials, including the ACCORD trial [20], have cautioned against the risk of hypoglycemia

when attempting to produce normoglycemia [21]. Glucose levels are an important variable in the response of the vascular wall to injury.

Early pharmacologic approaches to the prevention of restenosis after angioplasty have been ineffective. A variety of drugs including heparin, acetylsalicylic acid, coumadin, and dipyridamole and thromboxane A2 synthesis inhibitors failed to show a reduction in restenosis rates in randomized trials [22]. Calcium entry blockers, which were shown to decrease coronary spasm following angioplasty, decreased restenosis in patients who exhibited spasm but not in those who did not experience spasm [23]. A role for prostaglandins was thought to be central, as agents such as aspirin, the irreversible inhibitor of cyclooxygenase activity, and high-dose fish oil, a competing inhibitor of cyclooxygenase products formed from arachidonic acid by cyclooxygenase, were thought to be promising. It should be noted that the approach from early on was to attenuate the tendency for thromboembolic events with combinations of various drugs with aspirin [24]. This hypothesis was attractive due to the growing recognition of the role of aspirin in the secondary prevention of myocardial prevention. However, the limiting factor in the use of aspirin is the risk of increased incidence of cardiovascular bleeding [25, 26]. The use of aspirin is a still the basic therapeutic approach employed in patients with coronary artery disease [27]. This is in addition to the use of lipid lowering therapy and physical exercise.

Salicylates are widely used nonsteroidal anti-inflammatory drugs [28]. Initially the beneficial effect on the rate of cardiovascular complications following angioplasty and/or stent emplacement was thought to be due to irreversible inhibition of cyclooxygenase activity due to acetylation of the active site coupled with the subsequent downstream inhibition of thromboxane-mediated platelet aggregation, thrombosis, and release of growth factors [29]. Later, the anti-inflammatory activity of aspirin was ascribed a role in the treatment of postangioplasty vascular events. More recently, other effects have been reported for aspirin at the level of gene expression where it was shown aspirin alters pro- and antiapoptotic gene expression, e.g., BCL2L1 [30]. However, some patients exhibit aspirin resistance, and the mechanisms for this are not clear. It has been suggested to be related to bioavailability, interactions with other nonsteroidal anti-inflammatory drugs, comorbidities such as diabetes and hypercholesterolemia, genetic polymorphisms and increased platelet turnover [31]. In a recent overview of randomized controlled trials, it was reported aspirin reduced the risk of myocardial infarction and stroke by about 10% in those with type 2 diabetes; however, aspirin increased the risk of gastrointestinal bleeding [32]; it was concluded that low-dose aspirin is useful in those with type 2 diabetes and a 10 year risk of cardiovascular events over 10%. More recently, the prophylactic use of low- or high-dose aspirin for the primary prevention of cardiovascular disease has been suggested to be not indicated due to the potential for hemorrhagic stroke [33]. However, continued prophylactic use of aspirin is suggested in those who have experienced a myocardial infarction.

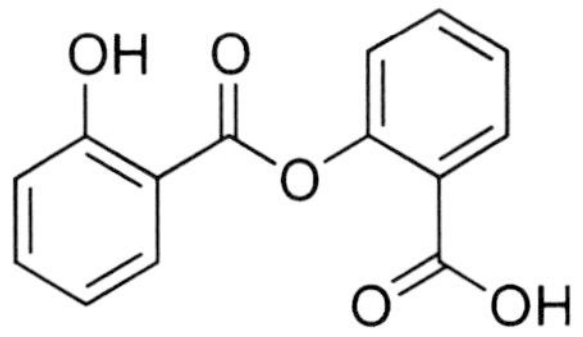

Salsalate

Fig. 3

On the contrary, salicylates are weak reversible inhibitors of cyclooxygenase activity in clinically relevant doses; therefore, the use of salicylates could avoid the potentially dangerous side effects of aspirin.

Sodium salicylate (5.0–7.5 g/day) has been reported to reduce glycosuria in diabetic patients [34, 35]. The molecular target for the hypoglycemic actions of high-dose sodium salicylate and aspirin have been identified as the inhibitory κB kinase (IKKβ)/NF-κB) pathway rather than cyclooxygenase [36, 37]. This pathway is a critical regulator of proinflammatory signals [9]. It has been reported that salicylate can exert these beneficial effects in the dose range of 3.0–4.5 g/day, which is within that achieved and tolerated by many patients with rheumatoid arthritis [38].

Salsalate is the dimeric form of salicylic acid (Fig. 3), and it has been used clinically for decades [39]. This agent has a good safety profile and does not significantly affect platelet aggregation/bleeding. It has been suggested that salsalate, which consists of two molecules of salicylate, may be a well-tolerated delivery method to achieve the beneficial effects of salicylate [38]. Salsalate has been shown to inhibit the synthesis of proinflammatory cytokines such as TNF-α, IL-6, and IL-7 [40] and the expression of vascular cell adhesion molecule, intercellular adhesion molecule, and endothelin-1, which are produced in response to balloon catheter injury. Inhibition of inflammatory cell migration to the intima would contribute to a decreased volume of fibrocellular mass or plaque volume in the wall (intimal hyperplasia). Salsalate has been reported to augment expression of the inhibitor of NF-κB and decrease total and nuclear expression of NF-κB in endothelial cells from overweight/obese

Study Design

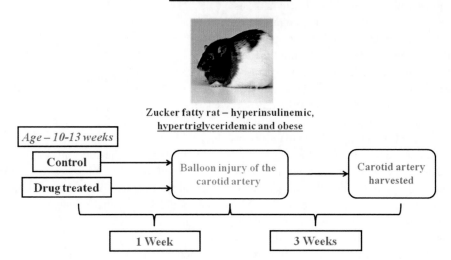

Zucker fatty rat – hyperinsulinemic,
hypertriglyceridemic and obese

Age – 10-13 weeks

Control

Drug treated

Balloon injury of the
carotid artery

Carotid artery
harvested

1 Week   3 Weeks

Fig. 4

middle-aged and older humans [41]. This effect was associated with increased flow-mediated dilation of the brachial artery, an in vivo determinant thought to reflect endothelial nitric oxide synthesis. Salsalate has been reported not to affect insulin levels in obese nondiabetic patients [39]. A large randomized trial [42] employing salsalate to reduce blood glucose levels in poorly controlled type 2 diabetes has been undertaken by the National Institutes of Health: Targeting Inflammation with Salsalate in Type 2 Diabetes (TINSAL-T2D); it has recently been concluded that salsalate lowers hemoglobin a (1c) levels and improves glycemic control in type 2 diabetics. Thus, there are data that support the efficacy of salsalate in treating metabolic syndrome and support the hypothesis that salsalate would attenuate intimal hyperplasia following catheter injury.

Increased intimal hyperplasia has been shown to be associated with increased expression of the mitogen vascular endothelial growth factor (VEGF) after angioplasty [43, 44]. In experimental studies stents coated with a VEGF inhibitor showed a decreased hyperplastic response [45]; however, this has not been extended to clinical trials. The expression of VEGF is stimulated by insulin and animals that exhibit insulin resistance and are hyperinsulinemic show an augmented

hyperplastic response associated with increased VEGF expression following catheter-induced injury [43]. The expression and secretion of VEGF has been reported to be mediated by NF-κB [46]. Thus, the hypothesis that salsalate inhibits VEGF-stimulated development of intimal hyperplasia following catheter-induced injury in association with decreased expression of NF-κB is reasonable.

We investigated the effect of salsalate treatment on the development of intimal hyperplasia and the inflammatory response that follows catheter-induced injury to the rat carotid artery [47]. The model employed, the obese female Fatty Zucker rat, exhibits normal glucose levels, hypertriglyceridemia, hyperinsulinemia, and reduced glucagon levels [48]. This model avoids the possibly cofounding issue of significant changes in glucose concentration. In addition, these animals develop intimal hyperplasia following catheter-induced injury independently of insulin deficiency or administration [49, 50]. Insulin levels have been reported to be 12.5 ± 2.7 and 3.4 ± 1, while triglycerides were $1,366 \pm 241$ and 641 ± 65 for Zucker fatty and control Zucker lean rats, respectively [50]. Catheter-mediated injury was published [48]; the study design was as in Fig. 4. We found salsalate treatment (300 mg/day 1 week

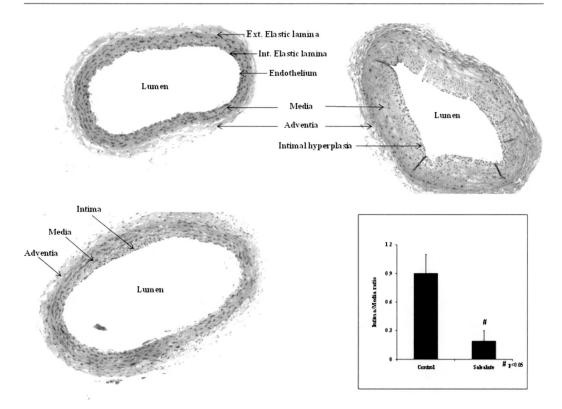

Fig. 5 Representative sections of carotid arteries of Zucker fatty rats: (**a**) control (uninjured); (**b**) injured and untreated; (**c**) injured and treated with salsalate. Salsalate significantly attenuated the catheter-induced hyperplastic response (**c**) as compared to that of rats that received catheter-induced injury but did not receive salsalate (**b**). Note the absence of little identifiable intima in the section (**a**) from a control animal (received no injury). (**d**) Quantitation of the hyperplastic response

prior to catheterization and for 3 weeks afterwards followed by sacrifice) significantly attenuated the development of intimal hyperplasia [intima–medial ratios 0.19 ± 0.11 versus 0.9 ± 0.2 $p < 0.05$ (Fig. 5)]. The hyperplastic response in these animals is associated with inflammation and insulin resistance but was independent of glucose levels [6]. Moreover, Western Blot analysis for the p65 subunit of NF-κB showed a significant decrease in protein expression. In addition, the expression of VEGF, which has been shown to be increased by NF-κB and to stimulate proliferation of vascular smooth muscle cells, was significantly decreased by 22% as determined by immunohistochemistry. Serum levels of IL-6 were significantly reduced; thus, the mediators of inflammation and proliferation were attenuated by salsalate. Conversely, the expression of inhibitors of proliferation, endothelial nitric oxide synthase (eNOS), and of inflammation, manganese superoxide dismutase, were upregulated, five- and twofold, respectively. More importantly, the expression of p-NOS, the phosphorylated active form of the enzyme [51], was also significantly increased tenfold. It was concluded salsalate may not only decrease insulin resistance as previously shown but also decrease inflammation by inhibiting NF-κB, which in turn produced a decrease in the proproliferative factor VEGF. Moreover, Goldfine et al. [52] and others [37] have reported decreased insulin clearance and decreased circulating C-peptide, the proinsulin cleavage product [28] in patients treated with 4.5 g of salsalate. It has been suggested that C-peptide deposition in the vascular wall can promote the recruitment of monocytes and CD4-positive lymphocytes in early lesions, thus promoting inflammation, atherosclerosis, and restenosis [53]. Goldfine et al. also suggested, based on the known inhibitory effects of salsalate on NF-κB, that it is possible that salsalate may decrease the expression of VEGF leading to decreased intimal hyperplasia after angioplasty; however, this hypothesis has not yet been tested. Thus, salsalate, a prodrug for salicylate therapy, is well tolerated over the dose range at which it exerts therapeutic effects. It does not exhibit gastrointestinal or bleeding problems as aspirin does. It inhibits the development of balloon catheter-induced intimal hyperplasia and inflammation in an animal model that exhibits characteristics of the metabolic syndrome. While glucose levels are not a variable in this model, salsalate has been shown to reduce hyperglycemia and increase insulin levels (decreased clearance) in type 2 diabetics [39].

Another possible mechanistic target of salicylate therapy is assymetric dimethyl l-arginine. This endogenous substance is a competitive inhibitor of nitric oxide synthase; thus, as the intracellular levels of this inhibitor rise, the formation/release of nitric oxide falls. Increased accumulation of this compound has been reported in the presence of hyperglycemia in association with augmented intimal hyperplasia follow endothelial denudation of the carotid artery in type 1 diabetic animals [54]. Aspirin has been reported to inhibit the formation of this inhibitor and increase nitric oxide and cGMP levels in endothelial cells [55].

As intimal–medial thickness is considered to be a surrogate marker for coronary events and atherosclerosis [4, 5], it is suggested that salicylates may have a beneficial effect on type 2 diabetics undergoing revascularization procedures. This possibility is very important based on the high rate of restenosis due to intimal hyperplasia seen in this population. Restenosis (intimal hyperplasia) following the placement of drug eluting stents is infrequent; however, it remains a problem especially in those with complex lesions [56]. Drug-eluting stents have been reported to produce restenosis rates similar to intravenous ultrasound-guided cutting angioplasty procedures; however, intimal hyperplasia remains the primary cause underlying increased restenosis rates [57].

Conclusions

It has been reported that in type 2 diabetic patients with stable coronary artery disease and controlled angina, intensive optimal medical therapy should the first-line therapy to reduce the incidence of myocardial infarction. However, in patients with advanced coronary disease, prompt coronary artery bypass surgery coupled with insulin sensitization is recommended [58]. While it is recognized that many therapies that are effective in animals for the attenuation of the development of intimal hyperplasia do not always translate to benefit in human trials, the effects of salsalate therapy on restenosis need investigation in a clinical trial.

Acknowledgments This work was supported in part by NIH grants HL 62000 and HL 77421.

References

1. Hall D, Gruentzig A. Percutaneous transluminal coronary angioplasty: current procedure and future direction. AJR Am J Roentgenol. 1984;142:13–6.
2. King SB. Percutaneous transluminal coronary angioplasty. J Am Coll Cardiol. 1999;34:615–7.
3. Gruberg L, Dangas G, Leon MB. Coronary artery stents: appropriate use of adjunctive pharmacology to prevent stent restenosis. Drugs Aging. 1999;15:341–8.
4. Hodis HN, Mack WJ, LaBree L, et al. The role of carotid arterial intima-media thickness in predicting clinical coronary events. Ann Intern Med. 1998;128:262–9.
5. Linhart A, Garlepy J, Massonneau M, et al. Carotid intima-media thickness: the ultimate surrogate endpoint of cardiovascular involvement in atherosclerosis. Appl Radiol. 2000;29:25–39.
6. McNamara DB, Murthy SN, Fonseca AN, et al. Animal models of catheter-induced intimal hyperplasia in type 1 and type 2 diabetes and the effects of pharmacologic intervention. Can J Physiol Pharmacol. 2009;87:37–50.
7. Mitra AK, Agrawal DK. Gene therapy of fibroproliferative vasculopathies: current ideas in molecular mechanisms and biochemical technology. Pharmacogenomics. 2006;7:1185–98.
8. Forte A, Della Corte A, De Feo M, et al. Role of myofibroblasts in vascular remodeling; focus on restenosis and aneurysm. Cardiovasc Res. 2010;88:395–405.
9. Shoelson SE, Lee J, Goldfine AB. Inflammation and insulin resistance. J Clin Invest. 2006;116:1793–801.
10. Newby AC, Zaltsman AB. Molecular mechanisms of intimal hyperplasia. J Pathol. 2000;190:300–9.

11. Brito L, Amiji M. Nanoparticulate carriers for the treatment of coronary restenosis. Int J Nanomed. 2007;2:143–61.

12. Christian T, Verin V, Bochaton-Piallat M, et al. Mechanisms of neointima formation and remodeling in the porcine coronary artery. Circulation. 2001;103: 882–8.

13. Schiller NK, Timothy AM, Aurora HS, et al. A selective somatostatin type-2 receptor agonist inhibits neointimal thickening and enhances endothelial cell growth and morphology following balloon injury in the rabbit. Mol Cell Biochem. 2002;240:31–7.

14. Jay D, Hitomi H, Griendling KK. Oxidative stress and diabetic cardiovascular complications. Free Radic Biol Med. 2006;40:183–92.

15. de Simone G, Devereux RB, Chinali M, et al. Diabetes and incident heart failure in hypertensive and normotensive participants of the Strong Heart Study. J Hypertens. 2010;28:353–60.

16. Preis SR, Pencina MJ, Hwang SJ, et al. Trends in cardiovascular disease risk factors in individuals with and without diabetes mellitus in the Framingham Heart Study. Circulation. 2009;120:212–20.

17. Arvanitakis Z, Wilson RS, Bienias J, et al. Diabetes mellitus and risk of Alzheimer's disease and decline in cognitive function. Arch Neurol. 2004;61:661–6.

18. Wilson PWF, Meigs JB. Cardiometabolic risk: a Framingham perspective. Int J Obes (Lond). 2008;32: S17–20.

19. Devici E, Yesil M, Akinci B, et al. Evaluation of insulin resistance in normoglycemic patients with coronary artery disease. Clin Cardiol. 2009;32:32–6.

20. Elam M, Lovato LC, Ginsberg H. Role of fibrates in cardiovascular disease prevention, the ACCORD-Lipid perspective. Curr Opin Lipidol. 2011;22(1):55–61.

21. Hamnvik OP, McMahion GT. Glycemic targets for patients with type 2 diabetes mellitus. Mt Sinai J Med. 2009;76:227–33.

22. Meier B. Prevention of restenosis after coronary angioplasty: a pharmacologic approach. Eur Heart J. 1989;10 Suppl G:64–8.

23. Schlant RC, King SB. Usefulness of calcium entry blockers during and after percutaneous transluminal coronary artery angioplasty. Circulation. 1989;80(6 Suppl):IV 88–92.

24. Chesebro JH, Fuster V. Platelet-inhibitor drugs before and after coronary artery bypass surgery and coronary angioplasty: the basis of their use, data from animal studies, clinical trial data, and current recommendations. Cardiology. 1986;73:292–305.

25. Willis AL, Smith DL. Therapeutic impact of eicosanoids in atherosclerotic disease. Eicosanoids. 1989;2:69–99.

26. Stein B, Fuster V, Israel DH, et al. Platelet inhibitor agents in cardiovascular disease: an update. J Am Coll Cardiol. 1989;14:813–36.

27. Baigent C, Blackwell L, Collins R, et al. Antithrombotic Trialists' (ATT) Collaboration. Aspirin in the primary and secondary prevention of vascular disease: collaborative meta-analysis of individual participant data from randomized trials. Lancet. 2009;373:1849–60.

28. Fleischman A, Shoelson SE, Bernier R, et al. Salsalate improves glycemia and inflammatory parameters in obese young adults. Diabetes Care. 2008;31:289–94.

29. Chesebro JH, Lam JY, Fuster V. The pathogenesis and prevention of aortocoronary vein bypass graft occlusion and restenosis after arterial angioplasty: role of vascular injury and platelet thrombus deposition. J Am Coll Cardiol. 1986;8(Suppl B):57B–66.

30. Elwood PC, Gallagher AM, Duthie GG, et al. Aspirin, salicylates and cancer. Lancet. 2009;373:1301–9.

31. Zimmermann N, Weber AA, Hohlfeld T. Aspirin resistance. Hertz. 2008;33:270–8.

32. Pignone M, Williams CD. Aspirin for primary prevention of cardiovascular disease in diabetes mellitus. Nat Rev Endocrinol. 2010;6:619–28.

33. Younis N, Williams S, Ammori B, et al. Role of aspirin in the primary prevention of cardiovascular disease in diabetes mellitus: a meta-analysis. Expert Opin Pharmacother. 2010;11:1459–66.

34. Ebstein W. Zur therapie des diabetes mellitus, insbesondere uber die anwendung des salicylsauren natron bei demselben. Berl Klin Wochenschr. 1877; 24:337–40.

35. Shoelson S. Invited comment on W Ebstein: on the therapy of diabetes mellitus, in particular the application of sodium salicylate. J Mol Med. 2002;80:618–9.

36. Yuan M, Konstantanpoulous N, Lee J, et al. Reversal of obesity- and diet-induced insulin resistance with salicylates or targeted disruption of IkB. Science. 2001;293:1673–7.

37. Hundal RS, Peterson KF, Mayerson AB, et al. Mechanism by which high-dose aspirin improves glucose metabolism in type 2 diabetes. J Clin Invest. 2002;109:1321–6.

38. McCarty MF. Salsalate may have broad utility in the prevention and treatment of vascular disorders and the metabolic syndrome. Med Hypotheses. 2010;75: 276–81.

39. Koska J, Ortega E, Blunt JC. The effect of salsalate on insulin action and glucose tolerance in obese nondiabetic patients: results of a randomized double-blind placebo-controlled study. Diabetologia. 2009;52: 385–93.

40. Tilg H, Moschen AR. Inflammatory mechanisms in the regulation of insulin resistance. Mol Med. 2008; 14:222–31.

41. Pierce GL, Lesniewski LA, Lawson BR, et al. Nulear factor-{kappa}B activation contributes to vascular endothelial dysfunction via oxidative stress in overweight/obese middle-aged and older humans. Circulation. 2009;119:1284–92.

42. Goldfine AB, Fonseca V, Jablonski KA, et al. TINSAL-T2D (Targeting Inflammation Using Salsalate in Type 2 Diabetes) Study Team. The effects of salsalate on glycemic control in patients with type 2 diabetes: a randomized trial. Am Int Med. 2010;152:346–57.

43. Desouza CV, Gerety M, Hamel FG. Neointimal hyperplasia and vascular endothelial growth factor expression are increased in normoglycemic, insulin resistant, obese fatty rats. Atherosclerosis. 2006;184:283–9.

44. Xinsheng XU, Huixia L, Huili L, et al. Aortic adven-
    titial angiogenesis and lymphogenesis promote inti-
    mal inflammation and hyperplasia. Cardiovasc Pathol.
    2009;18:269–78.
45. Stefanadis C, Toutouzas K, Stefanadi E, et al. Inhibition
    of plaque neovascularization and intimal hyperplasia
    by specific targeting vascular endothelial growth factor
    with bevacizumab-eluting stent: an experimental study.
    Atherosclerosis. 2007;195:269–76.
46. Novotny NM, Markel TA, Crisostomo PR, et al.
    Differential IL-6 and VEGF secretions in adult and
    neonatal mesenchymal stem cells: role of NFkB.
    Cytokine. 2008;43:215–9.
47. Murthy SN, Desouza CV, Bost NW, et al. Effects of
    salsalate therapy on recovery from vascular injury in
    female Zucker fatty rats. Diabetes. 2010;59:3240–6.
48. Bray GA. The Zucker-fatty rat: a review. Fed Proc.
    1977;36:148–53.
49. Park SH, Marso SP, Zhongmin Z, et al. Neointimal
    hyperplasia after arterial injury is increased in a rat
    model of non-insulin-dependent diabetes mellitus.
    Circulation. 2001;104:815–9.
50. Desouza C, Murthy SN, Diez J, et al. Differential
    effects of peroxisome proliferator activator-alpha and
    gamma ligands on intimal hyperplasia after balloon
    catheter-induced injury in Zucker rats. J Cardiovasc
    Pharmacol Ther. 2003;8:297–305.
51. Iwakiri Y, Tsai M-H, McCabe TJ, et al. Phosphorylation
    of eNOS initiates excessive NO production in early

phases of portal hypertension. Am J Physiol. 2002;282:
    H2084–90.
52. Goldfine AB, Silver R, Aldhahi W, et al. Use of salsalate
    to target inflammation in the treatment of insulin resis-
    tance and type 2 diabetes. Clin Transl Sci. 2008;1:36–43.
53. Walcher D, Marx N. C-Peptide in the vessel wall. Rev
    Diabet Stud. 2009;6:180–6.
54. Masuda H, Goto M, Tamaoki S, et al. Accelerated
    intimal hyperplasia and increased endogenous inhibi-
    tors for NO synthesis in rabbits with alloxan-induced
    hyperglycemia. Br J Pharmacol. 1999;126:211–8.
55. Bode-Boger SM, Martens-Lobenhoffer J, Tager M,
    et al. Aspirin reduces endothelial cell senescence.
    Biochem Biophys Res Commun. 2005;334:1226–32.
56. Vaknin-Assa H, Assali A, Lev E, et al. Characterization
    and clinical outcomes of drug-eluting in-stent rest-
    enosis. Isr Med Assoc J. 2010;12:273–6.
57. Ozaki Y, Lemos PA, Yamaguchi T, et al. A quantita-
    tive coronary angiography-matched comparison
    between a prospective randomized multicenter cutting
    balloon angioplasty and bare metal stent (REDUCE
    III) and the rapamycin-eluting stent evaluation at
    Rotterdam Cardiology Hospital (RESEARCH) study.
    Eurointervention. 2010;6:400–6.
58. Chairman BR, Hadid M, Laddu AA. Choice of initial
    medical therapy vs. prompt coronary revascularization
    in patients with type 2 diabetes and stable ischemic coro-
    nary artery disease with special emphasis on the BARI
    2D trial results. Curr Opin Cardiol. 2010;25:597–602.

Involvement of Growth Factor Receptor and Nonreceptor Protein Tyrosine Kinases in Endothelin-1 and Angiotensin II-Induced Signaling Pathways in the Cardiovascular System

George Vardatsikos and Ashok K. Srivastava

Abstract

Endothelin-1 (ET-1) and angiotensin II (Ang II) play important roles in maintaining blood pressure and vascular homeostasis, and a heightened activity of these vasoactive peptides are thought to contribute to the development of vascular pathologies, such as hypertension, atherosclerosis, hypertrophy, and restenosis. This is caused by an excessive activation of several growth and proliferative signaling pathways, which include members of the mitogen-activated protein kinase (MAPK) family, as well as the phosphatidylinositol 3-kinase (PI3-K)/protein kinase B (PKB) pathway. ET-1 and Ang II stimulate these pathways through the activation of transmembrane guanine nucleotide-binding protein-coupled receptors (GPCRs). While the activation of these signaling pathways is well elucidated, the upstream elements responsible for ET-1 and Ang II-induced MAPK and PI3-K/PKB activation remain poorly understood. During the last several years, the concept of transactivation of receptor protein tyrosine kinases (PTKs), such as EGFR, IGF-1R, and nonreceptor PTK, in triggering vasoactive peptide-induced signaling events has gained much recognition. As such, in this chapter, we provide an overview of the role of receptor and nonreceptor PTKs in modulating ET-1 and Ang II-induced PI3-K/PKB and MAPK signaling events in vascular smooth muscle cells (VSMC), and their potential implication in vascular pathology.

A.K. Srivastava (✉)
Laboratory of Cellular Signaling, Montreal Diabetes
Research Center, Research Center – Centre Hospitalier
de l'Université de Montréal (CRCHUM),
Montréal, Québec, Canada

Department of Medicine, Université de Montréal,
Montréal, Québec, Canada
e-mail: ashok.srivastava@umontreal.ca

N.S. Dhalla, M. Nagano, B. Ostadal (eds.), *Molecular Defects in Cardiovascular Disease*,
DOI 10.1007/978-1-4419-7130-2_23, © Springer Science+Business Media, LLC 2011

Keywords

Endothelin-1 • Angiotensin II • VSMC • PKB • ERK • IGF-1R • EGFR
• c-Src • PYK2

Introduction

According to the World Health Organization (WHO), more people die of cardiovascular diseases (CVD) yearly than any other cause or pathological condition, with approximately 17.4 million deaths due to CVDs in 2004, a number that is predicted to rise to 23.6 million by the year 2030 [1]. Alterations in vascular smooth muscle cell (VSMC) growth, migration, proliferation, and plasticity are believed to contribute to abnormal vascular functions associated with or leading to CVDs, such as hypertension, atherosclerosis, and stenosis after angioplasty [2–4]. Under normal physiological conditions, vasoactive peptides, such as angiotensin II (Ang II) and endothelin-1 (ET-1), normalize blood pressure through the regulation of salt and/or water homeostasis, sympathetic nervous system modulation, as well as VSMC contraction and relaxation [5–8]. Increased levels of both ET-1 and Ang II, present in certain pathophysiological states, such as essential hypertension, obesity, or advanced stages of diabetes, have been suggested to contribute to the pathogenesis of CVDs, by activating signaling events intimately linked to migration and proliferation of VSMC [5, 9–11]. Ang II and ET-1 both exert their biological actions through the activation of their respective guanine nucleotide-binding protein (G Protein)-coupled receptors (GPCRs).

Activation of growth factor receptor and/or nonreceptor protein tyrosine kinases (R-PTKs or NR-PTKs) has been implicated in transducing the downstream effects of GPCRs, leading to the stimulation of the PI3-K/PKB and MAPK cascades, which are involved in mediating the migratory, proliferative, and hypertrophic responses of ET-1 and Ang II [2]. GPCR ligands activate R- and/or NR-PTKs through a process termed "transactivation". Daub et al. first identified this process in 1996, by showing that ET-1 enhanced

the tyrosine phosphorylation of epidermal growth factor receptor (EGFR) [12]. Since that time, the transactivation of other R-PTKs, such as platelet derived growth factor receptor (PDGFR) and insulin-like growth factor type 1 receptor (IGF-1R), as well as NR-PTKs, such as proline-rich tyrosine kinase (PYK2), Janus Kinase (JAK), and c-Src, has been demonstrated in response to multiple GPCR agonists in a variety of cell types [13–19], and especially in the case of vasoactive peptide-induced signaling events [18, 20–22]. In this chapter, we provide an overview of the implication of R- and NR-PTKs in vasoactive peptide-induced signaling, focusing on PI3-K/PKB and MAPK pathways.

Angiotensin II and Endothelin-I

Ang II is a powerful vasoconstricting octapeptide cleaved from angiotensin I (Ang I) by angiotensin converting enzyme (ACE) and is an integral part of the renin–angiotensin system (RAS) [23]. The principal physiological function of Ang II is the acute regulation of vascular tone to regulate blood pressure. The cleavage of Ang II is a two-step process. In the first step, renin, produced by juxtaglomerular smooth muscle cells in the kidney in response to multiple stimuli (e.g., salt depletion), cleaves hepatically produced angiotensinogen (AGT), thereby producing Ang I, the inactive precursor of Ang II. Ang I is then cleaved by ACE in the luminal surface of the endothelium (primarily in the pulmonary vasculature) to produce Ang II [23]. Ang II acts primarily through the activation of its two main receptors, angiotensin type 1 receptor (AT1R) and angiotensin type 2 receptor (AT2R), which are both, as mentioned earlier, 7 transmembrane domain GPCRs [23]. These receptors are primarily found in blood vessels, but also in heart, lung, liver, and brain tissues [5].

ET-1 is one of the most potent vasoconstrictor peptides in circulation, responsible for regulating vascular tone and blood pressure through various mechanisms, such as salt and water homeostasis, as well as affecting the sympathetic nervous system [6–8]. ET exists in three isoforms, all sharing a common structure: ET-1, produced mainly by the cardiovascular system, ET-2, produced mainly in the intestine and kidneys, and ET-3, found mainly in the central nervous system (CNS) [24]. ET is produced primarily by endothelial cells in the vasculature [25], but is also produced by the heart, kidney, posterior pituitary, and central nervous system [26]. It is secreted as a preprohormone and cleaved several times by endothelin converting enzymes (ECE) to its final form [24]. ET-1 exerts its biological actions through the activation of its two receptor subtypes, ET_A and ET_B [27, 28], both of which, like the Ang II receptors, belong to the GPCR family. G proteins of the GPCRs are heterotrimetric proteins composed of three distinct subunits; α, β and γ subunits [29]. The GDP bound form of α binds tightly to $\beta\gamma$ and is inactive, whereas the GTP bound form of α dissociates from $\beta\gamma$ and serves as a regulator of effector proteins. Both α-GTP and $\beta\gamma$ subunits can interact with effectors. This activation cycle is terminated by intrinsic GTPase activity of α-subunit. The GDP-bound form of the α-subunit has a high affinity for $\beta\gamma$ subunit, with which it reassociates to form the heterotrimer in the basal resting state [29]. $G_{\alpha q}$ is associated to the activation of phospholipase C (PLC), leading to the formation of inositol 1,4,5-trisphosphate (IP3) and diacyglycerol (DAG), modulating downstream calcium signaling to activate calcium/calmodulin and protein kinase C (PKC), leading to the activation of the PI3-K/PKB and MAPK pathways (Fig. 1) [30, 31].

The Phosphatidylinositol 3-Kinase/Protein Kinase B Pathway

PI3-Ks are a family of lipid kinases that phosphorylate the D3 hydroxyl group (3′-OH) of the inositol ring in phosphatidyl inositol (PI) [32]. Products of the PI3-K reaction include phosphatidylinositol-3-monophosphate (PIP),

phosphatidylinositol-3,4-bisphosphate (PIP2), and phosphatidylinositol-3,4,5-trisphosphate (PIP3) [33]. This lipid kinase has been divided into classes I, II, and III. Class I PI3-Ks are heterodimeric proteins, each of which consists of a 110-kDa catalytic subunit and an associated regulatory subunit. This class is further divided into classes IA and IB, of which class IA has three isoforms (α, β, and δ) of the catalytic p110 subunit and several forms of regulatory subunits (p85α, p55α, p50α, p85β, and p55γ). Class IB, on the contrary, has only one member of the catalytic subunit called p110γ and one form of the regulatory subunit p101. Class IA is activated by R-PTK, while class IB is activated by GPCR [34]. In vitro, PI, PIP, and PIP2 are phosphorylated by class I PI3-K enzymes to form PIP, PIP2, and PIP3, yet phosphorylation of PIP2 is favored in vivo, which is responsible for the formation of PIP3 [34, 35].

Class II PI3-Ks, consisting of two major mammalian subclasses, α and β, contain a carboxy-terminal C2 domain, a protein module originally observed in PKC molecules, with phospholipid binding sites. There are no known regulatory subunits in this class, which may not even be necessary.

Class III PI3-Ks are thought to represent the primordial PI3-K that gave existence to the other classes due to the fact that it is the only class of PI3-K enzymes present in yeast. PI is the only substrate recognized by this class and is phosphorylated to generate PIP3 [36, 37]. Class III PI3-Ks induce local increases in PIP3, which are thought to be required for agonist-independent membrane trafficking processes [37].

Generally, the p85 subunit of PI3-K binds to and is activated by IRS-1, in turn activating the p110 catalytic subunit of PI3-K, which catalyzes the phosphorylation PI lipids, forming PIP3 and PIP2 (Fig. 1) [38]. The formation of PIP3 and PIP2 generates recognition sites for Pleckstrin Homology (PH) domain containing proteins, principally 3′-phosphoinositide-dependent kinase 1 (PDK1), which is translocated to the plasma membrane along with PKB [38, 39], and other and related serine/threonine protein kinases, which are responsible for phosphorylating and activating several downstream signaling protein kinases, such as PKB, protein kinase C-zeta

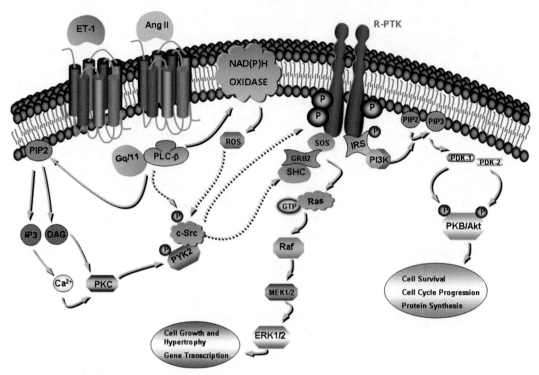

Fig. 1 Schematic model representing the activation of the MAPK and PI3-K/PKB pathways through R- and/or NR-PTK phosphorylation by ET-1 and Ang II. ET-1 and Ang II bind to their respective GPCRs, causing enhanced activity of PLCβ through $G_{\alpha q/11}$ activation. Activation of PLCβ causes the conversion of phosphatidylinositol 4,5 biphosphate (PIP2) to inositol 1, 4, 5 trisphosphate (IP3) and diacylglycerol (DAG). This increase in IP3 causes an elevation of intracellular calcium (Ca^{2+}) and DAG-dependent PKC activation. PKC/Ca^{2+} or other signaling intermediates activate R- and/or NR-PTKs, such as EGFR, IGF-1R, PYK2, and c-Src, by inducing their phosphorylation on target tyrosine residues. Activation of these PTKs leads to the phosphorylation of docking proteins, such as IRS-1, which serve as docking sites for Grb-2/SOS. The latter can bind directly to activated EGFR, triggering a conformational change in Ras, a GTP exchanger, resulting in its activation. Once activated, Ras binds to Raf, a Ser/Thr kinase, which binds to and phosphorylates the dual-specificity protein kinases MEK-1/2, which phosphorylate ERK1/2. ERK1/2 can then translocate to the nucleus and regulate cell growth, proliferation, and hypertrophy through phosphorylation of transcription factors. Phosphorylated IRS-1 and EGFR bind to the p85 subunit of PI3-K and lead to its activation. Activated PI3-K catalyzes the phosphorylation of PIP2 to phosphatidylinositol 3,4,5 triphosphate (PIP3). PIP3 recruits PKB and PDK-1/2, Pleckstrin homology (PH) domain-containing proteins, to the plasma membrane, where PDK-1 and -2 phosphorylate PKB on threonine and serine residues, which in turn phosphorylate several downstream effectors, which contribute to protein synthesis, cell growth, survival, and gene transcription

(PKC-ζ), and p70 ribosomal S6 kinase (p70^{s6k}) [40, 41]. PKB is a 57-kDa protein, and was finally given the name PKB due to its high homology with protein kinase A (PKA) and PKC. It is known to exist as three isoforms, PKBα/Akt1, PKBβ/Akt2 and PKBγ/Akt3 [42]. All PKB isoforms have an amino-terminal PH domain, a central catalytic Ser/Thr kinase domain, and a carboxy-terminal regulatory domain that contains the hydrophobic motif (HM) [43, 44]. PDK1, which is thought to be constitutively active, phosphorylates Thr 308 in PKB [45], stabilizing the activation loop in an active form. This phosphorylation is a prerequisite for kinase activation, but phosphorylation of Ser 473 is necessary for full PKB activation (Fig. 1). The nature of putative Ser 473-PKB kinase called PDK2 is still controversial [46], although several candidates have been suggested [47]. Aside from its well-characterized role as regulator of glucose transport, glycogen synthesis, gluconeogenesis, and lipogenesis, PKB also plays an important role in protein synthesis, cell growth, and cell survival [48–52].

Several studies have demonstrated a role of the PI3-K/PKB pathway in vasoactive peptide-induced signaling events in multiple cell types, including VSMC, cardiomyocytes and human umbilical cells, leading to increased cell survival, hypertrophy and proliferation, physiological responses contributing to the development of cardiovascular diseases, such as atherosclerosis and stenosis after angioplasty [18, 53–55].

The Mitogen-Activated Protein Kinase Pathway

MAPKs constitute a family of serine/threonine protein kinases, which are widely conserved among eukaryotes, and are involved in many cellular responses, such as cell proliferation, cell differentiation, cell movement, and cell death [56, 57]. In mammalian cells, 5 MAPK families have been identified, including ERK1/2, c-Jun N-terminal kinase 1, 2, and 3 (JNK1/2/3), also called stress-activated protein kinase (SAPK), p38α/β/γ/δ MAPK, ERK5, and ERK7 [56, 57].

The groups of vertebrate MAPK studied most extensively to date are ERK1/2, JNKs, p38 MAPK [56, 57]. ERK1/2 are stimulated by mitogens, such as polypeptide growth factors (IGF-1, platelet-derived growth factor (PDGF), colony stimulating factor-1 (CSF-1), etc.), as well as insulin and phorbol 12-myristate 13-acetate (PMA). By contrast, SAPKs and p38 MAPK are potently induced by a wide variety of stresses, including ultraviolet irradiation, gamma irradiation, anisomycin, heat shock, and chemotherapeutic drugs, yet recent studies have also implicated SAPK/JNK and p38 MAPK in vasoactive peptide-induced proliferative responses [58–64]. These two pathways are also activated by ischemia or reperfusion after ischemia, and by inflammatory cytokines [65].

These pathways follow a similar sequence of activation, in which a stimulus activates a MAPKKK, which will then activate a MAPKK, which is an upstream activator of MAPK, which leads to a cellular response. The MAPK is the final effector of the cellular response. MAPKKKs are Ser/Thr kinases and are activated through phosphorylation and/or as a result of their interaction with a small GTP-binding protein of the Ras/Rho family in response to extracellular stimuli. Activation of MAPKKKs phosphorylate and activate MAPKK, which then phosphorylates Thr and Tyr residues in the activation loop of the kinase, stimulating MAPK activity. Once activated, MAPKs phosphorylate target substrates on Ser or Thr residues followed by a proline. ERK1/2 is the primary MAPK activated. This pathway consists of the MAPKKKs (A-Raf, B-Raf, and Raf-1), the MAPKKs [mitogen and extracellular signal regulated kinase 1 and 2 (MEK1/2)], and the MAPKs (ERK1 and ERK2) (Fig. 1). Signals from activated receptor tyrosine kinase (RTK) or GPCR to Raf/MEK/ERK are transmitted through different isoforms of the small GTP-binding protein such as Ras. As mentioned earlier, IGF-1R transduces its effect through IRS proteins, where phosphorylated IRS serves as a docking site for Grb-2/SOS, whereas Grb-2/SOS binds directly on the activated EGFR to turn on MAPK signaling. This triggers a conformational change in Ras, a GTP exchanger, resulting in its activation. Once activated, Ras binds to a wide range of downstream effector proteins, including isoforms of the Ser/Thr kinase Raf (Fig. 1). Raf then binds to, and phosphorylates, the dual-specificity protein kinase MEK-1 and -2, the latter of which phosphorylates ERK1/2 within a conserved Thr-Glu-Tyr (TEY) motif in their activation loop. ERK1/2 can then be translocated to the nucleus where it can phosphorylate and activate a number of transcription factors involved in gene activation [57, 66]. It can also activate a number of cytosolic proteins, such as p90^{rsk} through its proline directed Ser/Thr kinase activity. Other members of the MAPK family, such as JNK and p38 MAPK, are activated in a similar fashion and mediate cellular functions by phosphorylating downstream targets.

Overwhelming evidence exists to support a vasoactive peptide-induced MAPK activation in multiple systems, including oligodendrocyte progenitor cells, pancreatic stellate cell, aortic and mesenteric artery-derived VSMC, increasing cell growth and hypertrophy, leading to complications such as atrial fibrillation due to left ventricle hypertrophy, vascular remodeling, cardiac hypertrophy, and coronary artery disease [19, 55, 67–70].

Vasoactive Peptide-Induced Transactivation of Protein Tyrosine Kinases

Receptor Protein Tyrosine Kinases

Epidermal Growth Factor Receptor

The EGFR is one of four members belonging to the Erythroblastic Leukemia Viral Oncogene (erbB) family of R-PTKs. As such, EGFR is also known as ErbB1 (ErbB2, ErbB3, and ErbB4 are the other three members of this family). This family of transmembrane receptors undergoes homodimerization or heterodimerization to induce autophosphorylation and receptor tyrosine kinase activation in response to ligand binding [71, 72]. The EGFR is universally expressed in a variety of cell types and is most abundant in epithelial cells and many cancer cells [71, 73, 74]. This receptor contains an extracellular ligand binding domain, a single transmembrane domain and a cytoplasmic tyrosine kinase autophosphorylation and regulatory domain (reviewed in ref. [75]). Recent work has shown that in basal conditions, the kinase domain of the EGFR exists in an autoinhibitory conformational state, and ligand binding-induced dimerization and changes in conformation allow its autophosphorylation, resulting in its activation [76]. This event activates the intrinsic tyrosine kinase activity of the intracellular domain, leading to receptor autophosphorylation on several key tyrosine residues located in the COOH-terminal tail of the receptor [77]. These phosphorylated tyrosine residues then act as docking sites for SH2 and phosphotyrosine-binding domain containing cytoplasmic proteins, such as Grb-2/SOS and the p85 subunit of PI3-K [78], involved in the activation of multiple signaling pathways, including MAPK and PKB. Both ligand-dependent and -independent mechanisms for its activation have been suggested [79]. To date, seven different ligands,

including EGF, are known to bind to the EGFR and cause its activation [80, 81].

Multiple studies have shown that Ang II, and more recently ET-1, can cause the activation, and subsequent phosphorylation of EGFR through receptor transactivation, a phenomenon stemming from the binding of Ang II to its AT1R [82], and ET-1 to the ET_A receptor [83]. More recently, a role of ET_B receptor in ET-1-induced EGFR transactivation has also been demonstrated in VSMC, through the use of the N-terminally truncated or full-length ET_B receptor [83]. ET-1 and Ang II-induced EGFR activation has been demonstrated in multiple cell types, including VSMC, cardiomyocytes, intestinal epithelial cells, preglomerular VSMC, C9 cells, and pancreatic stellate cells [14, 70, 84–90]. Ang II and ET-1-induced ERK1/2 and PKB phosphorylation were also found to be EGFR-dependent based on studies using pharmacological inhibitors of EGFR, like AG 1478 (Figs. 2 and 3). For example, Ang II-induced p38 MAPK and ERK1/2 phosphorylation was attenuated by AG1478 [59]. Furthermore, Ang II-induced PKB phosphorylation was associated with EGFR transactivation in rat aorta VSMC and in intestinal epithelial IEC-18 cells [87, 91]. ET-1-induced ERK1/2 phosphorylation through EGFR activation was also demonstrated in rat cardiomyocytes and more recently, in rat renal tubular cells [14, 92]. More importantly, the transactivation of EGFR by ET-1 and Ang II has been suggested to play an important role in vasoactive peptide-induced physiological responses linked to MAPK and PKB signaling, such as growth, hypertrophy, and proliferation, in multiple cell types, including VSMC [14, 82, 85, 93]. For example, ET-1-induced EGFR transactivation has been implicated in protein and DNA synthesis and c-Fos gene transcription in VSMC [90, 94]. In addition, a role of EGFR in vascular contraction in mouse aortic ring segments and rabbit basilar artery rings has been reported [95, 96].

It is well known that VSMC from spontaneously hypertensive rats (SHR) exhibit exaggerated cell proliferation compared to VSMC from normotensive Wistar Kyoto (WKY) rats [97]. This was thought to occur due to elevated levels of $Gi\alpha$

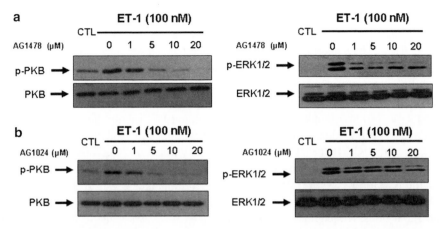

Fig. 2 Pharmacological blockade of EGFR or IGF-1R abolishes ET-1-induced ERK1/2 and PKB phosphorylation in A-10 VSMCs. Serum-starved quiescent A-10 VSMC were pretreated in the absence (0) or presence of the indicated concentrations of AG1478 (**a**) and AG1024 (**b**) for 30 min, followed by stimulation with 100 nM of ET-1 or Ang II for 5 min. Cell lysates were immunoblotted with phospho-specific-Ser 473-PKB and phospho-specific-Thr202/Tyr204-ERK1/2 antibodies. Blots were also analyzed for total ERK1/2 and PKB

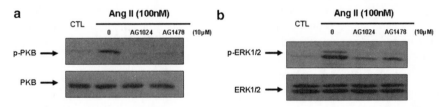

Fig. 3 Pharmacological blockade of EGFR and IGF-1R abolishes Ang II-induced ERK1/2 and PKB phosphorylation in A-10 VSMCs. Serum-starved quiescent A-10 VSMC were pretreated in the absence (0) or presence of 10 μM AG1024 or AG1478 for 30 min, followed by stimulation with 100 nM of Ang II for 5 min. Cell lysates were immunoblotted with phospho-specific-Ser 473-PKB (**a**) and phospho-specific-Thr202/Tyr204-ERK1/2 (**b**) antibodies. Blots were also analyzed for total ERK1/2 and PKB

proteins in VSMC from SHR, yet recent reports suggest for the first time that endogenously produced ET-1 and Ang II contribute to the enhanced proliferation of VSMC from SHR, through EGFR transactivation [98], linking growth factor receptor transactivation to the deleterious hypertrophic effects of elevated ET-1 and Ang II levels found in hypertensive states. In these studies, EGFR, AT1R, ET_A, and ET_B receptor inhibition decreased exaggerated ERK1/2 phosphorylation found in VSMC from SHR to levels found in VSMC from WKY, suggesting that endogenous ET-1 and Ang II-induced MAPK signaling contributes to the enhanced cell growth of VSMC in SHR through EGFR transactivation [98].

Insulin-Like Growth Factor Type 1 Receptor

IGF-1R, another transmembrane R-PTK, is a tetrameric protein consisting of 2α- and 2β-subunits and has a high degree of homology with the insulin receptor [99]. IGF-1R is activated by IGF-1 and associated growth factors, such as IGF-2, albeit with lower affinity. IGF-1R differs from other R-PTKs in that it exists on the cell surface as a covalent dimeric structure, which requires domain rearrangement for activation [100], whereas other R-PTKs, like the EGFR described earlier, dimerize or oligomerize on ligand binding to trigger receptor activation [101]. The α-subunit of IGF-1R contains the IGF-1-binding site, whereas the β-subunit comprises an intracellular PTK domain that is critical for transducing most of the downstream signaling [99]. The α-chain and the 195 residues of the β-chain make up the extracellular part of the IGF-1R [100]. The mature α2β2 receptor also has a single transmembrane sequence (906–929 residues) and a 408-residue cytoplasmic domain, which possesses tyrosine kinase activity. The N-terminal half of the IGF-1R also contains two homology domains, L1 and L2, separated by the Cys-rich region (Cys148 to Cys298). It has been shown that residues 131–315 (Cys-rich and L1 and L2 flanking regions) are required for binding IGF-1 [102]. This cytoplasmic domain is flanked by two regulatory regions: a juxtamembrane region, which plays a major role in docking of IR substrates (IRSs), Shc and receptor internalization [103], and a 108-residue long carboxy-terminal tail consisting of two phosphotyrosine-binding sites [103, 104]. IGF-1-binding to extracellular α-subunits triggers a conformational change in the β-subunit, resulting in its transautophosphorylation in multiple tyrosine residues and evoking the PTK catalytic activity of the receptor [105]. Activated IGF-1R phosphorylates several downstream substrates, such as Shc and IRSs 1–4, in multiple tyrosine residues [106, 107]. Phosphorylated IRSs serve as docking proteins for many SH2 domain-containing molecules, including growth factor receptor-binding protein 2 (Grb2), the p85 subunit of PI3-K, NcK and SH-phosphatase 2 Grb2 binding to the activated receptor, which recruits the son of sevenless (SOS), leading to the subsequent activation of the MAPK and/or PI3-K/PKB pathways [108, 109].

While EGFR transactivation by vasoactive peptides has been well described, the requirement of IGF-1R in vasoactive peptide-induced signaling is only more recently coming to light, in studies showing a requirement of IGF-1R activation in Ang II-induced downstream signaling [110], bridging the gap with studies done over a decade ago, demonstrating the stimulatory effect of Ang II on the tyrosine phosphorylation of IGF-1R β-subunit as well as on IRS-1 rat aortic VSMC [111]. These studies were confirmed more recently, when it was reported that Ang II treatment enhanced tyrosine phosphorylation of the β-subunit of IGF-1R in smooth muscle cells (SMC) isolated from porcine hearts [112]. IGF-1 neutralizing antibody was also used in these experiments, confirming that Ang II-induced IGF-1R phosphorylation was in fact ligand-independent [112]. While this study also showed that Ang II-induced phosphorylation of p85 and p70[s6k] was significantly attenuated by pretreatment of SMC with AG1024, a selective pharmacological inhibitor of IGF-1R-PTK activity, this drug failed to attenuate Ang II-induced ERK1/2 activation [112]. By contrast, however, recent studies have shown that AG1024 attenuated Ang II-induced phosphorylation of ERK1/2/5 (Figs. 2 and 3) and p38MAPK in mesenteric VSMC [113, 114]. Further consolidating the potential cross talk of between the Ang II and IGF-1/IGF-1R systems are studies showing that Ang II increases IGF-1mRNA and protein in heart tissue and VSMC [115, 116], and that IGF-1 can increase AT1R expression in VSMC [117]. Moreover, Nguyen et al. have also demonstrated that IGF-1R antisense-induced reduction in IGF-1R was associated with an inhibition of Ang II-induced vascular responses, as well as AT1R expression and functionality, in spontaneously hypertensive rats (SHR) and WKY rats [118, 119]. These, and studies showing that dominant negative or antisense oligonucleotide of IGF-1R are able to attenuate neointima formation in an injured carotid artery rat model [120], support a potential pathogenic role of upregulated IGF-1R signaling in vascular disease.

More recent studies have demonstrated a role of IGF-1R transactivation in both ET-1 and Ang II-induced PKB phosphorylation in VSMC, as well as in cell hypertrophy and proliferation induced by these vasoactive peptides [18]. These studies show that ET-1 and Ang II treatment induced the phosphorylation of key tyrosine residues in the auto-phosphorylation sites of IGF-1R and PKB, which was blocked by AG1024 pretreatment of VSMC (Figs. 2 and 3) [18]. AG1024 also attenuated ET-1 and Ang II-induced protein and DNA synthesis in A10 VSMC in these studies, which were among the first to identify an involvement of IGF-1R in transducing the downstream effects of ET-1 and Ang II in activating PKB in VSMC [18].

It was also recently reported for the first time that the transactivation of IGF-1R induced by enhanced levels of endogenous ET-1 contributes to the enhanced expression of Giα proteins in VSMC from SHR [121]. Previous studies had shown that VSMC from SHR exhibited enhanced levels of Giα proteins as compared to VSMC from normotensive WKY rats [122]. Inhibition of IGF-1R by AG1024 decreased Giα-2 and Giα-3 protein expression in SHR VSMC to levels found in WKY rats, suggesting the implication of IGF-1R in enhanced expression of Giα proteins in VSMC from SHR [121]. This work suggests that growth factor receptor transactivation causing enhanced Giα expression may be one of the mechanisms responsible for increased blood pressure in SHR [121].

Nonreceptor Protein Tyrosine Kinases

c-Src

c-Src, also known as Src or p60[c-Src], is a NR-PTK and is the cellular homologue of the v-Src avian oncogene of the Rous sarcoma virus, a chicken tumor virus, discovered by Peyton Rous [123]. It is a member of the Src family of NR-TK, which contains ten other members, including Blk, Brk, Fgr, Frk, Fyn, Hck, Lck, Lyn, Src, Srm, and Yes [124]. Src family of NR-TK plays a vital role in cell differentiation, proliferation, and survival signaling mechanisms, as well as in cell adhesion, morphology, and motility (reviewed in ref. [125]). Src, Yes, and Fyn are ubiquitously expressed in all cells, yet expression levels vary among certain cell types, such as platelets, neurons, and osteoclasts, which have been found to express 5- to 200-fold higher levels of Src protein than other cells [126]. Structurally, each member of the Src family contains a short N-terminal membrane anchor, or SH4 domain, which contains a 14 carbon myristoyl group. This domain is followed by a poorly conserved "unique" region of 40 to 70 residues, a SH3 domain of 50 residues, which can bind to specific proline-rich sequences, a SH2 domain of 100 residues, which can bind to Tyr phosphorylation sites, a SH2-linker domain rich in proline residues, a SH1, 250-residue

tyrosine kinase catalytic domain, and a short C-terminal regulatory region containing conserved tyrosine residues [126]. Each domain of the Src structure plays an important role in Src function. For example, studies have demonstrated that myristoylation allows for Src membrane localization and seems to be required for proper functioning of Src in cells [126], yet others have demonstrated that myristoylated Src is found free in the cytosol, and as such, does not guarantee Src binding to the cell membrane [125]. Myristoylation takes place on the myristoyl-rich SH4 (N-terminal) domain, which then binds to the cell membrane. The SH1 domain is the most conserved domain in all the tyrosine kinases, and contains an ATP-binding domain. Tyr 416/418 (416 in chicken and 418 in human) and Tyr 527/530 (527 in chicken and 530 in human) are the two major tyrosine phosphorylation sites that regulate Src activity. Phosphorylation of Tyr 416/418, through an autophosphorylation mechanism, is required for full c-Src activity, while phosphorylation of Tyr 527/530, a site located in the C-terminal regulatory region, is a negative regulator, whose phosphorylation will inhibit c-Src activity [127]. In a physiologically normal state, c-Src is found in an inactive state, or "closed" conformation, where the phosphorylated Tyr 527/530 site is linked to the SH2 domain, and the SH2-linker domain is bound to the SH3 domain, keeping the Tyr 416/418 dephosphorylated. Dephosphorylation of Tyr 527/530 causes a conformational change and disrupts the bond of this site with the SH2 domain, thus "opening" the conformation of the c-Src molecule, allowing for access of ATP to the catalytic site and release of ADP, leading to its autophosphorylation on Tyr 416/418, and causing c-Src activation [128]. In growth factor receptor signaling, the SH2 domain of c-Src binds to Tyr phosphorylated subunits of the growth factor receptor in question, leading to a conformational change and allowing for Tyr 416/418 phosphorylation and subsequent c-Src activation.

In the vasculature, especially VSMC, GPCR-linked contractile responses, induced by Ang II and phenylephrine, have been associated with c-Src activation [129, 130]. Furthermore, the use

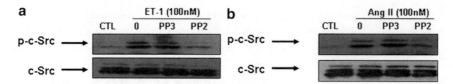

Fig. 4 Pharmacological blockade of c-Src attenuates ET-1 and Ang II-induced c-Src phosphorylation in A-10 VSMCs. Serum-starved quiescent A-10 VSMC were pretreated in the absence (0) or presence of 10 μM PP3 or 10 μM PP2 for 30 min, followed by stimulation with 100 nM for 5 min of ET-1 (**a**) or Ang II (**b**). Cell lysates were immunoblotted with phospho-specific-Tyr 418-c-Src and total c-Src antibodies (adapted from ref. [18])

of PP1 and PP2, pyrazolopyrimidine-based selective inhibitors of Src family tyrosine kinases [131], has indicated a role of Src in mediating H_2O_2, ET-1 and Ang II-induced transactivation of the EGFR, IGF-1R and PDGFR in several cell types [18, 132–135]. ET-1 and Ang II-induced MAPK activation has also been reported to be primarily dependent on the activation of c-Src in different cell types, including VSMC [22]. In Src-deficient VMSC derived from c-Src knockout mice, activation of ERK1/2 by Ang II was significantly decreased, as compared to VSMC from wild type mice [136, 137]. c-Src rescue in these cells through retroviral vector transfection caused a significant increase in Ang II-induced ERK1/2 phosphorylation, demonstrating that c-Src activation is necessary for Ang II-induced signal transduction in VSMC [137]. More recent studies have shown a role of c-Src in mediating ET-1 and Ang II-induced PKB phosphorylation [18]. In these studies, it was demonstrated that both vasoactive peptides can induce the Tyr 418 phosphorylation of c-Src in VSMC (Fig. 4), and that pharmacological inhibition of c-Src by PP-2 not only inhibited ET-1 and Ang II-induced c-Src phosphorylation, but also inhibited IGF-1R tyrosine phosphorylation, suggesting that c-Src is an upstream mediator of ET-1 and Ang II-induced IGF-1R transactivation, leading to PKB phosphorylation in VSMC [18]. These studies imply that c-Src activation is essential in triggering IGF-1R phosphorylation by ET-1, and therefore provide a molecular basis by which the ligand-independent transactivation of IGF-1R occurs in VSMC, in response to vasoactive peptides (Fig. 1).

Recent studies have also suggested the implication of c-Src in enhanced expression of Giα proteins in SHR, as PP2 was able to decrease the exaggerated Giα protein levels found in SHR to levels found in the normotensive WKY rats [121]. PP2 treatment also reduced exaggerated IGF-1R phosphorylation, as well as ERK1/2 phosphorylation to WKY levels, suggesting and further supporting the notion that c-Src is an upstream regulator of growth factor receptor activation [18, 121].

Both c-Src and IGF-1R have been implicated in the activation of NAD(P)H oxidase system [113], and since both ET-1 and Ang II trigger their effect through the generation of ROS [55], activation of IGF-1R and c-Src may be an early event in transducing vasoactive peptide-induced ROS generation, leading to the activation of growth promoting and hypertrophic signaling pathways. In fact, c-Src has also been shown to be activated in response to ROS, including H_2O_2, in different cell types [133, 135, 138–140]. Furthermore, through the use of PP1 and PP2, a role of c-Src in mediating H_2O_2-induced ERK1/2 phosphorylation in VSMCs derived from mesenteric arteries [141], in CHO-IR cells [140] and in renal cells [133, 142] has been shown. A requirement of c-Src has also been shown in H_2O_2-induced PKB phosphorylation in CHO-IR cells [140], renal cells [133], rat-2 fibroblasts [143] and, more recently, in A10 VSMCs [139]. Thus, c-Src appears to play a key role in signaling the effects of both H_2O_2, as well as vasoactive peptides.

Proline-Rich Tyrosine Kinase

PYK2 is a cytosolic Ca^{2+}-dependent, proline-rich tyrosine kinase [144], also known as calcium-dependent tyrosine kinase, cell adhesion kinase β, or related adhesion focal tyrosine kinase (RAFTK), as it has a similar overall structural organization to the FAK nonreceptor tyrosine kinases [145]. Like FAK, PYK2 has a C-terminal focal-adhesion targeting domain, a catalytic tyrosine kinase domain which is centrally located, an unstructured proline-rich region, and a N-terminal FERM domain, which can bind and autoinhibit the kinase activity of the tyrosine kinase domain [146]. However, recent reports demonstrate that the PYK2 FERM domain and the FAK FERM domain regulate the activity of PYK2 and FAK, respectively, but do so in different ways [147], indicating a role of the PYK2 FERM domain in the regulation of PYK2 activity [147]. PYK2 is activated by autophosphorylation in Tyr 402, located in its catalytic domain.

PYK2 has been proposed to facilitate the linkage between integrin receptors and the activation of signaling pathways, such as the PI3-K/PKB and MAPK pathways [144, 148]. Additionally, G-protein-associated ERK signaling was shown to be enhanced by PYK2 overexpression [144], which is further supported by studies showing that PYK2 inactivation, or mutation of its autophosphorylation sites, attenuates G-protein-induced ERK phosphorylation [149]. Moreover, the increases in intracellular Ca^{2+} and PKC activation via $G_{\alpha q}$ activation by Ang II have been well characterized and appear to be the main mechanism by which PYK2 is phosphorylated on Tyr 402, and thus fully activated by, Ang II [150]. The activated PYK2 forms a complex with shc and Grb/SOS, resulting in the activation of the Ras/MAPK and PI3-K pathways [151]. ET-1 was also shown to induce PYK2 phosphorylation in several cell types, including rabbit and rat VSMC [19, 55, 152]. This phosphorylation was blocked by BQ123, an ET_A receptor inhibitor, but not by BQ788, an ET_B receptor blocker, demonstrating that ET-1-induced PYK2 phosphorylation is dependent of ET_A receptor activation [152]. Furthermore, this study also showed that the Ca^{2+} channel blocker SK&F 96365 inhibited ET-1-induced PYK2 phosphorylation, linking ET-1-induced PYK2 phosphorylation to an increase in Ca^{2+} levels caused by ET_A receptor G-protein activation [152], similar to Ang II-induced PYK2

phosphorylation [153]. Furthermore, vasoactive peptide-induced MAPK and PKB activation have been linked to c-Src and PYK2 complex formation with either EGFR and/or IGF-1R, leading to their subsequent activation and downstream signaling [17, 154]. However, a recent report has suggested that Ang II activates MAPK signaling through a c-Src-dependent mechanism, while ET-1 activates MAPK signaling through a c-Src-independent mechanism [136]. Thus, PYK2 may activate EGFR signaling in a c-Src-independent fashion, yet the mechanism through which ET-1 signals MAPK activation still remains controversial. Nevertheless, it is quite evident that PYK2 plays an important role in mediating vasoactive peptide-induced signaling pathways involved in cell migration, proliferation, and hypertrophy (Fig. 1).

While the precise events that trigger the transactivation of R-/NR-PTK in response to vasoactive peptides are not clear, several mechanisms have been suggested. Studies have shown that inhibitors of matrix metalloproteinases (MMP), such as GM6001 and doxycyclin, attenuated ET-1 and Ang II-induced EGFR transactivation [155, 156]. MMPs act mainly by disrupting the link between growth factors and their transmembrane precursors, as is the case for heparin-bound-EGF (HB-EGF), allowing EGF to bind to EGFR, and leading to tyrosine kinase activation and stimulation of hypertrophic and growth promoting signaling cascades [157].

Another proposed mechanism of R-PTK transactivation by vasoactive peptides is through their capacity to induce the generation of reactive oxygen species (ROS) (Fig. 5). ET-1 has been shown to activate reduced nicotinamide adenine dinucleotide phosphate (NAD(P)H) oxidase, resulting in ROS generation in endothelial cells [158], and increased H_2O_2 levels via ET_A receptor binding in pulmonary smooth muscle cells [159]. This increase in ROS generation has been linked with the ET-1-induced activation of ERK1/2, JNK, p38mapk, PKB and PYK2 [55, 160]. For its part, Ang II has also been shown to induce ROS generation in multiple cell types, including cardiomyocytes, endothelial cells and VSMC [161–163], which appears to play a direct role in Ang II-induced

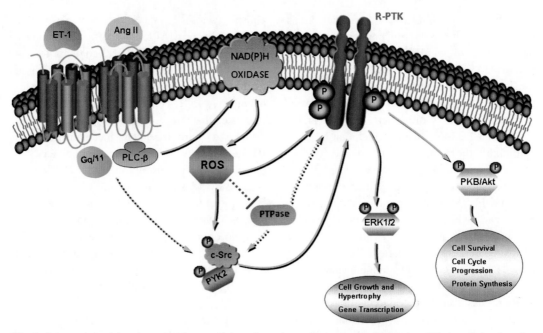

Fig. 5 Schematic model representing the potential mechanism through which R-/NR-PTKs are phosphorylated by vasoactive peptides. ET-1 and/or Ang II receptor activation is known to generate reactive oxygen species (ROS) through NAD(P)H oxidase system. ROS are able to inhibit protein tyrosine phosphatases (PTPase) through the oxidation of cysteine residues in their catalytic domain. Inhibition of PTPases favors a net increase in the tyrosine phosphorylation of c-Src, PYK2, and R-PTKs, such as EGFR and IGF-1R, resulting in the ligand-independent activation of EGFR and/or IGF-1R-which triggers PI3-K/PKB and MAPK signaling cascades

vascular hypertrophy through the activation of hypertrophic signaling pathways [164, 165]. ET-1-induced ROS generation in VSMC was suppressed by *N*-Acetylcysteine (NAc), a ROS scavenger, and diphenyleneiodonium (DPI), an inhibitor of NAD(P)H oxidase [55]. DPI and NAc pretreatment of VSMC also inhibited ET-1-induced ERK1/2, PKB, and PYK2 phosphorylation, demonstrating that ROS are critical mediators of ET-1-induced signaling events linked to growth-promoting proliferative and hypertrophic pathways in VSMCs. Observations that both ROS, e.g., H_2O_2, and vasoactive peptides induce the tyrosine phosphorylation of IGF-1R and EGFR, and pharmacological blockade or genetic ablation of the R- and/or NR-PTK activity resulted in the attenuation of ET-1 and Ang II-induced ERK1/2 and PKB phosphorylation have suggested that ROS may serve as intermediates to enhance the tyrosine phosphorylation of R- and NR-PTKs [18, 134, 139, 141, 166]. It should be noted that ROS molecules have been shown to inhibit the activity of protein tyrosine phosphatases (PTPases), such as PTP-1B [167] and SH-2 domain-containing tyrosine phosphatase-2 (SHP-2) [168]. PTPase inhibition can cause a shift in the phosphorylation–dephosphorylation cycle, leading to a net increase of tyrosine phosphorylation of R- and/or NR-PTKs [139, 140], which may contribute to the activation of the ERK1/2 and PKB signaling cascades (Fig. 5). It has also been reported that PTEN, which catalyzes PIP3 dephosphorylation, becomes inactivated by oxidation of Cys 124 in its catalytic domain subsequent to treatment with H_2O_2 or ROS-generating peptides [169–172], leading to an increase of PIP3 levels and a subsequent increase in PKB activation.

Conclusions

Although EGFR transactivation has been studied in detail with regard to vasoactive peptide-induced signaling, the transactivation of other receptor and/or nonreceptor tyrosine kinases is only recently coming to light as an important mechanism implicated in ET-1 and Ang II-induced migratory, hypertrophic, and proliferative signaling, leading to the deleterious effects of hypertensive states. While the precise mechanism of vasoactive peptide-induced R-/NR-PTK transactivation remains unclear, evidence points toward the implication of signal intermediates, such as matrix metalloproteinase and the generation of ROS, in inducing the activation and subsequent phosphorylation of R-/NR-PTKs, through either ligand-dependent or –independent mechanisms. Examples of this are the inhibition of protein tyrosine phosphatases by ROS, allowing for EGFR or IGF-1R phosphorylation, or the cleavage of heparin from EGF to allow for EGF-induced EGFR activation. Despite the lack of a clear explanation as to how R-/NR-PTK transactivation occurs, evidence is accumulating to indicate that activation of R-/NR-PTK plays a critical role in triggering the vasoactive peptide-induced signaling that mediates the hypertrophic, proliferative, and migratory responses in VSMC. Further research using pharmacological or genetic approaches will likely help to decipher the exact mechanisms by which R-/NR-PTK transactivation occurs, leading to potential developments in therapeutic tools to help restore dysregulated signaling events associated with vascular disorders.

Acknowledgments The work in the authors' laboratory is supported by funding from the Canadian Institutes of Health Research (CIHR) operating grant number 67037 to A.K.S. G.V. is the recipient of PhD studentships from the Faculty of Medicine, Université de Montréal and the Centre de Recherche du Centre Hospitalier de l'Université de Montréal (CRCHUM).

References

1. World Health Organisation. Cardiovascular diseases (CVDs) Fact sheet No. 317. World Health Organisation. 2009.

2. Bouallegue A, Daou GB, Srivastava AK. Endothelin-1-induced signaling pathways in vascular smooth muscle cells. Curr Vasc Pharmacol. 2007;5:45–52.

3. Schwartz SM. Smooth muscle migration in atherosclerosis and restenosis. J Clin Invest. 1997;100 (11 Suppl):S87–9.

4. Cordes KR, Sheehy NT, White MP, et al. miR-145 and miR-143 regulate smooth muscle cell fate and plasticity. Nature. 2009;460:705–10.

5. Mehta PK, Griendling KK. Angiotensin II cell signaling: physiological and pathological effects in the cardiovascular system. Am J Physiol Cell Physiol. 2007;292:C82–97.

6. Bobik A, Grooms A, Millar JA, et al. Growth factor activity of endothelin on vascular smooth muscle. Am J Physiol Cell Physiol. 1990;258:C408–15.

7. Rabelink TJ, Kaasjager KA, Boer P, et al. Effects of endothelin-1 on renal function in humans: implications for physiology and pathophysiology. Kidney Int. 1994;46:376–81.

8. Schiffrin EL. Endothelin: potential role in hypertension and vascular hypertrophy. Hypertension. 1995;25:1135–43.

9. Iglarz M, Schiffrin EL. Role of endothelin-1 in hypertension. Curr Hypertens Rep. 2003;5:144–8.

10. Touyz RM, Schiffrin EL. Signal transduction mechanisms mediating the physiological and pathophysiological actions of angiotensin II in vascular smooth muscle cells. Pharmacol Rev. 2000;52:639–72.

11. Touyz RM, Schiffrin EL. Role of endothelin in human hypertension. Can J Physiol Pharmacol. 2003;81:533–41.

12. Daub H, Weiss FU, Wallasch C, et al. Role of transactivation of the EGF receptor in signalling by G-protein-coupled receptors. Nature. 1996;379:557–60.

13. Hua H, Munk S, Whiteside CI. Endothelin-1 activates mesangial cell ERK1/2 via EGF-receptor transactivation and caveolin-1 interaction. Am J Physiol Renal Physiol. 2003;284:F303–12.

14. Kodama H, Fukuda K, Takahashi T, et al. Role of EGF Receptor and Pyk2 in endothelin-1-induced ERK activation in rat cardiomyocytes. J Mol Cell Cardiol. 2002;34:139–50.

15. Marrero MB, Schieffer B, Paxton WG, et al. Direct stimulation of Jak/STAT pathway by the angiotensin II AT1 receptor. Nature. 1995;375:247–50.

16. Marrero MB, Schieffer B, Li B, et al. Role of Janus kinase/signal transducer and activator of transcription and mitogen-activated protein kinase cascades in angiotensin II- and platelet-derived growth factor-induced vascular smooth muscle cell proliferation. J Biol Chem. 1997;272:24684–90.

17. Andreev J, Galisteo ML, Kranenburg O, et al. Src and Pyk2 mediate G-protein-coupled receptor activation of epidermal growth factor receptor (EGFR) but are not required for coupling to the mitogen-activated protein (MAP) kinase signaling cascade. J Biol Chem. 2001;276:20130–5.

18. Bouallegue A, Vardatsikos G, Srivastava AK. Role of insulin-like growth factor 1 receptor and c-Src in

endothelin-1- and angiotensin II-induced PKB phosphorylation, and hypertrophic and proliferative responses in vascular smooth muscle cells. Can J Physiol Pharmacol. 2009;87:1009–18.

19. Bouallegue A, Daou GB, Srivastava AK. Nitric oxide attenuates endothelin-1-induced activation of ERK1/2, PKB, and Pyk2 in vascular smooth muscle cells by a cGMP-dependent pathway. Am J Physiol Heart Circ Physiol. 2007;293:H2072–9.

20. Mehdi MZ, Vardatsikos G, Pandey SK, et al. Involvement of insulin-like growth factor type 1 receptor and protein kinase Cdelta in bis(maltolato) oxovanadium(IV)-induced phosphorylation of protein kinase B in HepG2 cells. Biochem. 2006;45:11605–15.

21. Pandey NR, Vardatsikos G, Mehdi MZ, et al. Cell-type-specific roles of IGF-1R and EGFR in mediating Zn2+–induced ERK1/2 and PKB phosphorylation. J Biol Inorg Chem. 2010;15:399–407.

22. Touyz RM, He G, Wu XH, et al. Src is an important mediator of extracellular signal-regulated kinase 1/2-dependent growth signaling by angiotensin II in smooth muscle cells from resistance arteries of hypertensive patients. Hypertension. 2001;38:56–64.

23. Hunyady L, Catt KJ. Pleiotropic AT1 receptor signaling pathways mediating physiological and pathogenic actions of angiotensin II. Mol Endocrinol. 2006;20:953–70.

24. Attina T, Camidge R, Newby DE, et al. Endothelin antagonism in pulmonary hypertension, heart failure, and beyond. Heart. 2005;91:825–31.

25. Inoue A, Yanagisawa M, Kimura S, et al. The human endothelin family: three structurally and pharmacologically distinct isopeptides predicted by three separate genes. Proc Natl Acad Sci USA. 1989;86:2863–7.

26. Gray GA. Generation of endothelin. In: Gray GA, Webb D, editors. Molecular biology and pharmacology of the endothelins. Austin: RG Landes; 1995. p. 13–32.

27. Arai H, Hori S, Aramori I, et al. Cloning and expression of a cDNA encoding an endothelin receptor. Nature. 1990;348:730–2.

28. Sakurai T, Yanagisawa M, Takuwa Y, et al. Cloning of a cDNA encoding a non-isopeptide-selective subtype of the endothelin receptor. Nature. 1990;348:732–5.

29. Ratnala VR, Kobilka B. Understanding the ligand-receptor-G protein ternary complex for GPCR drug discovery. Methods Mol Biol. 2009;552:67–77.

30. Harris DM, Cohn HI, Pesant S, et al. GPCR signalling in hypertension: role of GRKs. Clin Sci (Lond). 2008;115:79–89.

31. Rhee SG. Regulation of phosphoinositide-specific phospholipase C. Annu Rev Biochem. 2001;70:281–312.

32. Avruch J. Insulin signal transduction through protein kinase cascades. Mol Cell Biochem. 1998;182:31–48.

33. Leevers SJ, Vanhaesebroeck B, Waterfield MD. Signalling through phosphoinositide 3-kinases: the lipids take centre stage. Curr Opin Cell Biol. 1999; 11:219–25.

34. Deleris P, Gayral S, Breton-Douillon M. Nuclear PtdIns(3,4,5)P3 signaling: an ongoing story. J Cell Biochem. 2006;98:469–85.

35. Hawkins PT, Anderson KE, Davidson K, et al. Signalling through Class I PI3Ks in mammalian cells. Biochem Soc Trans. 2006;34:647–62.

36. Wymann MP, Zvelebil M, Laffargue M. Phosphoinositide 3-kinase signalling – which way to target? Trends Pharmacol Sci. 2003;24:366–76.

37. Fruman DA, Meyers RE, Cantley LC. Phosphoinositide kinases. Ann Rev Biochem. 1998;67:481–507.

38. Kanzaki M. Insulin receptor signals regulating GLUT4 translocation and actin dynamics. Endocr J. 2006;53:267–93.

39. Cantley LC. The phosphoinositide 3-kinase pathway. Science. 2002;296:1655–7.

40. Toker A, Newton AC. Cellular signaling: pivoting around PDK-1. Cell. 2000;103:185–8.

41. Downward J. Mechanisms and consequences of activation of protein kinase B/Akt. Curr Opin Cell Biol. 1998;10:262–7.

42. Coffer PJ, Jin J, Woodgett JR. Protein kinase B (c-Akt): a multifunctional mediator of phosphatidylinositol 3-kinase activation. Biochem J. 1998;335:1–13.

43. Alessi DR, Andjelkovic M, Caudwell B, et al. Mechanism of activation of protein kinase B by insulin and IGF-1. EMBO J. 1996;15:6541–51.

44. Chan TO, Rittenhouse SE, Tsichlis PN. AKT/PKB and other D3 phosphoinositide-regulated kinases: kinase activation by phosphoinositide-dependent phosphorylation. Annu Rev Biochem. 1999;68:965–1014.

45. Alessi DR, James SR, Downes CP, et al. Characterization of a 3-phosphoinositide-dependent protein kinase which phosphorylates and activates protein kinase Balpha. Curr Biol. 1997;7:261–9.

46. Dong LQ, Liu F. PDK2: the missing piece in the receptor tyrosine kinase signaling pathway puzzle. Am J Physiol Endocrinol Metab. 2005;289:E187–96.

47. Fayard E, Tintignac LA, Baudry A, et al. Protein kinase B/Akt at a glance. J Cell Sci. 2005;118:5675–8.

48. Hanada M, Feng J, Hemmings BA. Structure, regulation and function of PKB/AKT – a major therapeutic target. Biochim Biophys Acta. 2004;1697:3–16.

49. Cross DA, Alessi DR, Cohen P, et al. Inhibition of glycogen synthase kinase-3 by insulin mediated by protein kinase B. Nature. 1995;378:785–9.

50. Barthel A, Schmoll D. Novel concepts in insulin regulation of hepatic gluconeogenesis. Am J Physiol Endocrinol Metab. 2003;285:E685–92.

51. Rena G, Guo S, Cichy SC, et al. Phosphorylation of the transcription factor forkhead family member FKHR by protein kinase B. J Biol Chem. 1999;274:17179–83.

52. Hixon ML, Muro-Cacho C, Wagner MW, et al. Akt1/PKB upregulation leads to vascular smooth muscle cell hypertrophy and polyploidization. J Clin Invest. 2000;106:1011–20.

53. Pham FH, Cole SM, Clerk A. Regulation of cardiac myocyte protein synthesis through phosphatidylinositol 3′ kinase and protein kinase B. Adv Enzyme Regul. 2001;41:73–86.

54. Dong F, Zhang X, Wold LE, et al. Endothelin-1 enhances oxidative stress, cell proliferation and reduces apoptosis in human umbilical vein endothelial cells: role of ETB receptor, NADPH oxidase and caveolin-1. Br J Pharmacol. 2005;145:323–33.

55. Daou GB, Srivastava AK. Reactive oxygen species mediate Endothelin-1-induced activation of ERK1/2, PKB, and Pyk2 signaling, as well as protein synthesis, in vascular smooth muscle cells. Free Radic Biol Med. 2004;37:208–15.

56. Seger R, Krebs EG. The MAPK signaling cascade. Faseb J. 1995;9:726–35.

57. Kyosseva SV. Mitogen-activated protein kinase signaling. Int Rev Neurobiol. 2004;59:201–20.

58. Ohtsu H, Mifune M, Frank GD, et al. Signal-crosstalk between Rho/ROCK and c-Jun NH2-terminal kinase mediates migration of vascular smooth muscle cells stimulated by angiotensin II. Arterioscler Thromb Vasc Biol. 2005;25:1831–6.

59. Eguchi S, Dempsey PJ, Frank GD, et al. Activation of MAPKs by angiotensin II in vascular smooth muscle cells. Metalloprotease-dependent EGF receptor activation is required for activation of ERK and p38 MAPK but not for JNK. J Biol Chem. 2001;276:7957–62.

60. Araki S, Haneda M, Togawa M, et al. Endothelin-1 activates c-Jun NH2-terminal kinase in mesangial cells. Kidney Int. 1997;51:631–9.

61. Touyz RM, He G, El Mabrouk M, et al. Differential activation of extracellular signal-regulated protein kinase 1/2 and p38 mitogen activated-protein kinase by AT1 receptors in vascular smooth muscle cells from Wistar-Kyoto rats and spontaneously hypertensive rats. J Hypertens. 2001;19:553–9.

62. Zhou MS, Schulman IH, Chadipiralla K, et al. Role of c-Jun N-terminal kinase in the regulation of vascular tone. J Cardiovasc Pharmacol Ther. 2010;15:78–83.

63. Izumi Y, Kim S, Zhan Y, et al. Important role of angiotensin II-mediated c-Jun NH(2)-terminal kinase activation in cardiac hypertrophy in hypertensive rats. Hypertension. 2000;36:511–6.

64. Ding G, Zhang A, Huang S, et al. ANG II induces c-Jun NH2-terminal kinase activation and proliferation of human mesangial cells via redox-sensitive transactivation of the EGFR. Am J Physiol Renal Physiol. 2007;293:F1889–97.

65. Clark JE, Sarafraz N, Marber MS. Potential of p38-MAPK inhibitors in the treatment of ischaemic heart disease. Pharmacol Therap. 2007;116:192–206.

66. Chang F, Steelman LS, Lee JT, et al. Signal transduction mediated by the Ras//Raf//MEK//ERK pathway from cytokine receptors to transcription factors: potential targeting for therapeutic intervention. Leukemia. 2003;17:1263–93.

67. Touyz RM, Yao G, Viel E, et al. Angiotensin II and endothelin-1 regulate MAP kinases through different redox-dependent mechanisms in human vascular smooth muscle cells. J Hypertens. 2004;22:1141–9.

68. Daigle C, Martens FM, Girardot D, et al. Signaling of angiotensin II-induced vascular protein synthesis in conduit and resistance arteries in vivo. BMC Cardiovasc Disord. 2004;4:6.

69. Gadea A, Aguirre A, Haydar TF, et al. Endothelin-1 regulates oligodendrocyte development. J Neurosci. 2009;29:10047–62.

70. Hama K, Ohnishi H, Yasuda H, et al. Angiotensin II stimulates DNA synthesis of rat pancreatic stellate cells by activating ERK through EGF receptor transactivation. Biochem Biophys Res Commun. 2004;315:905–11.

71. Mendelson J. Blockade of receptors for growth factors: an anticancer therapy – the fourth annual Joseph H Burchenal American Association of Cancer Research Clinical Research Award Lecture. Clin Cancer Res. 2000;6:747–53.

72. Schlessinger J. Ligand-induced, receptor-mediated dimerization and activation of EGF receptor. Cell. 2002;110:669–72.

73. Carpenter G. The EGF receptor: a nexus for trafficking and signaling. Bioessays. 2000;22:697–707.

74. Prenzel N, Fischer OM, Streit S, et al. The epidermal growth factor receptor family as a central element for cellular signal transduction and diversification. Endocr Relat Cancer. 2001;8:11–31.

75. Normanno N, Bianco C, Strizzi L, et al. The ErbB receptors and their ligands in cancer: an overview. Curr Drug Targets. 2005;6:243–57.

76. Zhang X, Gureasko J, Shen K, et al. An allosteric mechanism for activation of the kinase domain of epidermal growth factor receptor. Cell. 2006;125:1137–49.

77. Burgess AW, Cho HS, Eigenbrot C, et al. An open-and-shut case? Recent insights into the activation of EGF/ErbB receptors. Mol Cell. 2003;12:541–52.

78. Yarden Y, Sliwkowski MX. Untangling the ErbB signalling network. Nat Rev Mol Cell Biol. 2001;2:127–37.

79. Scaltriti M, Baselga J. The epidermal growth factor receptor pathway: a model for targeted therapy. Clin Cancer Res. 2006;12:5268–72.

80. Linggi B, Carpenter G. ErbB receptors: new insights on mechanisms and biology. Trends Cell Biol. 2006;16:649–56.

81. Wu SL, Kim J, Bandle RW, et al. Dynamic profiling of the post-translational modifications and interaction partners of epidermal growth factor receptor signaling after stimulation by epidermal growth factor using Extended Range Proteomic Analysis (ERPA). Mol Cell Proteomics. 2006;5:1610–27.

82. Bokemeyer D, Schmitz U, Kramer HJ. Angiotensin II-induced growth of vascular smooth muscle cells requires an Src-dependent activation of the epidermal growth factor receptor. Kidney Int. 2000;58:549–58.

83. Grantcharova E, Reusch HP, Grossmann S, et al. N-terminal proteolysis of the endothelin B receptor abolishes its ability to induce EGF receptor transactivation and contractile protein expression in vascular smooth muscle cells. Arterioscler Thromb Vasc Biol. 2006;26:1288–96.

84. Eguchi S, Iwasaki H, Inagami T, et al. Involvement of PYK2 in angiotensin II signaling of vascular smooth muscle cells. Hypertension. 1999;33:201–6.

85. Eguchi S, Iwasaki H, Hirata Y, et al. Epidermal growth factor receptor is indispensable for c-Fos expression and protein synthesis by angiotensin II. Eur J Pharmacol. 1999;376:203–6.

86. Moriguchi Y, Matsubara H, Mori Y, et al. Angiotensin II-induced transactivation of epidermal growth factor receptor regulates fibronectin and transforming growth factor-beta synthesis via transcriptional and posttranscriptional mechanisms. Circ Res. 1999;84:1073–84.

87. Chiu T, Santiskulvong C, Rozengurt E. EGF receptor transactivation mediates ANG II-stimulated mitogenesis in intestinal epithelial cells through the PI3-kinase/Akt/mTOR/p70S6K1 signaling pathway. Am J Physiol Gastrointest Liver Physiol. 2005;288:G182–94.

88. Andresen BT, Linnoila JJ, Jackson EK, et al. Role of EGFR transactivation in angiotensin II signaling to extracellular regulated kinase in preglomerular smooth muscle cells. Hypertension. 2003;41:781–6.

89. Shah BH, Catt KJ. Calcium-independent activation of extracellularly regulated kinases 1 and 2 by angiotensin II in hepatic C9 cells: roles of protein kinase Cdelta, Src/proline-rich tyrosine kinase 2, and epidermal growth receptor trans-activation. Mol Pharmacol. 2002;61:343–51.

90. Iwasaki H, Eguchi S, Ueno H, et al. Endothelin-mediated vascular growth requires p42/p44 mitogen-activated protein kinase and p70 S6 kinase cascades via transactivation of epidermal growth factor receptor. Endocrinology. 1999;140:4659–68.

91. Li F, Malik KU. Angiotensin II-induced Akt activation through the epidermal growth factor receptor in vascular smooth muscle cells is mediated by phospholipid metabolites derived by activation of phospholipase D. J Pharmacol Exp Ther. 2005;312:1043–54.

92. Cheng-Hsien C, Yung-Ho H, Yuh-Mou S, et al. Src homology 2-containing phosphotyrosine phosphatase regulates endothelin-1-induced epidermal growth factor receptor transactivation in rat renal tubular cell NRK-52E. Pflugers Arch. 2006;452:16–24.

93. Ohtsu H, Dempsey PJ, Frank GD, et al. ADAM17 mediates epidermal growth factor receptor transactivation and vascular smooth muscle cell hypertrophy induced by angiotensin II. Arterioscler Thromb Vasc Biol. 2006;26:e133–7.

94. Iwasaki H, Eguchi S, Marumo F, et al. Endothelin-1 stimulates DNA synthesis of vascular smooth-muscle cells through transactivation of epidermal growth factor receptor. J Cardiovasc Pharmacol. 1998;31 Suppl 1:S182–4.

95. Flamant M, Tharaux PL, Placier S, et al. Epidermal growth factor receptor trans-activation mediates the tonic and fibrogenic effects of endothelin in the aortic wall of transgenic mice. FASEB J. 2003;17:327–9.

96. Kawanabe Y, Masaki T, Hashimoto N. Involvement of epidermal growth factor receptor-protein tyrosine kinase transactivation in endothelin-1-induced vascular contraction. J Neurosurg. 2004;100:1066–71.

97. Paquet JL, Baudouin-Legros M, Marche P, et al. Enhanced proliferating activity of cultured smooth muscle cells from SHR. Am J Hypertens. 1989;2:108–10.

98. Li Y, Levesque LO, Anand-Srivastava MB. Epidermal growth factor receptor transactivation by endogenous vasoactive peptides contributes to hyperproliferation of vascular smooth muscle cells of SHR. Am J Physiol Heart Circ Physiol. 2010;299:H1959–67.

99. Vardatsikos G, Sahu A, Srivastava A. The insulin-like growth factor family: molecular mechanisms, redox regulation and clinical implications. Antioxid Redox Signal. 2009;11:1165–90.

100. Ullrich A, Gray A, Tam AW, et al. Insulin-like growth factor I receptor primary structure: comparison with insulin receptor suggests structural determinants that define functional specificity. EMBO J. 1986;5:2503–12.

101. Heldin CH, Ostman A. Ligand-induced dimerization of growth factor receptors: variations on the theme. Cytokine Growth Factor Rev. 1996;7:3–10.

102. Ward CW, Garrett TPJ, McKern NM, et al. The three dimensional structure of the type I insulin-like growth factor receptor. Mol Pathol. 2001;54:125–32.

103. De Meyts P, Whittaker J. Structural biology of insulin and IGF1 receptors: implications for drug design. Nat Rev Drug Discov. 2002;1:769–83.

104. Adams TE, Epa VC, Garrett TP, et al. Structure and function of the type 1 insulin-like growth factor receptor. Cell Mol Life Sci. 2000;57:1050–93.

105. Gronborg M, Wulff BS, Rasmussen JS, et al. Structure-function relationship of the insulin-like growth factor-I receptor tyrosine kinase. J Biol Chem. 1993;268:23435–40.

106. Tsuruzoe K, Emkey R, Kriauciunas KM, et al. Insulin receptor substrate 3 (IRS-3) and IRS-4 impair IRS-1- and IRS-2-mediated signaling. Mol Cell Biol. 2001;21:26–38.

107. White MF. IRS proteins and the common path to diabetes. Am J Physiol Endocrinol Metab. 2002;283: E413–22.

108. LeRoith D, Werner H, Beitner-Johnson D, et al. Molecular and cellular aspects of the insulin-like growth factor I receptor. Endocr Rev. 1995;16: 143–63.

109. Saltiel AR, Kahn CR. Insulin signalling and the regulation of glucose and lipid metabolism. Nature. 2001;414:799–806.

110. Touyz RM, Tabet F, Schiffrin EL. Redox-dependent signalling by angiotensin II and vascular remodelling in hypertension. Clin Exp Pharmacol Physiol. 2003;30:860–6.

111. Du J, Sperling LS, Marrero MB, et al. G-protein and tyrosine kinase receptor cross-talk in rat aortic smooth muscle cells: thrombin- and angiotensin II-induced tyrosine phosphorylation of insulin receptor substrate-1 and insulin-like growth factor 1 receptor. Biochem Biophys Res Commun. 1996; 218:934–9.

112. Zahradka P, Litchie B, Storie B, et al. Transac-tivation of the insulin-like growth factor-I receptor by angiotensin II mediates downstream signaling from the angiotensin II type 1 receptor to phosphatidylinositol 3-kinase. Endocrinology. 2004;145:-2978–87.

113. Touyz RM, Cruzado M, Tabet F, et al. Redox-dependent MAP kinase signaling by Ang II in vascular smooth muscle cells: role of receptor tyrosine kinase transactivation. Can J Physiol Pharmacol. 2003;81:159–67.

114. Cruzado MC, Risler NR, Miatello RM, et al. Vascular smooth muscle cell NAD(P)H oxidase activity during the development of hypertension: effect of angiotensin II and role of insulinlike growth factor-1 receptor transactivation. Am J Hypertens. 2005;18:81–7.

115. Delafontaine P, Lou H. Angiotensin II regulates insulin-like growth factor I gene expression in vascular smooth muscle cells. J Biol Chem. 1993;268:16866–70.

116. Brink M, Chrast J, Price SR, et al. Angiotensin II stimulates gene expression of cardiac insulin-like growth factor I and its receptor through effects on blood pressure and food intake. Hypertension. 1999;34:1053–9.

117. Muller C, Reddert A, Wassmann S, et al. Insulin-like growth factor induces up-regulation of AT(1)-receptor gene expression in vascular smooth muscle cells. J Renin Angiotensin Aldosterone Syst. 2000;1:273–7.

118. Nguyen TT, White PJ. Intravenous IGF-I receptor antisense reduces IGF-IR expression and diminishes pressor responses to angiotensin II in conscious normotensive rats. Br J Pharmacol. 2005;146:935–41.

119. Nguyen TT, Cao N, Short JL, et al. Intravenous insulin-like growth factor-I receptor antisense treatment reduces angiotensin receptor expression and function in spontaneously hypertensive rats. J Pharmacol Exp Ther. 2006;318:1171–7.

120. Lim HJ, Park HY, Ko YG, et al. Dominant negative insulin-like growth factor-1 receptor inhibits neointimal formation through suppression of vascular smooth muscle cell migration and proliferation, and induction of apoptosis. Biochem Biophys Res Commun. 2004;325:1106–14.

121. Gomez Sandoval YH, Anand-Srivastava MB. Enhanced levels of endogenous endothelin-1 contribute to the over expression of Gialpha protein in vascular smooth muscle cells from SHR: role of growth factor receptor activation. Cell Signal. 2011;23:354–62.

122. Lappas G, Daou GB, Anand-Srivastava MB. Oxidative stress contributes to the enhanced expression of Gialpha proteins and adenylyl cyclase signaling in vascular smooth muscle cells from spontaneously hypertensive rats. J Hypertens. 2005;23:2251–61.

123. Rous P. A transmissible avian neoplasm (Sarcoma of the common fowl). J Exp Med. 1979;150:738–53.

124. Wheeler DL, Iida M, Dunn EF. The role of Src in solid tumors. Oncologist. 2009;14:667–78.

125. Roskoski Jr R. Src protein-tyrosine kinase structure and regulation. Biochem Biophys Res Commun. 2004;324:1155–64.

126. Brown MT, Cooper JA. Regulation, substrates and functions of src. Biochim Biophys Acta. 1996;1287:121–49.

127. Alvarez RH, Kantarjian HM, Cortes JE. The role of Src in solid and hematologic malignancies: development of new-generation Src inhibitors. Cancer. 2006;107:1918–29.

128. Rucci N, Susa M, Teti A. Inhibition of protein kinase c-Src as a therapeutic approach for cancer and bone metastases. Anticancer Agents Med Chem. 2008;8:342–9.

129. Lu R, Alioua A, Kumar Y, et al. c-Src tyrosine kinase, a critical component for 5-HT2A receptor-mediated contraction in rat aorta. J Physiol. 2008;586:3855–69.

130. Touyz RM, Wu XH, He G, et al. Role of c-Src in the regulation of vascular contraction and Ca^{2+} signaling by angiotensin II in human vascular smooth muscle cells. J Hypertens. 2001;19:441–9.

131. Hanke JH, Gardner JP, Dow RL, et al. Discovery of a novel, potent, and Src family-selective tyrosine kinase inhibitor. Study of Lck- and FynT-dependent T cell activation. J Biol Chem. 1996;271:695–701.

132. Prenzel N, Zwick E, Leserer M, et al. Tyrosine kinase signalling in breast cancer. Epidermal growth factor receptor: convergence point for signal integration and diversification. Breast Cancer Res. 2000;2:184–90.

133. Zhuang S, Schnellmann RG. H_2O_2-induced transactivation of EGF receptor requires Src and mediates ERK1/2, but not Akt, activation in renal cells. Am J Physiol Renal Physiol. 2004;286:F858–65.

134. Saito S, Frank GD, Mifune M, et al. Ligand-independent trans-activation of the platelet-derived growth factor receptor by reactive oxygen species requires protein kinase C-delta and c-Src. J Biol Chem. 2002;277:44695–700.

135. Catarzi S, Biagioni C, Giannoni E, et al. Redox regulation of platelet-derived-growth-factor-receptor: role of NADPH-oxidase and c-Src tyrosine kinase. Biochim Biophys Acta. 2005;1745:166–75.

136. Yogi A, Callera GE, Montezano AC, et al. Endothelin-1, but not Ang II, activates MAP kinases through c-Src independent Ras-Raf dependent pathways in vascular smooth muscle cells. Arterioscler Thromb Vasc Biol. 2007;27:1960–7.

137. Ishida M, Ishida T, Thomas SM, et al. Activation of extracellular signal-regulated kinases (ERK1/2) by angiotensin II is dependent on c-Src in vascular smooth muscle cells. Circ Res. 1998;82:7–12.

138. Rosado JA, Redondo PC, Salido GM, et al. Hydrogen peroxide generation induces pp 60src activation in human platelets: evidence for the involvement of this pathway in store-mediated calcium entry. J Biol Chem. 2004;279:1665–75.

139. Azar ZM, Mehdi MZ, Srivastava AK. Activation of insulin-like growth factor type-1 receptor is required for H2O2-induced PKB phosphorylation in vascular smooth muscle cells. Can J Physiol Pharmacol. 2006;84:777–86.

140. Mehdi MZ, Pandey NR, Pandey SK, et al. H_2O_2-induced phosphorylation of ERK1/2 and PKB requires tyrosine kinase activity of insulin receptor and c-Src. Antioxid Redox Signal. 2005;7:1014–20.

141. Tabet F, Schiffrin EL, Touyz RM. Mitogen-activated protein kinase activation by hydrogen peroxide is mediated through tyrosine kinase-dependent, protein

kinase C-independent pathways in vascular smooth muscle cells: upregulation in spontaneously hypertensive rats. J Hypertens. 2005;23:2005–12.

142. Lee JS, Kim SY, Kwon CH, et al. EGFR-dependent ERK activation triggers hydrogen peroxide-induced apoptosis in OK renal epithelial cells. Arch Toxicol. 2005;80:1–10.

143. Esposito F, Chirico G, Montesano GN, et al. Protein kinase B activation by reactive oxygen species is independent of tyrosine kinase receptor phosphorylation and requires SRC activity. J Biol Chem. 2003;278:20828–34.

144. Lev S, Moreno H, Martinez R, et al. Protein tyrosine kinase PYK2 involved in Ca^{2+}-induced regulation of ion channel and MAP kinase functions. Nature. 1995;376:737–45.

145. Avraham H, Park SY, Schinkmann K, et al. RAFTK/Pyk2-mediated cellular signalling. Cell Signal. 2000;12:123–33.

146. Schaller MD. Cellular functions of FAK kinases: insight into molecular mechanisms and novel functions. J Cell Sci. 2010;123:1007–13.

147. Riggs D, Yang Z, Kloss J, Loftus JC. The Pyk2 FERM regulates Pyk2 complex formation and phosphorylation. Cell Signal. 2011;23:288–96.

148. Sieg DJ, Ilic D, Jones KC, et al. Pyk2 and Src-family protein-tyrosine kinases compensate for the loss of FAK in fibronectin-stimulated signaling events but Pyk2 does not fully function to enhance FAK- cell migration. EMBO J. 1998;17:5933–47.

149. Dikic I, Tokiwa G, Lev S, et al. A role for Pyk2 and Src in linking G-protein-coupled receptors with MAP kinase activation. Nature. 1996;383:547–50.

150. Frank GD, Saito S, Motley ED, et al. Requirement of Ca^{2+} and PKCdelta for Janus kinase 2 activation by angiotensin II: involvement of PYK2. Mol Endocrinol. 2002;16:367–77.

151. Ivey ME, Osman N, Little PJ. Endothelin-1 signalling in vascular smooth muscle: pathways controlling cellular functions associated with atherosclerosis. Atherosclerosis. 2008;199:237–47.

152. Kawanabe Y, Hashimoto N, Masaki T. Involvements of voltage-independent Ca2+ channels and phosphoinositide 3-kinase in endothelin-1-induced PYK2 tyrosine phosphorylation. Mol Pharmacol. 2003;63:808–13.

153. Sabri A, Govindarajan G, Griffin TM, et al. Calcium- and protein kinase C-dependent activation of the tyrosine kinase PYK2 by angiotensin II in vascular smooth muscle. Circ Res. 1998;83:841–51.

154. Van KK, Gilany K, Moens L, et al. P2Y12 receptor signalling towards PKB proceeds through IGF-I receptor cross-talk and requires activation of Src, Pyk2 and Rap1. Cell Signal. 2006;18:1169–81.

155. Hao L, Nishimura T, Wo H, et al. Vascular responses to alpha1-adrenergic receptors in small rat mesenteric arteries depend on mitochondrial reactive oxygen species. Arterioscler Thromb Vasc Biol. 2006;26:819–25.

156. Saito S, Frank GD, Motley ED, et al. Metalloprotease inhibitor blocks angiotensin II-induced migration through inhibition of epidermal growth factor receptor transactivation. Biochem Biophys Res Commun. 2002;294:1023–9.

157. Nagareddy PR, Chow FL, Hao L, et al. Maintenance of adrenergic vascular tone by MMP transactivation of the EGFR requires PI3K and mitochondrial ATP synthesis. Cardiovasc Res. 2009;84:368–77.

158. Duerrschmidt N, Wippich N, Goettsch W, et al. Endothelin-1 induces NAD(P)H oxidase in human endothelial cells. Biochem Biophys Res Commun. 2000;269:713–7.

159. Wedgwood S, Black SM. Endothelin-1 decreases endothelial NOS expression and activity through ETA receptor-mediated generation of hydrogen peroxide. Am J Physiol Lung Cell Mol Physiol. 2005;288:L480–7.

160. Cheng CM, Hong HJ, Liu JC, et al. Crucial role of extracellular signal-regulated kinase pathway in reactive oxygen species-mediated endothelin-1 gene expression induced by endothelin-1 in rat cardiac fibroblasts. Mol Pharmacol. 2003;63:1002–11.

161. Wenzel S, Taimor G, Piper HM, et al. Redox-sensitive intermediates mediate angiotensin II-induced p38 MAP kinase activation, AP-1 binding activity, and TGF-beta expression in adult ventricular cardiomyocytes. FASEB J. 2001;15:2291–3.

162. Mahrouf M, Ouslimani N, Peynet J, et al. Metformin reduces angiotensin-mediated intracellular production of reactive oxygen species in endothelial cells through the inhibition of protein kinase C. Biochem Pharmacol. 2006;72:176–83.

163. Griendling KK, Sorescu D, Ushio-Fukai M. NAD(P)H oxidase: role in cardiovascular biology and disease. Circ Res. 2000;86:494–501.

164. Zafari AM, Ushio-Fukai M, Akers M, et al. Role of NADH/NADPH oxidase-derived H2O2 in angiotensin II-induced vascular hypertrophy. Hypertension. 1998;32:488–95.

165. Zhang Y, Griendling KK, Dikalova A, et al. Vascular hypertrophy in angiotensin II-induced hypertension is mediated by vascular smooth muscle cell-derived H_2O_2. Hypertension. 2005;46:732–7.

166. Frank GD, Mifune M, Inagami T, et al. Distinct mechanisms of receptor and nonreceptor tyrosine kinase activation by reactive oxygen species in vascular smooth muscle cells: role of metalloprotease and protein kinase C-delta. Mol Cell Biol. 2003;23:1581–9.

167. Lee SR, Kwon KS, Kim SR, et al. Reversible inactivation of protein-tyrosine phosphatase 1B in A431 cells stimulated with epidermal growth factor. J Biol Chem. 1998;273:15366–72.

168. Meng TC, Fukada T, Tonks NK. Reversible oxidation and inactivation of protein tyrosine phosphatases in vivo. Mol Cell. 2002;9:387–99.

169. Leslie NR, Bennett D, Lindsay YE, et al. Redox regulation of PI 3-kinase signalling via inactivation of PTEN. EMBO J. 2003;22:5501–10.

170. Lee SR, Yang KS, Kwon J, et al. Reversible inactivation of the tumor suppressor PTEN by H2O2. J Biol Chem. 2002;277:20336–42.

171. Seo JH, Ahn Y, Lee SR, et al. The major target of the endogenously generated reactive oxygen species in response to insulin stimulation is phosphatase and tensin homolog and not phosphoinositide-3 kinase (PI-3 kinase) in the PI-3 kinase/Akt pathway. Mol Biol Cell. 2005;16:348–57.

172. Kwon J, Lee SR, Yang KS, et al. Reversible oxidation and inactivation of the tumor suppressor PTEN in cells stimulated with peptide growth factors. Proc Natl Acad Sci USA. 2004;101:16419–24.

Sarco/Endoplasmic Reticulum Ca²⁺ Pump Damage by Oxidative Stress: Implications for Ca²⁺ Entry

Gauri Akolkar and Ashok K. Grover

Abstract

Oxidative stress has been implicated in a number of pathologies including ischemia–reperfusion. During ischemia–reperfusion, excess amounts of different types of reactive oxygen species accumulate and can cause tissue damage. In the coronary artery smooth muscle, one of the proteins readily affected by reactive oxygen species is the sarco/endoplasmic reticulum Ca^{2+} pump. This leads to an inability of cells to sequester Ca^{2+} into the sarco/endoplasmic reticulum and release it from this organelle for cell activation during signal transduction. Here, we present the hypothesis that the damage by reactive oxygen species to sarco/endoplasmic reticulum Ca^{2+} pump affects the Ca^{2+} refilling into the SER. The role of Na^+–Ca^{2+} exchanger and store-depletion-dependent channels is discussed in this context.

Keywords

Oxidative stress • Reactive oxygen species • Peroxide • Superoxide • Peroxynitrite • Peroxyl • SERCA • Orai • TRPC • TRPM • Stim • NCX • SOCE • Ischemia–reperfusion

Introduction

Ca^{2+} is an essential regulator of physiological responses in living cells. It is a ubiquitous second messenger that modulates diverse functions such as cell division, cell growth, electrical signaling, contraction, secretion, transcription, and apoptosis [1]. In resting smooth muscle cells, intracellular free Ca^{2+} concentration (Ca_i^{2+}) is maintained at 100–200 nM, whereas extracellular Ca^{2+} concentration is between 1 and 2 mM. A small increase in Ca_i^{2+} may cause large changes in cell function. Therefore, Ca_i^{2+} is maintained at a low level and to provide a transient signal, it is altered by Ca^{2+} entry, Ca^{2+} exit, release of sequestered Ca^{2+}, and/or Ca^{2+} binding to various proteins. This signaling uses a variety of Ca^{2+} regulatory mechanisms including various channels, pumps, exchangers, and binding proteins. Any defects in these processes

A.K. Grover (✉)
Department of Medicine, McMaster University, Hamilton, Ontario, Canada

Department of Biology, McMaster University, Hamilton, Ontario, Canada
e-mail: groverak@mcmaster.ca

may have dire consequences. Here, we focus on how excess accumulation of reactive oxygen species (ROS) during ischemia–reperfusion in coronary artery may alter these Ca^{2+} regulation mechanisms. One of the processes altered by ROS is the Ca^{2+} transport into the sarco/endoplasmic reticulum (SER) by the SER Ca^{2+} pump (SERCA) [2]. Our opinion is that ROS would also affect the entry of extracellular Ca^{2+} to be used in refilling the SER. Potential therapeutic impacts of this knowledge are also be presented.

Mechanisms of Decreasing Ca_i^{2+}

Elevated Ca_i^{2+} is required for only brief periods after which it is decreased to the basal levels. The decrease in Ca_i^{2+} is brought about by Ca^{2+} extrusion by the plasma membrane (PM) Ca^{2+} pump (PMCA) and the Na^+–Ca^{2+} exchanger (NCX) or by Ca^{2+} sequestration into SER by the SERCA pump [1, 3, 4]. SERCA and NCX play a crucial role in the removal of Ca_i^{2+} in smooth muscle cells; 92% of Ca_i^{2+} is removed by SERCA, 7% by NCX, and 1% by PMCA and mitochondria [5]. Ca_i^{2+} also is lowered by binding to Ca^{2+} binding proteins such as calsequesterin, calreticulin, and calnexin. Calsequesterin and calreticulin in the SER bind Ca^{2+}. They increase the Ca^{2+} storage capacity of SER and modulate the function of SERCA [6]. There are several recent reviews on these pathways [1, 3, 4].

Mechanisms of Increasing Ca_i^{2+}

An increase in Ca_i^{2+} can occur either by Ca^{2+} influx from extracellular fluid through channels in PM or by release of Ca^{2+} sequestered in the SER or other organelles [1]. Ca^{2+} channels that are operated by voltage (VOCC) or receptor action (ROCC) may cause entry of extracellular Ca^{2+}. In addition to these channels, NCX can operate in Ca^{2+} entry mode and hence increase the cytosolic Ca^{2+}. Ca_i^{2+} can also be increased by the release of Ca^{2+} from the SER through Ca^{2+} channels activated by inositol 1,4,5-triphosphate

(IP3) or Ca^{2+} (or the plant alkaloid ryanodine). Depletion of Ca^{2+} from intracellular stores activates Ca^{2+} entry from the extracellular space for refilling of the SER by store-depletion-dependent or store-operated calcium entry (SOCE) [7–9]. Inwardly rectifying Ca^{2+} current (I_{CRAC}) is a form of SOCE and has been associated with two families of proteins: the SER resident stromal interaction molecules (Stim) and the Orai proteins in the PM. In addition to Stim and Orai, members of transient receptor protein (TRP) family may be involved in SOCE. In contrast to the Orai channels, the TRP channels are not very selective for Ca^{2+}. Other than SOCE function, some members of TRP family can increase Ca_i^{2+} by receptor-induced Ca^{2+} entry [10–12]. NCX, Stim, Orai, and TRP are discussed further.

NCX

NCX are electrogenic transporters with a stoichiometry of 3 Na^+:1 Ca^{2+}. Depending on the electrochemical gradients, they can either expel Ca^{2+} from the cell (forward or extrusion mode) or cause Ca^{2+} entry (reverse or entry mode) [13]. NCX are encoded by genes NCX1, 2, and 3. Alternative splicing results in additional NCX isoforms, which differ in their regulation. Commonly used NCX inhibitors are XIP, dichlorobenzamil, KB-R7943, and SEA 0400. XIP is most selective, but it cannot be used extracellularly [14]. Amiloride derivatives such as dichlorobenzamil are least selective. Both KB-R7943 and SEA 0400 also block VOCC, but SEA 0400 is more selective for NCX. In pig coronary artery, smooth muscle and endothelium express NCX1 [15]. NCX-mediated Ca^{2+} entry was observed in both cultured PCSMC and PCEC. Ca^{2+} entry via NCX may be important in Ca^{2+} refilling into the SER. The role of NCX in vascular smooth muscle and endothelium has been shown by various methods including contractility experiments, by Ca_i^{2+} measurements and by NCX knock down [13, 15, 16]. NCX-mediated Ca^{2+} entry in smooth muscle cells leads to contraction and may also play a role in endothelium dependent relaxation.

A linkage between NCX and SERCA has been reported in blood vessels. The following is the experimental evidence for a *functional linkage* between NCX and SERCA in pig coronary artery smooth muscle cells. Na^+-loaded smooth muscle or endothelial cells show NCX-mediated Ca^{2+} entry when placed in a Na^+-free solution. In smooth muscle, but not in endothelial cells, this Ca^{2+} entry is decreased by inhibition of SERCA with thapsigargin [15]. Immunofluorescence microscopy and biochemical experiments also suggest a proximity between NCX and SERCA in smooth muscle cells cultured from this artery [17]. Several models have been proposed to explain the NCX-SERCA relationship in various cells. One of them is a "junctional cytoplasmic space model" in which NCX and SERCA occur in close complex within a narrow cytoplasmic space between subsurface sarco/endoplasmic reticulum and the PM [18].

SOCE, Stim, and Orai

Ca^{2+} depletion in the SER acts as a trigger for Ca^{2+} entry to refill the SER by a pathway termed SOCE. It is suggested that the activation of SOCE may be due to altered interactions between SER and PM. Two families of proteins play an important role in this process: Stim and Orai [8, 19–21]. These proteins mediate three important steps in SOCE: sensing Ca^{2+} levels in the SER lumen, transduction of the signal to PM, and opening of highly selective Ca^{2+} channels in the PM. After the SOCE-mediated increase, cytosolic Ca^{2+} is sequestered into the ER by SERCA protein.

Stim1 protein is found in tubular SER and to some degree in the PM. Its role in SOCE has been shown by suppression of Stim1 expression that prevents SOCE [22, 23]. Stim1 is N-glycosylated at its luminal side [21, 24]. It acts a sensor of SER luminal Ca^{2+} concentration. When luminal Ca^{2+} concentration decreases below 100–200 μM, Stim1 undergoes a conformational change. In basal state when ER Ca^{2+} stores are filled, Stim1 is a dimer stabilized by C-terminal coiled – coil interaction. The C-terminal portion forms dimers, whereas the N-terminal ER domain is monomeric

at basal SER Ca^{2+} concentration. When the SER Ca^{2+} store is depleted, Stim1 oligomerization occurs and triggers its translocation toward PM. Total internal reflection microscopy (TIRF) measurements indicate that the aggregated Stim1 in the SER approaches as close as 10–20 nm to the PM and interacts directly with Orai1 and possibly with other PM proteins [25]. Other members of the Stim family may also play a role, but currently the nature of this role is not clear.

Orai is an integral PM protein and forms the channel component of SOCE [8, 9, 21, 26]. Three different Orai proteins, 1, 2, and 3, display notable differences in their function. Orai1 is the most potent in reconstituting Ca^{2+} influx in most cells. It is highly selective for Ca^{2+}. The working model is that Stim1 clustering and translocation begins when SER luminal Ca^{2+} concentration falls below 300 μM and results in reorganization of Orai subunits in the PM to form Ca^{2+} channels. Part of the evidence is that expression of Orai1 and 2 alone decreases the SOCE, while their coexpression with Stim1 leads to an increase in this activity [21]. Another piece of evidence is the movement of Stim1 toward PM. Finally, an increase in FRET between Stim1 and Orai1 has been demonstrated under the conditions that activate SOCE [27].

TRP Channels

TRP family of proteins includes nonselective cation channels and has been divided into several subfamilies: TRPC, TRPM, and TRPV. TRPC is the classical or the canonical protein family with the members TRPC1-7. In some smooth muscles, TRPC1 is abundant and plays an important role in SOCE; other members of TRPC have also been implicated in this role [10–12, 18, 28–31]. TRPC have been shown to act as ROCC since they may be activated by metabolites such as diacylglycerol produced upon receptor activation or by direct linkage to IP3 activated channels in the SER [29]. Stim1 can also bind TRPC proteins. Association between TRPC1 and stim1 has been reported in platelets and vascular smooth muscle cells [10–12, 29]. Stim1-TRPC channel complexation may lead to SOCE. The role of TRPC in SOCE is controversial with some studies supporting this role, while others challenge it. In A549 endothelial cell line store-operated and thapsigargin-induced Ca^{2+} entry decreased by 50 and 25% respectively, when TRPC1 expression was suppressed selectively by antisense oligonucleotides directed against this protein [32]. By contrast, TRPC1 was not obligatory for SOCE because vascular smooth muscle cells from TRPC1 null mice showed similar SOCE induced as those from wild-type mice [33]. To complicate matters, TRPC are also seen to physically and functionally interact with Orai1 protein [31]. TRPC1 may also form a ternary complex with Orai1 to perform the SOCE function. The role of TRPC in SOCE may be complicated by their ability to allow influx of Na^+. Hence, in actuality the subject of SOCE may be far more complex. In one model, TRPC, NCX, and SERCA may form a signal linkage. The nonselective cation transport through TRPC would locally modulate Na^+-gradients (LNats), thereby altering the NCX-mediated Ca^{2+} entry [18]. In addition, TRPM family has also been implicated in SOCE [34].

Reactive Oxygen Species and the Oxidant–Antioxidant Balance

Cells maintain a balance of oxidants and antioxidants, and a disturbance in this balance leads to disorders [2]. ROS are normally formed in cells for physiological functions with mitochondria being the main source of ROS formation. Under normal conditions, ROS are destroyed once their function is over. However, in conditions such as ischemia–reperfusion, excessive accumulation of ROS such as peroxides, superoxide, hydroxyl radical, hypochlorite, and peroxynitrite causes oxidative stress. The excessive ROS accumulation occurs, in part due to iron liberated from hemoglobin during ischemia reperfusion and in part due to decreased activities of antioxidants. The damage by excessive ROS may involve peroxidation reaction of membrane and circulating lipids, oxidation of sulfhydryl groups in proteins,

and damage to nucleic acids including DNA. The lipid oxidation can cause an increase in PM permeability, a breakdown of transmembrane ion gradients, a loss of secretory functions, and an inhibition of certain metabolic processes. Here, we focus on the ischemia–reperfusion in the vasculature with an emphasis on the coronary artery.

Cardiovascular Damage by ROS

Excess ROS such as hydrogen peroxide, superoxide, hydroxyl anions, and peroxynitrite accumulate during atherosclerosis with the consequence of myocardial injury during ischemia or the reperfusion when the atherosclerotic plaque is removed [2]. The injury involves several cell types including coronary endothelial and smooth muscle cells, circulating blood cells (leukocytes, neutrophils, platelets), and cardiac myocytes. In cardiac muscle, ROS may cause contractile abnormalities by producing a Ca^{2+} overload. The most common cause of progressive coronary artery disease during adult life is artherosclerosis, which is associated with a number of risk factors, especially those associated with lifestyles. Classically, an atherosclerotic lesion in an arterial wall is considered to be a lipid disorder causing an influx of excess lipid deposits and macrophages contributing as lipid scavengers. Today, atherosclerosis is considered to be an inflammatory disease with macrophages interacting with other cells such as lymphocytes and mast cells. Macrophages produce large amounts of superoxide and NO, which together form the highly toxic reactive oxygen species peroxynitrite. There is a direct relationship between the number of inflammatory cells, markers of inflammation, and the severity of the coronary syndrome. Systemic infection and inflammation can also induce low-density lipoprotein oxidation in vivo and promote atherogenesis, thus contributing to increased incidence of coronary artery disease. Renin–angiotensin system may contribute to inflammatory processes within the vascular wall and to the development of acute coronary syndromes. Elevated levels of angiotensin II may also be associated with the generation of oxidative stress and may thus play a significant role in the early phase of atherosclerosis.

Actions of ROS on SERCA Pumps in Coronary Artery

Although ROS may damage a number of ion transporters and other pathways, only the SERCA pumps in coronary artery are discussed here with a further focus on coronary artery. SERCA pumps are encoded by the genes: SERCA1, 2, and 3 [3]. The effects of ROS on SERCA have been examined in endothelium, SERCA2 and 3, and smooth muscle SERCA2 of the coronary artery [2, 35–38]. The effects of peroxide, superoxide, and peroxynitrite on SERCA in this artery have been examined at various organizational levels: arterial contractility, changes in Ca_i^{2+}, and pump activity in isolated membranes and permeabilized cells. All three species of ROS irreversibly damage SERCA2 dependent Ca^{2+} transport in the isolated membranes but the effect on SERCA3 is less severe. The mechanism of the damage involves inhibition of an initial step in the reaction cycle of SERCA2. The reaction cycle of SERCA involves the formation of a high-energy intermediate acylphosphate, and this step is inhibited by all the ROS examined. A functional consequence of the SERCA2 damage in this tissue is the decrease in contraction in response to the SERCA2 inhibitors cyclopiazonic acid and thapsigargin [37]. The force produced in response to the actions of angiotensin II and endothelin B is also decreased, possibly because these agents depend on the Ca^{2+} stores in the SER. The smooth muscle cells cultured from this tissue produce an increase in Ca_i^{2+} with substances such as angiotensin II, cyclopiazonic acid, and thapsigargin. Exposure to ROS decreases these responses. An interesting observation is the heterogeneity of the effects of peroxide and superoxide in the permeabilized cells. Peroxide is equipotent in inhibiting loading into the IP3-sensitive and -insensitive Ca^{2+} pools. By contrast, superoxide pretreatment inhibits loading into the IP3-sensitive pool, but not into the IP3-insensitive pool [39]. The exact significance of this observation remains to be determined.

Effect of ROS on NCX, SOCE, and TRP Channels

The effects of ROS on NCX, SOCE, and TRP channels vary from tissue to tissue. Elevated NCX1 levels using an adenoviral system predispose rabbit ventricular cardiomyocytes to ROS-induced injury, a mechanism likely contributing to myocyte dysfunction and death in heart failure [40]. The effects of ROS have been associated with oxidative modification of thiols on both SERCA and NCX [41]. The effects on NCX may depend on the splice variants and hence the effects may vary between tissues. In a patch clamp study, H_2O_2 irreversibly increased the NCX-mediated Ca^{2+} entry in cells overexpressing NCX1.1 (cardiac variant) without affecting Ca^{2+} efflux. By direct contrast, H_2O_2 decreased the Ca^{2+} entry by NCX1.3 (vascular variant) [42]. The NCX modulation by ROS may be complicated further due to the interactions with other pathways. In guinea pig ventricular myocytes, H_2O_2 increases the NCX current via two signal transduction pathways: one involves Na^+–H^+-exchanger and PI3K-dependent mechanism, while the other involves activation of a Src family tyrosine kinase [43]. The effects may also vary with the types of ROS. In brain synaptic vesicles and in transfected CHO-K1 cells, H_2O_2 (up to 800 μM) has no effect, but peroxyl radical and peroxynitrite inhibit NCX by causing its oligomerization and fragmentation [44]. ROS may also cause regulation of NCX at the RNA level [45].

SOCE have been linked to NO synthase activation and ROS in endothelial cells. In one study, a 60-min exposure of calf pulmonary artery endothelial cells to tert-butyl-hydroperoxide did not affect intracellular Ca^{2+} release, but inhibited SOCE. Both were inhibited after 120 min of the exposure. The effect was prevented by the antioxidant Trolox [46]. In human platelets, H_2O_2 inhibits SOCE by causing an abnormal actin reorganization pattern involving both Ras- and tyrosine kinases-dependent pathways [47]. Glucose-induced eNOS expression and NO production in mesangial cells may contribute to hyperfiltration in diabetes, and retinoic acid may exert beneficial effects by downregulation of STIM1 and SOCE [48]. However, S-glutathionylation of cysteine 56 of Stim1 may also evoke Ca^{2+} entry via this protein independent of intracellular Ca^{2+} stores [49]. Orai may also be sensitive to ROS. In human T cell helper lymphocytes, the cells expressing Orai1 are more sensitive to H_2O_2 than those expressing Orai 3. Thus, SOCE can be modulated by ROS by several different mechanisms [50]. H_2O_2 may also activate TRPM2 directly via store depletion dependent pathways [51]. The net effect of the activation of this pathway can be an increase in the transmonolayer transendothelial permeability. Therefore, manipulating TRPM2 function in the endothelium may represent a novel strategy aimed to prevent oxidative stress-related vascular dysfunction [34, 52]. Ca^{2+} signaling of lipopolysaccharide-stimulated microglia to H_2O_2 may also be related to TRPM2 [53]. TRPM2 may also play a role in H_2O_2-induced neuronal death as redox-sensitive a Ca^{2+} permeable pathway [54].

TRPC channels may serve as redox sensors in the vascular endothelium. Heterologously expressed TRPC3 and TRPC4 in HEK293 cells are able to form redox-sensitive cation channels via ROS-induced promotion of protein tyrosine phosphorylation and stimulation of phospholipase C activity [55]. Another aspect of oxidative stress has been suggested to be the involvement of the cytochrome P450 metabolite 5,6-EET. In a study using human platelets, 5,6-EET induced divalent cation entry without having any detectable effect on Ca^{2+} store depletion. The entry was sensitive to the SOCE blockers and impaired by incubation with anti-hTRPC1 antibody. This entry required basal levels of H_2O_2, which might maintain a redox state favorable for this event [56]. TRPC6 that is involved in receptor operated Ca^{2+} entry may be activated by oxidation of a cysteine residue. This cysteine oxidation-dependent pathway not only stimulates the TRPC6 channel by itself but also sensitizes the channels to diacylglycerol and promotes TRPC6 trafficking to the cell surface [57].

Conclusions

During signal transduction, Ca^{2+} is released from the SER, and the depletion of Ca^{2+} stores leads to entry of extracellular Ca^{2+} to allow SER refilling. SOCE may involve the SER-resident proteins of the STIM family and the PM-resident ion channels and exchangers: NCX, Orai, TRPM, and TRPC. During ischemia–reperfusion, different types of ROS accumulate in excess and can cause tissue damage. In the coronary artery smooth muscle, SERCA is readily damaged by ROS, and this leads to an inability of these cells to sequester Ca^{2+} into the SER. SOCE may also be affected by ROS, but the effects depend on the types of pathways responsible for the entry. The effects of ROS on these pathways and their dependence on SER are an emerging topic.

Several different types of agents are used to prevent damage during ischemia and after reperfusion: voltage-operated Ca^{2+} channel blockers, inhibitors of NCX-mediated Ca^{2+} entry, antioxidants, and SOCE inhibitors. These treatments are used primarily to prevent damage due to Ca^{2+} overload. However, none of the therapies are fully effective. These therapies can be significantly improved by understanding interactions between SERCA and the various SOCE pathways in a tissue- and pathology-dependent manner. Even newer therapeutic targets can be developed with the discovery of how these pathways are physically and metabolically linked.

Acknowledgments This work was supported by a Grant-in-Aid from the Heart & Stroke Foundation of Ontario.

References

1. Clapham DE. Calcium signaling. Cell. 2007;131: 1047–58.
2. Walia M, Kwan CY, Grover AK. Effects of free radicals on coronary artery. Med Princ Pract. 2003;12:1–9.
3. Misquitta CM, Mack DP, Grover AK. Sarco/endoplasmic reticulum Ca^{2+} (SERCA)-pumps: link to heart beats and calcium waves. Cell Calcium. 1999;25:277–90.
4. Strehler EE, Caride AJ, Filoteo AG, et al. Plasma membrane Ca^{2+} ATPases as dynamic regulators of

cellular calcium handling. Ann N Y Acad Sci. 2007;1099:226–36.

5. Shin SY, Choo SM, Woo SH, et al. Cardiac systems biology and parameter sensitivity analysis: intracellular Ca²⁺ regulatory mechanisms in mouse ventricular myocytes. Adv Biochem Eng Biotechnol. 2008;110:25–45.

6. Lee D, Michalak M. Membrane associated Ca²⁺ buffers in the heart. BMB Rep. 2010;43:151–7.

7. Cahalan MD. STIMulating store-operated Ca²⁺ entry. Nat Cell Biol. 2009;11:669–77.

8. Hewavitharana T, Deng X, Soboloff J, et al. Role of STIM and Orai proteins in the store-operated calcium signaling pathway. Cell Calcium. 2007;42:173–82.

9. Parekh AB. Store-operated CRAC channels: function in health and disease. Nat Rev Drug Discov. 2010;9:399–410.

10. Ambudkar IS, Ong HL, Liu X, et al. TRPC1: the link between functionally distinct store-operated calcium channels. Cell Calcium. 2007;42:213–23.

11. Ng LC, McCormack MD, Airey JA, et al. TRPC1 and STIM1 mediate capacitative Ca²⁺ entry in mouse pulmonary arterial smooth muscle cells. J Physiol. 2009;587:2429–42.

12. Worley PF, Zeng W, Huang GN, et al. TRPC channels as STIM1-regulated store-operated channels. Cell Calcium. 2007;42:205–11.

13. Blaustein MP, Lederer WJ. Sodium/calcium exchange: its physiological implications. Physiol Rev. 1999; 79:763–854.

14. Iwamoto T. Forefront of Na⁺/Ca²⁺ exchanger studies: molecular pharmacology of Na⁺/Ca²⁺ exchange inhibitors. J Pharmacol Sci. 2004;96:27–32.

15. Davis KA, Samson SE, Hammel KE, et al. Functional linkage of Na⁺-Ca²⁺-exchanger to sarco/endoplasmic reticulum Ca²⁺ pump in coronary artery: comparison of smooth muscle and endothelial cells. J Cell Mol Med. 2009;13:1775–83.

16. Hurtado C, Prociuk M, Maddaford TG, et al. Cells expressing unique Na⁺/Ca²⁺ exchange (NCX1) splice variants exhibit different susceptibilities to Ca²⁺ overload. Am J Physiol Heart Circ Physiol. 2006;290:H2155–62.

17. Kuszczak I, Kuner R, Samson SE, et al. Proximity of Na⁺-Ca²⁺-exchanger and sarco/endoplasmic reticulum Ca²⁺ pump in pig coronary artery smooth muscle: fluorescence microscopy. Mol Cell Biochem. 2010;339:293–300.

18. Poburko D, Fameli N, Kuo KH, et al. Ca²⁺ signaling in smooth muscle: TRPC6, NCX and LNats in nanodomains. Channels (Austin). 2008;2:10–2.

19. Abdullaev IF, Bisaillon JM, Potier M, et al. Stim1 and Orai1 mediate CRAC currents and store-operated calcium entry important for endothelial cell proliferation. Circ Res. 2008;103:1289–99.

20. Bird GS, DeHaven WI, Smyth JT, et al. Methods for studying store-operated calcium entry. Methods. 2008;46:204–12.

21. Cahalan MD, Zhang SL, Yeromin AV, et al. Molecular basis of the CRAC channel. Cell Calcium. 2007;42:133–44.

22. Aubart FC, Sassi Y, Coulombe A, et al. RNA interference targeting STIM1 suppresses vascular smooth muscle cell proliferation and neointima formation in the rat. Mol Ther. 2009;17:455–62.

23. Lu W, Wang J, Peng G, et al. Knockdown of stromal interaction molecule 1 attenuates store-operated Ca²⁺ entry and Ca²⁺ responses to acute hypoxia in pulmonary arterial smooth muscle. Am J Physiol Lung Cell Mol Physiol. 2009;297:L17–25.

24. Dziadek MA, Johnstone LS. Biochemical properties and cellular localisation of STIM proteins. Cell Calcium. 2007;42:123–32.

25. Walker S, Cunniffe N, Bootman M, et al. Dynamic imaging of calcium and STIM1 in the same cell using wide-field and TIRF microscopy. Biotechniques. 2008;45:347–8.

26. Feske S. ORAI1 and STIM1 deficiency in human and mice: roles of store-operated Ca²⁺ entry in the immune system and beyond. Immunol Rev. 2009;231:189–209.

27. Calloway N, Vig M, Kinet JP, et al. Molecular clustering of STIM1 with Orai1/CRACM1 at the plasma membrane depends dynamically on depletion of Ca²⁺ stores and on electrostatic interactions. Mol Biol Cell. 2009;20:389–99.

28. Adebiyi A, Zhao G, Narayanan D, et al. Isoform-selective physical coupling of TRPC3 channels to IP3 receptors in smooth muscle cells regulates arterial contractility. Circ Res. 2010;106:1603–12.

29. Alicia S, Angelica Z, Carlos S, et al. STIM1 converts TRPC1 from a receptor-operated to a store-operated channel: moving TRPC1 in and out of lipid rafts. Cell Calcium. 2008;44:479–91.

30. DeHaven WI, Jones BF, Petranka JG, et al. TRPC channels function independently of STIM1 and Orai1. J Physiol. 2009;587:2275–98.

31. Liao Y, Plummer NW, George MD, et al. A role for Orai in TRPC-mediated Ca²⁺ entry suggests that a TRPC:Orai complex may mediate store and receptor operated Ca²⁺ entry. Proc Natl Acad Sci USA. 2009;106:3202–6.

32. Brough GH, Wu S, Cioffi D, et al. Contribution of endogenously expressed Trp1 to a Ca²⁺-selective, store-operated Ca²⁺ entry pathway. FASEB J. 2001;15:1727–38.

33. Dietrich A, Kalwa H, Storch U, et al. Pressure-induced and store-operated cation influx in vascular smooth muscle cells is independent of TRPC1. Pflugers Arch. 2007;455:465–77.

34. Hecquet CM, Ahmmed GU, Malik AB. TRPM2 channel regulates endothelial barrier function. Adv Exp Med Biol. 2010;661:155–67.

35. Grover AK, Samson SE. Effect of superoxide radical on Ca²⁺ pumps of coronary artery. Am J Physiol Cell Physiol. 1988;255:C297–303.

36. Grover AK, Samson SE, Fomin VP. Peroxide inactivates calcium pumps in pig coronary artery. Am J Physiol Heart Circ Physiol. 1992;263:H537–43.

37. Grover AK, Samson SE, Fomin VP, et al. Effects of peroxide and superoxide on coronary artery: ANG II

response and sarcoplasmic reticulum Ca^{2+} pump. Am J Physiol Cell Physiol. 1995;269:C546–53.

38. Grover AK, Samson SE, Robinson S, et al. Effects of peroxynitrite on sarcoplasmic reticulum Ca^{2+} pump in pig coronary artery smooth muscle. Am J Physiol Cell Physiol. 2003;284:C294–301.

39. Elmoselhi AB, Samson SE, Grover AK. SR Ca^{2+} pump heterogeneity in coronary artery: free radicals and IP3-sensitive and -insensitive pools. Am J Physiol Cell Physiol. 1996;271:C1652–9.

40. Wagner S, Seidler T, Picht E, et al. Na$^+$-Ca^{2+} exchanger overexpression predisposes to reactive oxygen species-induced injury. Cardiovasc Res. 2003;60:404–12.

41. Kuster GM, Lancel S, Zhang J, et al. Redox-mediated reciprocal regulation of SERCA and Na$^+$-Ca^{2+} exchanger contributes to sarcoplasmic reticulum Ca^{2+} depletion in cardiac myocytes. Free Radic Biol Med. 2010;48:1182–7.

42. Soliman D, Hamming KS, Matemisz LC, et al. Reactive oxygen species directly modify sodium-calcium exchanger activity in a splice variant-dependent manner. J Mol Cell Cardiol. 2009;47:595–602.

43. Hinata M, Matsuoka I, Iwamoto T, et al. Mechanism of Na$^+$/Ca^{2+} exchanger activation by hydrogen peroxide in guinea-pig ventricular myocytes. J Pharmacol Sci. 2007;103:283–92.

44. Huschenbett J, Zaidi A, Michaelis ML. Sensitivity of the synaptic membrane Na$^+$/Ca^{2+} exchanger and the expressed NCX1 isoform to reactive oxygen species. Biochim Biophys Acta. 1998;1374:34–46.

45. Kip SN, Strehler EE. Rapid downregulation of NCX and PMCA in hippocampal neurons following H$_2$O$_2$ oxidative stress. Ann N Y Acad Sci. 2007;1099: 436–9.

46. Florea SM, Blatter LA. The effect of oxidative stress on Ca^{2+} release and capacitative Ca^{2+} entry in vascular endothelial cells. Cell Calcium. 2008;43:405–15.

47. Redondo PC, Salido GM, Pariente JA, et al. Dual effect of hydrogen peroxide on store-mediated calcium entry in human platelets. Biochem Pharmacol. 2004;67:1065–76.

48. Zhang W, Meng H, Li ZH, et al. Regulation of STIM1, store-operated Ca^{2+} influx, and nitric oxide generation by retinoic acid in rat mesangial cells. Am J Physiol Renal Physiol. 2007;292:F1054–64.

49. Hawkins BJ, Irrinki KM, Mallilankaraman K, et al. S-glutathionylation activates STIM1 and alters mitochondrial homeostasis. J Cell Biol. 2010;190: 391–405.

50. Bogeski I, Kummerow C, Al Ansary D, et al. Differential redox regulation of ORAI ion channels: a mechanism to tune cellular calcium signaling. Sci Signal. 2010;3:ra24.

51. Grupe M, Myers G, Penner R, et al. Activation of store-operated I(CRAC) by hydrogen peroxide. Cell Calcium. 2010;48:1–9.

52. Hecquet CM, Ahmmed GU, Vogel SM, et al. Role of TRPM2 channel in mediating H$_2$O$_2$-induced Ca^{2+} entry and endothelial hyperpermeability. Circ Res. 2008;102:347–55.

53. Kraft R, Grimm C, Grosse K, et al. Hydrogen peroxide and ADP-ribose induce TRPM2-mediated calcium influx and cation currents in microglia. Am J Physiol Cell Physiol. 2004;286:C129–37.

54. Kaneko S, Kawakami S, Hara Y, et al. A critical role of TRPM2 in neuronal cell death by hydrogen peroxide. J Pharmacol Sci. 2006;101:66–76.

55. Groschner K, Rosker C, Lukas M. Role of TRP channels in oxidative stress. Novartis Found Symp. 2004;258:222–30.

56. Ben Amor N, Redondo PC, Bartegi A, et al. A role for 5,6-epoxyeicosatrienoic acid in calcium entry by de novo conformational coupling in human platelets. J Physiol. 2006;570:309–23.

57. Graham S, Ding M, Ding Y, et al. Canonical transient receptor potential 6 (TRPC6), a redox-regulated cation channel. J Biol Chem. 2010;285: 23466–76.

Obesity–Hypertension: Leptin as the Common Link to Cardiovascular and Renal Dysregulation

Shilpa Kshatriya, Hani Kozman, Danish Siddiqui, Luna Bhatta, Kan Liu, Ali Salah, Timothy Ford, Robert Michiel, Robert Carhart, and Daniel Villarreal

Abstract

Leptin is a 16-kDa peptide hormone that is primarily synthesized and secreted by adipose tissue. One of the major actions of this hormone is the control of energy balance by binding to receptors in the hypothalamus, leading to reduction in food intake, elevation in temperature, and energy expenditure. In addition, increasing evidence suggests that leptin, through both direct and indirect mechanisms, may play an important role in cardiovascular and renal regulation. While the relevance of endogenous leptin needs further clarification, it appears to function as a pressure and volume-regulating factor under conditions of health. However, in abnormal situations characterized by chronic hyperleptinemia such as obesity, it may function pathophysiologically for the development of hypertension and possibly also for direct renal, vascular, and cardiac damage.

Keywords

Diuresis • Hemodynamics • Natriuresis • Nitric oxide • Cardiac hypertrophy

Introduction

The prevalence of obesity in the adult population of USA has risen markedly in the last three decades, contributing to the increased incidence of diabetes, hypertension, and heart disease [1–3]. Indeed, epidemiological studies suggest that 65–75% of the risk for hypertension is attributed to excess weight [4, 5]. Recently, a novel and most promising area of research in obesity and hypertension that links these two pathologic conditions is the endocrinology of adipose tissue. It is now apparent that adipose tissue is a prolific organ that secretes several immunomodulators and bioactive molecules [3, 6]. Of these various factors, leptin has emerged as an important hormone with significant pleiotropic actions on several organ systems [7, 8].

The first described major action of leptin was on the hypothalamus to control body weight and fat deposition through its effects on appetite

D. Villarreal (✉)
Department of Internal Medicine, SUNY
Upstate Medical University, Syracuse, NY, USA

Veterans Affairs Medical Center, Syracuse, NY, USA
e-mail: Villarrd@upstate.edu

N.S. Dhalla, M. Nagano, B. Ostadal (eds.), *Molecular Defects in Cardiovascular Disease*,
DOI 10.1007/978-1-4419-7130-2_25, © Springer Science+Business Media, LLC 2011

inhibition, as well as stimulation of the metabolic rate and thermogenesis [9, 10]. However, increasing evidence suggests that the biology of leptin extends to other organs including the kidney, the heart, the sympathetic nervous system, and the systemic vasculature, areas in which it may have prominent effects [7, 8, 11–14].

Biology of Leptin Receptors

The leptin receptor (LR), a product of the *lepr* gene, is a member of the extended class I cytokine receptor family having at least six splice variants LR (a-f) [15–19]. Significant expression of the lepr gene occurs in the lung and adipocytes, while only moderate levels appear in the kidney, with relatively lower levels demonstrated in other tissues such as the heart, brain, spleen, liver, and muscle [20]. Though the extracellular domain of the leptin receptor and the short splice variant (LRa) have been detected in many peripheral tissues, the long splice variant (LRb) is expressed in fewer organ systems including the adrenal gland, kidney and heart [20]. This long splice variant leads to activation of the Janus Kinases (a family of tyrosine kinases) to promote transcription through activation of the STAT-3 (signal transduction and activator of transcription), PI3K (phosphoinositol-3 kinase) and inhibition of AMPK (AMP-activated protein kinase) [15–20]. LRa and LRb can also stimulate MAPK (mitogen-activated protein kinase), which may be involved in the induction of hypertrophy [21]. Finally, SOCS-3 (suppression of cytokine signaling protein) and PTB1b (protein tyrosine phosphatase 1b) have been identified as negative regulators of leptin signaling [15–19].

Leptin, Sympathetic Nervous System, and Arterial Blood Pressure

It is now well established that leptin can activate the sympathetic nervous system both by local peripheral actions as well as through centrally

mediated effects on the hypothalamus [22]. Studies with direct infusion of leptin into the cerebral ventricles of normal rats have demonstrated a slow increase of mean arterial pressure (MAP) of approximately 10% [13]. Moreover, recent investigations have suggested that leptin signaling in the nucleus tracti solitarii increased renal sympathetic flow in normal rats, but not in obese Zucker rats, indicating that intact leptin receptors are essential for this vasoactive response [22].

However, it is important to point out that in other investigations conducted both in normotensive as well as hypertensive rats [12, 14, 23], the acute systemic administration of leptin was associated with the peripheral activation of the sympathetic nervous system without elevation in MAP. This raises the possibility of the simultaneous local activation of counterregulatory vasodilatory mechanisms [14, 24, 25]. In vitro studies have demonstrated a dose-dependent leptin-induced vasorelaxation in the aortic rings of Wistar-Kyoto rats [24] which is mediated by nitric oxide (NO) and possibly by endothelial derived hyperpolarizing factor (EDHF). An elevation in plasma NO with intravenous administration of synthetic leptin in normal rats has also been demonstrated [25]. In these studies blockade of NO led to a leptin-induced enhancement of arterial blood pressure while blockade of the sympathetic nervous system led to leptin-mediated reduction in blood pressure [25]. Thus, leptin's lack of effect on arterial blood pressure in normal subjects may represent a balanced action of vasodilatation primarily mediated by NO, and vasoconstriction primarily mediated by the sympathetic nervous system, with a resultant neutral hemodynamic effect [25, 26]. This concept requires further validation because the vasodilatory actions of leptin in other vascular beds have been found to be inconsistent [27, 28]. In high-calorie-fed obese rats, however, recent studies by Beltowski et al. have indicated that acutely infused leptin was associated with a hypertensive effect, related, at least in part, to impaired vascular NO and EDHF production characteristic of obesity [29].

Chronic Hyperleptinemia, Leptin Resistance, and Hypertension

In chronic hyperleptinemic conditions such as obesity, the potential neutral effect of leptin on peripheral vascular resistance may no longer be present. It has been previously demonstrated that the agouti yellow obese mouse model is resistant to the satiety actions of leptin but not to the effects of leptin on the sympathetic nervous system [30, 31], although this stimulation may be attenuated with the progression of obesity [32]. From these findings, the concept of "selective leptin resistance" as a mechanism for the development of hypertension in obesity has emerged [30, 31]. The precise factors behind this selectivity are yet to be fully defined [31, 33], but may involve alterations in the SOCS3 signaling pathway or IRS-1 (insulin receptor substrate-1) serine residue phosphorylation [29, 34, 35].

Independent of the possibility of selective leptin resistance in obesity, studies in normal rats have demonstrated that chronic hyperleptinemia leads to a persistent elevation in MAP and this hypertensive effect is rapidly reversed upon cessation of the hormone administration [36]. Similar increases in systolic blood pressure have been demonstrated in transgenic mice overexpressing leptin where the endogenous level of the hormone was elevated twenty fold [37]. In this regard, it is pertinent to point out that hyperleptinemia may increase vascular smooth muscle cell proliferation [38], an effect that could contribute to the development and/or perpetuation of hypertension. Moreover, mice with leptin deficiency (ob/ob) or with a leptin receptor defect (db/db) exhibit significant obesity but do not develop hypertension, suggesting that at least in animal models, leptin may play a role in the regulation of systemic hemodynamics [31]. In humans, emerging evidence suggests a direct relationship between hyperleptinemia and hypertension in both men and women [39, 40], and this effect may be independent of BMI and insulin resistance.

Leptin and the Regulation of Sodium-Volume Balance

Previous studies have indicated that the LRb leptin receptor is localized in the renal medulla [20, 41] which suggests a functional role of this hormone in renal biology. In the last 5–10 years, numerous studies have demonstrated that acute administration of synthetic leptin in the rat produces a significant elevation in urinary sodium and water excretion [14, 41–43].

Villarreal et al. [14] demonstrated that in normotensive rats, an intravenous bolus of leptin produced a robust six to seven fold elevation in urinary sodium excretion and fractional excretion of sodium; by contrast, hypertensive rats were refractory to the renal effects of leptin. Interestingly, the natriuretic effect was attenuated in obese Zucker rats [14]. MAP and creatinine clearance remained unchanged in all of the rat strains with the acute infusion of the hormone. Collectively, these findings were interpreted to suggest that leptin might be a natriuretic hormone primarily acting at the tubular level for promotion of sodium and water excretion in normal rats, and that leptin may function pathophysiologically in obesity and hypertension, where chronic hyperleptinemia may contribute to a preferential stimulation of the sympathetic nervous system with further elevation in blood pressure and reduced sodium and water excretion [2, 7, 44]. Moreover, in a rat model of diet-induced obesity, initial studies by Patel et al. have shown markedly attenuated natriuretic and diuretic effects of synthetic leptin, as well as reduced urinary excretion of NO [45]. These findings suggest that in obesity, alterations in leptin-induced renal NO production and/or metabolism may account, at least in part, for the blunted natriuretic effects. However, additional observations in diet-induced obese rats indicate that caloric restriction was associated with the restoration of the natriuretic actions of leptin as well as with the renal generation of NO [45]. Aggregately, these studies are consistent with the concept that obesity is associated with renal leptin resistance [14, 46], and this resistance, at least in part, is reversible with caloric restriction and weight loss.

The significance of NO in the direct modulation of leptin-induced sodium excretion has been investigated in rats chronically treated with L-NAME to inhibit NO production [47]. L-NAME treated rats failed to produce significant natriuresis. However, there was a two to threefold elevation in sodium excretion induced by leptin with the restoration of NO by sodium nitroprusside [47], indicating that NO may play an important role in mediating or modulating the tubular natriuretic effects of leptin. These observations are supported by the studies of Beltowski et al. [46] which demonstrated that leptin produces a time- and dose-dependent reduction of renal medullary Na-K-ATPase, which may in part be regulated by NO [47, 48]. Beltowski et al. [46] also reported that in diet-induced obese rats, leptin-induced stimulation of plasma NO, reduction of renal Na-K-ATPase, and natriuresis are all significantly impaired.

The mechanisms for renal resistance to leptin in obesity and hypertension are not completely defined but may include receptor downregulation [12, 45], post-receptor signaling alterations [12, 16, 17], excessive degradation of NO produced by oxidative stress [49], or increased activation of the efferent renal sympathetic nervous system leading to antinatriuresis [43]. Indeed, studies that [43] have examined the latter hypothesis using an animal model of renal denervation indicate that the renal efferent sympathetic nervous system is an important counterregulatory mechanism impeding leptin-induced sodium excretion in hypertension, and perhaps also during obesity, which is similarly characterized by a heightened sympathetic nervous tone [2, 7].

The relevance of endogenous leptin as a distinct sodium-volume regulatory hormone has been examined in normal Sprague Dawley rats that were in a state of mild sodium/volume expansion [50]. Urinary sodium and volume excretion were significantly reduced by approximately 20–25% after blockade of leptin with a polyclonal antibody, indicating an important physiologic role for this hormone in the daily renal control of salt and water balance. The importance of leptin as a regulator of sodium and volume is further supported by recent investigations [51, 52], which have demonstrated that leptin expression in adipose tissue is directly proportional to dietary sodium, a response that would be expected for mechanisms regulating sodium balance.

Thus, the available information to date suggests that leptin's net effect on renal sodium metabolism may reflect both direct natriuretic and indirect antinatriuretic actions. The responsiveness to leptin at various sites that regulate natriuresis may differ under diverse physiological and pathophysiological conditions, and this in turn will be a determinant for the overall magnitude of leptin-induced urinary sodium excretion.

Leptin and Chronic Kidney Disease

Leptin's role in renal physiology and pathophysiology is complex. As previously discussed, leptin may play a significant role in the regulation of sodium and water balance in normal situations. However, in conditions of chronic hyperleptinemia, the hormone has been linked to renal structural changes that specifically have been associated with obesity [53]. Elegant studies by Wolf et al. [54] have determined that in glomerular endothelial cells, leptin can stimulate cellular proliferation, expression of TGF-β1, and type IV collagen synthesis leading to fibrosis. Indeed, chronic infusion of leptin in normal rats promoted the development of glomerulosclerosis and proteinuria [54]. It is of interest that similar renal abnormalities have been found in mice with chronic high-fat diet and the metabolic syndrome [55], which is characterized by sustained elevations of circulating leptin [56].

Inappropriate elevation in serum leptin levels has been demonstrated in patients with chronic kidney disease [57–59]. The origin and significance of hyperleptinemia in these patients is not completely defined, but it is important to emphasize that the marked elevation of leptin is out of proportion to obesity and persists after correction for body mass index [60]. Since the kidney is involved in clearance of leptin, its elevated levels in renal insufficiency are primarily due to reduced renal filtration and metabolism [57, 61]. It remains to be determined whether an increased rate of leptin production also contributes to the high serum leptin levels in renal insufficiency.

Leptin levels appear to be higher in patients receiving peritoneal dialysis (PD) compared to hemodialysis (HD) [62]. The reasons for this phenomenon are multifactorial. It is likely that the elevated body fat mass in patients with PD contributes to the increase in serum leptin [62]. However, other factors are probably involved. For instance, the continuous glucose load in PD results in chronic hyperinsulinemia, an important finding considering that insulin upregulates *lepr* gene expression [58]. In this regard, it is of interest that even higher leptin levels are observed in patients with renal insufficiency with elevated insulin levels compared to patients with low insulin levels [58, 63].

The pathophysiological significance of hyperleptinemia in renal insufficiency is not completely understood. High levels of leptin have been associated with weight loss in dialysis patients [60, 64–66], and therefore, it has been suggested that hyperleptinemia may be a contributing factor in uremic-induced cachexia [59, 64–68]. Other suggested actions in patients with end-stage renal disease include leptin-induced reduction in erythropoiesis [69, 70], promotion of renal osteodystrophy [71, 72], and chronic inflammation [58, 73, 74].

Leptin and the Heart

It is now well recognized that the role of leptin in energy homeostasis extends into cardiac metabolism. The effects of leptin mediated by the LRb receptor include a reduction of insulin signaling with enhanced lipid oxidation and, therefore, inhibition of anabolic pathways [75]. Similar to the kidney, chronic hyperleptinemia indirectly may be important in the development of cardiac disease via sympathetic activation, pressor effects, enhancement of platelet aggregation, impairment of fibrinolysis as well as proangiogenic actions [12, 35, 76, 77]. In addition, and

although still controversial, leptin may be involved in the pathogenesis of myocyte hypertrophy and cardiac dysfunction [78–80] through direct effects. Indeed, leptin can proliferate, differentiate, and functionally activate hemopoietic and embryonic cells to promote myocyte growth [81–83]. Moreover, in rats with myocardial infarction, cardiac hypertrophy has been shown to be attenuated with the blockade of leptin receptors [84]. Among the suggested mechanisms of leptin-induced hypertrophy is the stimulation of endothelin-1, angiotensin II [85], and reactive oxygen species [86]. Additional studies in rats with myocardial infarction have also indicated that long-term continuous administration of leptin promoted the development of eccentric cardiac hypertrophy [87].

In contrast to these investigations, studies in leptin-deficient mice (ob/ob) with [87, 88] or without myocardial infarction [89], have suggested that leptin can exert protective cardiac effects with reversal of baseline myocyte hypertrophy during leptin supplementation [89]. Also, Tajmir et al. [90] have indicated that leptin can activate ERK 1/2 (extracellular signal-regulated kinase) and phosphoinositol-3 kinase dependent signaling pathways in cardiomyocytes to promote physiological repair of myocardium. Presently, the reasons for the apparent discrepant effects of leptin on myocyte growth are unclear, but may be related to different experimental conditions, including the variable response of leptin in neonatal compared to adult cells [77–90].

In addition to its potential actions on myocardial cell growth, leptin has been shown to exert direct negative inotropic effects on adult rat ventricular myocytes [91]. The suggested mechanisms involve activation of fatty acid oxidation leading to decreased triglyceride content or an altered adenylate cyclase function [89, 92]. Alternatively, Nickola et al. [91] reported that leptin may abnormally increase expression of nitric oxide synthases in cardiac myocytes, promoting oxidative stress and depressed cardiac function. However, similar to the controversy related to cardiac hypertrophy, more recent studies in ob/ob mice [88] or rats [87] with myocardial infarction have suggested that leptin may

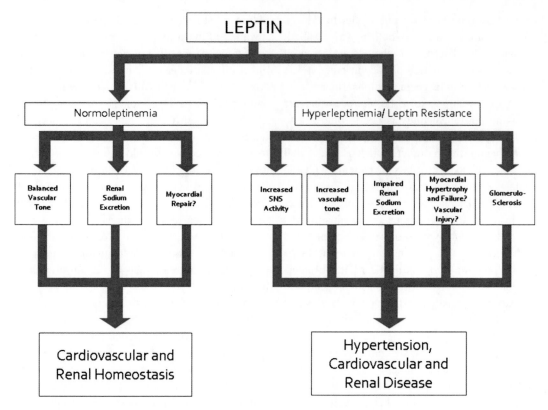

Fig. 1 Cardiovascular and renal actions of leptin. *SNS* sympathetic nervous system. Kshatriya S, Reams GP, Spear RM, Freeman RH, Dietz JR, Villarreal D. Obesity hypertension: the emerging role of leptin in renal and cardiovascular dyshomeostasis. Curr Opin Nephrol Hypertens. 2010;19(1):72–8. Reproduced with permission from Wolters Kluwer/Lippincott, Willilams & Wilkins

attenuate adverse cardiac remodeling by reducing apoptosis [88], which may improve left ventricular contractile function, and, at least in part, increase survival [87–89].

The relevance of these studies in humans is unclear. Although there is evidence to suggest a direct relationship between the hyperleptinemia of obesity with cardiac hypertrophy [89, 93], and possibly heart failure [94], they are not consistent findings [8, 11]. Additional in vitro and in vivo studies are needed to define and characterize the potential beneficial or deleterious effects of leptin in cardiac physiology and pathophysiology.

Conclusions

It is well established that cardiovascular and renal functions require the activation of multiple neurohormonal mechanisms designed to maintain homeostasis. The hormone leptin has multiple actions that may be important not only for energy metabolism but also in physiological and pathophysiological cardiovascular and renal regulation (Fig. 1). Potentially prominent are its effects on renal sodium excretion, NO, sympathetic nervous system activation, and vascular tone. The interaction among the vasoconstricting, vasodilatory, and natriuretic effects of leptin to help achieve volume and pressure homeostasis in normal conditions may be disrupted during chronic hyperleptinemia, and this effect could likely contribute to hypertension and possible cardiac and renal dysfunction. Further research awaits the additional characterization of both direct and indirect mechanisms of action of leptin, including its interface with other important hormonal sodium-volume-pressure regulatory systems, in both health and disease states, particularly obesity and related comorbidities.

Acknowledgments The authors wish to acknowledge the expert technical assistance Jeffrey Montalbano. Supported in part by the Veteran Affairs Research Program (Merit Review), the Joseph C. Georg Research Award, and the Hendricks Research Award.

References

1. Ogden CL, Carroll MD, Curtin LR, et al. Prevalence of overweight and obesity in the United States, 1999–2004. JAMA. 2006;295:1549–55.
2. Hall JE, Crook ED, Jones DW, et al. Mechanisms of obesity associated cardiovascular and renal disease. Am J Sci. 2002;324:27–37.
3. Hajer G, van Haeften TW, Visseren FLJ. Adipose tissue dysfunction in obesity, diabetes, and vascular diseases. Eur Heart J. 2008;29:2959–71.
4. Garrison RJ, Kannel WB, Stokes 3rd J, et al. Incidence and precursors of hypertension in young adults: The Framingham Offspring Study. Prev Med. 1987;16: 235–51.
5. Wofford MR, Hall JE. Pathophysiology and treatment of obesity hypertension. Curr Pharm Des. 2004;10: 3621–37.
6. Hutley L, Prins J. Fat as an endocrine organ: Relationship to the metabolic syndrome. Am J Med Sci. 2005;330:280–9.
7. Guha PK, Villarreal D, Reams GP, et al. Role of leptin in the regulation of body fluid volume and pressures. Am J Ther. 2003;10:211–8.
8. Sharma V, McNeill J. The emerging roles of leptin and ghrelin in cardiovascular physiology and pathophysiology. Curr Vasc Pharmacol. 2005;3:169–80.
9. Misra A, Garg A. Leptin: Its receptor and obesity. J Investig Med. 1996;44:540–8.
10. Lonnqvist F. The obese (ob) gene and its product leptin: A new route towards obesity treatment in man? J Med. 1996;89:327–32.
11. Beltowski J. Role of leptin in blood pressure regulation and arterial hypertension. J Hypertens. 2006;24:789–801.
12. Haynes WG, Morgan DA, Walsh SA, et al. Receptor-mediated regional sympathetic nerve activation by leptin. J Clin Invest. 1997;100:270–8.
13. Dunbar JC, Hu Y, Lu H. Intracerebroventricular leptin increases lumbar and renal sympathetic nerve activity and blood pressure in normal rats. Diabetes. 1997;46:2040–3.
14. Villarreal D, Reams G, Freeman RH, et al. Renal effects of leptin in normotensive, hypertensive and obese rats. Am J Physiol Regul Integr Comp. 1998; 275:R2056–60.
15. Chen H, Charlat O, Tartaglia LA, et al. Evidence that diabetes gene encodes leptin receptor: Identification of a mutation in the leptin receptor gene in db/db mice. Cell. 1996;84:491–5.
16. Banks AS, Davis SM, Bates SH, et al. Activation of downstream signals by the long form of the leptin receptor. J Biol Chem. 2000;275:14563–72.
17. Munzberg H, Myers Jr MG. Molecular and anatomical determinants of central leptin resistance. Nature. 2005;8:566–70.
18. Tartaglia LA, Dembski M, Weng X, et al. Identification and expression of cloning of a leptin receptor, OB-R. Cell. 1995;83:1263–71.
19. Wang M-Y, Zhou YT, Neward CB, et al. A novel leptin receptor isoform in rat. FEBS Lett. 1996;392:87–90.
20. Hoggard N, Mercer JG, Rayner DV, et al. Localization of leptin receptor mRNA splice variants in murine peripheral tissues by RT-PCR and in situ hybridization. Biochem Biophys Res Commun. 1997;232:383–7.
21. Anubhuti, Arora S. Leptin and its metabolic interactions: an update. Diabetes Obes Metab. 2008;10:973–93.
22. Mark AL, Agassandian K, Morgan DA, et al. Leptin signaling in the nucleus tractus solitarii increases sympathetic nerve activity to the kidney. Hypertension. 2009;53:375–80.
23. Beltowski J, Jochem J, Wojcicka G, et al. Influence of intravenously administered leptin on nitric oxide production, renal hemodynamics and renal function in the rat. Regul Pept. 2004;120:59–67.
24. Lembo L, Vecchione C, Fratta L. Leptin induces direct vasodilation through distinct endothelial mechanisms. Diabetes. 2000;49:293–7.
25. Fruhbeck G. Pivotal role of nitric oxide in the control of blood pressure after leptin administration. Diabetes. 1999;48:903–8.
26. Brook RD, Bard RL, Bodary PF, et al. Blood pressure and vascular effects of leptin in humans. Metab Synd Relat Dis. 2007;5:270–4.
27. Mitchell JL, Morgan DA, Correia ML, et al. Does leptin stimulate nitric oxide to oppose the effects of sympathetic activation? Hypertension. 2001;38:1081–6.
28. Gardiner SM, Kemp PA, March JE, et al. Regional hemodynamic effects of recombinant murine or human leptin in conscious rats. Br J Pharmacol. 2000;130:805–10.
29. Beltowski J, Wojcicka G, Jamroz-Wisniewska A, et al. Resistance to acute NO-mimetic and EDHF-mimetic effects of leptin in the metabolic syndrome. Life Sci. 2009;85:557–67.
30. Mark AL, Shaffer RA, Correia ML. Contrasting blood pressure effects of obesity in leptin-deficient ob/ob mice and agouti yellow obese mice. J Hypertension. 1999;17:1949–53.
31. Correia MI, Haynes WG, Rahmouni K. The concept of selective leptin resistance: evidence from agouti yellow obese mice. Diabetes. 2002;51:439–42.
32. Morgan DA, Thedens DR, Weiss R, et al. Mechanisms mediating renal sympathetic activation to leptin in obesity. Am J Physiol Regul Integr Comp Physiol. 2008;295:R1730–6.
33. Rahmouni K, Correia LG, Haynes WG, et al. Obesity-Associated Hypertension, new insights into mechanisms. Hypertension. 2005;45:9–14.
34. Tune JD, Consodine R. Effects of leptin on cardiovascular physiology. J Am Soc Hypertens. 2007;14:231–41.
35. Bjorbaek C, Elmquist JK, Frantz JD, et al. Identification of SOCS-3 as a potential mediator of central leptin resistance. Mol Cell. 1998;191:619–25.

36. Shek EW, Brands MW, Hall JE. Chronic leptin infusion increases arterial pressure. Hipertensión. 1998;31:409–14.

37. Aizawa-Abe M, Ogawa Y, Masuzaki H, et al. Pathophysiological role of leptin in obesity-related hypertension. J Clin Invest. 2000;105:1243–52.

38. Huang F, Xiong X, Wang H, et al. Leptin-induced vascular smooth muscle cell proliferation via regulating cell cycle, activating ERK ½ and NF-KB. Acta Biochim Biophys Sin. 2010;42:325–31.

39. Galletti F, D'Elia L, Barba G, et al. High-Circulating leptin Levels are associated with a greater risk of hypertension in men independently of body mass and insulin resistance: Results of an eight-year follow-up study. J Clin Endocrinol Metab. 2008;93:3922–6.

40. Ma D, Feitosa MF, Wilk JB, et al. Leptin is associated with blood pressure and hypertension in women from the National Heart, Lung, and Blood Institute Family Heart Study. Hypertension. 2009;53:473–9.

41. Serradeil-Le G, Raufaste D, Brossard G, et al. Characterization and localization of leptin receptors in the rat kidney. FEBS Lett. 1997;404:185–91.

42. Jackson EK, Li P. Human leptin has natriuretic activity in the rat. Am J Physiol Renal Physiol. 1997;272:F333–8.

43. Villarreal D, Reams G, Freeman RH. Effects of renal denervation on the sodium excretory action of leptin in hypertensive rats. Kidney Int. 2000;58:989–94.

44. DiBona GF. The kidney in the pathogenesis of hypertension: The role of renal nerves. Am J Kidney Dis. 1985;5:A27–31.

45. Patel S, Villarreal D, Kundra A, et al. Cardiovascular and renal actions of leptin. Cardiac Hormones. 2008;111–27.

46. Beltowski J, Wojcicka G. Human leptin administered intraperitoneally stimulates natriuresis and decreases renal medullary Na+, K+-ATPase activity in the rat-impaired effect in dietary-induced obesity. Med Sci Monit. 2002;8:BR221–9.

47. Villarreal D, Reams G, Samar H, et al. Effects of chronic nitric oxide inhibition on the renal excretory response to leptin. Obes Res. 2004;12:1006–10.

48. Lin L, Martin R, Schaffenhauier AO, et al. Acute changes in the response to peripheral leptin with alteration in the diet composition. Am J Physiol Regul Integ Comp Physiol. 2001;280:R504–9.

49. Bouloumine A, Marumo T, Lofanton M. Leptin induces oxidative stress in human endothelial cells. FASEB J. 1999;13:1231–8.

50. Villarreal D, Reams G, Samar H. Leptin blockade attenuates sodium excretion in saline-loaded normotensive rats. Mol Cell Biochem. 2006;283:153–7.

51. Dobrian AD, Schriver SD, Lynch T, et al. Effect of salt on hypertension and oxidative stress in rat model on diet-induced obesity. Am J Physiol. 2003;285:F619–28.

52. Adomczak M, Koleot F, Chutek J, et al. Effect of renin angiotensin system activation by dietary sodium restriction and upright position on plasma leptin concentration in patients with essential hypertension. Med Sci Monit. 2002;8:CR473–7.

53. Wolf G, Ziyadeh FN. Leptin and renal fibrosis. Contrib Nephrol. 2006;151:175–83.

54. Wolf G, Chen S, Han DC, et al. Leptin and renal disease. Am J Kidney Dis. 2002;39:1–11.

55. Deji N, Kume S, Araki S-I, et al. Structural and functional changes in the kidneys of high-fat diet-induced mice. Am J Physiol Renal Physiol. 2008;296:F118–26.

56. Gannagé-Yared M-H, Khalife S, Semaan M, et al. Serum adiponectin and leptin levels in relation to the metabolic syndrome, androgenic profile and somatotropic axis in healthy non-diabetic elderly men. Europ J Endocrinol. 2006;155:167–76.

57. Sharma K, Considine RV, Michael B, et al. Plasma leptin is partly cleared by the kidney and is elevated in hemodialysis patients. Kidney Int. 1997;51:1980–5.

58. Nordfors L, Lönnqvist F, Heimbürger O, et al. Low leptin gene expression and hyperleptinemia in chronic renal failure. Kidney Int. 1998;54:1267–75.

59. Stenvinkel P, Lönnqvist F, Schalling M. Molecular basis of renal disease. Molecular studies of leptin: implications for renal disease. Nephrol Dial Transplant. 1999;4:1103–12.

60. Heimburger O, Lönnqvist F, Danielsson A, et al. Serum immunoreactive leptin concentration and its relation to the body fat content in chronic renal failure. J Am Soc Nephrol. 1997;8:1423–30.

61. Cumin F, Baum HP, de Gasparo M, et al. Removal of endogenous leptin from the circulation by the kidney. Int J Obes Relat Metab Disord. 1997;21:495–504.

62. Johansen KL, Mulligan K, Tai V, et al. Leptin, body composition, and indices of malnutrition in patients on dialysis. J Am Soc Nephrol. 1998;9:1080–4.

63. Stenvinkel P, Heimbürger O, Lönnqvist F. Serum leptin concentrations correlate to plasma insulin concentrations independent of body fat content in chronic renal failure. Nephrol Dial Transplant. 1997;12:1321–5.

64. Fontan PM, Rodriguez-Carmona R, Cordido F, et al. Hyperleptinemia in uremic patients undergoing conservative management, peritoneal dialysis, and hemodialysis: A comparative analysis. Am J Kidney Dis. 1999;34:824–31.

65. Bossola M, Tazza L, Giungi S, et al. Anorexia in hemodialysis patients: an update. Kidney Int. 2006;70:417–22.

66. Stenvinkel P, Lindholm B, Lönnqvist F, et al. Increases in serum leptin levels during peritoneal dialysis are associated with inflammation and a decrease in lean body mass. J Am Soc Nephrol. 2000;11:1303–9.

67. Odamaki M, Furuya R, Yoneyama T. Association of the serum leptin concentration with weight loss in chronic hemodialysis patients. Am J Kidney Dis. 1999;33:361–8.

68. Mak RH, Cheung W, Cone RD, et al. Leptin and inflammation-associated cachexia in chronic kidney disease. Kidney Int. 2006;69:794–7.

69. Cheung W, Yu PX, Little BM, et al. Role of leptin and melanocortin signaling in uremia-associated cachexia. J Clin Invest. 2005;115:1659–65.

70. Axelsson J, Qureshi AR, Heimbürger O, et al. Body fat mass and serum leptin levels influence epoetin

sensitivity in patients with ESRD. Am J Kidney Dis. 2005;46:628–34.

71. Hung S-C, Tung T-Y, Yang C-S, et al. High-calorie supplementation increases serum leptin levels and improves response to rHuEPO in long-term hemodialysis patients. Am J Kidney Dis. 2005;45:1073–83.

72. Coen G, Ballanti P, Fischer M, et al. Serum leptin in dialysis renal osteodystrophy. Am J Kidney Dis. 2003;42:1036–42.

73. Mallamaci F, Tripepi G, Zoccali C. Leptin in end stage renal disease (ESRD): a link between fat mass, bone and the cardiovascular system. J Nephrol. 2005;18:464–8.

74. Zoccali C, Mallamaci F, Tripepi G. Adipose tissue as a source of inflammatory cytokines in health and disease: Focus on end-stage renal disease. Kidney Int. 2003;63:S65–6.

75. Emilsson V, Liu Y-L, Cawthorne M, et al. Expression of the functional leptin receptor mRNA in pancreatic islets and direct inhibitory action of leptin on insulin secretion. Diabetes. 1997;46:313–6.

76. Konstantinides S, Schafer K, Koschnick S, et al. Leptin-dependent platelet aggregation and arterial thrombosis suggests a mechanism for atherothrombotic disease in obesity. J Clin Invest. 2001;108:1533–40.

77. Sierra-Honigmann MR, Nath AK, Murakami C. Biological action of leptin as an angiogenic factor. Science. 1998;281:1683–6.

78. Karmazyn M, Purdham DM, Rajapurohitam V, et al. Leptin as a cardiac hypertrophic factor: A potential target for therapeutics. Trends Cardiovasc Med. 2007;17:206–11.

79. Rajapurohitam V, Gan XT, Kirshenbaum LA, et al. The obesity-associated peptide leptin induces hypertrophy in neonatal rat ventricular myocytes. Circ Res. 2003;93:277–9.

80. Selthofer-Relatic K, Radivoje R, Vedrana V, et al. Hyperleptinemia-non-haemodynamic risk factor for the left ventricular hypertrophy development in hypertensive overweight females. Coll Antropol. 2008;32:681–5.

81. Umemoto Y, Tsuji K, Yang FC, et al. Leptin stimulates the proliferation of murine myelocytic and primitive haematopoietic progenitor cells. Blood. 1997;90:3438–43.

82. Paolisso G, Tangliamonte MR, Galderisi M, et al. Plasma leptin level is associated with myocardial wall thickness in hypertensive insulin resistant men. Hypertension. 1999;34:1047–52.

83. Leyva F, Anker SD, Egerer K, et al. Hyperleptinemia in chronic heart failure. Relationship with insulin. Eur Heart J. 1998;19:1547–51.

84. Purdham DM, Rajapurohitam V, Zeidan A, et al. A neutralizing leptin receptor antibody mitigates hypertrophy and hemodynamic dysfunction in the postinfarcted rat heart. Am J Physiol Heart Circ Physiol. 2008;295:H441–6.

85. Rajapurohitam V, Javadov S, Purdham DM. An autocrine role for leptin in mediating the cardiomyocyte hypertrophic effects of angiotensin II and endothelin-1. J Mol Cell Cardiol. 2006;41:265–74.

86. Nagae A, Fujita M, Kawarazaki H, et al. Sympathoexcitation by oxidative stress in the brain mediates arterial pressure elevation in obesity-induced hypertension. Circulation. 2009;119:978–86.

87. Abe Y, Ono K, Kawamura T, et al. Leptin induces elongation of cardiac myocytes and causes left ventricular dilatation with compensation. Am J Physiol Heart Circ Physiol. 2007;292:H2387–96.

88. McGaffin K, Zou B, McTiernan CF, et al. Leptin attenuates cardiac apoptosis after chronic ischaemic injury. Cardiovasc Res. 2009;83:313–24.

89. Barouch LA, Berkowitz DE, Harrison RW, et al. Disruption of leptin signaling contributes to cardiac hypertrophy independently of body weight in mice. Circulation. 2003;108:754–9.

90. Tajmir P, Ceddia RB, Li RK, et al. Leptin increases cardiomyocyte hyperplasia via extracellular signal-regulated kinase- and phosphatidylinositol 3-kinase-dependent signaling pathways. Endocrinology. 2004;145:1550–5.

91. Nickola M, Wold L, Colligan P, et al. Leptin attenuates cardiac contraction in rat ventricular myocytes: Role of NO. Hypertension. 2000;36:501–5.

92. Luo J, Zhang G, Chen M. Leptin and cardiovascular diseases. Drug News Perspect. 2005;18:427–31.

93. Tritos NA, Manning WJ, Danias PG, et al. Role of leptin in the development of cardiac hypertrophy in experimental animals and humans. Circulation. 2004;109:e67.

94. Schulze PC, Kratzsch J, Linke A, et al. Elevated serum levels of leptin and soluble leptin receptor in patients with advanced chronic heart failure. Eur J Heart Fail. 2003;5:33–40.

Cardiorenal Protection in Diabetes Mellitus

Himanshu Vashistha, Leonard G. Meggs,
and Ashwani Malhotra

Abstract

Diabetic cardiomyopathy is a major complication of diabetes that is independent of high blood pressure or atherosclerosis. In addition to diastolic dysfunction, the diabetic heart is more susceptible to oxidative stress. Hyperglycemia (HG) dominates the pathophysiology and clinical course of type 1 and type 2 Diabetes. An important question concerns the signals used by high concentrations of extracellular glucose to alter the biochemical and mechanical properties of cardiac muscle cells. Recruitment of the Protein Kinase C (PKC) family of serine–threonine kinases is an integral component of the signaling events that direct the cardiac phenotype expressed during postnatal cardiac development and in response to pathological stimuli. We have described that genetically engineered mice with cardiac-specific expression of an isozyme-specific PKC-ε translocation activator exhibit protection from hyperglycemia-induced apoptosis and LV dysfunction. The $\psi\varepsilon$-RACK peptide facilitated the intracellular trafficking of PKC-ε, and thereby prevented hyperglycemia-mediated decreases in immunoreactivity in both membrane and mitochondrial compartments. A unifying hypothesis has been proposed for the development of diabetic complications, based on the overproduction of Reactive Oxygen Species (ROS). The adapter protein p66Shc A is a part of a signal transduction pathway and may be a key component of the cell signal response to oxidative stress contributing to the lifespan in mammals. p66ShcA functions as a potentially harmful regulatory gene, which is required for the generation of HG-induced oxidative stress and apoptosis. At high ambient glucose (HG), p66ShcA-deficient cells exhibit resistance to HG-induced ROS generation and attenuation in the amplitude of the

A. Malhotra (✉)
Division of Nephrology, Department of Medicine
Long Island Jewish Medical Center, New Hyde Park,
NY, USA
e-mail: malhotas@yahoo.com

N.S. Dhalla, M. Nagano, B. Ostadal (eds.), *Molecular Defects in Cardiovascular Disease*,
DOI 10.1007/978-1-4419-7130-2_26, © Springer Science+Business Media, LLC 2011

kinetic curves for intracellular ROS metabolism, indicative of the pivotal role of WTp66ShcA in the generation of HG oxidant stress. Inhibition of WTp66ShcA function shuts down HG-induced ROS production in cytosolic and mitochondrial compartments.

Keywords

Diabetes mellitus • PKC • P66Shc • Cardiomyopathy • Oxidative stress

Introduction

Diabetes Mellitus (DM) is a major public health concern that afflicts more than 170 million people worldwide, a number projected to increase to 370 million by 2030 [1]. DM is a major risk factor for cardiovascular disease, but is also complicated by a primary cardiomyopathy. Diabetic cardiomyopathy is a major complication of diabetes that is independent of high blood pressure or atherosclerosis. In addition to diastolic dysfunction, the diabetic heart is more susceptible to oxidative stress. Hyperglycemia dominates the pathophysiology and clinical course of type 1 and type 2 Diabetes. Compelling evidence from the Diabetes Control and Complications Trial has indicated that rigorous control of blood glucose reduces the risk of long-term microvasculature complications [2]. Although the cardiac myocyte is not a principal target cell for insulin, several lines of investigation support the notion that a primary myocardial defect exists in diabetes [2–4]. An important question concerns the signals used by high concentrations of extracellular glucose to alter the biochemical and mechanical properties of cardiac muscle cells. Recruitment of the protein kinase C (PKC) family of serine–threonine kinases is an integral component of the signaling events that direct the cardiac phenotype expressed during postnatal cardiac development [5] and in response to pathological stimuli [6–10].

High-Glucose-Induced PKC Translocation

Although in vivo models of human disease have served as paradigms to study pathophysiology, limitations exist with respect to establishing cause and effect. Adult cardiac myocytes coexpress multiple PKC isozymes [10, 11], increasing the complexity of determining the in vivo functional implications of PKC activation. A well-documented feature of experimental diabetes is the development of progressive cardiomyopathy that is independent of the vasculopathy [2–4]. Our group has demonstrated that hyperglycemia, independent of counter regulatory hormones, promotes the translocation of multiple PKC isozymes (β_1, β_2, δ, ε, and ζ) in a homogeneous population of adult rat ventricular myocytes. Glucose-induced PKC translocation was characterized by a delayed onset, requiring more than 1 h of exposure to high glucose. The latter property may serve to protect cardiac myocytes from transient glucose elevations or may reflect the time required for glucose-induced activation of signaling pathways involved in PKC translocation [12].

In adult rat ventricular myocytes, high glucose (25 mM) promotes PKC translocation via the activation of multiple intracellular signal transduction pathways and through the release of endogenous angiotensin II (ANG II). The latter peptide, by means of an autocrine signaling pathway, selectively promotes the translocation of PKC-β_1, -β_2, -δ, and -ε, which target critical serine residues, implicated in the activation of thin filamental protein troponin I. This demonstrated that endogenous release of ANG II by cardiac muscle cells activates an AT-1R-dependent signaling pathway that phosphorylates a myofilament regulatory protein implicated in the biochemical and mechanical abnormalities that characterize the diabetic myocardium. In summary, a high ambient glucose concentration is a potent stimulus for the translocation/activation of cardiac PKC isozymes. Further, AT-1R blockade may offer a selective advantage in the clinical management of diabetic cardiomyopathy [12].

PKC-ε-Dependent Survival Signals in Diabetic Hearts

The protein kinase C (PKC) family of isozymes plays a key role in the cardiac phenotype expressed during postnatal development and in response to pathological stimuli. Hyperglycemia is an activating signal for cardiac PKC isozymes that modulate a myriad of cell events including cell death and survival. The ε-isozyme of the PKC family transmits a powerful survival signal in cardiac muscle cells. In a streptozotocin (STZ)-induced type-1 diabetic model (genetically engineered mice with cardiac-specific expression of the PKC-ε translocation activator [$\psi\varepsilon$-receptors for activated C kinase ($\psi\varepsilon$-RACK)]), cardiac-specific expression of the PKC-ε translocation activator $\psi\varepsilon$-RACK (an ε-agonist) protected cardiac muscle cells from hyperglycemia-induced apoptosis signals. The survival phenotype was coupled with preserved parameters of LV function and resistance to hyperglycemia-mediated oxidative stress. Our data suggested that PKC-ERK signaling modules at the level of mitochondria preserved the integrity and function of this critical organelle via phosphorylation and/or inactivation of Bad and inhibition of hyperglycemia-induced cytochrome c release.

In summary, genetically engineered mice with cardiac-specific expression of an isozyme-specific PKC-ε translocation activator exhibited protection from hyperglycemia-induced apoptosis and LV dysfunction. The $\psi\varepsilon$-RACK peptide facilitated the intracellular trafficking of PKC-ε, and thereby prevented hyperglycemia-mediated decreases in immunoreactivity in both membrane and mitochondrial compartments. Importantly, PKC-ε-ERK signaling modules targeted the mitochondrial Bad protein to result in inactivated proapoptotic function and inhibited cytochrome c release. The described study has certain limitations; among these was the excess mortality in mice with cardiac-specific expression of the PKC-ε translocation inhibitor, which precludes detailed analysis of this group. Finally, it must be acknowledged that modest activation of cardiac PKC-ε may recruit additional survival programs [3] that are not explored here. The application of therapeutic interventions directed at selective activation of PKC-ε could offer a novel approach to preserve cell number and function in the hearts of diabetic patients.

PKCε Cardioprotection

PKCε transmits a powerful survival signal in cardiac muscle cells [13–17]. Mitochondria are the primary source of Reactive Oxygen Species (ROS) and critical determinants of cell death and cell survival. Hyperglycemia (HG) increases the generation of superoxide anion ($O_2^{\cdot-}$) in cells by interfering with the flow of electrons along the mitochondrial electron transport chain [18]. An essential component of PKCε cardioprotection is redistribution to mitochondria, where in association with the ERK family of MAPKs, it shifts the balance from cell death to cell survival. A critical event in translocation to the mitochondrial compartment is the recognition and binding of PKCε to isozyme specific anchor proteins, RACKS, facilitating the localization of activated PKCε in close proximity to target substrates [13–16]. The Bcl$_2$ family of proteins constitutes a critical checkpoint in both the susceptibility to apoptosis and mitochondrial dysfunction. This highly conserved family of proteins is distinguished by the presence of Bcl$_2$ homology (BH) domains, which are variably expressed aiming the different members [19–23]. The BH-3 domain is a prerequisite for the proapoptosis function of Bad, Bak and Bax proteins [20]. Several kinases including PKC-ε have been reported to phosphorylate the Bad protein at Ser112 and neutralize its function as a cell death protein [21–23]. The dephosphorylated Bad protein is capable of forming heterodimers with Bcl-$_{XL}$ and Bcl$_2$ at the level of mitochondria, neutralizing their anti-apoptotic function and promoting cytochrome c release. After release from the mitochondria intermembrane space, cytochrome c binds to Apaf-1 to form a macromolecular complex known as the apoptosome, which recruits and activates caspase-9, initiating the terminal apoptosis program [24].

Stress-Induced miRNA and Cardiac Phenotype

Micro-RNAs (miRNAs) are small noncoding RNAs that have been shown to be powerful regulators of CMC phenotype and the adaptive response of myocardium to stress stimuli [25]. miRNAs arise from primary transcripts of several thousand bases long (Pri-miRNA) that are processed in the nucleus by the RNase Drosha into Pre-miRNAs, which are hairpin-shaped precursors of 70–100 nt.; Pre-miRNAs are exported to the cytoplasm, where Dicer produces double stranded mi-RNA of 18–25 nt. One strand is selected as mature-mi-RNA, while the other strand is rapidly removed and degraded. MiRNAs that base pair perfectly with target mRNA sequences result in mRNA degradation; whereas those that display imperfect sequence complementarity with target mRNAs generally result in translational inhibition. miRNAs have been reported to be differentially expressed in various pathological and physiological states. MiRNA are characterized by having multiple targets, that are suppressed either through inhibition of translation or mRNA degradation. Therefore, it is possible that certain selective genes might be deregulated in the diabetic hearts. A unique aspect of miRNA function is that it serves as a molecular switch that triggers an immediate change in gene expression, in response to a stimulus [26].

Inhibition of p66ShcA Redox Activity Attenuates Hyperglycemia-Induced Oxidative Stress and Apoptosis

The p66ShcA protein is one of three isoforms encoded at the mammalian ShcA locus. The three overlapping Shc proteins, p66ShcA, p52ShcA, and p46ShcA, all share a COOH-terminal SH2 domain, central collagen homology region (CH), and NH$_2$-terminal phosphotyrosine-binding domain. p46ShcA and p52ShcA are the products of alternative translation initiation sites within the same transcript, whereas p66ShcA is distinguished by a unique NH$_2$-terminal region (CH2), generated by alternative splicing [27, 28]. The ShcA family of proteins is the cytoplasmic substrates for the activated IGF-1/insulin receptors. p46 and p52 participate in mitogenesis via the recruitment of the Ras signaling pathway [28], whereas p66ShcA by virtue of its unique NH$_2$-terminal region is a genetic determinant of longevity [29, 30] that controls mitochondrial metabolism [29]. Phosphorylation at a critical Ser36 (phospho-Ser36) residue position activates p66ShcA redox function by facilitating its translocation to mitochondria where p66ShcA generates ROS via the oxidation of cytochrome c. The latter redox reactions result in the opening of the mitochondrial transition pore, a collapse of mitochondrial transmembrane potential ($\Delta\Psi$m), and a cytochrome-c release. Shutting down the redox function of p66ShcA interrupting HG-induced phosphorylation at the critical Ser36 residue, prevents its translocation to mitochondria where p66ShcA functions as a ROS producer, resulting in organelle dysfunction and cell death.

Adult rat ventricular myocytes (ARVMs) transduced with dominant negative mutant-36 (p66ShcA) construct exhibit an oxidant-resistant phenotype, as judged by the inhibition of HG-induced ROS production, the stabilization of mitochondrial energetics, and the expression of the survival program [31]. The order of progression for phospho-Ser36 and downstream p66ShcA signaling events in diabetic hearts of Akita mouse were identical to that detected in in vitro studies with ARVMs at HG. Akita mice treated with the potent blood glucose-lowering hormone Leptin (LEP) showed an order of progression of p66ShcA signaling, identical to that detected in mu-36 ARVMs, indicative that HG stress signals target phospho-Ser36 in the diabetic myocardium to turn on p66ShcA redox activity. p66ShcA acts as a molecular switch whose redox function is turned on by HG-induced phosphorylation at Ser36 and turned off by interventions that prevented this modification.

At the organismal level, the p66ShcA$^{-/-}$ mouse is the unique genetic model of increased resistance to oxidative stress, aging, and apoptosis [29, 32]. Adenoviral transduction of ARVMs with dominant negative mu-36 (p66ShcA) protein would confer a dominant-interfering phenotype, attenuating or preventing the transmission of HG danger signals. mu-36 ARVMs exhibited an oxidant-resistant phenotype, as judged by the inhibition of HG-induced ROS production, the attenuation of phospho-Ser36 levels, and the maintenance of ΔΨm. A marked increase in ROS production at HG, an upregulation in phospho-Ser36 levels, and a collapse of ΔΨm was observed. mu-36 ARVMs were resistant to HG-induced component of apoptosis, whereas ARVMs exhibited a 40% increase in this parameter. Together, p66ShcA plays a pivotal role for redox function as a precursor to HG-induced free radical injury in ARVMs.

A dominant mutation in the Ins2 gene due to an amino-acid change results in HG and DM in the Akita mouse. Akita mice have several advantages over inbred mouse strains that require streptozotocin treatment [33, 34], including a better-defined etiology (endoplasmic reticulum stress and proteotoxicity in pancreatic β-cells), along with a more pronounced and durable hyperglycemia [33, 34]. Akita diabetic mice developed significant HG along with the upregulation in phospho-Ser36 levels that were accompanied by a translocation of p66ShcA protein to mitochondria and an increased formation of p66ShcA/cytochrome-c complexes. Similar to ARVMs at HG, the expression of cleaved caspase-3 and the apoptosis-related proteins p53 and Bax was found to be upregulated in hearts of Akita mice. Akita mice treated with leptin were euglycemic, and their hearts showed no detectable alteration in phospho-Ser-36, in p66ShcA/cytochrome-c complexes, or in the expression of terminal components of the apoptosis program. A single injection of leptin in the hypothalamus reversed the effect of HG on the phosphorylation status and redox function of the p66ShcA protein [31].

Redox Function of WTp66ShcA Protein

The p66ShcA protein is one of three isoforms encoded by the mammalian ShcA locus [28]. The three overlapping Shc protein (Fig. 1), p66ShcA, p52ShcA, and p46ShcA all share C-terminal Src homology 2 (SH2) domain, central

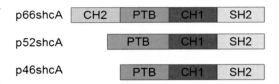

Fig. 1 Modular organization of ShcA isoforms

collagen-homologous (CH) region, and N-terminal phophotyrosine binding domain (PTB).

p66ShcA functions as a potentially harmful regulatory gene, which is required for the generation of HG-induced oxidative stress and apoptosis. A unifying hypothesis has been proposed for the development of diabetic complications, based on the overproduction of ROS. In support of this hypothesis, Rota et al. [35] reported that following the induction of experimental DM, p66ShcA−/− mice express a cardioprotection phenotype characterized by decreased markers of cell senescence and the preservation of cardiac muscle cells (CMC) number and LV function, whereas wild-type diabetic mice exhibited cardiac stem cell aging, myocyte apoptosis, and develop heart failure. Whether gene-based strategies that incorporate small-interfering RNA to silence disease-causing genes [36] such as p66ShcA can be applied in vivo to selectively target cardiac muscle cells remains to be determined.

P66Shc and p52ShcA are products of alternative translation initiation sites within the same transcript, whereas p66ShcA is distinguished by a unique N-terminal region (CH2), generated from alternative splicing [37, 38]. The ShcA family of proteins is cytoplasmic substrates for tyrosine kinase family of receptors that participate in mitogenesis via the recruitment of the adaptor protein Grb2 and subsequent activation of Ras signaling pathway. Recently, a clearer understanding of p66ShcA gene has emerged, based on evidence the WTp66ShcA protein functionally interacts with the mammalian Forkhead homolog FOXO3a [37, 38]. In the proposed scheme (Fig. 2), ROS induce phosphorylation at a critical CH2 Ser-36 residue, of the p66ShcA protein, a modification that serves to promote the intracellular generation of ROS and the recruitment of Akt/PKB, which directly phosphorylates and inactivates members of the FOXO family [37, 38].

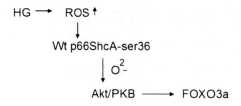

Fig. 2 Redox signaling by WT p66ShcA

FOXO3a is a potent stress response regulator, linked to the transcription of genes involved in such diverse biological processes as cell cycle progression, apoptosis, and antioxidant defense [39, 40].

Hyperglycemia and DM are associated with an exponential increase in ROS production at the cellular level, which has been linked to the development of diabetic complications. In DM, the two major sources of intracellular ROS are mitochondria and NADPH oxidase system [41, 42]. Mitochondria are critical determinants of cell survival and cell death [43, 44]. Collapse of mitochondrial transmembrane potential ($\Delta\Psi m$) triggers the release of cytochrome c and other aptogenic proteins, activating the terminal apoptosis program. Emerging evidence indicates that ROS-dependent phosphorylation at Ser-36 of the p66ShcA protein results in translocation of p66ShcA to mitochondria [31], where it plays a key role in the opening of the mitochondrial permeability transition pore (PTP) with the subsequent collapse of $\Delta\Psi m$. In the cytosolic compartment, the multicomponent NADPH oxidase system generates O_2^-, in response to the stress of HG [41, 42]. Activation of the conventional PKC isozymes (and β) have been shown to modulate HG induced upregulation of NADPH activity. Data from our laboratory indicated that the inhibition of WTp66ShcA function shuts down HG-induced ROS production in cytosolic and mitochondrial compartments [31].

Diabetes Accumulates ROS

ROS are recognized as important mediators of biological responses, including cell death by apoptosis [45, 46]. Hyperglycemia promotes the

intracellular generation of superoxide anion and hydrogen peroxide. In several cell lines, oxidant stress has been linked to the activation of death programs. Evidence suggests that high-glucose concentration triggers the generation of ROS in mesangial cells [47, 48] raised questions concerning the effect of oxidant stress on mesangial cell survival. The enhanced production of free radicals has been linked to increased mesangial matrix deposition, increased glomerular volume, and urinary transforming growth factor-β excretion [47]. The mitochondria are the primary source of reactive oxygen intermediates and critical determinants of cell death and cell survival [45, 49]. Hyperglycemia increases the generation of superoxide anion (O_2^-) by interfering with the flow of electrons along the mitochondrial electron transport chain [19]. The Bcl-2 family of proteins constitutes a critical checkpoint in both the susceptibility to apoptosis and mitochondrial dysfunction. These alterations in the growth phenotype and biochemical properties of mesangial cells are suppressed in genetically engineered mice [47] with constitutively activated SOD. ROS have also been implicated in the activation of death programs [46] and ischemic preconditioning [50, 51].

Mesangial Cell Apoptosis by Oxidant-Dependent Mechanism

Diabetic glomerulopathy is characterized by the loss of resident glomerular cells, sclerosis of glomeruli, and occlusion, events that correlate strongly with the decline in glomerular filtration rate (GFR) [52]. Mesangial cells possess the genetic program for apoptosis [53–56], and this mechanism of cell death has been reported during the resolution phase of inflammatory glomerular lesions [57, 58]. Recruitment of the redox-sensitive transcription factor NF-κB plays a pivotal role in the regulation of cell survival [59–65]. Hyperglycemia has been reported to promote nuclear translocation and activation of NF-κB in several cell lines [19, 65]. The generation of ROS has been implicated in the activation of cell death programs [51], providing a rationale to examine the effect of oxidant stress on the fate of mesangial cells exposed to a high-glucose environment. The signaling cascade activated by glucose-induced oxidant stress included the heterodimeric redox-sensitive transcription factor NF-kappaB, which exhibited an upregulation in p65/c-Rel binding activity and suppresses the binding activity of the p50 dimer. Antioxidants inhibit the recruitment of NF-kappaB and mesangial cell apoptosis by implicating oxidant-induced activation of NF-kappaB in the transmission of the death signal. The genetic program for glucose-induced mesangial cell apoptosis is characterized by an upregulation of the Bax/Bcl-2 ratio. These perturbations in the expression and phosphorylation of the Bcl-2 family are coupled with the release of cytochrome c from mitochondria and caspase activation. In mesangial cells, exposed to high ambient glucose concentration, oxidant stress is a proximate event in the activation of the death program, which culminates in mitochondrial dysfunction and caspase-3 activation, as the terminal event [66].

IGF-1 Inhibits the Mitochondrial Apoptosis Program in Mesangial Cells

The activated insulin-like growth factor-1 receptor (IGF-1R) protects several cell lines including normal human mesangial cells (NHMC) and mouse mesangial cells (MMC) from a wide range of apoptotic stimuli [67–71]. Ligand binding to the IGF-1R results in the phosphorylation of specific tyrosine residues at the IGF-1R β-subunit, activating the signaling cascade. The phosphorylated IGF-1R transmits intracellular signals via tyrosyl phosphorylation of the insulin receptor substrate (IRS) family and Shc, adaptor proteins that interact with a myriad of signaling molecules [72]. The recruitment of IRS-1 results in the activation of phosphatidylinositol 3-kinase (PI-3K), which in turn activates Akt/protein kinase B (Akt/PKB) [73]. The latter signaling cascade is generally regarded as the main pathway used by the IGF-1R for protection against apoptotic cell death [72, 74, 75]. The IGF-1R via its interaction with the

adaptor protein Shc [72, 76] promotes activation of the ERK subfamily. IGF-1R-dependent signals inactivate the proapoptosis protein Bad by phosphorylating Ser112 and Ser136 [72]. The non-phosphorylated Bad protein is capable of forming heterodimers with Bcl-$_{XL}$ and Bcl-2 at the level of mitochondria; neutralizing their antiapoptotic function and promoting cytochrome c release [17, 20, 23]. After release from the mitochondrial intermembrane space, cytochrome c binds to Apaf-1 to form a macromolecular complex known as the apoptosome [24], which recruits and activates caspase-9, initiating the terminal apoptosis program. IGF-1 activates a survival program that maintains the integrity of mitochondria and prevents the expression of the genetic program for apoptosis in mesangial cells maintained at high ambient glucose concentration [77].

IGF-1R Inhibits Hyperglycemia-Induced DNA Damage and Promotes DNA Repair

ROS-dependent signals have also been linked to defects in genomic maintenance systems and the aging process [44]. The novel IGF-1R antioxidant function is closely coupled with expression of the survival phenotype and inhibition of the apoptosis program. These observations are in keeping with genetic experiments, in which longevity in mice was directly linked to increased resistance to oxidant stress [19, 56]. Interestingly, the IGF-1R [19] and the adaptor protein p66Shc, a key IGF-1R signaling molecule, have both emerged as major genetic determinants of longevity and oxidative stress, in mammals. The DNA double helix is a target for ROS-dependent signals, which inflict more than 100 different types of DNA lesions, ranging from base modifications to single-strand breaks (SSB) and potentially lethal double-strand breaks (DSB) [44, 78]. DNA repair is a fundamental mechanism by which cells protect themselves from oxidative stress. Failure to repair DSB commits a cell to a death sentence or malignant transformation [79–81]. The insulin receptor substrate (IRS) family is a major cytoplasmic substrate for the activated IGF-1R [72]. Recent investigations have suggested a novel function of the IGF-1R/IRS-1 pathway is the intracellular trafficking of Rad51 to the nucleus [81]. In that proposed model, Rad51 is sequestered in the cytoplasm, bound to the NH_2-terminal domain of IRS-1. Ligand activation of the IGF-1R results in phosphorylation at IRS-1 tyrosine residues, which in turn, attenuates this protein–protein interaction, facilitating translocation of Rad51 to foci of damaged DNA. IGF-1R-dependent signals prevent genotoxic stress by suppressing hyperglycemic O_2^- danger signals and enhancing the repair of DSB by HRR in MMC and NHMC [82].

p66ShcA Prevents Glycooxidant-Dependent FOXO3a Regulation

The ShcA family of proteins are cytoplasmic substrates for the tyrosine kinase family of receptors [83], which participate in mitogenesis via the recruitment of the adaptor protein Grb2 [84] and subsequent activation of the Ras signaling pathway. Several lines of evidence support a dominant role for wild-type (WT) p66ShcA protein in the intracellular pathways that convert oxidative stress to apoptosis [30, 38, 85], whereas homozygous mutation of the *WTp66Shc* gene in mice confers increased resistance to oxidative stress, aging, and apoptosis [28, 78]. Recently, a clearer understanding of the *WTp66ShcA* gene has emerged, based on evidence WTp66ShcA protein functionally interacts with the mammalian Forkhead homolog FKHRL1 (FOXO3a) [38]. ROS induce phosphorylation of WTp66ShcA protein at a critical CH2 Ser-36 residue, a modification that serves to promote the intracellular generation of ROS [30, 38] and the recruitment of Akt/PKB, which directly phosphorylates and inactivates members of the FOXO family [86]. Silencing the expression of the *WTp66ShcA* gene by transfecting MMC and NHMC with either mutant 36 p66ShcA or p66ShcA short-intervening RNA (siRNA) maintained at HG exhibit the oxidant-resistant phenotype and protection from HG-induced DNA damage [40]. At high ambient glucose (HG), p66ShcA-deficient cells exhibit resistance to HG-induced ROS generation and attenuation in the amplitude of the kinetic curves for intracellular ROS metabolism, indicative of the pivotal role of WTp66ShcA in the generation of HG oxidant stress. FKHRL1 (FOXO3a), a potent stress response regulator and downstream target of WTp66ShcA redox function. At hyperglycemic conditions, p66ShcA-deficient cells, compared to the control cells, showed attenuation of FOXO3a phosphorylation at Thr-32, and nuclear localization of FOXO3a. p66ShcA-deficient cells exhibit increased resistance to DSB and apoptosis, while parental cells show a striking increase in both parameters. Knockdown of WTp66ShcA redox function prevents HG-dependent FOXO3a regulation and promotes the survival phenotype [40].

Conclusions

We have described that genetically engineered mice with cardiac-specific expression of an isozyme-specific PKC-ε translocation activator exhibits protection from hyperglycemia-induced apoptosis and LV dysfunction. The $\psi\varepsilon$-RACK peptide facilitated the intracellular trafficking of PKC-ε, and thereby prevented hyperglycemia-mediated decreases in immunoreactivity in both membrane and mitochondrial compartments. p66ShcA functions as a potentially harmful regulatory gene, which is required for the generation of HG-induced oxidative stress and apoptosis. At high ambient glucose (HG), p66ShcA-deficient cells exhibit resistance to HG-induced ROS generation and attenuation in the amplitude of the kinetic curves for intracellular ROS metabolism, indicative of the pivotal role of WTp66ShcA in the generation of HG oxidant stress. A unifying hypothesis has been proposed for the development of diabetic complications, based on the overproduction of ROS (Fig. 3). Inhibition of WTp66ShcA function shuts down HG-induced ROS production in cytosolic and mitochondrial compartments.

In mesangial cells, exposed to high ambient glucose concentration, oxidant stress is a proximate

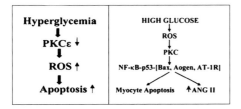

Fig. 3 Unifying hypothesis proposed for the development of diabetic complications based on the overproduction of ROS

event in the activation of the death program, which culminates in mitochondrial dysfunction and caspase-3 activation, as the terminal event. IGF-1 activates a survival program that maintains the integrity of mitochondria and prevents the expression of the genetic program for apoptosis in mesangial cells maintained at high ambient glucose concentration. The application of therapeutic interventions directed at selective activation of PKC-ε could offer a novel approach to preserve cell number and function in the hearts of diabetic patients. We suggest that the studies reported in this chapter are fundamental to the development of gene-based strategies to induce cardiorenal protection in DM and may be relevant to other myopathies and nephropathies, where ROS have been implicated in inflammatory, metabolic, and toxic insults.

References

1. The Diabetes Control and Complications Trial Research Group. The effect of intensive treatment of diabetes on the development and progression of long-term complications in insulin-dependent diabetes mellitus. N Engl J Med. 1993;329:977–86.
2. Rodrigues B, Cam MC, McNeill JH. Metabolic disturbances in diabetic cardiomyopathy. Mol Cell Biochem. 1998;180:53–7.
3. Rodrigues B, McNeill JH. The diabetic heart: metabolic causes for the development of a cardiomyopathy. Cardiovasc Res. 1992;26:913–22.
4. Bell DS. Diabetic cardiomyopathy. A unique entity or a complication of coronary artery disease? Diabetes Care. 1995;18:708–14.
5. Rybin VO, Steinberg SF. Protein kinase C isoform expression and regulation in the developing rat heart. Circ Res. 1994;74:299–309.
6. Gu X, Bishop SP. Increased protein kinase C and isozyme redistribution in pressure-overload cardiac hypertrophy in the rat. Circ Res. 1994;75:926–31.
7. Zou Y, Komuro I, Yamazaki T, et al. Protein kinase C, but not tyrosine kinases or Ras, plays a critical role in angiotensin II-induced activation of Raf-1 kinase and extracellular signal-regulated protein kinases in cardiac myocytes. J Biol Chem. 1996;271:33592–7.
8. Qiu Y, Ping P, Tang XL, et al. Direct evidence that protein kinase C plays an essential role in the development of late preconditioning against myocardial stunning in conscious rabbits and that epsilon is the isoform involved. J Clin Invest. 1998;101:2182–98.
9. Goto M, Cohen MV, Downey JM. The role of protein kinase C in ischemic preconditioning. Ann N Y Acad Sci. 1996;793:177–90.
10. Steinberg SF, Goldberg M, Rybin VO. Protein kinase C isoform diversity in the heart. J Mol Cell Cardiol. 1995;27:141–53.
11. Takeishi Y, Jalili T, Ball NA, et al. Responses of cardiac protein kinase C isoforms to distinct pathological stimuli are differentially regulated. Circ Res. 1999;85:264–71.
12. Malhotra A, Kang BP, Cheung S, et al. Angiotensin II promotes glucose-induced activation of cardiac protein kinase C isozymes and phosphorylation of troponin I. Diabetes. 2001;50:1918–26.
13. Malhotra A, Begley R, Kang BP, et al. PKC-{epsilon}-dependent survival signals in diabetic hearts. Am J Physiol Heart Circ Physiol. 2005;289:H1343–50.
14. Mochly-Rosen D, Wu G, Hahn H, et al. Cardiotrophic effects of protein kinase C epsilon: analysis by in vivo modulation of PKCepsilon translocation. Circ Res. 2000;86:1173–9.
15. Wu G, Toyokawa T, Hahn H, et al. Epsilon protein kinase C in pathological myocardial hypertrophy. Analysis by combined transgenic expression of translocation modifiers and Galphaq. J Biol Chem. 2000;275:29927–30.
16. Wild S, Roglic G, Green A, et al. Global prevalence of diabetes: estimates for the year 2000 and projections for 2030. Diabetes Care. 2004;27:1047–53.
17. Baines CP, Zhang J, Wang GW, et al. Mitochondrial PKCepsilon and MAPK form signaling modules in the murine heart: enhanced mitochondrial PKCepsilon-MAPK interactions and differential MAPK activation in PKCepsilon-induced cardioprotection. Circ Res. 2002;90:390–7.
18. Baines CP, Song CX, Zheng YT, et al. Protein kinase Cepsilon interacts with and inhibits the permeability transition pore in cardiac mitochondria. Circ Res. 2003;92:873–80.
19. Nishikawa T, Edelstein D, Du XL, et al. Normalizing mitochondrial superoxide production blocks three pathways of hyperglycaemic damage. Nature. 2000;404:787–90.
20. Haunstetter A, Izumo S. Apoptosis: basic mechanisms and implications for cardiovascular disease. Circ Res. 1998;82:1111–29.
21. Green DR, Chipuk JE. Apoptosis: Stabbed in the BAX. Nature. 2008;455:1047–9.
22. Heidkamp MC, Bayer AL, Martin JL, et al. Differential activation of mitogen-activated protein kinase cascades

and apoptosis by protein kinase C epsilon and delta in neonatal rat ventricular myocytes. Circ Res. 2001; 89:882–90.

23. Harada H, Becknell B, Wilm M, et al. Phosphorylation and inactivation of BAD by mitochondria-anchored protein kinase A. Mol Cell. 1999;3:413–22.

24. Nicholson DW, Thornberry NA. Apoptosis. Life and death decisions. Science. 2003;299:214–5.

25. van Rooij E, Sutherland LB, Qi X, et al. Control of stress-dependent cardiac growth and gene expression by a microRNA. Science. 2007;316:575–9.

26. Rane S, He M, Sayed D, et al. Downregulation of miR-199a derepresses hypoxia-inducible factor-1alpha and Sirtuin 1 and recapitulates hypoxia preconditioning in cardiac myocytes. Circ Res. 2009;104:879–86.

27. Graiani G, Lagrasta C, Migliaccio E, et al. Genetic deletion of the p66Shc adaptor protein protects from angiotensin II-induced myocardial damage. Hypertension. 2005;46:433–40.

28. Migliaccio E, Giorgio M, Mele S, et al. The p66shc adaptor protein controls oxidative stress response and life span in mammals. Nature. 1999;402:309–13.

29. Giorgio M, Migliaccio E, Orsini F, et al. Electron transfer between cytochrome c and p66Shc generates reactive oxygen species that trigger mitochondrial apoptosis. Cell. 2005;122:221–33.

30. Orsini F, Migliaccio E, Moroni M, et al. The life span determinant p66Shc localizes to mitochondria where it associates with mitochondrial heat shock protein 70 and regulates trans-membrane potential. J Biol Chem. 2004;279:25689–95.

31. Malhotra A, Vashistha H, Yadav VS, et al. Inhibition of p66ShcA redox activity in cardiac muscle cells attenuates hyperglycemia-induced oxidative stress and apoptosis. Am J Physiol Heart Circ Physiol. 2009;296:H380–8.

32. Pinton P, Rimessi A, Marchi S, et al. Protein kinase C beta and prolyl isomerase 1 regulate mitochondrial effects of the life-span determinant p66Shc. Science. 2007;315:659–63.

33. Kakoki M, Kizer CM, Yi X, et al. Senescence-associated phenotypes in Akita diabetic mice are enhanced by absence of bradykinin B2 receptors. J Clin Invest. 2006;116:1302–9.

34. Kakoki M, Takahashi N, Jennette JC, et al. Diabetic nephropathy is markedly enhanced in mice lacking the bradykinin B2 receptor. Proc Natl Acad Sci USA. 2004;101:13302–5.

35. Rota M, LeCapitaine N, Hosoda T, et al. Diabetes promotes cardiac stem cell aging and heart failure, which are prevented by deletion of the p66shc gene. Circ Res. 2006;99:42–52.

36. Santiago Y, Chan E, Liu PQ, et al. Targeted gene knockout in mammalian cells by using engineered zinc-finger nucleases. Proc Natl Acad Sci USA. 2008;105:5809–14.

37. Nemoto S, Fergusson MM, Finkel T. Nutrient availability regulates SIRT1 through a forkhead-dependent pathway. Science. 2004;306:2105–8.

38. Nemoto S, Finkel T. Redox regulation of forkhead proteins through a p66shc-dependent signaling pathway. Science. 2002;295:2450–2.

39. You H, Jang Y, You-Ten AI, Okada H, et al. p53-dependent inhibition of FKHRL1 in response to DNA damage through protein kinase SGK1. Proc Natl Acad Sci USA. 2004;101:14057–62.

40. Chintapalli J, Yang S, Opawumi D, et al. Inhibition of wild-type p66ShcA in mesangial cells prevents gly-cooxidant-dependent FOXO3a regulation and promotes the survival phenotype. Am J Physiol Renal Physiol. 2007;292:F523–30.

41. Hua H, Munk S, Goldberg H, et al. High glucose-suppressed endothelin-1 Ca^{2+} signaling via NADPH oxidase and diacylglycerol-sensitive protein kinase C isozymes in mesangial cells. J Biol Chem. 2003;278: 33951–62.

42. Rajagopalan S, Kurz S, Munzel T, et al. Angiotensin II-mediated hypertension in the rat increases vascular superoxide production via membrane NADH/NADPH oxidase activation. Contribution to alterations of vaso-motor tone. J Clin Invest. 1996;97:1916–23.

43. Campisi J. Cellular senescence and apoptosis: how cellular responses might influence aging phenotypes. Exp Gerontol. 2003;38:5–11.

44. Hasty P, Campisi J, Hoeijmakers J, et al. Aging and genome maintenance: lessons from the mouse? Science. 2003;299:1355–9.

45. Akao M, Ohler A, O'Rourke B, et al. Mitochondrial ATP-sensitive potassium channels inhibit apoptosis induced by oxidative stress in cardiac cells. Circ Res. 2001;88:1267–75.

46. von Harsdorf R, Li PF, Dietz R. Signaling pathways in reactive oxygen species-induced cardiomyocyte apoptosis. Circulation. 1999;99:2934–41.

47. Craven PA, Melhem MF, Phillips SL, et al. Overexpression of Cu2+/Zn2+ superoxide dismutase protects against early diabetic glomerular injury in transgenic mice. Diabetes. 2001;50:2114–25.

48. Jaimes EA, Galceran JM, Raij L. Angiotensin II induces superoxide anion production by mesangial cells. Kidney Int. 1998;54:775–84.

49. Green DR, Reed JC. Mitochondria and apoptosis. Science. 1998;281:1309–12.

50. Gottlieb RA, Burleson KO, Kloner RA, et al. Reperfusion injury induces apoptosis in rabbit cardiomyocytes. J Clin Invest. 1994;94:1621–8.

51. Zweier JL, Flaherty JT, Weisfeldt ML. Direct measurement of free radical generation following reperfusion of ischemic myocardium. Proc Natl Acad Sci USA. 1987;84:1404–7.

52. Osterby R, Schmitz A, Nyberg G, et al. Renal structural changes in insulin-dependent diabetic patients with albuminuria. Comparison of cases with onset of albuminuria after short or long duration. APMIS. 1998;106:361–70.

53. Sandau K, Pfeilschifter J, Brune B. Nitric oxide and superoxide induced p53 and Bax accumulation during mesangial cell apoptosis. Kidney Int. 1997;52:378–86.

54. Sharma P, Reddy K, Franki N, et al. Native and oxidized low density lipoproteins modulate mesangial cell apoptosis. Kidney Int. 1996;50:1604–11.

55. Singhal PC, Franki N, Kumari S, et al. Extracellular matrix modulates mesangial cell apoptosis and mRNA

expression of cathepsin-B and tissue transglutaminase. J Cell Biochem. 1998;68:22–30.

56. Singhal PC, Gibbons N, Franki N, et al. Simulated glomerular hypertension promotes mesangial cell apoptosis and expression of cathepsin-B and SGP-2. J Investig Med. 1998;46:42–50.

57. Baker AJ, Mooney A, Hughes J, et al. Mesangial cell apoptosis: the major mechanism for resolution of glomerular hypercellularity in experimental mesangial proliferative nephritis. J Clin Invest. 1994;94:2105–16.

58. Mooney A, Jobson T, Bacon R, et al. Cytokines promote glomerular mesangial cell survival in vitro by stimulus-dependent inhibition of apoptosis. J Immunol. 1997;159:3949–60.

59. Karin M, Ben-Neriah Y. Phosphorylation meets ubiquitination: the control of NF-[kappa]B activity. Annu Rev Immunol. 2000;18:621–63.

60. Kirch HC, Flaswinkel S, Rumpf H, et al. Expression of human p53 requires synergistic activation of transcription from the p53 promoter by AP-1, NF-kappaB and Myc/Max. Oncogene. 1999;18:2728–38.

61. Lawrence T, Gilroy DW, Colville-Nash PR, et al. Possible new role for NF-kappaB in the resolution of inflammation. Nat Med. 2001;7:1291–7.

62. Ryan KM, Ernst MK, Rice NR, et al. Role of NF-kappaB in p53-mediated programmed cell death. Nature. 2000;404:892–7.

63. Sun X, Shimizu H, Yamamoto K. Identification of a novel p53 promoter element involved in genotoxic stress-inducible p53 gene expression. Mol Cell Biol. 1995;15:4489–96.

64. Wu H, Lozano G. NF-kappa B activation of p53. A potential mechanism for suppressing cell growth in response to stress. J Biol Chem. 1994;269:20067–74.

65. Yerneni KK, Bai W, Khan BV, et al. Hyperglycemia-induced activation of nuclear transcription factor kappaB in vascular smooth muscle cells. Diabetes. 1999;48:855–64.

66. Kang BP, Frencher S, Reddy V, et al. High glucose promotes mesangial cell apoptosis by oxidant-dependent mechanism. Am J Physiol Renal Physiol. 2003;284:F455–66.

67. Dudek H, Datta SR, Franke TF, et al. Regulation of neuronal survival by the serine-threonine protein kinase Akt. Science. 1997;275:661–5.

68. Jin K, Mao XO, Zhu Y, et al. MEK and ERK protect hypoxic cortical neurons via phosphorylation of Bad. J Neurochem. 2002;80:119–25.

69. Leri A, Liu Y, Claudio PP, et al. Insulin-like factor-1 induces Mdm2 and down-regulates p53, attenuating the myocyte renin-angiotensin system and stretch-mediated apoptosis. Am J Pathol. 1999;154:567–80.

70. Leri A, Liu Y, Wang X, et al. Overexpression of insulin-like growth factor-1 attenuates the myocyte renin-angiotensin system in transgenic mice. Circ Res. 1999;84:752–62.

71. Nakamura S, Watanabe H, Miura M, et al. Effect of the insulin-like growth factor I receptor on ionizing radiation-induced cell death in mouse embryo fibroblasts. Exp Cell Res. 1997;235:287–94.

72. Peruzzi F, Prisco M, Dews M, et al. Multiple signaling pathways of the insulin-like growth factor 1 receptor in protection from apoptosis. Mol Cell Biol. 1999;19:7203–15.

73. Myers Jr MG, Grammer TC, Wang LM, et al. Insulin receptor substrate-1 mediates phosphatidylinositol 3′-kinase and p70S6k signaling during insulin, insulin-like growth factor-1, and interleukin-4 stimulation. J Biol Chem. 1994;269:28783–9.

74. Kennedy SG, Wagner AJ, Conzen SD, et al. The PI 3-kinase/Akt signaling pathway delivers an anti-apoptotic signal. Genes Dev. 1997;11:701–13.

75. Kulik G, Klippel A, Weber MJ. Antiapoptotic signalling by the insulin-like growth factor I receptor, phosphatidylinositol 3-kinase, and Akt. Mol Cell Biol. 1997;17:1595–606.

76. Pronk GJ, McGlade J, Pelicci G, et al. Insulin-induced phosphorylation of the 46- and 52-kDa Shc proteins. J Biol Chem. 1993;268:5748–53.

77. Kang BP, Urbonas A, Baddoo A, et al. IGF-1 inhibits the mitochondrial apoptosis program in mesangial cells exposed to high glucose. Am J Physiol Renal Physiol. 2003;285:F1013–24.

78. Napoli C, Martin-Padura I, de Nigris F, et al. Deletion of the p66Shc longevity gene reduces systemic and tissue oxidative stress, vascular cell apoptosis, and early atherogenesis in mice fed a high-fat diet. Proc Natl Acad Sci USA. 2003;100:2112–6.

79. Baumann P, West SC. Role of the human RAD51 protein in homologous recombination and double-stranded-break repair. Trends Biochem Sci. 1998; 23:247–51.

80. Tombline G, Fishel R. Biochemical characterization of the human RAD51 protein. I. ATP hydrolysis. J Biol Chem. 2002;277:14417–25.

81. Trojanek J, Ho T, Del Valle L, et al. Role of the insulin-like growth factor I/insulin receptor substrate 1 axis in Rad51 trafficking and DNA repair by homologous recombination. Mol Cell Biol. 2003;23: 7510–24.

82. Yang S, Chintapalli J, Sodagum L, et al. Activated IGF-1R inhibits hyperglycemia-induced DNA damage and promotes DNA repair by homologous recombination. Am J Physiol Renal Physiol. 2005;289: F1144–52.

83. Gotoh N, Toyoda M, Shibuya M. Tyrosine phosphorylation sites at amino acids 239 and 240 of Shc are involved in epidermal growth factor-induced mitogenic signaling that is distinct from Ras/mitogen-activated protein kinase activation. Mol Cell Biol. 1997;17:1824–31.

84. Lowenstein EJ, Daly RJ, Batzer AG, et al. The SH2 and SH3 domain-containing protein GRB2 links receptor tyrosine kinases to ras signaling. Cell. 1992;70:431–42.

85. Baynes JW, Thorpe SR. Role of oxidative stress in diabetic complications: a new perspective on an old paradigm. Diabetes. 1999;48:1–9.

86. Tran H, Brunet A, Griffith EC, et al. The many forks in FOXO's road. Science. 2003;STKE 172:RE5.

Molecular Mechanisms in the Pathogenesis of Diabetic Cardiomyopathy

Subrata Chakrabarti

Abstract

Diabetic population continues to increase all over the world. With improved longevity, diabetic patients increasingly suffer from morbidity and mortality due to chronic secondary complications affecting the lower limbs, nervous system, eyes, kidneys, and heart. Long-standing diabetes leads to structural and functional alterations in the cardiovascular system compromising the expectancy of life. Hyperglycemia has been identified as the key determinant for the development of diabetic heart disease. The symphony of biochemical and signaling anomalies that govern the development of chronic diabetic complications are further subjected to cross-interaction and complex interplays. Alteration several vasoactive effector molecules may be instrumental in mediating diabetes-induced structural and functional deficits. This review discusses the molecular mechanisms leading to structural and functional changes in diabetic cardiomyopathy.

Keywords

Diabetes • Heart • Cardiomyocytes • Molecular mechanisms

Introduction

As diabetes reaches epidemic magnitude worldwide, more diabetics face the problems of morbidity and mortality due to chronic complications

[1, 2]. Nearly, three-fourths of the deaths associated with diabetes are due to cardiovascular complications [3]. Diabetic individuals are two to four times more likely to have heart disease compared to the normal population, and 75% of diabetes related deaths are due to heart diseases [4–6]. Diabetic patients develop congestive heart failure more readily with worse prognosis than the non-diabetic counterparts once they develop coronary disease, presumably due to myocardial abnormalities [4–6].

S. Chakrabarti (✉)
Department of Pathology, University of Western Ontario, London, Ontario, Canada
e-mail: Subrata.Chakrabarti@lhsc.on.ca

Cardiac Consequences of Diabetes

Cardiac involvement in diabetes includes coronary atherosclerosis, diabetic cardiomyopathy, and autonomic neuropathy [6, 7]. Although coronary atherosclerosis and autonomic neuropathy have been identified as disease entities for a long time, recognition of diabetic cardiomyopathy as a disease process is relatively new and was first described in 1972 [8]. Diabetic patients demonstrate increased susceptibility to develop heart failure [6, 7]. Furthermore, following a myocardial infraction, they demonstrate increased mortality and tendency to develop cardiac failure [5–7]. Clinically, diabetic cardiomyopathy causes systolic and/or diastolic dysfunction leading to heart failure [5–7]. Over the last several years, contribution of diabetic cardiomyopathy leading to functional and structural cardiac damage has been well recognized. Forty to 50% of diabetics without any known cardiac disease manifest left ventricular functional abnormalities affecting diastolic properties and present clinically as a failure of left ventricular contractile function and prolonged relaxation [6, 7]. Pathological findings include cardiomyocyte hypertrophy, interstitial and perivascular fibrosis, myocyte necrosis, and microangiopathic lesions such as capillary basement membrane (BM) thickening [5–7, 9]. Coronary atherosclerosis, hypertension, and autonomic neuropathy may exert additional effects [6, 7, 9, 10]. This review delineates cellular and molecular mechanisms of tissue damage in diabetic cardiomyopathy. Furthermore, transcriptional regulation of gene expression is elaborated in this review.

The Triggers and the Cellular Targets

A large numbers of changes at the molecular, cellular, and organ level occur secondary to diabetes. Both in type 1 and in type 2 diabetes, the initial insult is hyperglycemia. In addition, in type 2 diabetes, both hyperlipidemia and hyperinsulinemia may have additional deleterious effects. These biochemical triggers target both endothelial cells (ECs) and cardiomyocytes in the heart. In the heart, cardiomyocytes constitute about 70% of the volume but only 30% in terms of cell number [11, 12]. ECs outnumber the cardiomyocytes by a ratio of 3:1 [11, 12]. A significant number of cardiac fibroblasts are also present in the heart which may be responsible for extracellular matrix protein (ECM) deposition in addition to the ECs. ECs, however, form a dynamic unit and are critical for the maintenance of the integrity of the vascular system. They play important roles in regulating vascular tone, permeability, blood fluidity, thrombotic/fibrinolytic balance, and leukocyte traffic [13]. Owing to their location, ECs are first to get exposed to high levels of glucose and respond to increased glucose by initiating a number of intracellular events and may cause increased extracellular matrix protein production and stiffness. ECs incorporate glucose via facilitative diffusion [14, 15] and changes in the level of glucose does not lead to altered expression of the primary EC glucose transporter, glucose transporter-1 (Glut1) [14, 15]. Hence, increased plasma glucose causes augmented intracellular glucose levels in the ECs. In addition, hyperglycemia further affects the metabolism of the cardiomyocytes. The cardiomyocytes respond to hyperglycemia by substrate switching and demonstrate impaired calcium homeostasis ultimately manifesting defective contractility [16]. Altered myocardial energy metabolism is an important contributor to diabetic cardiomyopathy. Cardiomyocytes demonstrate increased fatty acid metabolism and reduced glucose metabolism in diabetes [17, 18]. Reduced bioavailability of insulin as well as activation of peroxisome proliferator-activated receptor-α (PPAR-α)-mediated signaling is major contributor in such pathways. Such increased use of fatty acids leads to mitochondrial uncoupling and reduce contractile efficiency of the heart [17–19]. The accumulation of intermediate products of lipid metabolism may also augment lipotoxicity on the heart [20, 21]. Furthermore, altered Ca^{2+} handling causes impaired contractility of the cardiomyocytes [22, 23]. Secondary effects of all such abnormalities lead to alterations of vasoactive and cardioactive factor production, causing cellular structural and functional abnormalities and ultimately clinically manifesting as diabetic cardiomyopathy.

Alteration of Vasoactive and Cardioactive Factors in Diabetic Cardiomyopathy

Altered production of vasoactive and cardioactive factors in chronic diabetic complications precede the structural changes [24–27]. An increase in expression/activity of vasoconstrictors and a concurrent decrease in expression/activity of vasodilators are charactertistic of early diabetes. A major vasoactive and cardioactive factor that is altered in diabetes is endothelin-1 (ET-1). ET-1, the most potent endogenous vasoconstrictor, is a short peptide that is primarily produced by the ECs [28, 29]. Dysfunction and/or activation of the ECs increase the levels of ET-1 production. Augmented ET-1 levels have been reported in diabetes and have been shown to mediate vasoconstriction and reduced blood flow [30]. Increased activity of ETs has also been shown in the resistance arteries of diabetic patients [31]. Moreover, administration of exogenous ET-1 in humans reduces coronary and renal blood flow and increases vasoconstriction [32–34]. We have demonstrated upregulation of ET-1 and its receptors in the heart in diabetes and that diabetes induced functional and structural changes in the heart can be prevented by a dual ET receptor antagonist [35]. We have further showed that ET-1 interacts with other cardiocative factors such as sodium–hydrogen exchanger-1 and obesity associated peptide leptin, in mediating its effects [36, 37].

Concurrently, alteration in the vasodilators leads to functional deficits in diabetes. Nitric oxide synthase (NOS) enzymes have been suggested to play important roles in acetylcholine-induced paradoxical vasoconstriction in atherosclerotic coronary arteries [38]. NOS are a family of enzymes that produce the vasodilator, nitric oxide (NO). There are three members of the family: neuronal NOS (type I), inducible NOS (type II), and endothelial NOS (type III). Acute exposure of ECs to glucose decreases NO generation by agonists such as bradykinin and A23187 [39]. Purified ECs when assayed in the presence of glucose also shows significantly lower level of NO production [39]. In addition to reduced generation, NO may also be sequestered by glucose-induced oxidative stress [30, 40, 41]. This creates an imbalance in the counteractivity of ETs and NO [42]. Alterations in NO have been demonstrated in the heart in diabetes [43]. Furthermore, renin–angiotensin system (RAS) is known to be altered in diabetic cardiomyopathy as evidenced by increased angiotensin II receptor density and mRNA production in the heart in diabetes [44, 45]. Activation of RAS has been causally associated with Ca^{2+} abnormalities, reactive oxygen species (ROS) production, cardiomyocyte and EC apoptosis [46–49].

Among other vasoactive factors, alteration in vascular endothelial growth factor (VEGF) is of significant importance in several chronic diabetic complications. VEGF is an EC-specific mitogen and has been demonstrated to cause angiogenesis in a number of disease models [40, 41]. In noncardiac diabetic complications, such as in diabetic retinopathy, the oxygenation state regulates various growth factors that promote angiogenesis in response to reduced blood flow and capillary nonperfusion [50]. Similar to the retina, structural changes in the kidney in diabetes, may also include increased angiogenesis. An increased glomerular filtration rate which may, in part, be due to an increased surface area has been reported in experimental diabetes [51]. However, in contrast to the retina [41, 52] and possible kidney [51], diabetes leads to impairment in the neovascularization of the heart. It has been reported that diabetes causes reduced expression of VEGF and its receptors in the myocardium [53]. The reduced VEGF expression in the heart is in sharp contrast to the retina, where high levels of VEGF have been shown [52]. In addition, collateral vessel formation has also been reported to be impaired in the hearts in diabetes [54–56]. One possible explanation could underlie defective VEGF signaling in monocytes, which are important for the process of arteriogenesis [55]. Activated monocytes have been shown in ischemic tissues [57, 58]. Monocytes migrate in response to VEGF through the activation of VEGFR1 (also known as Flt-1). In vitro assays have shown that monocytes isolated from diabetic patients fail to migrate in response to VEGF [59]. Taken together, these findings suggest that reduced expression of growth factors and growth factor receptors and impaired signaling may, in concert, lead to inadequate neovascularization in the myocardium. However, further studies are required to delineate the role of such processes in the pathogenesis of diabetic cardiomyopathy.

Interestingly, cardiac fibroblasts are possibly responsible for the cardiac ECM deposition in addition to the cardiac ECs. Angiotensin II is able to cause cardiac fibroblast proliferation and collagen deposition [60, 61]. Studies have also indicated that angiotensin II exerts the action on cardiac fibroblasts through the induction of ET-1 [62, 63]. In addition to ECs, fibroblasts also express ET receptors [64]. In vitro studies reveal that isolated rat fibroblasts increase production of ECM components upon ET administration [64–66]. These changes can be readily blocked by ET antagonists. It has further been shown that endocardial capillary ECs (in culture) show a 25% higher growth index as compared to other vascular ECs. These findings indicate that tissue microenvironment is an important regulator of impaired angiogenic response in the heart which could be mediated by increased ECM deposition. In clinical trials, ET antagonists have shown promise in short-term studies as indexed by improved cardiac index and pulmonary capillary pressure [67, 68]. However, long-term studies have yet to show beneficial effects [69].

Molecular Pathways

High levels of glucose cause biochemical changes in the ECs, which are reminiscent of early molecular alterations in the target organs of diabetes [30, 40]. Under physiological conditions, in the ECs glucose is primarily metabolized by the glycolytic pathway with the hexose monophosphate pathway and Krebs cycle accounting for less than 2% of total glucose metabolism [70, 71]. In hyperglycemic state, there is increased glucose oxidation through the Krebs cycle, which leads to augmented mitochondrial superoxide production [72]. There is also activation of additional pathways of glucose metabolism, e.g., polyol pathway, hexosamine pathway, and protein kinase C (PKC) as well as formation of advanced glycated end products [72–75]. PKC activation, in particular that of PKCβ and PKCε isoforms, leads to upregulation of several vasoactive and cardioactive factors [75–77]. In addition to intracellular changes, the ECM is also modified by glycation. Glycation decreases the turnover rate of the proteins and thus provide an efficient means of chronic signaling to the vascular ECs. Glucose reacts with proteins via Maillard reaction to produce advanced glycation end products (AGEs) [78]. AGE products have been reported to cause NO scavenging [79]. Furthermore, AGEs interact with cell surface receptors (RAGEs) to increase cytokine/growth factor expression [70]. All these pathways lead to increased intracellular oxidative stress, which is an early change in the ECs. Acute exposure to high ambient glucose causes glucose autooxidation [72]. Other hyperglycemia-induced pathways causing oxidative stress include oxidized-low lipoprotein and heme oxygenase pathways [43, 80]. It is to be pointed out that the pathways demonstrate intricate relationships. It has, however, been shown that prevention of increased mitochondrial superoxide production inhibits major pathways in chronic diabetic complication such as PKC activation, hexosamine and polyol pathways, and AGE formation [72, 81].

Along with ECs, increased ROS production has been demonstrated in the cardiomyocytes, and such increased ROS production may lead to apoptosis of the cardiomyocytes [82, 83]. Reduced expression of proteins involved in the electron transport chain and increased expression of proteins in β-oxidation, as demonstrated in the heart, cause increased superoxide production, mitochondrial uncoupling, and reduced ATP generation [16, 82–85]. Oxidative stress and the subsequent metabolic abnormalities cause DNA damage and alteration of gene transcription of several specific vasoactive and cardioactive factors.

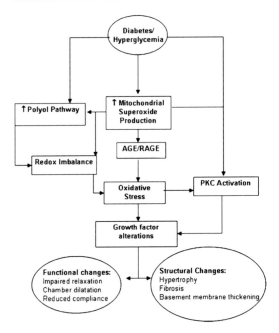

Fig. 1 Diagram showing various interactive biochemical processes secondary to hyperglycemia, leading to functional and structural changes in diabetic cardiomyopathy (please see the text for abbreviations)

Oxidative stress, together with generation of cardioactive and vasoactive factors, represents major avenues that can lead to functional and structural defects in the organs [40–42]. A diagrammatic representation of such various processes has been represented in Fig. 1.

In addition to intracellular mechanisms, the ECM is equally if not more important than growth factor alteration and may provide a more sustained signaling environment [40, 41]. Modification of ECM proteins also represents an important event in chronic stimulation of biochemical pathways such as protein kinase C and NF-κB [72, 75, 86, 87]. One consistent and continual structural change that accompanies diabetes in vivo and exposure to glucose in vitro is ECM protein deposition [86, 89]. Experimental evidence shows that the amount and the composition (type of ECM proteins) of ECM changes in diabetes. This matrix serves as a reservoir of growth factors and other signaling proteins. With continued exposure to high levels of glucose, the ECs accumulate growth factors and other mitogens in the matrix. These accumulated factors may provide continual signaling to the ECs. We have demonstrated that high glucose produces a splice variant of FN, namely, extra domain B (EDB+) containing FN, which produces outside-in signaling and VEGF upregulation [87–89]. We have also shown that the mRNA of VEGF is upregulated as early as 24 h following exposure to high levels of glucose [88, 89]. In addition to providing growth factors itself as a reservoir, the changing matrix may also regulate how ECs perceive and respond to the growth factors [88]. Subsequent to such cellular dysfunction, the target tissues in diabetes exhibit poor blood flow and ischemia [40, 41, 52, 89]. This is brought upon by the combined effect of functional and structural alterations in the cardiac microvasculature, which is further augmented in the heart due to impaired vessel formation [54–56].

Transcriptional Pathways in Diabetic Cardiomyopathy

As discussed above, hyperglycemia-induced molecular and biochemical changes upregulate several growth factors, vasoactive molecules, and hypertrophic and cardioactive factors causing tissue damage. Activation of specific transcription factors play important roles in the production of these growth factors [41, 77] We have previously shown that ET-1 causes activation of transcription factors such as nuclear factor kappaB (NF-κB) and activating protein-1 (AP-1) in the heart of diabetic animals [88, 89]. However, it has also been demonstrated that ET-1 is also regulated by NF-κB [90]. Oxidative DNA damage also leads to activation of poly (ADP ribose) polymerase (PARP). PARP causes depletion of NAD$^+$ and ATP and cellular dysfunction in diabetic vasculopathy [91]. Furthermore, PARP modulates the activity of NF-κB through transcription coactivators p300 (see later) [91]. We have shown that PARP activation and p300 upregulation play a major role in diabetic heart disease through NF-κB and AP-1 [92, 93]. p300 also regulates other transcription factors, e.g., myocyte enhancing factor 2 (MEF2) [93].

Transcription Factors in Diabetic Cardiomyopathy

Recently, we have demonstrated that cells exposed to high glucose level show alteration of multiple transcription factors [94]. From a functional standpoint, the altered transcription factors included both constitutively active and conditional factors. The latter group consisted of cell-specific developmental factors and signal-dependent factors such as steroid receptor and intracellular ligand-dependent factors, cell-membrane receptor–ligand-dependent latent cytoplasmic factors, and cell-membrane receptor–ligand-dependent resident nuclear factors [94]. The altered transcription factors included GATA1, GATA4, MEF2, NF-κB, AP-1 and CREB, SRF, MyoD, etc. These factors are known to mediate glucose-induced upregulation of vasoactive factors, ECM proteins, and structural changes in the organs affected by chronic diabetic complications such as cardiomyopathy as well as other chronic diabetic complications [95–97]. In this context, discussion of certain key transcription factors is needed.

NF-κB

NF-κB plays a pivotal role in the regulation of several genes [98, 99]. In nonstimulated cells, NF-κB exists in a latent dimer form in the cytoplasm being bound to IκB, an inhibitor protein. Several subunits of NF-κB (p50, p65, c-rel, p52, rel B, and IκB) are present. The main form of activated NF-κB is p50/p65. Upon stimulation, IκB is phosphorylated on its serine residues and is ubiquitinated by E3 ligase, releasing p50/p65, which then translocates to the nucleus and affects target gene expression by binding with κB elements in their promoters [99]. Two main kinases affecting IκBα are IκKα and IκKβ. Oxidative stress is one of the main activators of NF-κB [100, 101]. In diabetes, redox modulation as well as nonenzymatic glycation may result in oxidative stress and NF-κB activation [97, 98]. We have shown that diabetes causes NF-κB activation in several organs including the heart [87, 97].

AP-1

DNA-binding transcription factor proteins that form AP-1 dimers are activated by multiple stimuli and mediate cell proliferation and cell death. These proteins include the Jun, Fos, and ATF subgroups of transcription factors [102, 103]. AP-1 proteins, especially those that belong to the Jun group, control cell survival through regulation (expression and function) of cell cycle regulators such as Cyclin D1, p53, p21(cip1/waf1), p19(ARF), and p16 [104, 105]. c-Jun is unique in its ability to positively regulate cell proliferation through the repression of tumor suppressor gene expression and induction of cyclin D [105]. We have demonstrated activation of AP-1 in diabetic cardiomyopathy, suggesting an important role in disease pathogenesis [87, 97].

MEF2

MEF2 is an important transcription factor in myocyte hypertrophy [106]. MEF2 is associated with class II histone deacetylases (HDACs, discussed later). Translocation of HDAC to the cytoplasm frees up MEF2 and allows its association with HATs such as p300 to regulate transcription of effector genes [106, 107]. MEF2 controls the expression of many fetal cardiac genes. The normal adult heart exhibits no MEF2-dependent gene expression [108]. However, MEF2 gene expression is reactivated in cardiac hypertrophy. Moreover, blockade of MEF2-dependent gene expression completely inhibits cardiac hypertrophy caused by a variety of prohypertrophic stimuli [109].

GATA-4

GATA transcription factors consist of six proteins that regulate expression of several genes. GATA-4 is one of the early factors to be expressed in the embryo and is an important factor in cardiomyocyte hypertrophy. DNA binding of GATA-4 increases in hypertrophy [110]. Treatment of cells with hypertrophic factors such as ET-1 causes increased DNA binding activity of GATA4 [111–114]. It has been suggested that MAPK/ERK regulates basal GATA-4 activity in cardiomyocytes, whereas p38 mediates its nuclear binding [115]. Transcription coactivator p300 has also been shown to play an important role in regulating GATA-4 activity [115]. In a recent study, we have shown that cardiomyocyte hypertrophy, in animals and cultured cells, is associated with MEF2 and GATA-4 upregulation [93].

Regulation at the Nuclear Level

The activity of the transcription factors are further regulated in the nucleus by transcriptional coactivators and other epigenetic factors such as miRNAs. The epigenetic regulation of gene expression has just started to unravel in diabetic cardiomyopathy. Such alterations include histone acetylation, DNA methylation, phosphorylation, ubiquitination, and microRNA alteration. Some of the salient features are discussed below.

P300 and Histone Acetylation

At the chromosomal level, histone-dependent packaging of genomic DNA is a key mechanism of gene regulation [116, 117]. Chromatin remodeling by acetylation/deacetylation of histone residues is important in allowing access of transcription factors for DNA binding. Nuclear histone acetylation is a reversible process regulated by acetyltransferases (HATs) promoting acetylation and deacetylases (HDACs) promoting deacetylation [117, 118]. Transcriptional coactivator p300 is a well-known HAT and regulates several cellular processes [119]. p300 was first described as a protein associated with adenovirus E1a oncoprotein [120, 121]. p300 regulates a number of transcription factors such as AP-1 and NF-κB [122]. Association of NF-κB with p300 is essential for transcriptional activation, and without such association, NF-κB remains transcriptionally silent [123]. p300 regulates both MEF2 and GATA-4 [124]. p300 acts by (a) acetylation of histones allowing RNA polymerase II access,

(b) promoting interaction between transcription factors and the preinitiation complex, and c) promoting DNA–protein and protein–protein interactions acting as an adapter [119, 124]. p300 plays a crucial role in differentiation, growth, and myocyte hypertrophy [125]. We have previously shown an important role of p300 in cardiac hypertrophy in diabetes [93, 97]. We have also shown that oxidative stress and PARP activates p300 and HDACs. p300-mediated nuclear acetylation may play a key role in ET-1 induced cardiomyocyte hypertrophy in diabetes [126]. We have shown that in cells exposed to high glucose, p300 regulates a large number of transcription factors including MEF2, AP-1, GATA-4, NF-κB, and SRF and several vasoactive factors [94]. Studies have further shown that a regulatory relationship exists between p300 and MEF2 upregulation with miR133a downregulation [93, 127].

Histone acetylation activity of p300 and related proteins is balanced by histone deacetylases (HDACs) [128, 129]. Three classes of HDACs have been identified. Class II HDACs, by virtue of their binding sites for transcriptional regulators and possession of phosphorylation sites, connect signals to the genomes. HDACs 4, 5, and 9 of this class play a key role in cardiomyocyte hypertrophy [128, 129]. Class II HDACs, via an 18 aminoacid motif, present only on HDACs, normally represses MEF2 pathway [128–130]. Both HDAC5 and 9 knockouts develop activation of MEF2 and myocardial hypertrophy in response to stimulus, whereas overexpression of HDACs prevents such hypertrophy [131, 132]. Furthermore, recently it has been demonstrated that HDAC actions are regulated by several miRNAs and vice versa [133–135]. HDAC inhibition has been demonstrated to alter the action of several miRNAs [136].

miRNAs in Diabetes and in Heart Failure

MicroRNAs are small (~20–25 nucleotide long) RNA molecules that have significant effects on the regulation of gene expression [133]. The transcription of the miRNA occurs through RNA polymerase II. Subsequent processing to precursor miRNAs (70–100 nucleotides, hairpin-shaped) in the nucleus is mediated by RNAse III Dorsha and DGCR8. Following synthesis, they are exported to the cytoplasm by exportin 5. In the cytoplasm, they are processed by Dicer into functionally active mature miRNA [133, 137]. miRNA bind to the specific mRNA targets causing degradation of specific mRNA or translational inhibition [133, 137]. Several investigators, using overexpression experiments, have shown the importance of miRNA in diverse cellular processes [133]. miRNAs also play important roles in controlling histone modification [133, 134]. A significant number of miRNA coding regions are located in the intron of the protein coding gene and are coregulated with their host genes. However, they may also be regulated by their own promoters [133]. Several oncogenic miRNA have been demonstrated to regulate a wide variety of factors, e.g., oncogenes (c-*MYC*), transcription factors (NF-κB), etc. [133, 137]. Epigenetic mechanism may play a fundamental role in the regulation of miRNAs [133, 137, 138].

Recently, some investigators have examined miRNA in the context of heart failure. Using miRNA microarrays, alteration of 11 miRNAs (seven upregulated and four downregulated) were reported in the mouse heart following aortic banding [139]. The same study also showed that overexpression of miR195 may lead to cardiomyocyte hypertrophy [139]. Another study has demonstrated alteration of 19 miRNA in the mouse heart following similar insult (7 upregulated and 12 downregulated). They further demonstrated that miR21 may play a key role in phenylephrine- or angiotensin II-induced hypertrophy of neonatal cardiomyocytes [140]. In neonatal cardiomyocytes, studies have shown that α myosin heavy chain (αMHC) may regulate cardiac growth and gene expression in response to stress and hormonal signaling through miR208, which is encoded by α MHC intron [141, 142]. It has also been postulated that the altered miRNA expression may hold a clue to fetal gene programming in heart failure [138, 140]. Although there are some discrepancies as to specific miRNA alteration in cardiomyocyte hypertrophy (largely due various approaches and arrays used), several

studies demonstrated downregulation of miR1 and miR133 in cardiac hypertrophy [141, 143]. Furthermore, infusion of antagonists of miR133 (antagomir) in normal animals have produced hypertrophy [143]. One study has demonstrated that miR133 modulates HERG K+ channel causing QT prolongation in diabetic rabbits [144]. However, miRNA alterations in diabetic cardiomyopathy may be different from other causes of cardiac hypertrophy. Upregulation of miR320 has been demonstrated in isolated cardiac microvascular endothelial cells in diabetic rats [145]. This finding differs from our studies in the whole heart from chronically diabetic mice [127]. We further found that miR195 is repressed in diabetes [127]. However, it has been reported to be increased during nondiabetic cardiac hypertrophy [139]. Interestingly, in a study of pressure overload hypertrophy, miR133a was shown to regulate fibrosis without altering hypertrophy [146]. Studies from our laboratory show that several miRNAs are altered in the myocardium of chronically diabetic rats with functional evidence of diabetic cardiomyopathy. Among these, miR133a was downregulated. This downregulation was associated with SGK1 and IGF1 upregulation and cardiomyocyte hypertrophy [127].

Methylation

A fascinating aspect of molecular changes that mediate the adverse effects of high glucose levels is that the phenotypic changes produced in the vascular cells are long-term effects. This is dubbed as diabetic or hyperglycemic memory [147]. Recent studies attribute this memory to chromatin remodeling. According to this postulate, glucose-induced alteration of enzymes regulating methylation/demethylation causes long-term increases or decreases in target gene expression. Most recently, smooth muscle cells isolated from diabetic animals showed increased monocyte chemotactic protein-1 and interleukin expression, which was mediated by methylation of histone-3 lysine-4 near the nuclear factor-κB (NF-κB) response element [148] and reduced histone-3 lysine-9 trimethylation at the promoter region of these target genes [149]. A similar phenomenon is also seen in the ECs [150, 151]. A brief exposure of aortic ECs to high glucose levels was associated with increased NF-κB p65 expression and histone-3 lysine-4 monomethylation at the NF-κB p65 promoter region [151].

Conclusions

As evidenced from the previous discussion, a symphony involving a large number of abnormalities secondary to hyperglycemia is responsible for specific pathogenetic abnormalities in diabetic cardiomyopathy. Several interactive and intertwined pathways contribute to the pathogenesis of diabetic cardiomyopathy. A simplified overview of such molecular pathways, causing alterations of transcriptional machinery, secondary to hyperglycemia leading to cardiomyocyte hypertrophy, has been diagrammatically depicted in Fig. 2. In addition, other metabolic derangements such as hyperlipidemia and hyperinsulinemia may trigger additional pathogenetic mechanisms. Such intricate pathways pose a significant

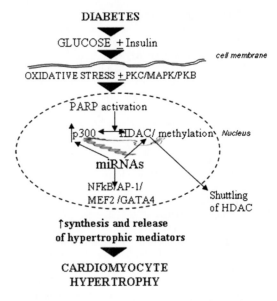

Fig. 2 Diagram showing various molecular pathways causing alterations of transcriptional machinery, secondary to hyperglycemia, leading to cardiomyocyte hypertrophy and other changes in diabetic cardiomyopathy (please see the text for abbreviations)

challenge for the development of specific adjuvant treatment for diabetic cardiomyopathy, as targeting one factor may not produce desired effects. Hence, along with control of hyperglycemia, simultaneous blockade of multiple pathways may provide a more rational approach. However, further investigations are needed to identify and establish such specific targets.

References

1. Zimmet P, Alberti KG, Shaw J. Global and societal implications of the diabetes epidemic. Nature. 2001;414:782–7.
2. Zimmet P. Globalization, coca-colonization and the chronic disease epidemic: can the Doomsday scenario be averted? J Intern Med. 2000;247:301–10.
3. Geiss LS, Herman WH, Smith PJ. Mortality in non-insulin-dependent diabetes. In: Harris MI, editor. Diabetes in America. Bethesda: National Health Institute; 1995. p. 233–57. Publication 95–1468.
4. American Diabetes Association. Economic consequences of diabetes mellitus in the U.S. in 1997. Diabetes Care. 1998;21:296–309.
5. Savage MP, Krolewski AS, Kenien GG, et al. Acute myocardial infarction in diabetes mellitus and significance of congestive heart failure as a prognostic factor. Am J Cardiol. 1988;62:665–9.
6. Raman M, Nesto RW. Heart disease in diabetes mellitus. Endocrinol Metab Clin North Am. 1996;25:425–38.
7. Shehadeh A, Regan TJ. Cardiac consequences of diabetes mellitus. Clin Cardiol. 1995;18:301–5.
8. Rubler S, Dlugash J, Yuceoglu YZ, et al. New type of cardiomyopathy associated with diabetic glomerulosclerosis. Am J Cardiol. 1972;30:595–602.
9. LeWinter MM. Diabetic cardiomyopathy: an overview. Coron Artery Dis. 1996;7:95–8.
10. Nunoda S, Genda A, Sekiguchi M, et al. Left ventricular endomyocardial biopsy findings in patients with essential hypertension and hypertrophic cardiomyopathy with special reference to the incidence of bizarre myocardial hypertrophy with disorganization and biopsy score. Heart Vessel. 1985;1:170–5.
11. Jugdutt BI. Ventricular remodeling after infarction and the extracellular collagen matrix: when is enough enough? Circulation. 2003;108:1395–403.
12. Weber KT. Cardiac interstitium in health and disease: the fibrillar collagen network. J Am Coll Cardiol. 1989;13:1637–52.
13. Cines DB, Pollak ES, Buck CA, et al. Endothelial cells in physiology and in the pathophysiology of vascular disorders. Blood. 1998;91:3527–61.
14. Mandarino LJ, Finlayson J, Hassell JR. High glucose downregulates glucose transport activity in retinal

capillary pericytes but not endothelial cells. Invest Ophthalmol Vis Sci. 1994;35:964–72.

15. Kaiser N, Sasson S, Feener EP, et al. Differential regulation of glucose transport and transporters by glucose in vascular endothelial and smooth muscle cells. Diabetes. 1993;42:80–9.

16. Boudina S, Abel D. Diabetic cardiomyopathy revisited. Basic Sci Clin. 2007;115:3213–23.

17. Lopaschuk GD. Metabolic abnormalities in the diabetic heart. Heart Fail Rev. 2002;7:149–59.

18. Taegtmeyer H, McNulty P, Young ME. Adaptation and maladaptation of the heart in diabetes, part I: general concepts. Circulation. 2002;105:1727–33.

19. Stanley WC, Lopaschuk GD, McCormack JG. Regulation of energy substrate metabolism in the diabetic heart. Cardiovasc Res. 1997;34:25–33.

20. McGavock JM, Victor RG, Unger RH, et al. Adiposity of the heart, revisited. Ann Intern Med. 2006;144:517–24.

21. Sharma S, Adrogue JV, Golfman L, et al. Intramyocardial lipid accumulation in the failing human heart resembles the lipotoxic rat heart. FASEB J. 2004;18:1692–700.

22. Endoh M. Signal transduction and Ca^{2+} signaling in intact myocardium. J Pharmacol Sci. 2006;100:525–37.

23. Cesario DA, Brar R, Shivkumar K. Alterations in ion channel physiology in diabetic cardiomyopathy. Endocrinol Metab Clin North Am. 2006;35:601–10.

24. Johnstone MT, Creager SJ, Scales KM, et al. Impaired endothelium-dependent vasodilation in patients with insulin-dependent diabetes mellitus. Circulation. 1993;88:2510–6.

25. Nitenberg A, Valensi P, Sachs R, et al. Impairment of coronary vascular reserve and ACh-induced coronary vasodilation in diabetic patients with angiographically normal coronary arteries and normal left ventricular systolic function. Diabetes. 1993;42:1017–25.

26. Steinberg HO, Chaker H, Leaming R, et al. Obesity/insulin resistance is associated with endothelial dysfunction. Implications for the syndrome of insulin resistance. J Clin Invest. 1996;97:2601–10.

27. Ting HH, Timimi FK, Boles KS, et al. Vitamin C improves endothelium-dependent vasodilation in patients with non-insulin-dependent diabetes mellitus. J Clin Invest. 1996;97:22–8.

28. Yanagisawa M, Kurihara H, Kimura S, et al. A novel potent vasoconstrictor peptide produced by vascular endothelial cells. Nature. 1988;332:411–5.

29. Inoue A, Yanagisawa M, Kimura S, et al. The human endothelin family: three structurally and pharmacologically distinct isopeptides predicted by three separate genes. Proc Natl Acad Sci USA. 1989;86:2863–7.

30. Khan ZA, Chakrabarti S. Endothelins in chronic diabetic complications. Can J Physiol Pharmacol. 2003;81:622–34.

31. Cardillo C, Campia U, Bryant MB, et al. Increased activity of endogenous endothelin in patients with

type II diabetes mellitus. Circulation. 2002;106:1783–7.

32. Ahlborg G, Ottosson-Seeberger A, Hemsen A, et al. Big ET-1 infusion in man causes renal ET-1 release, renal and splanchnic vasoconstriction, and increased mean arterial blood pressure. Cardiovasc Res. 1994;28:1559–63.

33. Ahlborg G, Weitzberg E, Lundberg JM. Circulating endothelin-1 reduces splanchnic and renal blood flow and splanchnic glucose production in humans. J Appl Physiol. 1995;79:141–5.

34. Pernow J, Kaijser L, Lundberg JM, et al. Comparable potent coronary constrictor effects of endothelin-1 and big endothelin-1 in humans. Circulation. 1996;94:2077–82.

35. Chen S, Evans T, Mukherjee K, et al. Diabetes-induced myocardial structural changes: role of endothelin-1 and its receptors. J Mol Cell Cardiol. 2000;32:1621–9.

36. Hileeto M, Cukiernik M, Mukherjee S, et al. Contributions of endothelin-1 and sodium hydrogen exchanger-1 in the diabetic myocardium. Diabetes Metab Res Rev. 2002;18:386–94.

37. Majumdar P, Chen S, George B, et al. Leptin and endothelin-1 mediated increased extracellular matrix protein production and cardiomyocyte hypertrophy in diabetic heart disease. Diab Metabol Res Rev. 2009;25:452–63.

38. Ludmer PL, Selwyn AP, Shook TL, et al. Paradoxical vasoconstriction induced by acetylcholine in atherosclerotic coronary arteries. N Engl J Med. 1986;315:1046–51.

39. Giugliano D, Marfella R, Coppola L, et al. Vascular effects of acute hyperglycemia in humans are reversed by L-arginine. Evidence for reduced availability of nitric oxide during hyperglycemia. Circulation. 1997;95:1783–90.

40. Khan ZA, Chakrabarti S. Therapeutic targeting of endothelial dysfunction in chronic diabetic complications. Recent Pat Cardiovasc Drug Discov. 2006;1:167–75.

41. Khan ZA, Farhangkhoee H, Chakrabarti S. Towards newer molecular targets for chronic diabetic complications. Curr Vasc Pharmacol. 2006;4:45–57.

42. Zanetti M, Sato J, Katusic ZS, et al. Gene transfer of endothelial nitric oxide synthase alters endothelium-dependent relaxations in aortas from diabetic rabbits. Diabetologia. 2000;43:340–7.

43. Farhangkhoee H, Khan ZA, Mukherjee S, et al. Heme oxygenase in diabetes-induced oxidative stress in the heart. J Mol Cell Cardiol. 2003;35:1439–48.

44. Fiordaliso F, Li B, Latini R, et al. Myocyte death in streptozotocin-induced diabetes in rats in angiotensin II-dependent. Lab Invest. 2000;80:513–27.

45. Khatter JC, Sadri P, Zhang M, et al. Myocardial angiotensin II (Ang II) receptors in diabetic rats. Ann N Y Acad Sci. 1996;793:466–72.

46. Frustaci A, Kajstura J, Chimenti C, et al. Myocardial cell death in human diabetes. Circ Res. 2000;87:1123–32.

47. Liu X, Suzuki H, Sethi R, et al. Blockade of the renin-angiotensin system attenuates sarcolemma and sarcoplasmic reticulum remodeling in chronic diabetes. Ann N Y Acad Sci. 2006;1084:141–54.

48. Yaras N, Bilginoglu A, Vassort G, et al. Restoration of diabetes-induced abnormal local Ca2+ release in cardiomyocytes by angiotensin II receptor blockade. Am J Physiol Heart Circ Physiol. 2007;292:H912–20.

49. Fiordaliso F, Cuccovillo I, Bianchi R, et al. Cardiovascular oxidative stress is reduced by an ACE inhibitor in a rat model of streptozotocin induced diabetes. Life Sci. 2006;79:121–9.

50. Patz A. Clinical and experimental studies on retinal neovascularization. XXXIX Edward Jackson Memorial Lecture. Am J Ophthalmol. 1982;94:715–43.

51. Nyengaard JR, Flyvbjerg A, Rasch R. The impact of renal growth, regression and regrowth in experimental diabetes mellitus on number and size of proximal and distal tubular cells in the rat kidney. Diabetologia. 1993;36:1126–31.

52. Khan ZA, Chakrabarti S. Growth factors in proliferative diabetic retinopathy. Exp Diabesity Res. 2003;4:287–301.

53. Chou E, Suzuma I, Way KJ, et al. Decreased cardiac expression of vascular endothelial growth factor and its receptors in insulin-resistant and diabetic states: a possible explanation for impaired collateral formation in cardiac tissue. Circulation. 2002;105:373–9.

54. Abaci A, Oguzhan A, Kahraman S, et al. Effect of diabetes mellitus on formation of coronary collateral vessels. Circulation. 1999;99:2239–42.

55. Waltenberger J. Impaired collateral vessel development in diabetes: potential cellular mechanisms and therapeutic implications. Cardiovasc Res. 2001;49:554–60.

56. Weihrauch D, Lohr NL, Mraovic B, et al. Chronic hyperglycemia attenuates coronary collateral development and impairs proliferative properties of myocardial interstitial fluid by production of angiostatin. Circulation. 2004;109:2343–8.

57. Arras M, Ito WD, Scholz D, et al. Monocyte activation in angiogenesis and collateral growth in the rabbit hindlimb. J Clin Invest. 1998;101:40–50.

58. Ito WD, Arras M, Winkler B, et al. Monocyte chemotactic protein-1 increases collateral and peripheral conductance after femoral artery occlusion. Circ Res. 1997;80:829–37.

59. Waltenberger J, Lange J, Kranz A. Vascular endothelial growth factor-A-induced chemotaxis of monocytes is attenuated in patients with diabetes mellitus: a potential predictor for the individual capacity to develop collaterals. Circulation. 2000;102:185–90.

60. Weber KT, Sun Y, Katwa LC, et al. Connective tissue: a metabolic entity? J Mol Cell Cardiol. 1995;27:107–20.

61. Weber KT, Sun Y, Tyagi SC, et al. Collagen network of the myocardium: function, structural remodeling and regulatory mechanisms. J Mol Cell Cardiol. 1994;26:279–92.

62. Alexander BT, Cockrell KL, Rinewalt AN, et al. Enhanced renal expression of preproendothelin mRNA during chronic angiotensin II hypertension. Am J Physiol Regul Integr Comp Physiol. 2001;280:R1388–92.

63. Bohlender J, Gerbaulet S, Kramer J, et al. Synergistic effects of AT(1) and ET(A) receptor blockade in a transgenic, angiotensin II-dependent, rat model. Hypertension. 2000;35:992–7.

64. Katwa LC, Guarda E, Weber KT. Endothelin receptors in cultured adult rat cardiac fibroblasts. Cardiovasc Res. 1993;27:2125–9.

65. Guarda E, Katwa LC, Myers PR, et al. Effects of endothelins on collagen turnover in cardiac fibroblasts. Cardiovasc Res. 1993;27:2130–4.

66. Harada M, Itoh H, Nakagawa O, et al. Significance of ventricular myocytes and nonmyocytes interaction during cardiocyte hypertrophy: evidence for endothelin-1 as a paracrine hypertrophic factor from cardiac nonmyocytes. Circulation. 1997;96:3737–44.

67. Luscher TF, Enseleit F, Pacher R, et al. Hemodynamic and neurohumoral effects of selective endothelin A (ET(A)) receptor blockade in chronic heart failure: the Heart Failure ET(A) Receptor Blockade Trial (HEAT). Circulation. 2002;106:2666–72.

68. Torre-Amione G, Young JB, Colucci WS, et al. Hemodynamic and clinical effects of tezosentan, an intravenous dual endothelin receptor antagonist, in patients hospitalized for acute decompensated heart failure. J Am Coll Cardiol. 2003;42:140–7.

69. Kalra PR, Moon JC, Coats AJ. Do results of the ENABLE (Endothelin Antagonist Bosentan for Lowering Cardiac Events in Heart Failure) study spell the end for non-selective endothelin antagonism in heart failure? Int J Cardiol. 2002;85:195–7.

70. Krutzfeldt A, Spahr R, Mertens S, et al. Metabolism of exogenous substrates by coronary endothelial cells in culture. J Mol Cell Cardiol. 1990;22:1393–404.

71. Florey. The endothelial cell. Br Med J. 1966;5512:487–90.

72. Brownlee M. Biochemistry and molecular cell biology of diabetic complications. Nature. 2001;414:813–20.

73. Lorenzi M. The polyol pathway as a mechanism for diabetic retinopathy: attractive, elusive, and resilient. Exp Diabetes Res. 2007;2007:61038.

74. Du XL, Edelstein D, Rossetti L, et al. Hyperglycemia-induced mitochondrial superoxide overproduction activates the hexosamine pathway and induces plasminogen activator inhibitor-1 expression by increasing Sp1 glycosylation. Proc Natl Acad Sci USA. 2000;97:12222–6.

75. Koya D, King GL. Protein kinase C activation and the development of diabetic complications. Diabetes. 1998;47:859–66.

76. Feener EP, King GL. Endothelial dysfunction in diabetes mellitus: role in cardiovascular disease. Heart Fail Monit. 2001;1:74–82.

77. Wakasaki H, Koya D, Schoen FJ, et al. Targeted overexpression of protein kinase C beta2 isoform in

myocardium causes cardiomyopathy. Proc Natl Acad Sci USA. 1997;94:9320–5.

78. Thornalley PJ. Cell activation by glycated proteins. AGE receptors, receptor recognition factors and functional classification of AGEs. Cell Mol Biol (Noisy-le-grand). 1998;44:1013–23.

79. Bucala R, Tracey KJ, Cerami A. Advanced glycosylation products quench nitric oxide and mediate defective endothelium-dependent vasodilatation in experimental diabetes. J Clin Invest. 1991;87:432–8.

80. Farhangkhoee Y, Khan ZA, Chakrabarti S. Glucose-induced upregulation of CD36 mediates oxidative stress and microvascular endothelial cell dysfunction. Diabetologia. 2005;48:1401–10.

81. Nishikawa T, Edelstein D, Du XL, et al. Normalizing mitochondrial superoxide production blocks three pathways of hyperglycaemic damage. Nature. 2000;404:787–90.

82. Cai L, Wang Y, Zhou G, et al. Attenuation by metallothionein of early cardiac cell death via suppression of mitochondrial oxidative stress results in a prevention of diabetic cardiomyopathy. J Am Coll Cardiol. 2006;48:1688–97.

83. Wold LE, Ren J. Streptozotocin directly impairs cardiac contractile function in isolated ventricular myocytes via a p38 map kinase dependent oxidative stress mechanism. Biochem Biophys Res Commun. 2004;318:1066–71.

84. Khullar M, Al-Shudiefat AA, Ludke A, et al. Oxidative stress: a key contributor to diabetic cardiomyopathy. Can J Physiol Pharmacol. 2010;88: 233–40.

85. Shen X, Zheng S, Metreveli NS, et al. Protection of cardiac mitochondria by overexpression of MnSOD reduces diabetic cardiomyopathy. Diabetes. 2006;55:798–805.

86. Chen S, Mukherjee S, Chakraborty C, et al. High glucose-induced, endothelin-dependent fibronectin synthesis is mediated via NF-kappa B and AP-1. Am J Physiol Cell Physiol. 2003;284:C263–72.

87. Chen S, Khan ZA, Cukiernik M, et al. Differential activation of NF-kappa B and AP-1 in increased fibronectin synthesis in target organs of diabetic complications. Am J Physiol Endocrinol Metab. 2003;284:E1089–97.

88. Khan ZA, Chan BM, Uniyal S, et al. EDB fibronectin and angiogenesis – a novel mechanistic pathway. Angiogenesis. 2005;8:183–96.

89. Khan ZA, Farhangkhoee H, Mahon JL, et al. Endothelins: regulators of extracellular matrix protein production in diabetes. Exp Biol Med (Maywood). 2006;231:1022–9.

90. Quehenberger P, Bierhaus A, Fasching P, et al. Endothelin 1 transcription is controlled by nuclear factor-kappaB in AGE-stimulated cultured endothelial cells. Diabetes. 2000;49:1561–70.

91. Garcia Soriano F, Virag L, Jagtap P, et al. Diabetic endothelial dysfunction: the role of poly(ADP-ribose) polymerase activation. Nat Med. 2001;7:108–13.

92. Chiu J, Xu BY, Chen S, et al. Oxidative stress-induced, poly(ADP-ribose) polymerase-dependent upregulation of ET-1 expression in chronic diabetic complications. Can J Physiol Pharmacol. 2008; 86:365–72.

93. Feng B, Chen S, Chiu J, et al. Regulation of cardiomyocyte hypertrophy in diabetes at the transcriptional level. Am J Physiol Endocrinol Metab. 2008;294:E1119–26.

94. Chen S, Feng B, George B, et al. Transcriptional co-activator p300 regulates glucose induced gene expression in the endothelial cells. Am J Physiol Endocrinol Metab. 2010;298:E127–37.

95. Rivanlou AH, Darnell JE. Signal transduction and the control of gene expression. Science. 2002; 295:813–8.

96. Wilson KD, Li Z, Wagner R, et al. Transcriptome alteration in the diabetic heart by rosiglitazone: implications for cardiovascular mortality. PLoS One. 2008;3:e2609.

97. Kaur H, Chen S, Xin X, et al. Diabetes-induced extracellular matrix protein expression is mediated by transcription coactivator p300. Diabetes. 2006;55:104–11.

98. Bowie A, O'Neill LA. Oxidative stress and nuclear factor-kappaB activation: a reassessment of the evidence in the light of recent discoveries. Biochem Pharmacol. 2000;59:13–23.

99. Baeuerle PA, Baltimore D. NF-kappa B: ten years after. Cell. 1996;87:13–20.

100. Suzuki YJ, Packer L. Inhibition of NF-kappa B DNA binding activity by alphatocopheryl succinate. Biochem Mol Biol Int. 1993;31:693–700.

101. Nadler JL, Winer L. Free radicals, nitric oxide, and diabetic complications. In: LeRoith D, Taylor SI, Olefsky JM, editors. Diabetes mellitus: a fundamental and clinical text. Philadelphia: Lippincott-Raven; 1996. p. 840–8.

102. Shaulian E, Karin M. AP-1 in cell proliferation and survival. Oncogene. 2001;20:2390–400.

103. Chinenov Y, Kerppola TK. Close encounters of many kinds: Fos-Jun interactions that mediate transcription regulatory specificity. Oncogene. 2001;20:2438–52.

104. Bakiri L, Lallemand D, Bossy-Wetzel E, et al. Cell cycle-dependent variations in c-Jun and JunB phosphorylation: a role in the control of cyclin D1 expression. EMBO J. 2000;19:2056–68.

105. Shaulian E, Schreiber M, Piu F, et al. The mammalian UV response: c-Jun induction is required for exit from p53-imposed growth arrest. Cell. 2000;103:897–907.

106. McKinsey TA, Zhang CL, Olson EN. MEF2: a calcium-dependent regulator of cell division, differentiation and death. Trends Biochem Sci. 2002;27:40–7.

107. Youn HD, Grozinger CM, Liu JO. Calcium regulates transcriptional repression of myocyte enhancer factor 2 by histone deacetylase 4. J Biol Chem. 2000;275:22563–7.

108. Youn HD, Chatila TA, Liu JO. Integration of calcineurin and MEF2 signals by the coactivator p300 during T-cell apoptosis. EMBO J. 2000; 19:4323–31.

109. Czubryt MP, Olson EN. Balancing contractility and energy production: the role of myocyte enhancer factor 2 (MEF2) in cardiac hypertrophy. Recent Prog Horm Res. 2004;59:105–24.

110. Pikkarainen S, Tokola H, Kerkela R, et al. GATA transcription factors in the developing and adult heart. Cardiovasc Res. 2004;63:196–207.

111. Morin S, Paradis P, Aries A, et al. Serum response factor-GATA ternary complex required for nuclear signaling by a G-protein-coupled receptor. Mol Cell Biol. 2001;21:1036–44.

112. He Q, Lapointe MC. Src and Rac mediate endothelin-1 and lysophosphatidic acid stimulation of the human brain natriuretic peptide promoter. Hypertension. 2001;37:478–84.

113. Morimoto T, Hasegawa K, Kaburagi S, et al. Phosphorylation of GATA-4 is involved in alpha 1-adrenergic agonist-responsive transcription of the endothelin-1 gene in cardiac myocytes. J Biol Chem. 2000;275:13721–6.

114. Wei JQ, Shehadeh LA, Mitrani JM, et al. Quantitative control of adaptive cardiac hypertrophy by acetyltransferase p300. Circulation. 2008;118:934–46.

115. Kerkela R, Pikkarainen S, Majalahti-Palviainen T, et al. Distinct roles of mitogen activated protein kinase pathways in GATA-4 transcription factor mediated regulation of B-type natriuretic peptide gene. J Biol Chem. 2002;277:13752–60.

116. Yanazume T, Morimoto T, Wada H, et al. Biological role of p300 in cardiac myocytes. Mol Cell Biochem. 2003;248:115–9.

117. McKinsey TA, Olson EN. Toward transcriptional therapies for the failing heart: chemical screens to modulate genes. J Clin Invest. 2005;115:538–46.

118. McKinsey TA, Olson EN. Cardiac histone acetylation – therapeutic opportunities abound. Trends Genet. 2004;20:206–13.

119. Goodman RH, Smolik S. CBP/p300 in cell growth, transformation, and development. Genes Dev. 2000;14:1553–77.

120. Avantaggiati ML, Carbone M, Graessmann A, et al. The SV40 large T antigen and adenovirus E1a oncoproteins interact with distinct isoforms of the transcriptional co-activator, p300. EMBO J. 1996;15: 2236–48.

121. Arias J, Alberts AS, Brindle P, et al. Activation of cAMP and mitogen responsive genes relies on a common nuclear factor. Nature. 1994;370:226–9.

122. Chen LF, Greene WC. Regulation of distinct biological activities of the NF-kappaB transcription factor complex by acetylation. J Mol Med. 2003;81:549–57.

123. Zhong H, May MJ, Jimi E, et al. The phosphorylation status of nuclear NF-kappa B determines its association with CBP/p300 or HDAC-1. Mol Cell. 2002;9:625–36.

124. Giordano A, Avantaggiati ML. p300 and CBP: partners for life and death. J Cell Physiol. 1999; 181:218–30.

125. Yanazume T, Hasegawa K, Morimoto T, et al. Cardiac p300 is involved in myocyte growth with decompensated heart failure. Mol Cell Biol. 2003;23:3593–606.

126. Yamashita K, Discher DJ, Hu J, et al. Molecular regulation of the endothelin-1 gene by hypoxia: contributions of hypoxia-inducible factor-1, activator protein-1, GATA-2, and p300/CBP. J Biol Chem. 2001;276:12645–53.

127. Feng B, Chen S, George B, et al. miR133a regulates cardiomyocyte hypertrophy in diabetes. Diabetes Metab Res Rev. 2010;26:40–9.

128. Zhang CL, McKinsey TA, Chang S, et al. Class II histone deacetylases act as signal-responsive repressors of cardiac hypertrophy. Cell. 2002;110:479–88.

129. Fischle W, Wang Y, Allis CD. Histone and chromatin cross-talk. Curr Opin Cell Biol. 2003;15:172–83.

130. Verdin E, Dequiedt F, Kasler HG. Class II histone deacetylases: versatile regulators. Trends Genet. 2003;19:286–93.

131. Chang S, McKinsey TA, Zhang CL, et al. Histone deacetylases 5 and 9 govern responsiveness of the heart to a subset of stress signals and play redundant roles in heart development. Mol Cell Biol. 2004;24:8467–76.

132. Bush E, Fielitz J, Melvin L, et al. A small molecular activator of cardiac hypertrophy uncovered in a chemical screen for modifiers of the calcineurin signaling pathway. Proc Natl Acad Sci USA. 2004;101:2870–5.

133. Chuang JC, Jones PA, et al. Epigenetics and microRNAs. Pediatr Res. 2007;61:24R–9.

134. Chen JF, Mandel EM, Thomson JM, et al. The role of microRNA-1 and microRNA-133 in skeletal muscle proliferation and differentiation. Nat Genet. 2006;38:228–33.

135. Saito Y, Liang G, Egger G, et al. Specific activation of microRNA-127 with downregulation of the proto-oncogene BCL6 by chromatin-modifying drugs in human cancer cells. Cancer Cell. 2006;9:435–43.

136. Scott GK, Mattie MD, Berger CE, et al. Rapid alteration of microRNA levels by histone deacetylase inhibition. Cancer Res. 2006;66:1277–81.

137. Bartel DP. MicroRNAs: genomics, biogenesis, mechanism, and function. Cell. 2004;116:281–97.

138. Egger G, Liang G, Aparicio A, et al. Epigenetics in human disease and prospects for epigenetic therapy. Nature. 2004;429:457–63.

139. van Rooij E, Sutherland LB, Liu N, et al. A signature pattern of stress-responsive microRNAs that can evoke cardiac hypertrophy and heart failure. Proc Natl Acad Sci USA. 2006;103:18255–60.

140. Cheng Y, Ji R, Yue J, et al. MicroRNAs are aberrantly expressed in hypertrophic heart: do they play a role in cardiac hypertrophy? Am J Pathol. 2007;170:1831–40.

141. van Rooij E, Sutherland LB, Qi X, et al. Control of stress-dependent cardiac growth and gene expression by a microRNA. Science. 2007;316:575–9.

142. Callis TE, Pandya K, Seok HY, et al. MicroRNA-208a is a regulator of cardiac hypertrophy and conduction in mice. J Clin Invest. 2009;119: 2772–86.

143. Carè A, Catalucci D, Felicetti F, et al. MicroRNA-133 controls cardiac hypertrophy. Nat Med. 2007;13: 613–8.

144. Xiao J, Luo X, Lin H, et al. MicroRNA miR-133 represses HERG K$^+$ channel expression contributing to QT prolongation in diabetic hearts. J Biol Chem. 2007;282:12363–7.

145. Wang XH, Qian RZ, Zhang W, et al. MicroRNA-320 expression in myocardial microvascular endothelial cells and its relationship with insulin-like growth factor-1 in type 2 diabetic rats. Clin Exp Pharmacol Physiol. 2009;36:181–8.

146. Matkovich SJ, Wang W, Tu Y. MicroRNA-133a protects against myocardial fibrosis and modulates electrical repolarization without affecting hypertrophy in pressure-overloaded adult hearts. Circ Res. 2010;106:166–75.

147. Engerman RL, Kern TS. Progression of incipient diabetic retinopathy during good glycemic control. Diabetes. 1987;36:808–12.

148. Reddy MA, Villeneuve LM, Wang M, et al. Role of the lysine-specific demethylase 1 in the proinflammatory phenotype of vascular smooth muscle cells of diabetic mice. Circ Res. 2008;103:615–23.

149. Villeneuve LM, Reddy MA, Lanting LL, et al. Epigenetic histone H3 lysine 9 methylation in metabolic memory and inflammatory phenotype of vascular smooth muscle cells in diabetes. Proc Natl Acad Sci USA. 2008;105:9047–52.

150. Brasacchio D, Okabe J, Tikellis C, et al. Hyperglycemia induces a dynamic cooperativity of histone methylase and demethylase enzymes associated with gene-activating epigenetic marks that coexist on the lysine tail. Diabetes. 2009;58:1229–36.

151. El-Osta A, Brasacchio D, Yao D, et al. Transient high glucose causes persistent epigenetic changes and altered gene expression during subsequent normoglycemia. J Exp Med. 2008;205:2409–17.

INDEX

N.S. Dhalla, M. Nagano, B. Ostadal (eds.), *Molecular Defects in Cardiovascular Disease*,
DOI 10.1007/978-1-4419-7130-2, © Springer Science+Business Media, LLC 2011